Trauma and Posttraumatic Stress Disorder

Trauma and Posttraumatic Stress Disorder

Global Perspectives from the WHO World Mental Health Surveys

Edited by

Evelyn J. Bromet
Stony Brook University

Elie G. Karam
St. George Hospital University Medical Center

Karestan C. Koenen
Harvard T. H. Chan School of Public Health

Dan J. Stein
University of Cape Town

CAMBRIDGE
UNIVERSITY PRESS

CAMBRIDGE
UNIVERSITY PRESS

University Printing House, Cambridge CB2 8BS, United Kingdom

One Liberty Plaza, 20th Floor, New York, NY 10006, USA

477 Williamstown Road, Port Melbourne, VIC 3207, Australia

314–321, 3rd Floor, Plot 3, Splendor Forum, Jasola District Centre, New Delhi – 110025, India

79 Anson Road, #06-04/06, Singapore 079906

Cambridge University Press is part of the University of Cambridge.

It furthers the University's mission by disseminating knowledge in the pursuit of education, learning, and research at the highest international levels of excellence.

www.cambridge.org
Information on this title: www.cambridge.org/9781107059696
DOI: 10.1017/9781107445130

First published 2018

Printed and bound in Great Britain by Clays Ltd, Elcograf S.p.A.

A catalogue record for this publication is available from the British Library.

Library of Congress Cataloging-in-Publication Data

Names: Bromet, Evelyn J., editor. | Karam, Elie, editor. | Koenen, Karestan C., editor. | Stein, Dan J., editor.
Title: Trauma and posttraumatic stress disorder : global perspectives from the WHO world mental health surveys / edited by Evelyn Bromet, Elie Karam, Karestan Koenen, Dan Stein.
Other titles: Global perspectives from the WHO world mental health surveys
Description: Cambridge, United Kingdom; New York, NY: Cambridge University Press, 2018. | Includes bibliographical references and index.
Identifiers: LCCN 2018012435 | ISBN 9781107059696 (hardback)
Subjects: | MESH: Stress Disorders, Post-Traumatic—epidemiology | Wounds and Injuries—epidemiology | Global Health | Health Surveys
Classification: LCC RC552.P67 | NLM WM 172.5 | DDC 362.196/8521—dc23
LC record available at https://lccn.loc.gov/2018012435

ISBN 978-1-107-05969-6 Hardback

Contents

Contributors

Sergio Aguilar-Gaxiola, MD, PhD
Center for Reducing Health Disparities, University of California Davis School of Medicine, Davis, CA, USA

Jordi Alonso, MD, PhD
Health Services Research Unit, IMIM-Hospital del Mar Medical Research Institute, Pompeu Fabra University (UPF), CIBER en Epidemiología y Salud Pública (CIBERESP), Barcelona, Spain

Laura Helena Andrade, MD, PhD
Section of Psychiatric Epidemiology – LIM 23, Institute of Psychiatry, University of São Paulo Medical School, São Paulo, Brazil

Lukoye Atwoli, MD, PhD
Department of Psychiatry and Mental Health, University of Cape Town, Cape Town, Republic of South Africa

Corina Benjet, PhD
Department of Epidemiologic & Psychosocial Research, National Institute of Psychiatry Ramón de la Fuente Muñiz, Mexico City, Mexico

Evelyn J. Bromet, PhD
Department of Psychiatry, Stony Brook University, Stony Brook, NY, USA

Ronny Bruffaerts, PhD
Universitair Psychiatrisch Centrum – Katholieke Universiteit Leuven (UPC-KUL), Campus Gasthuisberg, University of Leuven, Belgium

Brendan Bunting, PhD
School of Psychology, Ulster University, Londonderry, UK

José Miguel Caldas-de-Almeida, MD, PhD
Lisbon Institute of Global Mental Health and Chronic Diseases Research Center (CEDOC), NOVA Medical School, Universidade Nova de Lisboa, Lisbon, Portugal

Graça Cardoso, MD, PhD
Lisbon Institute of Global Mental Health and Chronic Diseases Research Center (CEDOC), NOVA Medical School, Universidade Nova de Lisboa, Lisbon, Portugal Somnath Chatterji, MD
Department of Information, Evidence and Research, World Health Organization, Geneva, Switzerland

Louisa Degenhardt, PhD
National Drug and Alcohol Research Centre, University of New South Wales, Sydney, Australia

Giovanni de Girolamo, MD
Istituti di Ricovero e Cura a Carattere Scientifico (IRCCS), St. John of God Clinical Research Centre, Brescia, Italy

Peter de Jonge, PhD
Department of Developmental Psychology, University of Groningen, University Medical Center Groningen, Groningen, The Netherlands

Koen Demyttenaere, MD, PhD
Department of Psychiatry, University Hospital Gasthuisberg, Katholieke Universiteit Leuven (KUL), Leuven, Belgium

Sara Evans-Lacko, PhD
Institute of Psychiatry, Psychology & Neuroscience, King's College London, PSSRU, London School of Economics and Political Science, London, UK

Matthew J. Friedman, MD, PhD
National Center for PTSD, US Department of Veterans Affairs, Washington, DC, Geisel School of Medicine at Dartmouth, Hanover, NH, USA

John Fayyad, MD
Institute for Development, Research, Advocacy & Applied Care (IDRAAC), Beirut, Lebanon

Silvia Florescu, MD, PhD
National School of Public Health, Management and Development, Bucharest, Romania

Oye Gureje, MD, PhD, FRCPsych
Department of Psychiatry, University of Ibadan, Ibadan, Nigeria

Josep Maria Haro, MD, PhD
Parc Sanitari Sant Joan de Déu, Universitat de Barcelona, CIBERSAM, Barcelona, Spain

Yanling He, MD
Shanghai Mental Health Center, Shanghai Jiao Tong University, School of Medicine, Shanghai, People's Republic of China

Steven G. Heeringa, PhD
Survey Research Center, Institute for Social Research, University of Michigan, Ann Arbor, MI, USA

Hristo Hinkov, MD, PhD
National Center for Public Health and Analyses, Sofia, Bulgaria

Yueqin Huang, MD, MPH, PhD
Institute of Mental Health, Peking University, Beijing, People's Republic of China

Elie G. Karam, MD
Department of Psychiatry and Clinical Psychology, St George Hospital University Medical Center, Balamand University, Faculty of Medicine, Institute for Development, Research, Advocacy and Applied Care (IDRAAC), Beirut, Lebanon

Norito Kawakami, MD, DMSc
Department of Mental Health, School of Public Health, The University of Tokyo, Tokyo, Japan

Ronald C. Kessler, PhD
Department of Health Care Policy, Harvard Medical School, Boston, MA, USA

Karestan C. Koenen, PhD
Department of Epidemiology, Harvard T.H. Chan School of Public Health, Boston, MA, USA

Viviane Kovess-Masfety, MD, PhD
Ecole des Hautes Etudes en Santé Publique (EHESP), EA 4057, Paris Descartes University, Paris, France

Sing Lee, MB, BS
Department of Psychiatry, Chinese University of Hong Kong, Tai Po, Hong Kong

Jean-Pierre Lépine, MD
Hôpital Lariboisière Fernand Widal, Assistance Publique Hôpitaux de Paris, Universités Paris Descartes-Paris Diderot, INSERM UMR-S 1144 Paris, France

Daphna Levinson, PhD
Mental Health Services, Ministry of Health, Jerusalem, Israel

Howard Liu, SM
Department of Health Care Policy, Harvard Medical School, Department of Epidemiology, Harvard T.H. Chan School of Public Health, Boston, MA, USA

John J. McGrath, MD, PhD
Queensland Brain Institute, Queensland Centre for Mental Health Research, University of Queensland, Australia, Aarhus University, Denmark

Katie A. McLaughlin, PhD
Department of Psychology, University of Washington, Seattle, WA, USA

Maria Elena Medina-Mora, DrPH
National Institute of Psychiatry, Ramón de la Fuente Muñiz, Mexico City, Mexico

Fernando Navarro-Mateu, PhD, MD
UDIF-SM, Subdirección General de Planificación, Innovación y Cronicidad, Servicio Murciano de Salud, IMIB-Arrixaca, CIBERESP-Murcia, Murcia, Spain

Beth-Ellen Pennell, MA
Survey Research Center, Institute for Social Research, University of Michigan, Ann Arbor, MI, USA

Marina Piazza, ScD, MPH
Universidad Cayetano Heredia, National Institute of Health, Lima, Peru

José Posada-Villa, MD
Faculty of Social Sciences, Colegio Mayor de Cundinamarca University, Bogota, Colombia

Andrew Ratanatharathorn, MA
Department of Epidemiology, Mailman School of Public Health, Columbia University New York, NY, USA

Sherri Rose, PhD
Department of Health Care Policy, Harvard Medical School, Boston, MA, USA

Anthony J. Rosellini, PhD
Department of Psychological & Brain Sciences, Boston University, Boston, MA, USA

Ayelet Meron Ruscio, PhD
Department of Psychology, University of Pennsylvania, Philadelphia, PA, USA

Kate M. Scott, PhD
Department of Psychological Medicine, University of Otago, Dundein, New Zealand

Victoria Shahly, PhD
Department of Health Care Policy, Harvard Medical School, Boston, MA, USA

Arieh Y. Shalev, MD
Department of Psychiatry, NYU Langone Medical Center, New York, NY, USA

David Spiegel, MD
Department of Psychiatry and Behavioral Sciences, Stanford University School of Medicine, Stanford, CA, USA

Paul Stang, PhD
Janssen Pharmaceutical R&D, Titusville, NJ, USA

Dan J. Stein, FRCPC, PhD
Department of Psychiatry and Mental Health University of Cape Town Cape Town, Republic of South Africa

Margreet ten Have, PhD
Trimbos-Instituut, Netherlands Institute of Mental Health and Addiction, Utrecht, The Netherlands

Graham Thornicroft, PhD
Centre for Global Mental Health, Institute of Psychiatry, Psychology and Neuroscience, King's College London, London, UK

Yolanda Torres, MPH, DraHC
Center for Excellence on Research in Mental Health, CES University, Medellin, Colombia

Maria Carmen Viana, PhD, MD
Department of Social Medicine, Federal University of Espirito Santo, Vitoria, Brazil

David R. Williams, MPH, PhD
Department of Social and Behavioral Sciences, Harvard T.H. Chan School of Public Health, Boston, MA, USA

Alan M. Zaslavsky, PhD
Department of Health Care Policy, Harvard Medical School, Boston, MA, USA

Foreword

Matthew J. Friedman

This remarkable volume represents the most comprehensive, detailed, and rigorous attempt ever undertaken to characterize the risk factors, clinical phenomenology, and global burden of posttraumatic stress disorder (PTSD). The World Mental Health (WMH) Survey Consortium has applied its powerful methodology and cross-national research network to investigate PTSD predictors, prevalence, population differences, and potential preventive strategies on such a large scale that there was sufficient statistical power to carry out many sub-analyses of great interest. Approximately 125,000 individuals were surveyed from 26 low- to high-income settings around the globe. Major topics include: the epidemiology of trauma and PTSD, factors influencing the onset and course of PTSD, the validity of the American Psychiatric Association's current diagnostic criteria for PTSD as described in the *Diagnostic and Statistical Manual Fifth Edition, DSM-5* (APA, 2013), and the clinical and public health implications of these findings with respect to preventive strategies and early case identification.

There is no need for me to attempt to use this brief introduction to summarize the wealth of findings presented in each chapter. Instead, I would like to focus on three major cross-cutting issues that have occupied my thoughts over the years: the global relevance of the PTSD diagnosis, the goodness-of-fit of the DSM-5 diagnostic criteria to the findings of the WMH survey, and how these findings might inform future clinical practice and public health policy.

The Cross-Cultural Applicability of the PTSD Construct

Ever since its introduction as an official diagnosis in the DSM-III (APA, 1980), PTSD has been criticized as a Western cultural construction with limited applicability to non-industrialized nations and cultures (Young, 1995; Summerfield, 1999; Jones et al., 2003; Lewis-Fernández et al., 2014). Another criticism has been that by medicalizing human suffering, the PTSD diagnosis has obscured the social and moral implications of catastrophic events such as war and genocide and narrowed the posttraumatic clinical focus from genuine culture-specific idioms of distress to the Western DSM diagnosis (Kleinman & Kleinman, 1991; Lewis-Fernández et al., 2014).

My personal experience of the intensity of this controversy occurred when Tony Marsella and I organized a conference more than 20 years ago (Marsella et al., 1996) that sought to integrate PTSD diagnostic criteria with cross-cultural and medical anthropological constructs of trauma. To me, this seemed to be an achievable and useful undertaking. But there was intense disagreement about the appropriateness of such an initiative.

This book does not, and cannot, address the question of whether PTSD might be a more useful construct in some settings than, for example, *ataque de nervios, khyal, ihahamuka, llaki,* or *masilango*. On the other hand, this book does show that PTSD occurs in low- as well as in high-income countries. Although prevalence may vary from one country to the next, such variation is not necessarily attributable to whether or not such countries are Western/industrialized. Furthermore, PTSD appears to remain PTSD. In many cases, the symptom characteristics, risk factors, clinical course, associated disorders, and burden of PTSD appear to be consistent from one country to the next.

In short, thanks to these findings, we can feel confident that PTSD is not restricted to Western populations although there is significant cross-cultural variability. As Lewis-Fernández et al. (2014) point out, such variability may, in part, be due to variability in trauma exposure as well as culturally driven differences in trauma expression. Much more research is needed to understand the relationship between culture, posttraumatic distress, PTSD, and culture-specific idioms of distress. Attention to underlying pathophysiology and identification of posttraumatic/PTSD-related biomarkers should help to sort this out. Finally, achieving the appropriate balance between culture-specific syndromes and the universal PTSD diagnosis should enable us to optimize clinical approaches and public health preventive policies in a wide variety of settings. This important path forward should be guided by these findings from the WMH Survey.

Did DSM-5 Get It Right?

As the chair of the DSM-5 sub-workgroup that developed the current PTSD criteria, I was, of course, very interested in the findings of the WMH Survey regarding the final PTSD diagnostic criteria. Most people do not realize that, in contrast to the DSM-IV (APA, 1994) process, there was no opportunity to field test the proposed DSM-5 criteria before they were finalized. Furthermore, although DSM-5 was an empirically driven process that was based on the most rigorous research, a number of key diagnostic questions had not been investigated as thoroughly as or carefully as we would have hoped. The WMH Survey has several specific chapters that focus on DSM-5 diagnostic criteria.

One major change between DSM-IV and DSM-5 was elimination of the subjective (Criterion A2) component of Criterion A which stipulated that in addition to exposure to the traumatic event itself (Criterion A1), an individual must have experienced an intense emotional response (e.g., "fear, helplessness, or horror"). DSM-5 eliminated the A2 criterion because it had little clinical utility and did not improve diagnostic accuracy. The WMH Survey results support that decision.

Another important change was the addition of a dissociative subtype (Lanius et al., 2012). Individuals diagnosed as such meet full DSM-5 criteria for PTSD but also exhibit dissociative symptoms, such as depersonalization or derealization. There is a long history of dissociative symptoms occurring after exposure to a traumatic event dating back to the classic work of Charcot and Janet. Again, the WMH Survey supports DSM-5 by showing that the dissociative subtype distinguished a significant minority of PTSD cases, that it was present throughout a diverse set of countries, and that it was associated with considerable morbidity, chronicity, and functional impairment.

In my opinion, one piece of unfinished business from DSM-5 is the lack of a diagnostic niche for people who suffer from extreme distress and functional impairment following exposure to a traumatic event, but who fail to meet full diagnostic criteria for PTSD. This has variously been called partial or sub-threshold PTSD. DSM-5 did not include a specific sub-threshold PTSD diagnosis because a standard case definition has never been achieved; therefore, it was not possible to pool and synthesize the growing literature on this topic. The WMH survey clearly supports earlier studies showing that traumatized individuals with some, but not all, requisite PTSD symptoms represent an important clinical population (Friedman et al., 2011). The WMH Survey's suggestion that people who meet two or three of the DSM-5 Criteria B–E should be diagnosed as having sub-threshold PTSD is a very good place to start toward developing a case definition of sub-threshold PTSD in order to guide and standardize future research.

The WMH survey addresses the differences in PTSD diagnostic criteria between DSM-IV, DSM-5, and the World Health Organization's (WHO) *International Classification of Disease 10th Edition* (ICD-10; WHO, 1993) and *11th Edition* (ICD-11; WHO, 2012). Although the Survey found results consistent with DSM-5 in distinguishing four PTSD symptom clusters, the most important result confirms previous findings regarding a lack of congruence between these four different diagnostic schemes. Given the differences between DSM-5 and ICD-11 (Friedman, 2013; Maercker et al., 2013), the finding that one-third of respondents met PTSD criteria only in DSM-5, DSM-IV, ICD-10, or ICD-11, but not in any other classification scheme, is very important. I believe that rather than confronting us with a conceptual problem, this is a golden opportunity to recognize that we should no longer try to fit all posttraumatic psychopathology under a single tent labeled "PTSD." It is time to recognize that different people will express posttraumatic distress differently. Perhaps it makes sense to identify different posttraumatic phenomenological phenotypes such as adrenergic/aroused, dysphoric/anhedonic, dissociative and externalizing (Friedman, 2016). Or more likely, it is time for PTSD to evolve into a spectrum disorder (as has depression) with a variety of phenotypes that include biomarkers among its diagnostic criteria. These WMH Survey results provide strong additional evidence that identification of posttraumatic phenotypes is one of the highest priorities in this field.

Clinical and Public Health Implications

To me, the most remarkable finding is the WMH survey PTSD risk algorithm based on machine learning models. We have known for a long time that most individuals exposed to a traumatic event will not develop PTSD. The clinical and public health challenge is how to identify those individuals at greatest risk in comparison with resilient others who will not develop PTSD. During mass casualty, war, genocide, and natural disaster scenarios, the problem has been that almost everyone exhibits severe distress during the acute aftermath of a trauma, but only a significant minority will exhibit a chronic PTSD clinical trajectory. Indeed, the WMH survey found that 95.6% of PTSD cases occurred among the 10% of respondents classified by the machine learning algorithms as having the greatest predicted PTSD risk. The model includes socio-demographics, type of trauma, prior trauma history, prior psychopathology, and social support. The predictive power of future models will definitely be improved by the identification of specific biomarkers as well as by the explication of specific posttraumatic phenotypes. But as with the importance of lipid profiles in assessing the risk of cardiovascular disease, refinement of the PTSD risk algorithm will play a major role in identification and management of individuals at greatest risk for PTSD in both traditional clinical and population-based public health settings.

In closing, the WMH survey of PTSD will greatly influence the future research agenda, diagnostic assessment, clinical management, and public health strategy regarding PTSD. It is a major achievement that should be mandatory reading for anyone concerned about trauma and its consequences.

References

American Psychiatric Association. (1980). *Diagnostic and Statistical Manual of Mental Disorders, Third Edition. DSM-III*. Washington, DC: American Psychiatric Association.

American Psychiatric Association. (1994). *Diagnostic and Statistical Manual of Mental Disorders, Fourth Edition. DSM-IV*. Washington, DC: American Psychiatric Association.

American Psychiatric Association. (2013). *Diagnostic and Statistical Manual of Mental Disorders, Fifth Edition. DSM-5*. Arlington, VA: American Psychiatric Association.

Friedman, M. J. (2013). Finalizing PTSD in DSM-5: getting here from there and where to go next. *Journal of Traumatic Stress*, 26, 548–56.

(2016). Deconstructing PTSD. In E. J. Bromet, ed., *Long Term Outcomes in Psychopathology Research: Rethinking the Scientific Agenda*. Oxford, England: Oxford University Press, pp. 123–39.

Friedman, M. J., Resick, P. A., Bryant, R. A., & Brewin, C. R. (2011). Considering PTSD for DSM-5. *Depression & Anxiety*, 28, 750–69.

Jones, E., Hodgins Vermaas, R., McCartney, H., et al. (2003). Flashbacks and post-traumatic stress disorder: the genesis of a 20th-century diagnosis. *British Journal of Psychiatry*, 182, 158–63.

Kleinman, A., & Kleinman, J. (1991). Suffering and its professional transformation: toward an ethnography of interpersonal experience. *Culture, Medicine, and Psychiatry*, 15, 275–301.

Lanius, R. A., Brand, B., Vermetten, E., Frewen, P. A., & Spiegel, D. (2012). The dissociative subtype of posttraumatic stress disorder: rationale, clinical and neurobiological evidence, and implications. *Depression and Anxiety*, 29, 701–8.

Lewis-Fernández, R., Hinton, D. E., Laria, A. J., & Marques, L. (2014). Culture and PTSD. In M. J. Friedman, T. M. Keane, & P. A. Resick, eds., *Handbook of PTSD: Science and Practice*, 2nd Edition. New York, NY: Guilford Publications, pp. 522–39.

Maercker, A., Brewin, C. R., Bryant, R. A., et al. (2013). Proposals for mental disorders specifically associated with stress in the International Classification of Diseases-11. *The Lancet*, 381, 1683–5.

Marsella, A. J., Friedman, M. J., Gerrity, E. T., & Surfield, R. M. (1996). Ethnocultural aspects of PTSD: some closing thoughts. In A. J. Marsella, M. J. Friedman, E. T. Gerrity, & R. M. Scurfield, eds., *Ethnocultural Aspects of Posttraumatic Stress Disorder: Issues, Research, and Clinical Applications*. Washington, DC: American Psychological Association, pp. 529–38.

Summerfield, D. A. (1999). A critique of seven assumptions behind psychological trauma programmes in war-affected areas. *Social Science and Medicine*, 48, 1449–62.

World Health Organization. (1993). *The ICD-10 Classification of Mental and Behavioral Disorders: Diagnostic Criteria for Research*. Geneva, Switzerland: World Health Organization.

World Health Organization. (2012). *ICD-11 Beta: Mental and Behavioral Disorders*. Geneva, Switzerland: World Health Organization. https://icd.who.int/dev11.

Young, A. (1995). *The Harmony of Illusions: Inventing Post-traumatic Stress Disorder*. Princeton, NJ: Princeton University Press.

Acknowledgments

The World Health Organization World Mental Health (WMH) Survey Initiative has been supported by the United States National Institute of Mental Health (NIMH; R01 MH070884), the John D and Catherine T. MacArthur Foundation, the Pfizer Foundation, the United States Public Health Service (R13-MH066849, R01-MH069864, and R01 DA016558), the Fogarty International Center (FIRCA R03-TW006481), the Pan American Health Organization, Eli Lilly and Company, Ortho-McNeil Pharmaceutical Inc., GlaxoSmithKline, and Bristol-Myers Squibb.

We thank the staff of the WMH Data Collection and Data Analysis Coordination Centres for assistance with instrumentation, fieldwork, and consultation on data analysis. None of the funders had any role in the design, analysis, interpretation of results, or preparation of this book. The views and opinions expressed in this report are those of the authors and should not be construed to represent the views of the World Health Organization, other sponsoring organizations, agencies, or governments.

The 2007 Australian National Survey of Mental Health and Wellbeing was funded by the Australian Government Department of Health and Ageing. The São Paulo Megacity Mental Health Survey has been supported by the State of São Paulo Research Foundation (FAPESP) Thematic Project Grant 03/00204-3. The Bulgarian Epidemiological Study of common mental disorders EPIBUL has been supported by the Ministry of Health and the National Center for Public Health Protection. The Chinese World Mental Health Survey Initiative has been supported by the Pfizer Foundation. The Colombian National Study of Mental Health (NSMH) has been supported by the Ministry of Social Protection. The Mental Health Study Medellín, Colombia, was carried out and supported jointly by the Center for Excellence on Research in Mental Health (CES University) and the Secretary of Health of Medellín. The ESEMeD project has been funded by the European Commission (Contracts QLG5-1999-01042, SANCO 2004123, and EAHC 20081308), (the Piedmont Region (Italy)), Fondo de Investigación Sanitaria, Instituto de Salud Carlos III, Spain (FIS 00/0028), Ministerio de Ciencia y Tecnología, Spain (SAF 2000-158-CE), Departament de Salut, Generalitat de Catalunya, Spain, Instituto de Salud Carlos III (CIBER CB06/02/0046, RETICS RD06/0011 REM-TAP), and other local agencies and by an unrestricted educational grant from GlaxoSmithKline. The Israel National Health Survey has been funded by the Ministry of Health with support from the Israel National Institute for Health Policy and Health Services Research and the National Insurance Institute of Israel. The World Mental Health Japan (WMHJ) Survey has been supported by the Grant for Research on Psychiatric and Neurological Diseases and Mental Health (H13-SHOGAI-023, H14-TOKUBETSU-026, H16-KOKORO-013, H25-SEISHIN-IPPAN-006) from the Japan Ministry of Health, Labour and Welfare. The Lebanese Evaluation of the Burden of Ailments and Needs of the Nation (L.E.B.A.N.O.N.) has been supported by the Lebanese Ministry of Public Health, the WHO (Lebanon), National Institute of Health/Fogarty International Center (R03 TW006481-01), anonymous private donations to IDRAAC, Lebanon, and unrestricted grants from Algorithm, AstraZeneca, Benta, Bella Pharma, Eli Lilly, GlaxoSmithKline, Lundbeck, Novartis, OmniPharma, Pfizer, Phenicia, Servier, UPO. The Mexican National Comorbidity Survey (MNCS) has been supported by the National Institute of Psychiatry Ramon de la Fuente (INPRFMDIES 4280) and by the National Council on Science and Technology (CONACyT-G30544-H), with supplemental support from the Pan American Health Organization (PAHO). Te Rau Hinengaro: The New Zealand Mental Health Survey (NZMHS) has been supported by the New Zealand Ministry of Health, Alcohol Advisory Council, and the Health Research Council. The

Nigerian Survey of Mental Health and Wellbeing (NSMHW) is supported by the WHO (Geneva), the WHO (Nigeria), and the Federal Ministry of Health, Abuja, Nigeria. The Northern Ireland Study of Mental Health was funded by the Health & Social Care Research & Development Division of the Public Health Agency. The Peruvian World Mental Health Study was funded by the National Institute of Health of the Ministry of Health of Peru. The Portuguese Mental Health Study was carried out by the Department of Mental Health, Faculty of Medical Sciences, NOVA University of Lisbon, with collaboration of the Portuguese Catholic University, and was funded by Champalimaud Foundation, Gulbenkian Foundation, Foundation for Science and Technology (FCT), and Ministry of Health. The Romania WMH study projects "Policies in Mental Health Area" and "National Study regarding Mental Health and Services Use" were carried out by National School of Public Health & Health Services Management (former National Institute for Research & Development in Health), with technical support of Metro Media Transylvania, the National Institute of Statistics-National Centre for Training in Statistics, SC, Cheyenne Services SRL, Statistics Netherlands and were funded by Ministry of Public Health (former Ministry of Health) with supplemental support of Eli Lilly Romania SRL. The South Africa Stress and Health Study (SASH) has been supported by the US National Institute of Mental Health (R01-MH059575) and National Institute of Drug Abuse with supplemental funding from the South African Department of Health and the University of Michigan. The Psychiatric Enquiry to General Population in Southeast Spain, Murcia (PEGASUS-Murcia) Project has been financed by the Regional Health Authorities of Murcia (ServicioMurciano de Salud and Consejería de Sanidad y Política Social) and Fundación para la Formación e Investigación-Sanitarias (FFIS) of Murcia. The Ukraine Comorbid Mental Disorders during Periods of Social Disruption (CMDPSD) study has been funded by the US National Institute of Mental Health (RO1-MH61905). The US National Comorbidity Survey Replication (NCS-R) has been supported by the National Institute of Mental Health (NIMH; U01-MH60220) with supplemental support from the National Institute of Drug Abuse (NIDA), the Substance Abuse and Mental Health Services Administration (SAMHSA), the Robert Wood Johnson Foundation (RWJF; Grant 044708), and the John W. Alden Trust.

Chapter 1 The Global Epidemiology of Trauma Exposure and Posttraumatic Stress Disorder

Evelyn J. Bromet, Elie G. Karam, Karestan C. Koenen, and Dan J. Stein

This volume is the result of a long-term collaboration by an international consortium of mental health researchers from over two dozen countries who participated in the World Mental Health (WMH) surveys. The WMH initiative is a coordinated series of epidemiological surveys conducted throughout the world that are designed to provide a comprehensive global portrait of the prevalence, risk factors, and consequences of common mental disorders. WMH survey results, which have been reported in numerous papers in leading scientific journals, have served as the basis for five previous books published by Cambridge University Press. The first volume in this series focused on the descriptive epidemiology of mental disorders (Kessler & Üstün, 2008), the second on mental–physical comorbidity (Von Korff et al., 2009), the third on suicidal behaviors (Nock et al., 2012), the fourth on the burdens of mental disorders (Alonso et al., 2013) and the fifth on facts about mental disorders around the world (Scott et al., 2018). The current volume addresses trauma and posttraumatic stress disorder (PTSD).

A Brief History of PTSD

The symptoms of PTSD have been recognized since the beginnings of recorded history, as exemplified by Homer's epic poem, *The Iliad* (Shay, 1994). However, PTSD was not fully acknowledged as a unique diagnostic entity until the publication of the third edition of the *Diagnostic and Statistical Manual of Mental Disorders* (DSM-III) (American Psychiatric Association, 1980). DSM-III defined PTSD as a set of re-experiencing, avoidance, and hyper-arousal symptoms in the wake of a trauma that was "outside the range of normal human experience." The DSM-III conceptualization, which was more inclusive than the acute stress reaction categories in DSM-I (American Psychiatric Association, 1952) and DSM-II (American Psychiatric Association, 1968), was influenced by a growing body of evidence about the distinctive features and comorbidity of posttraumatic symptoms in active-duty soldiers (Moskos, 1975), veterans (Kardiner & Spiegel, 1947; Figley, 1978; Helzer et al., 1979), prisoners of war (Strassman et al., 1956), as well as in other trauma-exposed groups, such as Holocaust victims (Klein, 1971), atomic bomb survivors (Lifton, 1967), and women subjected to child sexual abuse (Herman & Hirschman, 1977), rape (Burgess & Holmstrom, 1974), and physical assault (Walker, 1979). DSM-III assumed that PTSD was rare, and early epidemiological studies, which assessed trauma with two open-ended stem questions, reported lifetime prevalence rates of 1% to 3% (Shore et al., 1986; Helzer et al., 1987; Davidson et al., 1991). The low rates later proved to be underestimates, but the reported correlations of female sex, childhood trauma, and suicidality with DSM-III PTSD were consistently confirmed in later studies.

DSM-III-R (American Psychiatric Association, 1987), together with newly developed trauma checklists (Wolfe & Kimerling, 1997), facilitated epidemiological research on PTSD by clearly elucidating the nature of qualifying traumas, clarifying the required symptoms, and specifying a minimum duration for the diagnosis (Brett et al., 1988). DSM-IV (American Psychiatric Association, 1994) later reformulated the definition of trauma to include experiencing or witnessing events that involved actual or threatened death or serious injury or a threat to the physical integrity of self or others. Indeed, these revised criteria stimulated a new generation of epidemiological and public health research on PTSD in both general populations (Resnick et al., 1993; Finkelhor, 1994; Kessler et al., 1995) and in vulnerable groups (e.g., Kulka et al., 1990; Zerach et al., 2013). While ICD-10 also introduced PTSD as a separate diagnosis (Janca et al., 1994), most epidemiological studies of PTSD have been based on DSM criteria (Gradus, 2017). Finally, DSM-5 (American Psychiatric Association, 2013) added behavioral symptoms and a fourth symptom cluster involving negative cognition and mood, and recent studies are operationalizing PTSD using these new criteria.

Epidemiology of Trauma and PTSD

Since the publication of DSM-III, a number of epidemiological studies of trauma and PTSD have been conducted in North America and Europe. In contrast, far fewer epidemiological studies have been conducted in other countries and regions of the world. This chapter summarizes findings from surveys that examined lifetime PTSD diagnoses in representative samples drawn from the general population, high-risk regions of the world, and vulnerable groups, such as veterans. (Studies based on symptom checklists or child/adolescent samples are not considered here.) These surveys all use the respondent-selected worst or most stressful trauma as the focal trauma.

Table 1.1 provides examples of widely cited surveys of trauma and PTSD that took place primarily in select high-income countries. The WMH survey findings reported in this book thus fill in a large gap in knowledge about the global epidemiology of trauma and PTSD.

The first comprehensive study of trauma and PTSD in the general population was the highly influential National Comorbidity Survey (NCS), conducted in the United States in 1990–2 (Kessler et al., 1995). The NCS was a nationwide, in-person survey of 8,098 adults aged 15–54 who were administered a modified version of the Composite International Diagnostic Interview (CIDI). The CIDI inquired about 12 DSM-III-R-qualifying traumas (Kessler et al., 1995). To minimize embarrassment and stigma, the traumas were presented to respondents in a booklet and were asked about by number (*"Did you ever experience event number 1 on the list?"*). More than half of the sample (60.7% of men and 51.2% of women) reported exposure to at least one trauma, and the majority endorsed two or more. Comparable rates of lifetime trauma exposure have subsequently been found in other studies assessing a similar number of traumas, including research conducted in Kenya (48.2%, Jenkins et al., 2015), the Netherlands (52.2%, Bronner et al., 2009), and Australia (57.2%, Rosenman, 2002). However, rates have varied from less than 30% in Germany (Maercker et al., 2008) and South Korea (Jeon et al., 2007) to more than 70% in Mexico (Norris et al., 2003), Canada (Stein et al., 1997), and Portugal (Albuquerque et al., 2003). In contrast, studies that used longer trauma lists (20+ traumas) have typically found lifetime exposure rates of 75% to 85%. Examples include national surveys in Australia (Mills et al., 2011), Canada (Van Ameringen et al., 2008), and the Netherlands (de Vries & Olff, 2009), as well as regional surveys in Detroit, Michigan (Breslau et al., 1998; Goldmann et al., 2011). The most commonly reported traumas were unexpected death of a loved one, motor vehicle collisions, and being mugged (Norris, 1992; Breslau et al., 1998; Roberts et al., 2011). Overall, the most consistent risk factors for trauma exposure include younger age, male sex, lower socioeconomic status, and a history of prior traumas (Hatch & Dohrenwend, 2007; Shalev et al., 2017). Some traumas, such as severe motor vehicle collisions, appear to be more prevalent in high-income countries than in developing countries (World Health Organization, 2016). Cross-national comparisons of the rates and risk factors for specific trauma exposures in the WMH cohorts are explored in Chapters 3 and 4 as well as in Section 4 of this volume.

In addition to examining exposure to trauma, the NCS provided the first systematic portrait of the descriptive epidemiology of PTSD associated with respondents' most upsetting (i.e., worst) trauma. The lifetime rate of PTSD was 7.8% overall, ranking it lower than major depression (17.1%) but considerably higher than panic disorder (3.5%) and bipolar disorder (1.7%) (Kessler et al., 1994). Other US general population surveys of lifetime PTSD after respondent-nominated worst trauma have found similar rates of PTSD (e.g., Roberts et al., 2011; Alegria et al., 2013; Breslau et al., 2013) as did surveys conducted in the Netherlands (de Vries & Olff, 2009) and Canada (Van Amerigen et al., 2008). Of note, two national surveys found considerably lower rates of PTSD for respondents' most stressful event – namely, Zlotnik et al. (2006), which reported 4.4% in Chile and Jeon et al. (2007), which reported 1.7% in South Korea. As expected, regional studies of high-conflict areas have reported higher rates of PTSD than national surveys. Examples include the 13.6% rate of PTSD in the Detroit Area Survey of Trauma (Breslau et al., 2004) and the high rates found by de Jong et al. (2001) in Algeria (37.4%), Cambodia (28.9%), and Gaza (15.8%). Studies of high-risk samples, such as active-duty soldiers, veterans, and first-responders, most of which were conducted in high-income countries, have also reported rates that are higher (e.g., 17–20%) than those found in general population samples.

The lifetime risk of PTSD in conjunction with specific traumas (i.e., the conditional probability of PTSD) has been shown to vary widely, depending on the type of trauma (Shalev et al., 2017). In the NCS, the rates of PTSD in men for respondent-nominated worst trauma

Table 1.1 Major epidemiological surveys of PTSD based on worst lifetime trauma as the focal trauma[a]

Study	Country	Design[b]	(n)	Assessment instrument and criteria[c]	PTSD lifetime prevalence (%)
General					
Helzer et al. (1987)	United States	St. Louis site of the Epidemiologic Catchment Area study	(2,493)	DIS; DSM-III	1
Davidson et al. (1991)	United States	North Carolina site of the Epidemiologic Catchment Area study	(2,985)	DIS; DSM-III	1.3
Resnick et al. (1993)	United States	National Women's Study (18+)	(4,008)	DIS; DSM-III-R	12.3
Kessler et al. (1995)	United States	National Comorbidity Survey (15–54)	(8,098)	CIDI; DSM-III-R	7.8
Zlotnik et al. (2006)	Chile	Chile Psychiatric Prevalence Study (15+)	(2,978)	DIS; DSM-III-R	4.4
Jeon et al. (2007)	South Korea	National sample (18–64)	(6,258)	CIDI; DSM-IV	1.7
Van Ameringen et al. (2008)	Canada	National sample (18+)	(2,991)	CIDI; DSM-IV	9.2
De Vries & Olff (2009)	The Netherlands	National sample (18–80)	(1,087)	CIDI; DSM-IV	7.4
Hauffa et al. (2011)	Germany	National sample (14+)	(2,510)	PSS; DSM-IV	2.9
Pietrzak et al. (2011)	United States	National Epidemiological Survey of Alcohol & Related Conditions (18+)	(34,653)	AUDADIS; DSM-IV	6.4
Chapman et al. (2012)	Australia	Australian National Survey of Mental Health & Wellbeing, 2007 (18–65)	(8,841)	CIDI; DSM-IV	7.2
Alegria et al. (2013)	United States	Collaborative Psychiatric Epidemiology Studies (18+)	(16,238)	CIDI; DSM-IV	6.4
Puac-Polanco et al. (2015)	Guatemala	2009 Guatemalan National Mental Health Survey (18–65)	(1,452)	CIDI; DSM-IV	1.9
Lassemo et al. (2017)	Norway	Representative sample of Oslo and a rural area	(1,643)	CIDI; ICD-10	4.3
High-Stress Areas					
de Jong et al. (2001)	Asia, Middle East, and Africa	Random samples of areas of Algeria, Cambodia, Gaza	(653)	CIDI; DSM-IV	37.4 (Algeria) 28.4 (Cambodia) 17.8 (Gaza)
Breslau et al. (2004)	Detroit, Michigan	Detroit Area Survey of Trauma (18–46)	(2,181)	CIDI; DSM-IV	13.6
High-Risk Samples					
CDC (1988)	United States	Vietnam Experience Study. Random sample of Vietnam veterans	(2,490)	DIS; DSM-III; combat-related	14.7[d]
Kulka et al. (1988); Dohrenwend et al. (2006)	United States	National Vietnam Veterans Readjustment Study (NVVRS)	(2,348)	SCID	18.7 (veterans)
O'Toole et al. (1996)	Australia	Vietnam veterans	(641)	DIS; DSM-III	17.1
de Jong et al. (2001)	Eritrea	Random sample of refugees in shelters in Addis Ababa	(1,200)	CIDI; DSM-IV	15.8
Nelson et al. (2011); Fikretoglu & Liu (2012)	Canada	Representative sample of active members of Canadian forces (16–64)	(8,441)	CIDI; DSM-IV	6.5
Magruder et al. (2015)	United States	Vietnam Era veterans	(8,742)	CIDI; DSM-IV	20.1 (in Vietnam) 11.5 (nearby)
Marmar et al. (2015)	United States	NVVRS follow-up (theater veterans)	(400)	CAPS-5	17.0 (males) 15.2 (females)
Bromet et al. (2016)	United States	Monitoring sample of World Trade Center responders	(3,504)	SCID; DSM-IV World Trade Center connected	17.7

[a]Data from Lowe, S. R., Blachman-Forshay, J., & Koenen, K. C. (2015). Trauma as a public health issue: epidemiology of trauma and trauma-related disorders. In U. Schnyder & M. Cloitre, eds., *Evidence Based Treatments for Trauma-Related Psychological Disorders: A Practical Guide for Clinicians*. Cham, Switzerland: Springer International Publishing, pp. 11–40.
[b]Age in parenthesis.
[c]DIS is the Diagnostic Interview Schedule; AUDADIS is the Alcohol Use Disorders and Associated Disabilities Interview Schedule; SCID is the Structured Clinical Interview for DSM; PSS is the PTSD Symptom Scale; CAPS is the Clinician Administered PTSD Scale.
[d]Total prevalence not reported; value represents trauma with highest prevalence.

ranged from 1.8% (physical attack) to 65.0% (rape), while in women, the range was 5.4% (natural disaster) to 48.5% (physical abuse) (Kessler et al., 1995). In the Detroit Area Survey of Trauma, the trauma-specific rates of PTSD also ranged widely, with rates varying from a low of 1.5% (learning that a relative was attacked) to a high of 62.0% (being held captive/tortured/kidnapped) (Breslau et al., 2004). Overall, the severity of the threat associated with the trauma is strongly linked to the risk of PTSD. In line with this body of research, this volume reports the conditional risks of PTSD after 29 trauma types for survey participants residing in both high- and low-income countries. As discussed later in this chapter, the trauma for which PTSD was evaluated was a randomly selected trauma rather than the respondent-nominated worst trauma.

Various personal risk factors have also been shown to be associated with an elevated likelihood of PTSD. Meta-analyses (Brewin et al., 2000; Ozer et al., 2003) and a systematic review of prospective studies of PTSD (DiGangi et al., 2013) have shown that cognitive ability, prior traumas, and history of psychopathology are among the most important risk factors for developing PTSD (Koenen et al., 2007; Scott et al., 2010; Breslau et al., 2014). Demographic risk factors were also found to be associated with PTSD, especially female sex, younger age, being unmarried, lower socioeconomic status, and unemployment (Norris et al., 2002; Shalev et al., 2017). Notably, research from high-income countries has repeatedly shown that men are more likely to experience a trauma, but once exposed, women are more likely to develop PTSD (Kessler et al., 1995; Breslau et al., 1999; Breslau, 2002).

Since the earliest epidemiological studies, PTSD has been shown to be highly comorbid with both other types of mental disorders and a wide range of physical health disorders. Mood, anxiety, and substance use disorders have all been reliably linked to PTSD in general population samples (e.g., Kessler et al., 1995; Chilcoat & Breslau, 1998; Breslau, 2009) and vulnerable groups (e.g., Kulka et al., 1990; Smith et al., 2016). In a recent review, Flory and Yehuda (2015) noted that almost 50% of individuals with PTSD have comorbid depression. Similarly, McFarlane (2000) concluded that depression, anxiety, and substance use disorders accompany PTSD in the majority of cases. In general, prospective studies have also shown that preexisting psychopathology is a major risk factor for the development of PTSD after trauma exposure (Breslau, 2002; DiGangi et al., 2013; Smith et al., 2016), and longitudinal studies have shown that PTSD increases the risk of new onset psychiatric and substance use disorders (e.g., Breslau et al., 1997). PTSD is also comorbid with various physical health conditions (Eaton, 2006; Boscarino, 2008; Von Korff et al., 2009; Miller & Sadeh, 2014), particularly cardiovascular disease (Sumner et al., 2015; Edmonson & von Känel, 2017; Koenen et al., 2017) and chronic pain (Brennstuhl et al., 2015). In addition, preliminary evidence suggests that PTSD is also associated with signs of accelerated aging (Cohen et al., 2013; Clouston et al., 2016; Roberts et al., 2017; Wolf et al., 2017), dementia (Yaffe et al., 2010; Flatt et al., 2017), and premature mortality (Lohr et al., 2015). There is also growing awareness that medical diagnoses, especially cardiovascular disease, cancer, and degenerative neurological diseases, can cause medical-related PTSD symptoms, which worsen prognosis by interfering with treatment adherence (e.g., Hobfoll et al., 2015; Edmonson & von Känel, 2017). The same gap in knowledge about the prevalence of trauma and PTSD and their respective risk factors applies to studies on the comorbidity of mental and physical conditions – namely, that to date, the research has by and large taken place only in high-income countries.

One of the most highly cited findings from the NCS was that a third of individuals with PTSD failed to remit after many years, even with treatment (Kessler et al., 1995). This result was subsequently confirmed in a population-based survey of Australia (Chapman et al., 2012), in which approximately one-third of respondents with PTSD continued to experience symptoms more than 30 years after onset. In addition, more than half of the remitted PTSD cases in the Australian cohort still experienced symptoms after 14 years. Recent meta-analyses of epidemiological and clinical samples have placed the average rate of chronicity at closer to 50% (Morina et al., 2014; Steinert et al., 2015). The Morina et al. (2014) meta-analysis focused on prospective studies of clinical and community cases diagnosed with PTSD who had a minimum of 10 months of follow-up. Among the more than 80,000 participants, less than half (44.0%) were in remission at follow-up, although the range varied from 8% to 89%, depending on the trauma that triggered the PTSD, the length of the follow-up, and personal characteristics.

One of the most consistent findings in the literature is that women with PTSD are far more likely than men with PTSD to develop a chronic disorder. An early epidemiological study of 1,000 adults between 20 and 30 years of age found that the risk of chronicity in women was increased by a factor of four (Breslau & Davis, 1992). A partial explanation can be found in data from a national survey of American women in which PTSD chronicity was associated with reporting rape and physical assault before age 18 (Cougle et al., 2009). Other risk factors for chronicity found in surveys in high-income countries include those associated with PTSD onset noted earlier (i.e., history of childhood adversities, history of prior traumas, preexisting psychopathology, and intensity of the current trauma) as well as adverse circumstances that occur in the immediate aftermath of the trauma, such as trauma-linked stressful life events, inadequate emotional and practical support, new onset of psychiatric and substance disorders, and physical injury and illness (Steinert et al., 2015).

Despite the chronicity and impairment attached to PTSD, the vast majority of affected individuals do not receive any treatment, and only a small minority receive evidence-based treatments, such as cognitive-behavioral therapy (CBT), selective-serotonin uptake inhibitors (SSRIs), and serotonin-norepinephrine reuptake inhibitors (SNRIs), or a combination therapy (Bisson et al., 2013). In the United States, where mental health services are much more available than in most other countries (Roberts et al., 2011), only about half of those with PTSD seek treatment, and only 58% of those seeking treatment receive care from a mental health professional (Kessler, 2000). It is worth noting that the rates of treatment for PTSD in the United States are consistent with the rates of mental health treatment for severe mental and substance use disorders in general (Kessler et al., 2005). As expected, ethnic minorities are less likely and women are more likely to receive treatment than Whites and men (Roberts et al., 2011). Relatively little is known about treatment-seeking by individuals with PTSD in developing countries – another gap investigated in the WMH surveys (Chapter 8).

Research has shown that early treatment in first-response settings can help prevent the onset of PTSD (Foa et al., 1995; Kearns et al., 2012; Shalev et al., 2012). However, since a minority of trauma victims go on to develop PTSD (Kessler et al., 1995; Kessler, 2000; Roberts et al., 2010, 2011), and a substantial proportion of acute cases recover spontaneously (Shalev et al., 2017), researchers have been developing models to predict which individuals are most likely to develop PTSD and thus also most likely to benefit from expensive early interventions. One example is the PsySTART system adopted by the American Red Cross to target rapid delivery of psychological first aid and referral for mental health services to survivors judged to be at high risk of mental disorders in the immediate aftermath of a disaster (Schreiber et al., 2014). PsySTART differs from previous post-disaster risk evaluation schemes by focusing on evidence-based predictors of PTSD (severity of exposure, prior traumas, and history of prior mental disorders) and acute suicidality, rather than on current distress. Recent data-mining approaches aimed at detecting patterns of behavior in large data sets are also being applied to identify the highest risk groups for developing PTSD in the wake of specific types of traumas. This approach is discussed in Chapter 22 using relevant data from both high- and low-income countries.

Dissecting the Clinical Picture

Given that a majority of individuals with PTSD do not seek treatment, especially within the mental health sector, and treatment-seeking is not random (Kessler et al., 2005), respondents with PTSD identified in general population surveys provide the least biased source of clinical information available for examining phenomenological and nosological issues (Cohen & Cohen, 1984). One pressing issue best examined with epidemiological evidence involves differences in rates of PTSD across current criterion sets. As noted above, while most PTSD studies to date have been based on DSM-IV criteria, some European epidemiological studies have been based on ICD-10 criteria (e.g., Lassemo et al., 2017). In addition, recent studies have begun to examine PTSD using DSM-5 criteria. Potential differences in prevalence as well as in clinical and demographic characteristics of individuals diagnosed according to these different criterion sets are a central concern not just for meta-analyses that compare results across epidemiological studies, but also for recent national and international multicenter genetic and neurobiological studies of PTSD. Such genome-wide association studies (Logue et al., 2015) require massive sample sizes that are beyond the reach of a single research team. For example, the Psychiatric Genomics Consortium-Post-Traumatic Stress Disorder Working Group pools data globally to identify genes for PTSD. For the first pooled analysis, caseness was determined according to DSM-IV criteria as that was the criterion used in extant studies (Duncan et al., 2017). The specific instruments applied to diagnose PTSD caseness, however, varied across data sets. Moreover, future analyses will include PTSD diagnosed according to DSM-5, raising new challenges in terms of pooling phenotypes across studies. (Caseness based on symptom scale cut-points rather than gold standard diagnostic assessments presents another set of problems.) The CIDI was designed to make both ICD-10 and DSM-IV diagnoses and contains sufficient information to estimate DSM-5 and the likely features of ICD-11. Chapter 17 uses the WMH data to provide a rare glimpse into the relative prevalence and risk factors for PTSD based on different diagnostic criteria.

DSM-5 also eliminated the requirement that the trauma must immediately induce "fear, helplessness, or horror" (Criterion A2) in order to be considered a qualifying event. As noted above, this decision in DSM-5 is consistent with the Red Cross PsySTART risk criteria in which current distress is no longer a critical part of the triage process. The WMH surveys provided empirical evidence to the DSM-5 PTSD work group committee that supported the decision to remove the A2 criterion. These previously published findings (Karam et al., 2010), which serve as the basis for Chapter 18, illustrate the value of large epidemiological data sets for assessing the utility of specific diagnostic criteria.

Many studies of trauma-exposed populations have focused on partial or subthreshold PTSD, but these studies have applied different operational definitions. The criteria for subthreshold PTSD include fully endorsing a specific number of symptom clusters, requiring fewer symptoms from each cluster, or the narrower approach, namely, focusing on symptoms that are unique to PTSD, such as re-experiencing symptoms (Maercker et al., 2013). Clearly, the rates of subthreshold PTSD will vary according to the strictness of the criteria applied. Thus, for epidemiological purposes, a consensus definition of subthreshold PTSD would enable examination of the rates, risk factors, and consequences of subthreshold PTSD across multiple investigations. The WMH surveys attempted to determine an optimal criterion set for defining subthreshold PTSD (Chapter 19). Further replication is required before the issue can be settled, but given the growing attention to subthreshold PTSD, it is critical that the field develop an empirically based consensus classification system.

Epidemiological evidence can also inform discussions about subtypes of PTSD, particularly the dissociative subtype and complex PTSD. A few studies have suggested that PTSD characterized by dissociative symptoms is underpinned by somewhat different neurobiological mechanisms from most other PTSD symptom constellations and that patients with the dissociative subtype may require different interventions (Lanius et al., 2012). Similarly, the field has debated questions about the uniqueness of complex PTSD, a subtype characterized by dysfunction in self-organization or emotional regulation, with symptoms in the affective, self-concept, and relational domains (Herman, 1992). DSM-5 introduced a dissociative subtype, and ICD-11 has proposed including complex PTSD as a separate subtype. Epidemiological evidence on both issues is presented in Chapter 20 and in Chapter 21 of this volume.

Overall, the contributions to understanding the nature of PTSD included in Section 5 of this volume fulfill one of the basic functions of epidemiology, which is to complete the clinical picture (Morris, 1957). For PTSD and other psychiatric disorders, this is best accomplished with data from community samples composed of a mix of untreated and treated cases.

Strengths and Limitations of the WMH Surveys

PTSD clearly places a great burden on the population because of the ubiquity of trauma, the relatively high rate of PTSD, the high rate of chronicity after onset, and in many parts of the world, the scarcity of treatment interventions that might lead to prevention or early remission. The WMH studies discussed in this volume take a comprehensive approach to the global epidemiology and phenomenology of PTSD. The WMH initiative constitutes the largest cross-national series of population-based surveys of mental disorders ever conducted (Kessler & Üstün, 2008). The core strength of the WMH surveys is the standardization of every aspect of the study, from the comprehensive assessment of mental and substance use disorders to the broad selection of risk factors and consequences. Methodologically, these surveys employed uniform procedures for (1) translation and back-translation of the CIDI; (2) representative sampling strategies; (3) training and oversight of local trainers and supervisors; and (4) oversight of country-specific data collection, management, and analysis.

The heart of the study is the CIDI diagnostic interview schedule, which is described in detail in Chapter 2. The instrument has broad diagnostic coverage and special methods for determining age-of-onset, disability, service utilization, medical conditions, demographic histories, family history, and childhood adversities. Interviewers are given special training about best practices for keeping respondents focused and motivated throughout the assessment. Most importantly, the WMH surveys instituted unique methods to facilitate recall in order to create a database containing temporally ordered variables capable of disentangling antecedents from sequelae.

A critical feature of the CIDI is the assessment of PTSD for a randomly selected trauma in order to provide unbiased estimates of the prevalence of PTSD in general and the conditional risk of PTSD after specific traumas. Prior community surveys assessed PTSD for respondent-reported most stressful or worst trauma. For clinical samples, this approach is judicious. For epidemiological purposes, however, this approach overestimates the overall and conditional rates of PTSD because the traumas selected (DSM-IV Criterion A1) are not representative of the multiple traumas occurring over the course of the lifetime. In addition, the worst traumas are not representative of all traumas of a given type. Thus, the use of the random trauma method ensures that the conditional risks of PTSD reflect the full range of human experiences, not just the worst possible situations. This decision was based in part on a comparison of PTSD prevalence after random versus worst trauma in a general population sample, which, not surprisingly, found higher rates of PTSD after respondent-reported worst trauma (Breslau et al., 2004). Specifically, the overall rate of PTSD after worst traumas was 13.6%, while the rate after randomly selected traumas was 9.2%. This considerable disparity was found for PTSD in conjunction with each trauma assessed by the study. The biggest disparity occurred for one of the most commonly reported traumas – life-threatening illness. When selected as the worst trauma, the rate of PTSD was 31.2%. When selected as a random trauma, it was 1.1%. Similarly, when rape was chosen by respondents as their worst trauma, the rate of PTSD was 62.0%. When rape was chosen randomly, the rate was 49.0%. Such discrepancies suggest that for purposes of determining the prevalence and risk factors for PTSD in general population samples drawn from culturally and socioeconomically diverse settings, basing estimates of PTSD on a randomly selected trauma would provide a more unbiased portrait of the epidemiology of PTSD.

Another pivotal decision in designing the version of the CIDI used in the WMH surveys was to assess all of the DSM-IV PTSD criteria, without skipping out if the respondent failed to endorse the A2 criterion or the requisite number of re-experiencing, avoidance/numbing, or hyper-arousal symptoms. This was especially important for achieving the nosological aims described above. Due to the choice of a random trauma as the focal trauma for assessing PTSD as well as the rest of the WMH methodology, this volume brings together a fresh perspective on the epidemiology and phenomenology of PTSD.

Of course, cross-national studies such as the WMH surveys have built-in limitations, as is true of all cross-sectional surveys. Each chapter of this volume reflects on the limitations of the specific analyses of trauma and PTSD under consideration. Overall, we note that the WMH surveys made an effort to balance the standardization needed to compare and combine data from countries across the globe with inclusion of culturally relevant clinical, demographic, and psychosocial risk factors needed for clinically meaningful country-specific analyses of PTSD. The final chapter of this volume discusses the research and policy implications of the WMH findings.

As alluded to earlier in this chapter, PTSD and psychiatric epidemiology as a whole are both relatively new fields of research. It is thus noteworthy that since its inception, the WMH initiative has been a training ground for investigators from around the world with an interest in psychiatric epidemiology. In addition to annual WMH meetings where achievements, problems, and new ideas for research are discussed, WMH investigators receive feedback about framing research questions, carrying out analyses, writing, and making in-person presentations of research results from senior WMH colleagues and outside experts. WMH collaborators also have access to the basic tools, building blocks, and supports needed to build successful and productive careers in psychiatric epidemiology. Several researchers who initially joined the WMH initiative as junior investigators have since become internationally recognized leaders in mental health research in general and PTSD research specifically. This accomplishment is a tribute to the vision and consistent oversight by the WMH founders and their staff to whom the field of global mental health research owes an enormous debt.

Conclusion

This volume is the culmination of in-depth interviews with close to 70,000 adult participants from 24 countries on 6 continents who answered questions about exposure to 29 separate trauma types and the PTSD symptoms that occurred in their wake. This book represents the collective work of investigators from each country and their outstanding research teams. Section 1 provides an overview of key studies of the epidemiology of PTSD and details about the methodology implemented by the WMH surveys. Section 2 assesses the nature and extent of trauma exposure around the globe, socio-demographic risk factors, and two potent influences on the risk of exposure, childhood adversities and pre-existing psychopathology. Section 3, which is devoted to the descriptive epidemiology of PTSD, contains chapters on the prevalence and risk factors for PTSD, secondary psychiatric and medical morbidities, impairments, and use of mental health services as well as barriers to care. Section 4, the longest section of the book, explores a few critical drivers of the development and course of PTSD, such as childhood adversities and prior psychopathology, and examines four specific traumas in detail: sexual assault in women, motor vehicle collisions, unexpected death of a loved one, and disasters. Section 5 provides evidence from the WMH on key nosological issues, including the overlap in case identification across sets of diagnostic criteria, empirical findings supporting the DSM-5 decision to remove the DSM-IV A2 criterion, and WMH evidence on the prevalence and correlates of subthreshold, dissociative, and complex PTSD. Section 6 features a chapter describing a novel statistical strategy for identifying groups at high risk for developing PTSD, and a concluding chapter on the broad implications of the WMH results for both our current understanding of PTSD and for future research into this commonly occurring, seriously impairing, and severely undertreated disorder. Our deepest hope is that this volume will serve as a valuable resource for clinicians, researchers, and policy makers around the world for many years to come.

References

Albuquerque, A., Soares, C., De Jesus, P. M., & Alves, C. (2003). Post-traumatic stress disorder (PTSD). Assessment of its rate of occurrence in the adult population of Portugal. *Acta Medica Portugal*, 16, 309–20.

Alegria, M. R., Fortuna, L. Y., Lin, J. H., et al. (2013). Prevalence, risk and correlates of posttraumatic stress disorder across ethnic and racial minority groups in the United States. *Medical Care*, 51, 1114–23.

Alonso, J., Chatterje, S., & He, Y., eds. (2013). *The Burdens of Mental Disorders: Global Perspective from the WHO Mental Health Surveys*. New York, NY: Cambridge University Press.

American Psychiatric Association (1952). *Diagnostic and Statistical Manual of Mental Disorders, First Edition. DSM-1*. Washington, DC: American Psychiatric Association.

American Psychiatric Association (1968). *Diagnostic and Statistical Manual of Mental Disorders, Second Edition. DSM-II*. Washington, DC: American Psychiatric Association.

American Psychiatric Association (1980). *Diagnostic and Statistical Manual of Mental Disorders, Third Edition. DSM-III*. Washington, DC: American Psychiatric Association.

American Psychiatric Association (1987). *Diagnostic and Statistical Manual of Mental Disorders, Third Edition-Revised. DSM III-R*. Washington, DC: American Psychiatric Association.

American Psychiatric Association (1994). *Diagnostic and Statistical Manual of Mental Disorders, Fourth Edition. DSM-IV*. Washington, DC: American Psychiatric Association.

American Psychiatric Association (2013). *Diagnostic and Statistical Manual of Mental Disorders, Fifth Edition. DSM-5*. Arlington, VA: American Psychiatric Association.

Bisson, J. I., Roberts, N. P., Andrew, M., Cooper, R., & Lewis, C. (2013). Psychological therapies for chronic post-traumatic stress disorder (PTSD) in adults. *Cochrane Database Systematic Review*, 12, CD003388.

Boscarino, J. A. (2008). A prospective study of PTSD and early-age heart disease mortality among Vietnam veterans: implications for surveillance and prevention. *Psychosomatic Medicine*, 70, 668–76.

Brennstuhl, M. J., Tarquinio, C., & Montel, S. (2015). Chronic pain and PTSD: evolving views on their comorbidity. *Perspectives on Psychiatric Care*, 51, 295–304.

Brett, E. A., Spitzer, R. L., & Williams, J. B. (1988). DSM-III-R criteria for posttraumatic stress disorder. *American Journal of Psychiatry*, 145, 1232–6.

Breslau, N., & Davis, G. C. (1992). Posttraumatic stress disorder in an urban population of young adults: risk factors for chronicity. *American Journal of Psychiatry*, 149, 671–5.

Breslau, N., Davis, G. C., Peterson, E. L., & Schultz, L. (1997). Psychiatric sequelae of posttraumatic stress disorder in women. *Archives of General Psychiatry*, 54, 81–7.

Breslau, N., Kessler, R. C., Chilcoat, H. D., et al. (1998). Trauma and posttraumatic stress disorder in the community: the 1996 Detroit Area Survey of Trauma. *Archives of General Psychiatry*, 55, 626–32.

Breslau, N., Chilcoat, H. D., Kessler, R. C., Peterson, E. L., & Lucia, V. C. (1999). Vulnerability to assaultive violence: further specifications of the sex differences in post-traumatic stress disorder. *Psychological Medicine*, 29, 813–21.

Breslau, N. (2002). Gender differences in trauma and posttraumatic stress disorder. *Journal of Gender Specific Medicine*, 5, 34–40.
Breslau, N., Peterson, E. L., Poisson, L. M., Schultz, L. R., & Lucia, V. C. (2004). Estimating post-traumatic stress disorder in the community: lifetime perspective and the impact of typical traumatic events. *Psychological Medicine*, 34, 889–98.
Breslau, N. (2009). The epidemiology of trauma, PTSD, and other posttrauma disorders. *Trauma, Violence, & Abuse*, 10, 198–210.
Breslau, N., Troost, J. P., Bohnert, K., & Luo, Z. (2013). Influence of predispositions on post-traumatic stress disorder: does it vary by trauma severity? *Psychological Medicine*, 43, 381–90.
Breslau, N., Koenen, K. C., Luo, Z., et al. (2014). Childhood maltreatment, juvenile disorders, and adult post-traumatic stress disorder: a prospective investigation. *Psychological Medicine*, 44, 1937–45.
Brewin, C. R., Andrews, B., & Valentine, J. D. (2000). Meta-analysis of risk factors for posttraumatic stress disorder in trauma-exposed adults. *Journal of Consulting and Clinical Psychology*, 68, 748–66.
Bromet, E., Hobbs, M., Clouston, S. et al. (2016). DSM-IV post-traumatic stress disorder among World Trade Center responders 11–13 years after the disaster of 11 September 2001 (9/11). *Psychological Medicine*. 46(4), 771–83.
Bronner, M. B., Peek, N., Vries, M. D., et al. (2009). A community-based survey of posttraumatic stress disorder in the Netherlands. *Journal of Traumatic Stress*, 22, 74–8.
Burgess, A. W., & Holmstrom, L. L. (1974). Rape trauma syndrome. *American Journal of Psychiatry*, 131, 981–6.
Chapman, C., Mills, K., Slade, T., et al. (2012). Remission from post-traumatic stress disorder in the general population. *Psychological Medicine*, 42, 1695–703.
Chilcoat, H. D., & Breslau, N. (1998). Investigations of casual pathways between PTSD and drug use disorders. *Addictive Behaviors*, 23, 827–40.
Clouston, S. A., Kotov, R., Pietrzak, R. H., et al. (2016). Cognitive impairment among World Trade Center responders: long-term implications of re-experiencing the 9/11 terrorist attacks. *Alzheimer's and Dementia*, 4, 67–75.
Cohen, P., & Cohen, J. (1984). The clinician's illusion. *Archives of General Psychiatry*, 41, 1178–82.
Cohen, B. E., Neylan, T. C., Yaffe, K., et al. (2013). Posttraumatic stress disorder and cognitive function: findings from the mind your heart study. *The Journal of Clinical Psychiatry*, 74, 1063–70.
Cougle, J. R., Resnick, H., & Kilpatrick, D. (2009). PTSD, depression, and their comorbidity in relation to suicidality: cross-sectional and prospective analyses of a national probability sample of women. *Depression and Anxiety*, 26, 1151–7.
Davidson, J. R., Hughes, D., Blazer, D. G., & George, L. K. (1991). Post-traumatic stress disorder in the community: an epidemiological study. *Psychological Medicine*, 21, 713–21.
de Jong, J. T., Komproe, I. H., Van Ommeren, M., et al. (2001). Lifetime events and posttraumatic stress disorder in 4 postconflict settings. *JAMA*, 286, 555–62.
de Vries, G. J., & Olff, M. (2009). The lifetime prevalence of traumatic events and posttraumatic stress disorder in the Netherlands. *Journal of Traumatic Stress*, 22, 259–67.
DiGangi, J. A., Gomez, D., Mendoza, L., et al. (2013). Pretrauma risk factors for posttraumatic stress disorder: a systematic review of the literature. *Clinical Psychology Review*, 33, 728–44.
Dohrenwend, B. P., Turner, J. B., Turse, N. A., et al. (2006). The psychological risks of Vietnam for US veterans: a revisit with new data and methods. *Science*, 313(5789), 979–82.
Duncan, L., Ratanatharathorn, A., Aiello, A. E., et al. (2018). Largest GWAS of PTSD (N = 20 070) yields genetic overlap with schizophrenia and sex differences in heritability. *Molecular Psychiatry*, 23, 666–73.
Eaton, W. W., ed. (2006). *Medical and Psychiatric Comorbidity over the Course of Life*. Washington, DC: American Psychiatric Publishing.
Edmonson, D., & von Känel, R. (2017). Post-traumatic stress disorder and cardiovascular disease. *Lancet Psychiatry*, 4, 320–9.
Figley, C. R., ed. (1978). *Stress Disorders among Vietnam Veterans: Theory, Research, and Treatment*. New York, NY: Brunner/Mazel.
Fikretoglu, D., & Liu, A. (2012). Prevalence, correlates, and clinical features of delayed-onset posttraumatic stress disorder in a nationally representative military sample. *Social Psychiatry and Psychiatric Epidemiology*, 47(8), 1359–66.
Finkelhor, D. (1994). The international epidemiology of child sexual abuse. *Child Abuse and Neglect*, 18, 409–17.
Flatt, J. D., Gilsanz, P., Quesenberry, C. P. Jr., Albers, K. B., & Whitmer, R. A. (2018). Post-traumatic stress disorder and risk of dementia among members of a health care delivery system. *Alzheimer's and Dementia*, 14, 28–34.
Flory, J. D., & Yehuda, R. (2015). Comorbidity between post-traumatic stress disorder and major depressive disorder: alternative explanations and treatment considerations. *Dialogues in Clinical Neuroscience*, 17, 141–50.
Foa, E. B., Hearst-Ikeda, D., & Perry, K. J. (1995). Evaluation of a brief cognitive-behavioral program for the prevention of chronic PTSD in recent assault victims. *Journal of Consulting and Clinical Psychology*, 63, 948–55.
Goldmann, E., Aiello, A., Uddin, M., et al. (2011). Pervasive exposure to violence and posttraumatic stress

disorder in a predominantly African American Urban Community: the Detroit Neighborhood Health Study. *Journal of Traumatic Stress*, 24, 747–51.

Gradus, J. L. (2017). Prevalence and prognosis of stress disorders: a review of the epidemiologic literature. *Clinical Epidemiology*, 9, 251–60.

Hatch, S. L., & Dohrenwend, B. P. (2007). Distribution of trauma and other stressful life events by race/ethnicity, SES and age: a review of the research. *American Journal of Community Psychology*, 40, 313–32.

Hauffa, R., Rief, W., Brähler, E., et al. (2011) Lifetime traumatic experiences and posttraumatic stress disorder in the German population: results of a representative population survey. *The Journal of Nervous and Mental Disease*, 199(12), 934–9.

Helzer, J. E., Robins, L. N., Wish, E., & Hesselbrock, M. (1979). Depression in Viet Nam veterans and civilian controls. *American Journal of Psychiatry*, 136, 526–9.

Helzer, J. E., Robins, L, N., & McEvoy, L. (1987). Post-traumatic stress disorder in the general population. Findings of the epidemiologic catchment area survey. *New England Journal of Medicine*, 317, 1630–4.

Herman, J., & Hirschman, L. (1977). Incest between fathers and daughters. *The Sciences*, 17, 4–7.

Herman, J. L. (1992). Complex PTSD: a syndrome in survivors of prolonged and repeated trauma. *Journal of Traumatic Stress*, 5, 377–91.

Hobfoll, S. E., Gehart, J. I., Zaita, A. K., et al. (2015). Posttraumatic stress symptoms predict impaired neutrophil recovery in stem cell transplant recipients. *Psychooncology*, 24, 1529–35.

Janca, A., Üstün, T. B., & Sartorius, N. (1994). New version of World Health Organization instruments for the assessment of mental disorders. *Acta Psychiatrica Scandinavica*, 90, 73–83.

Jenkins, R., Otheieno, C., Omollo, R., et al. (2015). Probable posttraumatic stress disorder in Kenya and its associated risk factors: a cross-sectional household survey. *International Journal of Environmental Research and Public Health*, 12, 13494–509.

Jeon, H. J., Suh, T., Lee, H. J., et al. (2007). Partial versus full PTSD in the Korean community: prevalence, duration, correlates, comorbidity, and dysfunctions. *Depression and Anxiety*, 24, 577–84.

Karam, E., Andrews, G., Bromet, E., et al. (2010). The role of criterion A2 in the DSM-IV diagnosis of posttraumatic stress disorder. *Biological Psychiatry*, 68, 465–73.

Kardiner, A., & Spiegel, H. (1947). *War Stress and Neurotic Illness*, 2nd edn. New York, NY: Paul B. Hoeber.

Kearns, M. C., Ressler, K. J., Zatzick, D., & Rothbaum, B. O. (2012). Early interventions for PTSD: a review. *Depression and Anxiety*, 29, 833–42.

Kessler, R. C., McGonagle, K. A., Zhao, S., et al. (1994). Lifetime and 12-month prevalence of DSM III-R psychiatric disorders in the United States. Results from the National Comorbidity Survey. *Archives of General Psychiatry*, 51, 8–19.

Kessler, R. C., Sonnega, A., Bromet, E., Hughes, M., & Nelson, C. B. (1995). Posttraumatic stress disorder in the National Comorbidity Survey. *Archives of General Psychiatry*, 52, 1048–60.

Kessler, R. C. (2000). Posttraumatic stress disorder: the burden to the individual and to society. *Journal of Clinical Psychiatry*, 61, Suppl 5, 4–12.

Kessler, R. C., Demler, O., Frank, R. G., et al. (2005). Prevalence and treatment of mental disorders, 1990 to 2003. *New England Journal of Medicine*, 352, 2515–23.

Kessler, R. C., & Üstün, T. B., eds. (2008). *The WHO World Mental Health Surveys: Global Perspectives on the Epidemiology of Mental Disorders*. New York, NY: Cambridge University Press.

Klein, H. (1971). Families of holocaust survivors in the kibbutz: psychological studies. *International Psychiatry Clinics*, 8, 67–92.

Koenen, K. C., Moffitt, T. E., Poulton, R., Martin, J., & Caspi, A. (2007). Early childhood factors associated with the development of post-traumatic stress disorder: results from a longitudinal birth cohort. *Psychological Medicine*, 37, 181–92.

Koenen, K. C., Sumner, J. A., Gilsanz, P., et al. (2017). Post-traumatic stress disorder and cardiometabolic disease: improving causal inference to inform practice. *Psychological Medicine*, 47, 209–25.

Kulka, R., Schlenger, W. E., Fairbank, J. A., et al. (1988). *National Vietnam Veterans Readjustment Study (NVVRS): Description, current status, and initial PTSD prevalence estimates*. Washington, DC: Veterans Administration.

Kulka, R. A., Schlenger, W. E., Fairbanks, J. A., et al. (1990). *Trauma and the Vietnam War Generation: Report of Findings from the National Vietnam Veterans Readjustment Study*. New York, NY: Bruner/Mazel.

Lanius, R. A., Brand, B., Vermetten, E., Frewen, P. A., & Spiegel, D. (2012). The dissociative subtype of posttraumatic stress disorder: rationale, clinical and neurobiological evidence and implications. *Depression and Anxiety*, 29, 701–8.

Lassemo, E., Sandanger, I., Nygard, J. F., & Sorgaard, K. W. (2017). The epidemiology of post-traumatic stress disorder in Norway: trauma characteristics and pre-existing psychiatric disorders. *Social Psychiatry and Psychiatric Epidemiology*, 52, 11–19.

Lifton, R. J. (1967). *Death in Life: Survivors of Hiroshima*. New York, NY: Random House.

Logue, M. W., Amstadter, A. B., Baker, D. G., et al. (2015). The psychiatric genomics consortium posttraumatic stress disorder workgroup: posttraumatic stress disorder enters the age of large-scale genomic collaboration. *Neuropsychopharmacology*, 40, 2287–97.

Lohr, J. B., Palmer, B. W., Eidt, C. A., et al. (2015). Is Post-traumatic stress disorder associated with premature

senescence? A review of the literature. *American Journal of Geriatric Psychiatry*, 23, 709–25.
McFarlane, A. C. (2000). Posttraumatic stress disorder: a model of the longitudinal course and the role of risk factors. *Journal of Clinical Psychiatry*, 61, Suppl 5, 15–20.
Maercker, A., Forstmeier, S., Wagner, B., Glaesmer, H., & Brähler, E. (2008). Post-traumatic stress disorder in Germany. Results of a nationwide epidemiological study. *Der Nervenarzt*, 79, 577–86.
Maercker, A., Brewin, C. R., Bryant, R. A., et al. (2013). Diagnosis and classification of disorders specifically associated with stress: proposals for ICD-11. *World Psychiatry*, 12, 198–206.
Magruder, K., Serpi, T., Kimerling, R., et al. (2015) Prevalence of posttraumatic stress disorder in Vietnam-era women veterans: The health of Vietnam-era women's study (healthviews). *JAMA Psychiatry*, 72(11), 1127–34.
Marmar, C. R., Schlenger, W., Henn-Haase, C., et al. (2015) Course of posttraumatic stress disorder 40 years after the Vietnam War: Findings from the National Vietnam Veterans Longitudinal Study. *JAMA Psychiatry*, 72(9), 875–81.
Miller, M. W., & Sadeh, N. (2014). Traumatic stress, oxidative stress and post-traumatic stress disorder: neurodegeneration and the accelerated-aging hypothesis. *Molecular Psychiatry*, 19, 1156–62.
Mills, K. L., McFarlane, A. C., Slade, T., et al. (2011). Assessing the prevalence of trauma exposure in epidemiological surveys. *The Australian and New Zealand Journal of Psychiatry*, 45, 407–15.
Morina, N., Wicherts, J. M., Lobbrecht, J., & Priebe, S. (2014). Remission from post-traumatic stress disorder in adults: a systematic review and meta-analysis of long term outcome studies. *Clinical Psychology Review*, 34, 249–55.
Morris, J. N. (1957). *Uses of Epidemiology*, 3rd edn. Edinburgh, Scotland: Churchill Livingstone.
Moskos, C. C. (1975). The American combat soldier in Vietnam. *Journal of Social Issues*, 31, 25–37.
Nelson, C., Cyr, K. S., Corbett, B., et al. (2011). Predictors of posttraumatic stress disorder, depression, and suicidal ideation among Canadian Forces personnel in a National Canadian Military Health Survey. *Journal of Psychiatric Research*, 45(11), 1483–8.
Nock, M. K., Borges, G., & Ono, Y., eds. (2012). *Suicide: Global Perspectives from the WHO Mental Surveys.* New York, NY: Cambridge University.
Norris, F. H. (1992). Epidemiology of trauma: frequency and impact of different potentially traumatic events on different demographic groups. *Journal of Consulting and Clinical Psychology*, 60, 409–18.
Norris, F. H., Kaniasty, K., Conrad, M. L., Inman, G. L., & Murphy, A. D. (2002). Placing age differences in cultural context: a comparison of the effects of age on PTSD after disasters in the United States, Mexico and Poland. *Journal of Clinical Geropsychology*, 8, 153–73.
Norris, F. H., Murphy, A. D., Baker, C. K., et al. (2003). Epidemiology of trauma and posttraumatic stress disorder in Mexico. *Journal of Abnormal Psychology*, 112, 646–56.
Ozer, E. J., Best, S. R., Lipsey, T. L., & Weiss, D. S. (2003). Predictors of posttraumatic stress disorder and symptoms in adults: a meta-analysis. *Psychological Bulletin*, 129, 52–73.
O'Toole, B. I., Marshall, R. P., Grayson, D. A., et al. (1996) The Australian Vietnam veterans health study: III. Psychological health of Australian Vietnam veterans and its relationship to combat. *International Journal of Epidemiology*, 25(2), 331–40.
Pietrzak, R. H., Goldstein, R. B., Southwick, S. M., & Grant, B. F. (2011) Prevalence and Axis I comorbidity of full and partial posttraumatic stress disorder in the United States: results from Wave 2 of the National Epidemiologic Survey on Alcohol and Related Conditions. *Journal of Anxiety Disorders*, 25(3), 456–65.
Puac-Polanco, V. D., Lopez-Soto, V. A., Kohn, R., et al. (2015) Previous violent events and mental health outcomes in Guatemala. *American Journal of Public Health*, 105(4), 764–71.
Resnick, H. S., Kilpatrick, D. G., Danksy, B. S., Saunders, B. E., & Best, C. L. (1993). Prevalence of civilian trauma and posttraumatic stress disorder in a representative national sample of women. *Journal of Consulting and Clinical Psychiatry*, 61. 984–91.
Roberts, A. L., Austin, S. B., Corliss, H. L., Vandemorris, A. K., & Koenen, K. C. (2010). Pervasive trauma exposure among US sexual orientation minority adults and risk of posttraumatic stress disorder. *American Journal of Public Health*, 100, 2443–1.
Roberts, A. L., Gilman, S. E., Breslau, J., Breslau, N., & Koenen, K. C. (2011). Race/ethnic differences in exposure to traumatic events, development of post-traumatic stress disorder and treatment-seeking for post-traumatic stress disorder in the United States. *Psychological Medicine*, 41, 71–83.
Roberts, A. L., Koenen, K. C., Chen, Q., et al. (2017). Posttraumatic stress disorder and accelerated aging: PTSD and leukocyte telomere length in a sample of civilian women. *Depression and Anxiety*, 34, 391–400.
Rosenman, S. (2002). Trauma and posttraumatic stress disorder in Australia: findings in the population sample of the Australian National Survey of Mental Health and Wellbeing. *Australian and New Zealand Journal of Psychiatry*, 36, 515–20.
Schreiber, M. D., Yin, R., Omaish, M., & Broderick, J. E. (2014). Snapshot from Superstorm Sandy: American Red Cross mental health risk surveillance in lower New York State. *Annals of Emergency Medicine*, 64, 59–65.
Scott, K. M., Smith, D. R., & Ellis, P. M. (2010). Prospectively ascertained child maltreatment and its association with DSM-IV mental disorders in young adults. *Archives of General Psychiatry*, 67, 712–19.

Scott, K. M., de Jonge, P., Stein, D. J., & Kessler, R.C., eds. (2018). *Mental Disorders Around the World: Facts and Figures from the World Mental Health Surveys*. Cambridge: Cambridge University Press.

Shalev, A. Y., Ankri, Y., Israeli-Shalev, Y., et al. (2012). Prevention of posttraumatic stress disorder by early treatment: results from the Jerusalem Trauma Outreach and Prevention study. *Archives of General Psychiatry*, 69, 166–76.

Shalev, A., Liberzon, I., & Marmar, C. (2017). Post-traumatic stress disorder. *New England Journal of Medicine*, 376, 2459–69.

Shay, J. (1994). *Achilles in Vietnam: Combat Trauma and the Undoing of Character*. New York, NY: Simon and Schuster.

Shore, J. H., Tatum, E. L., & Vollmer, W. M. (1986). Psychiatric reactions to disaster: the Mount St. Helens experience. *American Journal of Psychiatry*, 143, 590–5.

Smith, B. C., Armelle, A. P., Boarts, J. M., Brazil, M., & Delahanty, D. L. (2016). PTSD, depression and substance use in relation to suicidality among traumatized minority lesbian, gay and bisexual youth. *Archives of Suicide Research*, 20, 80–93.

Stein, M. B., Walker, J. R., Hazen, A. L., & Forde, D. R. (1997). Full and partial posttraumatic stress disorder: findings from a community survey. *American Journal of Psychiatry*, 154, 1114–19.

Steinert, C., Hofmann, M., Leichsenring, F., & Kruse, J. (2015). The course of PTSD in naturalistic long-term studies: high-variability of outcomes. A systematic review. *Nordic Journal of Psychiatry*, 69, 483–96.

Strassman, H. D., Thaler, M. B., & Schein, E. H. (1956). A prisoner of war syndrome: apathy as a reaction to severe stress. *American Journal of Psychiatry*, 112, 998–1003.

Sumner, J. A., Kubranksy, L. D., Elkind, M. S., et al. (2015). Trauma exposure and posttraumatic stress disorder symptoms predict course of cardiovascular events in women. *Circulation*, 132, 251–9.

The Centers for Disease Control Vietnam Experience Study. (1988). Health status of Vietnam veterans: I. Psychosocial characteristics. *JAMA*, 259, 2701–7.

Van Ameringen, M., Mancini, C., Patterson, B., & Boyle, M. H. (2008). Post-traumatic stress disorder in Canada. *CNS Neuroscience and Therapeutics*, 14, 171–81.

Von Korff, M. R., Scott, K. M., & Gureje, O., eds. (2009). *Global Perspectives on Mental–Physical Comorbidity in the WHO World Mental Health Surveys*. New York, NY: Cambridge University Press.

Walker, L. E. (1979). *The Battered Woman*. New York, NY: HarperCollins.

World Health Organization (2016). *World Health Statistics 2016: Monitoring Health for the Sustainable Development Goals (SDGs)*. Geneva, Switzerland: WHO Press.

Wolfe, J., & Kimerling, R. (1997). Gender issues in the assessment of posttraumatic stress disorder. In J. P. Wilson & T. M. Keane, eds., *Assessing Psychological Trauma and PTSD*. New York, NY: Guilford Press, pp. 192–238.

Wolf, E. J., Logue, M. W., Stoop, T. B., et al. (2018). Accelerated DNA methylation age: associations with PTSD and mortality. *Psychosomatic Medicine*, 80, 42–8.

Yaffe, K., Vittinghoff, E., Lindquist, K., et al. (2010). Posttraumatic stress disorder and risk of dementia among US veterans. *Archives of General Psychiatry*, 67, 608–13.

Zerach, G., Solomon, Z., Cohen, A., & Ein-Dor, T. (2013). PTSD, resilience, and posttraumatic growth among ex-prisoners of war and combat veterans. *Israeli Journal of Psychiatry and Related Sciences*, 50, 91–9.

Zlotnik, C., Johnson, J., Kohn, R., et al. (2006). Epidemiology of trauma, post-traumatic stress disorder (PTSD) and co-morbid disorders in Chile. *Psychological Medicine*, 36, 1523–33.

Chapter 2

Methods of the World Mental Health Surveys

Ronald C. Kessler, Steven G. Heeringa, Beth-Ellen Pennell, and Alan M. Zaslavsky

The World Mental Health (WMH) Survey Initiative is a World Health Organization (WHO) initiative designed to help countries carry out and analyze epidemiological surveys of the burden of mental disorders in their populations (www.hcp.med.harvard.edu/wmh). This chapter provides a broad overview of the methods used in the surveys, with a particular focus on the assessment of traumas and posttraumatic stress disorder (PTSD). Throughout the chapter, we emphasize the standardized procedures of sampling, data collection, measurement, and analysis that were used across the WMH surveys, which are based on the WHO Composite International Diagnostic Interview (CIDI) Version 3.0 (Kessler & Üstün, 2004). The CIDI is a fully structured research diagnostic interview designed for use by trained lay interviewers who do not have clinical experience. The version of the CIDI used in the WMH surveys generates diagnoses of mental disorders according to the criteria of both the ICD-10 and DSM-IV systems, although only DSM-IV criteria are used in this volume. Consistent WHO translation, back-translation, and harmonization procedures were used to modify the CIDI for use in each WMH survey (Harkness et al., 2008). The same interviewer training materials, training programs, and quality control monitoring procedures were also used across WMH surveys to guarantee cross-survey comparability of data (Pennell et al., 2008).

The use of these standardized procedures has been critical for the success of the WMH initiative, as its main mission is to enable countries to implement mental health needs assessment surveys by building on the existing WMH survey infrastructure. The use of standardized materials reduces costs for each country and makes it easier to implement high-quality surveys by building on tried and true procedures. This applies not only to instrumentation and data collection, but also to analysis, as the WMH surveys use a centralized data processing and cross-national peer consultation model, which enables less experienced collaborators to work with world-class statisticians and psychiatric epidemiologists and to analyze, interpret, and write scientific reports about their data.

The WMH Samples

The sampling procedures used in the WMH surveys are closely related to those originally developed for the World Fertility Survey (WFS) program, one of the first efforts to coordinate a cross-national survey carried out across many countries (Verma et al., 1980). The sample designs for the WMH surveys drew heavily on the lessons of the WFS experience. Like the WFS and more recent successful international programs of community survey research, the WMH surveys required collaborating countries to employ probability sample designs to select nationally or regionally representative samples of adults for the survey interview. The WMH surveys aimed to obtain a representative sample of the household population in the country or region under study. This usually involved drawing a multi-stage clustered area probability sample of households in the population and then selecting one, or, in some cases, two respondents from each sampled household using probability methods without replacement. These sample designs were standardized across countries based on the principles of probability sampling, but with less emphasis placed on the specific probability sample design features employed across countries than on the use of some efficient probability sampling scheme rather than a quota or other nonprobability sampling scheme. This flexibility in design specifics was needed because countries varied widely in the information available to develop a sample frame from which the WMH sample could be selected.

In order to achieve the level of coordination in sampling required across countries, we established a WMH Data Collection Coordination Centre at the Institute for Social Research (ISR), University of Michigan in the United States. The Survey Research Center (SRC) at ISR is one of the leading academic survey research organizations in the world, with a long history of leadership in the development and implementation of large community surveys (www.src.isr.umich.edu). The Survey Sampling group at SRC, under the direction of Steve Heeringa, supervises WMH sampling, while the Survey Implementation group, under the direction of Beth-Ellen Pennell and more recently, Zeina Mneimneh, supervises WMH interviewer training and field implementation. The CIDI Training and Reference Centre at SRC, under the direction of Nancy Gebler and more recently, Stephanie Chardoul, is responsible for interviewer and supervisor train-the-trainer dissemination of CIDI training.

With regard to sampling, the SRC group developed a list containing a common set of requirements and performance standards that the probability sample design in each WMH survey is required to meet. Unique opportunities available in individual countries are then used to develop a sampling plan that achieves these requirements and meets the WMH standards. The staff of the WMH Data Collection Coordination Centre work closely with local collaborators to develop these sample design plans. The plans are reviewed by a panel of technical experts and then revised, based on feedback from this panel. Once the design is finalized, day-to-day oversight of implementation is the responsibility of the local research team, although SRC supervisors continue to provide consultation throughout the field period.

Most WMH survey countries develop a similar sampling plan that features multistage area probability sampling. Several countries, though, adopt an alternative probability sampling procedures, such as the use of a national registry or combined uses of area probability methods and registry sampling to achieve the required probability sampling of the designated target population. All these samples, though, are probability samples. No WMH survey uses a convenience sample, an interviewer-managed quota sample, or any other nonprobability method of sample selection.

The Target Populations

Probability sample surveys are designed to describe a target population of elements that spans a specific geographic space during a specific window of time. Although the definition of the target population might seem simple, a number of important questions arise as soon as one begins to consider the possibilities. Should persons who were temporary residents, guest workers, or those who had legal claim to medical treatment or services be included in the sample? What about individuals who were incapable of participating in the survey because they were institutionalized or cognitively or physically impaired, and what about individuals living in remote places who would require disproportionate amounts of survey resources to sample and interview? In the end, a decision was made to allow the answers to these questions to vary across countries within a range of options described below.

The survey population is defined as the subset of the target population that is eligible for sampling under the survey design (Groves et al., 2004). It is necessary to decide what restrictions would apply in each participating WMH country in order to establish a survey population definition that conforms to the survey's scientific objectives, available sample frames, and budget limitations. Multiple dimensions are taken into consideration here. One of these involves the age range of the sample. The WMH survey was designed to focus on adults. However, the age that defines adulthood (commonly referred to as the "age of majority") varies across countries (typically either 18 or 21). In addition, some countries decided to impose an upper age limit on the sample (usually 65). Other dimensions that define the survey population involve geographic scope limitations (typically excluding otherwise eligible people who live in remote areas of the country), language restrictions, citizenship requirements, and whether to include special populations such as persons living in military barracks and group quarters or persons who were institutionalized at the time of the survey (e.g., hospital patients, prison inmates). These vary somewhat across countries.

Table 2.1 provides a summary of the survey populations for the 26 WMH surveys included in this volume. The vast majority of the surveys had a minimum age of 18 years. The lowest minimum age was 16 in New Zealand (although analysis of the New Zealand data is restricted to respondents 18 and above in cross-national reports for comparability with other countries) and the oldest was 21 in Israel. For maximum age requirements, Colombia, Mexico, and the regional surveys carried out in Beijing and Shanghai mandated that respondents be no older than 65 or 70. Turning to the geographic scope of the survey population, 17 of the 26 surveys defined it as the entire country, and three others as all areas in the country besides very rural areas (Colombia, Mexico, and Peru). The six remaining surveys defined the geographic scope of the survey as specific regions (Murcia in Spain; five of the six regions

Table 2.1 WMH sample characteristics by World Bank income categories[a]

Country by income category	Survey[b]	Sample characteristics[c]	Field dates	Age range	Sample size		Assessed for traumas	Response rate[d]
					Part I	Part II		
I. Low- and lower-middle-income countries								
Colombia	NSMH	All urban areas of the country (approximately 73% of the total national population)	2003	18–65	4,426	2,381	2,068	87.7
Nigeria	NSMHW	21 of the 36 states in the country, representing 57% of the national population. Surveys were conducted in Yoruba, Igbo, Hausa, and Efik languages	2002–4	18–100	6,752	2,143	1,516	79.3
PRC – Beijing/ Shanghai	B-WMH/S-WMH	Beijing and Shanghai metropolitan areas	2001–3	18–70	5,201	1,628	929	74.7
Peru	EMSMP	Five urban areas of the country (approximately 38% of the total national population)	2004–5	18–65	3,930	1,801	1,530	90.2
Ukraine	CMDPSD	Nationally representative	2002	18–91	4,724	1,719	1,545	78.3
(Total)					(25,033)	(9,672)	(7,588)	81.0
II. Upper-middle-income countries								
Brazil – São Paulo	São Paulo Megacity	São Paulo metropolitan area	2005–8	18–93	5,037	2,942	2,330	81.3
Bulgaria	NSHS	Nationally representative	2002–6	18–98	5,318	2,233	776	72.0
Colombia – Medellin[e]	MMHHS	Medellin metropolitan area	2011–12	19–65	3,261	1,673	1,387	97.2
Lebanon	LEBANON	Nationally representative	2002–3	18–94	2,857	1,031	873	70.0
Mexico	M-NCS	All urban areas of the country (approximately 75% of the total national population)	2001–2	18–65	5,782	2,362	1,818	76.6
Romania	RMHS	Nationally representative	2005–6	18–96	2,357	2,357	997	70.9
South Africa[f]	SASH	Nationally representative	2002–4	18–92	4,315	4,315	3,085	87.1
(Total)					(28,927)	(16,913)	(11,266)	78.5
III. High-income countries								
Australia[f]	NSMHWB	Nationally representative	2007	18–85	8,463	8,463	6,519	60.0
Belgium	ESEMeD	Nationally representative. Sample was selected from a national register of Belgium residents	2001–2	18–95	2,419	1,043	710	50.6
France	ESEMeD	Nationally representative. Sample was selected from a national list of households with listed telephone numbers	2001–2	18–97	2,894	1,436	1,071	45.9
Germany	ESEMeD	Nationally representative	2002–3	19–95	3,555	1,323	928	57.8
Israel	NHS	Nationally representative	2003–4	21–98	4,859	4,859	3,679	72.6
Italy	ESEMeD	Nationally representative. Sample was selected from municipality resident registries	2001–2	18–100	4,712	1,779	1,064	71.3
Japan	WMHJ 2002–2006	Eleven metropolitan areas	2002–6	20–98	4,129	1,682	1,138	55.1
Netherlands	ESEMeD	Nationally representative. Sample was selected from municipal postal registries	2002–3	18–95	2,372	1,094	788	56.4
New Zealand[f]	NZMHS	Nationally representative	2004–5	18–98	12,790	7,312	6,089	73.3
Northern Ireland	NISHS	Nationally representative	2005–8	18–97	4,340	1,986	1,287	68.4

(cont.)

Table 2.1 *(cont.)*

Country by income category	Survey[b]	Sample characteristics[c]	Field dates	Age range	Sample size		Assessed for traumas	Response rate[d]
					Part I	Part II		
Portugal	NMHS	Nationally representative	2008–9	18–81	3,849	2,060	1,548	57.3
Spain	ESEMeD	Nationally representative	2001–2	18–98	5,473	2,121	1,284	78.6
Spain – Murcia	PEGASUS–Murcia	Murcia region. Regionally representative	2010–12	18–96	2,621	1,459	942	67.4
United States	NCS-R	Nationally representative	2001–3	18–99	9,282	5,692	4,954	70.9
(Total)					(71,758)	(42,309)	(32,001)	64.8
IV. Total					(125,718)	(68,894)	(50,855)	70.4

[a]The World Bank (2012) Data. Accessed May 12, 2012 at: http://data.worldbank.org/country. Some of the WMH countries have moved into new income categories since the surveys were conducted. The income groupings above reflect the status of each country at the time of data collection. The current income category of each country is available at the preceding URL.

[b]NSMH (The Colombian National Study of Mental Health); NSMHW (The Nigerian Survey of Mental Health and Wellbeing); B-WMH (The Beijing World Mental Health Survey); S-WMH (The Shanghai World Mental Health Survey); EMSMP (La Encuesta Mundial de Salud Mental en el Peru); CMDPSD (Comorbid Mental Disorders during Periods of Social Disruption); NSHS (Bulgaria National Survey of Health and Stress); MMHHS (Medellín Mental Health Household Study); LEBANON (Lebanese Evaluation of the Burden of Ailments and Needs of the Nation); M-NCS (The Mexico National Comorbidity Survey); RMHS (Romania Mental Health Survey); SASH (South Africa Health Survey); NSMHWB (National Survey of Mental Health and Wellbeing); ESEMeD (The European Study of the Epidemiology of Mental Disorders); NHS (Israel National Health Survey); WMHJ2002–2006 (World Mental Health Japan Survey); NZMHS (New Zealand Mental Health Survey); NISHS (Northern Ireland Study of Health and Stress); NMHS (Portugal National Mental Health Survey); PEGASUS–Murcia (Psychiatric Enquiry to General Population in Southeast Spain-Murcia); NCS-R (The US National Comorbidity Survey Replication).

[c]Most WMH surveys are based on stratified multistage clustered area probability household samples in which samples of areas equivalent to counties or municipalities in the United States were selected in the first stage followed by one or more subsequent stages of geographic sampling (e.g., towns within counties, blocks within towns, households within blocks) to arrive at a sample of households, in each of which a listing of household members was created and one or two people were selected from this listing to be interviewed. No substitution was allowed when the originally sampled household resident could not be interviewed. These household samples were selected from Census area data in all countries other than France (where telephone directories were used to select households) and the Netherlands (where postal registries were used to select households). Several WMH surveys (Belgium, Germany, Italy, Spain–Murcia) used municipal or universal health-care registries to select respondents without listing households. The Japanese sample is the only totally unclustered sample, with households randomly selected in each of the 11 metropolitan areas and 1 random respondent selected in each sample household. Of the 26 surveys, 17 are based on nationally representative household samples.

[d]The response rate is calculated as the ratio of the number of households in which an interview was completed to the number of households originally sampled, excluding from the denominator households known not to be eligible either because of being vacant at the time of initial contact or because the residents were unable to speak the designated languages of the survey. The weighted average response rate is 70.4%.

[e]Colombia moved from the "low- and lower-middle-income" to the "upper-middle-income" category between 2003 (when the Colombian National Study of Mental Health was conducted) and 2010 (when the Medellin Mental Health Household Study was conducted), hence Colombia's appearance in both income categories. For more information, please see footnote a.

[f]For the purposes of cross-national comparisons we limit the sample to those 18+.

in Nigeria, representing about 57% of the national population; and five metropolitan areas in Japan) or as one or two specific cities (Sao Paulo in Brazil, Medellin in Colombia, and Beijing and Shanghai in the People's Republic of China). Earlier analyses which are reported in a few chapters also include data obtained from a national survey in Iraq and a regional survey in Pondicherry, India, but these two surveys are not considered part of the surveys described here because of their lack of core variables included in the bulk of analyses.

Sampling Frames

Probability sampling requires a sampling frame that provides a high level of coverage for the defined survey population. The sampling frame is defined as a list or equivalent enumeration procedure that identifies all population elements and enables the sampler to assign non-zero selection probabilities to each element (Kish, 1965). We carefully reviewed the available choices of sample frames with the collaborators in each WMH survey country before deciding on a final frame. Options could have included population registries, new or existing area probability sampling frames, postal address lists, voter registration lists, and telephone subscriber lists. The final choice of the frame for each country was determined by a number of factors, including the extent of coverage and statistical efficiency of available frame alternatives, the cost of developing and using the frame for sample selection, and the experience of the data collection organization in the use of the sample frame. These final sampling frames were generally of three types: (1) a database of individual-level contact information provided in the form of national population registries, voter registration lists, postal address lists, or household telephone directories; (2) a multistage area probability sample frame (Kish, 1965); and (3) or a hybrid multistage frame that combined area probability methods in the initial stages and a registry or population list in the penultimate and/or final stages of sample selection. Table 2.1 identifies the sample frame type chosen in each of the participating surveys.

Complex Sample Designs for the WMH Surveys

The goal of all survey sample designs is either to minimize sampling variance and bias for a fixed total cost or to minimize total cost while meeting predetermined analysis objectives. The analysis objectives are typically formulated as fixed targets for the variance and bias components of the total survey error for key survey estimates or the parameter estimates for important population models. In the WMH survey program, there was no single path to this goal. The surveys shared a set of common analysis objectives, primarily centered on the estimation of the population prevalence and correlates of mental disorders. Survey cost structures were highly variable from one country to another, depending on factors such as availability and accessibility of survey infrastructure (government or commercial survey organizations), availability and costs for databases and map materials required to develop sample frames, labor rates for field interviewers and team leaders, and transportation costs for getting trained interviewers to distributed samples of households. Total funding for the surveys also varied widely across countries. In many cases, funding restrictions limited not only the total size of the interviewed sample but also the scope of the survey populations or the use of costly sample design options.

The individual WMH sample designs in the surveys considered in this volume employed the full range of probability sampling techniques that survey statisticians can use to improve sample precision and reduce costs. Stratification of the samples by geographic regions and demographic characteristics was used to increase sample precision and control sample allocation. Multistage designs with modest clustering in the initial stages of sampling were used to control travel time and expenses. A version of the "double sampling" technique (Cochran, 1977) was used in the vast majority of surveys to determine the subsample of initial Part I CIDI screening interview respondents who would complete the more intensive Part II CIDI diagnostic questionnaire. This two-part approach is discussed in more detail in the next section of this chapter.

The variety of designs used in different WMH surveys is a reflection of the differences in the essential survey conditions faced by the collaborators. With the exception of a small number of studies that sampled adults directly from high-quality population registries, the vast majority of the WMH surveys considered in this volume used a multistage area probability sampling method. The population registry approach is attractive because it avoids within-household selection and weighting. A few other countries chose a first-stage probability sample of households directly from national postal lists (e.g., the Netherlands) or telephone directories (e.g., France) and then chose random respondents within the selected households. Germany used a two-stage design that involved a first-stage sampling of municipalities and a second-stage sampling of adults from population registries available within each of the selected municipalities. A number of other countries used a similar design, but added an intermediate second-stage sampling of electoral or postal districts before selecting eligible adults from a district registry (e.g., Italy) or an enumerated list of residents within selected districts (e.g., Ukraine).

The vast majority of the WMH surveys in this volume, though, used three-stage or four-stage area probability designs. The three-stage designs began with a primary stage sample of census enumeration districts or neighborhood units selected with probabilities proportional to size followed by a second-stage sampling of households within the first-stage units and a third-stage random selection of one or sometimes two eligible adults within a sampled household. Countries that used four-stage designs expanded this same basic approach by beginning with the selection of large county or municipal units and then progressing to selection of area segment blocks, then to households, and then to respondents within households. All WMH surveys that used within-household selection of respondents did so with an objective household selection table method developed by Kish (1949). In a probability subsample of households in some countries, the spouses of certain respondents were also selected to take part in the survey.

Considerable effort was required to construct the frames for the WMH samples in countries where survey frames did not already exist. In Lebanon, for example, area probability methods were used to build the frame and select a multistage sample due to the fact that only limited population data existed in Lebanon. The primary stage of sampling consequently selected area segments (sectors) from a comprehensive list developed by the WMH collaborators stratified by region and urbanicity. From this list, 342 area segments were selected with probabilities proportional to size. Prior to the second stage of sampling, the Lebanese team sent trained field staff to each selected area segment to create a comprehensive list of all housing units in the segment. Once this enumerative list was completed for each area segment, a second-stage sample was selected of housing units and then of respondents within households.

The WMH survey guidelines specified a response rate target of 65%, based on a precise method required to calculate the response rate (the American Association for Public Opinion Research RR4 definition; American Association for Public Opinion Research, 2000; www.aapor.org). This target response rate was achieved by 19 of the 26 surveys, with 7 having response rates in the range of 70% to 75%, 4 in the range of 75% to 80%, and 5 over 80%. The seven surveys that failed to meet the target had response rates in the range of 45.9% to 60.0%. It is noteworthy that these seven surveys were all carried out in high-income countries (Australia, Belgium, France, Germany, Japan, Netherlands, and Portugal). This is consistent with other evidence showing that difficulties contacting respondents are greatest in high-income countries, where residents have a higher probability than elsewhere of being away from home in the evening and on weekends, and that marketing surveys have become so common in high-income countries that the willingness of individuals to participate in surveys has declined substantially over time (Couper & de Leeuw, 2003). As surveys remain relatively novel in lower-income countries, the response rates there are generally higher than in high-income countries. Survey response rates are, of course, also influenced by many other factors, including government privacy rules, population resistance to survey participation, the experience and norms of the chosen data collection organization, and the availability of financial resources to invest in incentives or other refusal aversion efforts.

The Two-Part Interview Design

As noted above, in the vast majority of WMH surveys (the exceptions being Iraq, Israel, Romania, and South Africa, where all respondents were administered the full interview), the interview was divided into two parts, with the questions in Part I administered to all respondents and the questions in Part II administered to a probability subsample of respondents based on responses to the Part I questions. The reason for this was that the interview was long and the interviewer sometimes had to return to the respondent's household a second or third time to complete it. As many respondents did not have any mental disorders, we did not need all of these non-cases to achieve maximum statistical power in comparing to cases. This meant that we could realize considerable cost saving by terminating the interview for a probability subsample of non-cases as soon as we learned that they did not meet criteria for any mental disorder. This was accomplished with the two-part interview design. The interview began with a series of basic descriptive warm-up questions and then evaluated lifetime presence of a wide range of core mental disorders. All (100%) of the respondents who met criteria for any of these disorders were continued into Part II, which included questions about a wide range of correlates of the core disorders and also assessed mental disorders of secondary interest. In addition, a probability subsample of other Part I respondents (i.e., those who did not meet criteria for any core disorder) were also selected to complete Part II, while interviews with the remaining non-cases were ended after the completion of the Part I questions.

There has been a good deal of confusion on the part of some journal article reviewers about this two-part design. A common criticism is that the Part II sample overestimates prevalence because it does not include all non-cases, but this concern is unwarranted due to the fact that the Part II data were weighted to adjust for the under-sampling of Part II cases. For example, if we included only a random one-fourth (0.25) of all Part I non-cases in the Part II sample in a given country, each of those Part II non-cases would be assigned a weight of 4.0 (1.0/0.25) to compensate for their under-sampling. This means that if the estimated prevalence of a given lifetime mental disorder was 10% in the Part I sample, it would still be 10% in the weighted Part II sample. In a similar way, estimates of the correlates of disorder would be expected to be unbiased in the Part II sample compared to the Part I sample.

However, the precision of these estimates might be lower in the Part II sample due to the fact that the denominator sample size on which estimates were based would be smaller. Four observations are relevant with regard to precision. First, the precision of estimates increases at a decreasing rate, as the number of non-cases increases relative to cases, with the optimal allocation 1:1 (Schlesselman, 1982). The number of non-cases selected for the Part II sample was generally in the range of 15% to 33%, yielding more non-cases than cases of every single disorder in every survey. Second, the Part II sample was post-stratified (a term described later in the chapter) in order to adjust for any discrepancies that existed between the measured characteristics of the non-cases selected into Part II and those not selected into Part II. Third, the certainty selections into Part II included 100% of respondents not only with any lifetime core disorder, but also with any sub-threshold manifestation of the core disorders, increasing power to distinguish cases from near-cases. Fourth, probability of selection into Part II among other non-cases was made in proportion to the number of eligible respondents in the sample household in all surveys that used household sampling.

The last of these four observations is subtle and refers to an issue that touches on the discussion of weighting later in this chapter. Briefly, the precision of estimates is inversely related to the variance of sample weights. Both the probability of selection into Part I and the conditional probability of selection into Part II among Part I respondents contributed to this total weight. The Part I weight is inversely proportional to the number of eligible respondents in each household due to the fact that we selected only one respondent per household (with the exception of the small couples sample mentioned above, which is described in detail in the next subsection of this chapter), no matter how many eligible people resided in the household. This led to an over-sampling of people living alone and an under-sampling of individuals living in married couples and an even greater under-sampling of individuals living in households with three or more eligible respondents. The Part I weight corrects for this differential representation. By sampling non-cases in Part II with probabilities proportional (rather than inversely proportional) to number of eligible household members, we were partially able to cancel out the variance in Part I weights for non-cases. So, for example, while individuals living alone were over-represented in the Part I sample (due to having a 100% chance of selection as the household respondent versus a 50% chance for individuals living with a spouse, a 33% chance for individuals living with a spouse and one other adult household resident, etc.), they were under-sampled in the selection of non-cases in the Part II sample, making their proportion in the unweighted Part II sample closer to their true population proportion than it was in the unweighted Part I sample. The vast majority of the analyses reported in this volume are based on the Part II sample.

Nonresponse Surveys

WMH collaborators in all countries were encouraged to carry out systematic nonresponse surveys in an effort to evaluate and, to the extent possible, correct the effects of systematic survey nonresponse. The basic design of the nonresponse survey was to select a stratified probability subsample of initial survey nonrespondents who were approached one last time and asked to participate in a brief (typically 10 to 20 minutes) interview that would provide the investigators with basic information about individuals who were not able to participate in the full survey. Respondents in these nonresponse surveys were typically offered a financial incentive to participate. The survey was typically carried out either by telephone or face-to-face. The questions in the survey included a small number about basic socio-demographics (e.g., age, sex, education, marital status) and diagnostic stem questions for diagnoses of core mental and substance use disorders. Importantly, identical questions were asked in the main survey. Comparison of responses to these questions in the main sample and the nonrespondent sample was used to make inferences about nonresponse bias, while weighting adjustments described below were used to adjust the main sample for these biases.

Weighting

Person-level analysis weights that incorporated factors for sample selection, nonresponse and poststratification (i.e., weighting the sample distributions on one or more variables or multivariate profiles to equal the distribution known to exist in the population, with the population targets typically coming from government Census data) were constructed for each WMH survey data set. In a number of cases, these weights were developed by survey statisticians on the individual country research teams, while weights were constructed in other cases by the staff of the WMH Data Analysis Coordination Centre at Harvard Medical School (HMS) using sample design and population control data supplied by the local project teams. The case-specific analysis weights were used in computing estimates of descriptive statistics for the survey population and for estimating the descriptive statistics reported in this volume.

Construction of Analysis Weights

In general, the final analysis weight for each WMH survey respondent was computed as the product of the three weight components:

$$W_{final,i} = W_{sel,i} \cdot W_{nr,i} \cdot W_{psc,i}$$

where

$W_{sel,i}$ = the selection weight factor for respondent $i = 1, \ldots, n$;

$W_{nr,i}$ = the nonresponse weight adjustment factor for respondent $i = 1, \ldots, n$; and

$W_{psc,i}$ = the poststratification factor for respondent $i = 1, \ldots, n$.

The exact sequence of weight calculation steps differed slightly across surveys. In some countries, a separate nonresponse adjustment step was skipped, and the final weight was derived as the product of the sample selection factor and a final, all-encompassing poststratification to external population controls.

The sample selection weight was designed to compensate for the differing sampling probabilities for selecting individuals as WMH respondents. The selection weight factor, W_{sel}, was generally the product of the reciprocals of three probabilities: $W_{sel,hh}$, the reciprocal of the multistage probability of selecting the respondent's housing unit selection from the sample frame; $W_{sel,resp}$, the reciprocal of the conditional probability of selecting the WMH respondent at random within the eligible household (Kish, 1965); and W_{sel}, Part II, the reciprocal of the probability that an eligible WMH survey respondent was subsampled to complete the in-depth Part II diagnostic section of the WMH interview.

The nonresponse adjustment weight, W_{nr}, could be computed to account for differential patterns of response across categories of eligible respondents for a country-specific survey. When this weight was applied, nonresponse adjustments to survey weights were based on endogenous data; that is, on data from the sample frame that was known for both sample respondents and nonrespondents. In baseline or cross-sectional surveys such as the WMH studies, the data available to develop nonresponse adjustments is often limited to geographic and demographic information available for respondents and nonrespondents in the sample frame, such as population census data collected by the government.

In cases where nonresponse adjustment was implemented, a nonrespondent survey of the sort described above was used to generate this weight. The nonresponse sample was first weighted to be representative of all nonrespondents using within-household probability of selections weights (see below) and then this weighted subsample was compared to the similarly weighted main sample in an effort to determine if the two samples differed meaningfully on the variables assessed in both the samples. When differences of this sort were found, either a weighting class method or a propensity modeling approach (Little & Rubin, 2002) was used to develop the adjustment factors.

The weight calculations for most of the WMH survey data sets, however, did not include a separate nonresponse adjustment. Instead, an adjustment for differential nonresponse and sample noncoverage of the survey population was integrated into one consolidated adjustment in the poststratification weighting step, which is described below. In such cases, the factor W_{nr} can be viewed as taking a value of 1.0 in the final composite weight calculation. Readers who are interested in detailed case studies of nonresponse adjustment weighting for selected WMH data sets are referred to Alonso et al. (2004) and Kessler and Üstün (2004).

The final component in the WMH individual analysis weight is a poststratification factor, W_{ps}. The poststratification weighting adjustment differs from the nonresponse adjustment factors in that poststratification weighting uses data that are exogenous to the survey design to calibrate the weights for survey estimation. The WMH poststratification used estimates of population values from external sources such as a recent national census or demographic population estimation program to standardize the sampling weights to known population distribution values, such as the distribution of the population of the cross-classification of age (in categories), sex, and education. The logic of the general procedure used in each country involved forming a matrix of adjustment cells by cross-classifying age, sex, and major geographic regions (data permitting) of the survey population. Within each cell of this matrix, the poststratification weight factors were computed as the ratio of the external population count for each cell to the sum of computed sample selection weights for the WMH survey cases assigned to that cell:

$$W_{pstrat,c,i} = \frac{\hat{N}_c}{\sum_{i \in c}^{n_c} W_{sel,i} \cdot W_{nr,i}}$$

where

$W_{pstrat,c,i}$ = the poststratification factor for all cases in cell c;

$\hat{N}_c$ = the WMH country population estimate for cell c;

n_c = WMH country sample size in cell c;

$W_{sel,i}$ = the composite sample selection weight for case $i = 1, \ldots, n_c$; and

$W_{nr,i}$ = the nonresponse adjustment for case $i = 1, \ldots, n_c$.

In some countries, it was possible to include much more information than a few socio-demographic and geographic variables due to the availability of much more detailed population data on a wide range of socio-demographic variables that were also assessed in the WMH survey. In cases of this sort, data analyses were carried out to compare the WMH survey data with other weights imposed on the data to the population data in an effort to pinpoint any variables that were meaningfully discrepant between the two. When the number of such variables was small, a modified poststratification table of the sort described in the last paragraph could have been carried out that constructed poststratification tables from only those variables. However, this procedure would run the risk of creating discrepancies between the weighted sample and the population on other variables that were originally non-discrepant. In order to guard against this possibility, propensity score adjustment was used whenever a large number of poststratification variables were present (Rosenbaum & Rubin, 1983). In this approach, logistic regression analysis was used to develop a multivariate prediction equation from the poststratification variables that discriminated between the WMH sample and the population, where a dichotomous outcome variable was used to distinguish the sample from the population in an analysis that combined both data files. This prediction equation allowed for interactions among the poststratification variables and sequentially evaluated a wide range of predictors, arriving at a final model that included core variables (i.e., age, sex, education, geography) and significant discriminating variables. Appropriately weighted, predicted probabilities generated from this final equation were used to adjust the final WMH sample to approximate the multivariate distribution of the population on these variables.

Although poststratification can potentially reduce sampling variances for survey estimates, the primary purpose of weighting is to eliminate potential sources of bias that would be present in an unweighted analysis. Those biases could arise due to differences in the original selection probabilities for respondents, differential nonresponse (probabilities of observation), and differential sample noncoverage for elements of the target population. However, the pursuit of "unbiasedness" can have a price in the form of increased variance of survey estimates compared to an unweighted estimate based on the same sample size. Weighting effects on standard errors arise due to several factors, including the association between the distributions of the weights and the variables of interest and variance of the weight values assigned to the individual cases. In the process of developing the final analysis weights for the WMH data sets, sensitivity analyses were conducted to determine the effect of extreme weight values on the estimated sampling errors and potential bias of key survey estimates. If sampling variances proved highly sensitive to the most extreme weight values, the computed weights in the extreme lower and upper ranges were trimmed using methods that retained the sum of weights but distributed those weights across cases at each tail of the distribution. This trimming was typically carried out for respondents with the highest and lowest 1% to 2% of weights and in extreme cases, for those in the highest and lowest 5% of weights. For a detailed example of how this was done in one WMH survey, see Kessler et al. (2004).

Sampling Error and Inference from the WMH Survey Data

The WMH surveys are based on a variety of probability sample designs, with each design adapted to the resources, experiences, and cost structures that are unique to the particular collaborating country. Despite the variations in probability sample design forms, each survey is designed to support robust, design-based estimation of population statistics such as the prevalence of mental health disorders in a chosen survey population.

The survey literature refers to designs such as the ones used in the WMH surveys as complex designs, a loosely defined term meant to denote that the sample incorporates special design features such as stratification, clustering, and differential selection probabilities (i.e., weighting) that analysts must consider in computing sampling errors and confidence intervals for sample estimates of descriptive statistics and model parameters. Standard programs in statistical analysis software packages assume simple random sampling (SRS) or independence of observations in computing standard errors for sample estimates. In general, the SRS assumption results in underestimation of variances of survey estimates of descriptive statistics and model parameters. This means that the confidence intervals based on computed variances that assume independence of observations will be biased (generally too narrow) and design-based inferences will be affected accordingly. This section focuses on sampling error estimation and construction of confidence intervals for WMH survey estimates of descriptive statistics such as means, proportions, ratios, and coefficients for linear and logistic regression models.

Over the past 50 years, advances in survey sampling theory have led to a number of methods for estimating variances from complex sample data sets correctly. Several sampling error programs that implement these complex sample variance estimation methods were available to WMH data analysts. The two most common approaches were the Taylor Series linearization method (and corresponding approximation to its variance) and resampling variance estimation methods such as the Balanced Repeated Replication (BRR) method and the Jackknife Repeated Replication (JRR) method (Rust, 1985). The sampling error estimates presented in subsequent chapters of this volume were for the most part estimated in SUDAAN Version 9 (Research Triangle Institute, 2002) using the Taylor Series Linearization method, although some of the more complex estimates required the use of the JRR method, which we implemented in special SAS macros (SAS Institute Inc., 2011) written by staff of the WMH Data Collection Coordination Centre.

As noted earlier in this chapter, the WMH surveys, like most other health-related surveys, use stratification and clustering. Stratification is introduced to increase the statistical and administrative efficiency of the sample. Sample elements are selected as clusters in multistage designs to reduce travel costs and improve interviewing efficiency. Disproportionate sampling of population elements may be used to increase the sample sizes for subpopulations of special interest, resulting in the need to employ weighting in the estimation of population prevalence or other descriptive statistics. Relative to simple random sampling, each of these complex sample design features influences the size of standard errors for survey estimates. Figure 2.1 illustrates the effects of these design features on standard errors of estimates. The curve plotted in this figure represents the SRS standard error of an estimate as a function of sample size. At any chosen sample size, the effect of sample stratification is generally a reduction in standard errors relative to SRS. Clustering of sample elements and designs that require weighting for unbiased estimation generally have larger standard errors than an SRS sample of equal size (Kish, 1965).

The combined effects of stratification, clustering, and weighting on the standard errors of estimates are termed the design effect (D^2) and are measured by the ratio:

$$D^2 = \frac{SE(p)^2_{complex}}{SE(p)^2_{srs}} = \frac{Var(p)_{complex}}{Var(p)_{srs}}$$

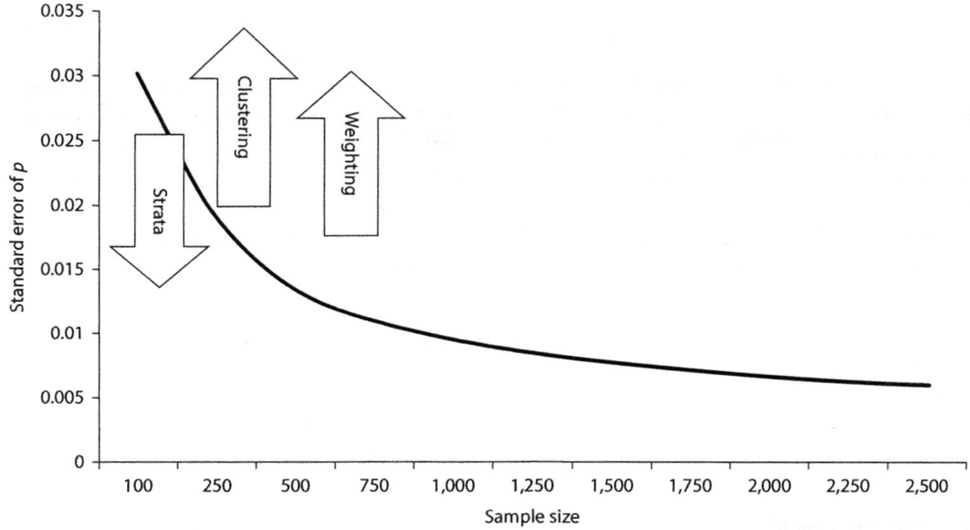

Figure 2.1 Complex sample design effects on standard errors of prevalence estimates (illustration for $p = 0.10$)

Originally appeared in Heeringa et al. (2008). Sample designs and sampling procedures. In R. C. Kessler & T. B. Üstün, eds., *The WHO World Mental Health Surveys: Global Perspectives on the Epidemiology of Mental Disorders*. New York, NY: Cambridge University Press, p. 29. ©2008, World Health Organization, used with permission.

where

D^2 = the design effect;

$Var(p)_{complex}$ = the complex sample design variance of the sample statistic p; and

$Var(p)_{srs}$ = the simple random variance of p.

Table 2.2 presents the design effects for estimates of lifetime, 12-month, 30-day, 12-month/lifetime, 30-day/12-month prevalence of DSM-IV PTSD. Close to two-thirds of the design effects are less than 1.0. And those that are greater than 1.0 are relatively modest in elevation, with a median of 1.5 across time frames and an inter-quartile range of 1.03–1.42. This pattern reflects the fact that PTSD was assessed in Part II of the samples, which was enriched for Part I cases. Given that PTSD is a highly comorbid disorder, this led to a considerably higher unweighted prevalence of PTSD in the Part II sample than in the Part I sample, reducing the design effect. The design effect is generally higher for lifetime prevalence than for more recent prevalence and lowest for conditional prevalence estimate. This pattern reflects the fact that the effects of sample clustering in increasing design effects are reduced when there are few cases within individual sample clusters, which is more likely when the outcome is rare and/or estimated in subsamples within clusters. Design effects are somewhat larger when results are pooled across countries than when they are estimated within countries. It needs to be remembered, though, that the sample size increases dramatically when data are combined across countries, resulting in substantial decreases in standard errors of estimates, despite the relatively small increases in design effects.

Measures

Traumas

DSM-IV defines trauma as a "stressor involving direct personal experience of an event that involves actual or threatened death or serious injury, or other threat to one's physical integrity; or witnessing an event that involves death, injury, or a threat to the physical integrity of another person; or learning about unexpected or violent death, serious harm, or threat of death or injury experienced by a family member or other close associate" (American Psychiatric Association, 1994). Twenty-nine types of trauma were assessed in the WMH surveys to operationalize this definition, with reports of lifetime exposure followed by questions about age at first occurrence of each type. As detailed in Chapter 3, exploratory factor analysis found six meaningful factors among these reports (referred to below as trauma groups) representing exposure to organized violence (e.g., civilian in war zone, relief worker in war zone, refugee); participation in organized violence

Table 2.2 Design effects of prevalence estimates of DSM-IV/CIDI PTSD in the WMH surveys

	Lifetime PTSD	12-month PTSD	30-day PTSD	12-month PTSD among those with lifetime PTSD	30-day PTSD among those with 12-month PTSD
I High-Income Countries					
Australia	0.841	0.675	0.871	0.617	0.848
Belgium	0.812	0.493	0.879	0.525	0.570
France	1.039	1.037	1.032	0.759	0.511
Germany	1.466	0.968	1.127	0.349	0.186
Israel	1.049	0.996	0.994	0.870	0.841
Italy	1.570	1.378	1.236	0.390	0.034
Japan	0.784	0.834	1.104	0.152	0.490
Netherlands	1.005	1.173	1.230	0.765	0.345
New Zealand	1.148	1.049	1.240	0.898	0.988
Northern Ireland	1.067	1.055	1.067	0.906	0.992
Portugal	1.102	1.094	0.986	0.893	0.549
Spain	0.996	0.923	0.689	0.900	0.267
Spain – Murcia	1.022	1.443	0.545	1.421	0.409
United States	1.398	1.404	1.456	1.148	1.479
II Upper-Middle-Income Countries					
Brazil – São Paulo	0.431	0.647	0.873	0.832	1.061
Bulgaria	1.179	0.630	0.807	0.262	0.975
Colombia – Medellin	1.102	0.997	1.004	0.848	1.011
Lebanon	0.670	0.894	0.968	0.916	0.010
Mexico	0.981	0.984	0.939	0.205	0.061
Romania	1.285	1.206	0.986	0.292	0.184
South Africa	1.348	1.425	0.999	0.756	0.125
III Low- and Lower-Middle-Income Countries					
Colombia	0.878	1.030	0.977	0.644	0.831
Nigeria[a]	0.995				
PRC – Beijing/Shanghai	1.009	0.942	1.025	0.042	0.164
Peru	0.753	1.399	1.990	0.097	0.003
Ukraine	1.440	1.425	1.411	0.812	0.645
IV Country Income Groups					
High-income countries	1.237	1.003	1.025	1.087	1.128
Upper-middle-income countries	1.010	0.962	0.933	0.588	0.490
Low- and lower-middle-income countries	1.074	1.315	1.262	0.749	0.625
V Total	**1.112**	**0.928**	**0.937**	**0.954**	**0.965**

[a]Nigeria only had 1 respondent with lifetime PTSD and none with 12-month or 30-day PTSD.

(e.g., combat experience, witnessed atrocities); physical violence victimization (witnessed violence at home as child; beaten by caregiver as child; beaten by someone else other than romantic partner); exposure to sexual violence victimization (e.g., raped, sexually assaulted, beaten by romantic partner); accidents/injuries (e.g., natural disaster, automobile accident); and three trauma types not loading with any others (mugged/threatened with weapon, human-made disaster, unexpected death of loved one).

Twenty-seven trauma types were assessed in the WMH surveys. Respondents were presented with a visual list of the trauma types (see Box 2.1) and asked to go down the list with the interviewer and answer yes or no about whether each trauma type ever occurred to them at any time in their life. Explicit yes–no responses were required to minimize the possibility of superficial negative responses. This possible problem was also addressed by training interviewers to use the contingent reinforcement feedback methods discussed below to encourage more active memory search (e.g., "*You said 'no' awfully quickly. Please take your time and think carefully about whether these things ever occurred to you. These are important questions for our research.*").

In addition to the 27 explicit trauma questions, the list included 2 final residual questions. The first one asked: "*Did you ever experience any other extremely traumatic or life-threatening event that I haven't asked you about?*" Verbatim responses to this question were back-coded into the other 27 categories whenever possible and the residual reports coded in an "other" category. The second residual question asked about a

Box 2.1 The traumas assessed in the WMH surveys

I **Experiences Involving Interpersonal Violence**
Combat experience (military or nonmilitary) in a war or sectarian violence (e.g., political, religious, or ethnic conflicts)
Relief worker or peacemaker in a war zone or region of sectarian violence
Civilian in a war zone
Civilian in a region of sectarian violence
Displaced refugee from a war zone or region of sectarian violence
Kidnapped or held captive
Beaten as a child by a caregiver
Beaten by a spouse or romantic partner
Beaten by someone else
Mugged or threatened with a weapon
Raped
Sexually assaulted or molested
Stalked

II **Other Threats to the Physical Integrity of the Respondent**
Natural disaster (e.g., flood, hurricane, earthquake)
Life-threatening automobile accident
Other life-threatening accident
Toxic chemical exposure
Other exposure to a human-made disaster (e.g., fire, explosion at a place of work)
Other life-threatening illness or injury

III **Threats to the Physical Integrity of Others**
UD of a loved one
Child with serious illness
Any other trauma experienced by a loved one
Witnessed repeated physical fights at home as a child
Witnessed any other injury or death
Accidentally caused injury or death to someone
Purposefully injured, tortured, or killed someone
Witnessed atrocities or carnage

IV **Open-Ended Questions about Other Potential Traumas**
Any other objectively qualifying experiences (respondents are asked to describe these experiences)
Private experiences (respondents are explicitly told in advance that they will not be asked to describe these experiences)

"private" trauma: "*Sometimes people have experiences they don't want to talk about in interviews. I won't ask you to describe anything like this but, without telling me what it was, did you ever have a traumatic event that you didn't tell me about because you didn't want to talk about it?*" As shown in Chapter 3, a surprisingly large number of respondents answered this question affirmatively.

Trauma Characteristics

Component stressors within traumas are known to be associated with PTSD risk. For example, risk of PTSD after motor vehicle collisions (MVCs) is known to be positively associated with severity, as indicated by the extent of injury or death of individuals involved in the MVC (Kazantzis et al., 2012), as well as with cognitions about who is perceived to be at fault (Nickerson et al., 2013). Rather extensive literatures document the associations of trauma characteristics and cognitions with PTSD-risk associated with a number of common types of trauma (e.g., Galea et al., 2005; Tiihonen Moller et al., 2014). However, these studies are based almost entirely on focused samples of individuals who were exposed only to one trauma type, such as MVCs, rapes that came to medical attention in emergency departments, or natural disasters. Studies of this sort are inherently incapable of comparing across trauma situations.

We wanted to address this limitation of previous studies in the WMH surveys by asking questions about trauma characteristics and cognitions in our general population samples so as to allow comparisons across different trauma situations. However, questions about the circumstances surrounding traumas can be time consuming; likewise, traumas are commonly occurring, making it infeasible to ask respondents about the circumstances surrounding each of the traumas that they have experienced. We resolved these problems by enumerating all occurrences of all lifetime traumas reported by each respondent and selecting one random occurrence of one randomly selected trauma type to be the focus of additional questions about trauma characteristics. As detailed in Chapter 3, we focused these questions on commonly occurring trauma types (MVC, natural disaster, sexual assault, unexpected death of a loved one) and asked questions about trauma characteristics and cognitions for each of these trauma types consistent with those found to be significant predictors of PTSD in prior studies.

For example, one of the trauma questions asked respondents: "*Did someone very close to you ever die unexpectedly; for example, were they killed in an auto accident, or murdered, or did they commit suicide, or have a fatal heart attack at an early age?*" At the end of the assessment of all traumas, respondents who reported the lifetime occurrence of this unexpected death were asked how many times they ever had this experience and their age the first time it happened. If unexpected death was then selected as the random trauma type, one particular instance of that type was then selected at random if the respondent reported more than one instance (e.g., the second time it happened, the most recent time it happened, etc.). The respondent's age at the time of this randomly selected occurrence of the randomly selected trauma type was then recorded and several additional questions were asked about the experience. These questions differed, depending on the type of trauma that was selected. In the case of unexpected death, the respondent was asked about his or her relationship to the deceased (spouse, parent, child, sibling, other relative, or nonrelative), the cause of death (homicide, suicide, accident/medical error, or illness), the length of the illness if the death was due to illness, the age of the person who died at the time of death; and the respondent's perception about the extent to which he or she could have done something to prevent the death. These trauma-specific questions are described in Chapter 14.

Random Traumas versus Worst Traumas

Of the 14 common mental disorders assessed in the WMH surveys, PTSD was the only one that was assessed more than once. Respondents who reported lifetime exposure to two or more traumas were assessed twice – once for the lifetime trauma nominated by the respondent as their worst lifetime trauma (i.e., the one associated with the largest number of "problems like upsetting memories or dreams, feeling emotionally distant or depressed, trouble sleeping or concentrating, and feeling jumpy or easily startled") and a second time for the random trauma operationalized as the randomly selected occurrence of the randomly selected lifetime trauma type experienced by the individual that was probed for trauma characteristics and cognitions.

We already noted one reason for selecting a random trauma: that we wanted to obtain information about trauma characteristics, but could not do this for every trauma ever experienced by respondents. The common data collection convention used in general population epidemiological studies of PTSD to address this problem is to ask respondents about lifetime exposure to a wide range of traumas, but then to assess PTSD only for the trauma nominated by the respondent as their worst or most upsetting lifetime trauma. This approach produces a realistic estimate of lifetime PTSD prevalence, based on the intuition, supported by some empirical evidence (Breslau, 2002), that lifetime PTSD is considerably more likely to be associated with these worst lifetime traumas than with other traumas and that individuals who did not develop PTSD after their worst traumas seldom do so after other traumas.

Unfortunately, this approach makes it impossible to obtain unbiased estimates of the conditional prevalence of PTSD associated with different types of trauma due to the fact that respondent reports about PTSD are associated with atypically severe traumas that they nominated as worst. This problem was first noted in a report on conditional trauma-specific PTSD risk in a U.S. national household survey where PTSD prevalence was roughly 50% among women who reported that a sexual assault was their worst lifetime trauma (Kessler et al., 1995). The authors noted that only a minority of the women with a lifetime history of sexual assault victimization in the survey nominated sexual assault as their worst lifetime trauma and that the prevalence of PTSD associated with the lifetime traumas nominated by other sexual assault victims as worst (i.e., as worse than their sexual assaults) was far less than 50%. Further analysis of the small amount of additional information collected about sexual assault characteristics in the survey (e.g., age of occurrence, the respondent's relationship to the perpetrator, whether the assault was a one-time occurrence or a repeated occurrence) showed that the sexual assault victims who nominated these as their worst lifetime traumas were considerably more likely than other sexual assault victims to report that their assaults were repeated occurrences in which a relative or step-relative was the perpetrator, demonstrating that traumas nominated as worst are atypical of all lifetime traumas of the same type. This raises a concern that estimates of conditional PTSD risk are upwardly biased when these estimates are based on surveys in which PTSD is assessed only for worst traumas.

Our main reason for developing the random trauma approach to assessing PTSD was to address this methodological problem in order to obtain accurate estimates of between-trauma differences in conditional risk of PTSD. We did this by weighting respondent reports involving the random trauma by the inverse of its probability of selection at the individual level and combining these weighted reports with reports about the worst lifetime trauma (or only lifetime trauma, in the case of respondents who reported lifetime exposure to only one occurrence of one trauma type). This generates a representative sample of all lifetime traumas experienced by all survey respondents. For example, if

20 individuals out of every 100 in the population with a trauma history experienced only one lifetime occurrence of one trauma type and the other 80 experienced an average of 3.5 occurrences of one or more trauma types, there would be 300 occurrences of a trauma in the lives of these 100 individuals ($20 \times 1 + 80 \times 3.5$), and we would assess PTSD associated with 180 (1 for each of the 20 individuals who experienced only one and 2 for each of the 80 individuals who experienced more than one) of these 300. Individuals who experienced many traumas would be under-represented in the PTSD assessment because the probability of selection of any one of their lifetime traumas other than their nominated worst trauma would be pit = 1/(1 − nit), where nit is the number of lifetime traumas experienced by respondent *i*. Our trauma weight adjusts for this differential representation by assigning a weight of 1/pit to each random trauma. In the example here, this would lead to the weights across the 180 traumas evaluated for PTSD summing to 300, the actual number of lifetime traumas that occurred in the population. This weighting introduces a rather substantial design effect because some respondents had a large number of lifetime traumas, but the very large WMH sample size to some extent compensates for this inefficiency.

Mental Disorders

PTSD and 13 other common mental disorders were assessed with the CIDI (Kessler & Üstün, 2004), a fully structured lay interview that assesses these disorders according to the definitions and criteria of both the DSM-IV and ICD-10 systems. DSM-IV criteria were used here. Organic exclusion and diagnostic hierarchy rules were not used in making diagnoses. The disorders assessed included two mood disorders (major depressive disorder/dysthymic disorder and broadly defined bipolar disorder [bipolar I and II and sub-threshold bipolar disorder, defined using criteria described elsewhere]) (Kessler et al., 2006), six anxiety disorders (generalized anxiety disorder, panic disorder and/or agoraphobia, PTSD, separation anxiety disorder, social phobia, specific phobia), four disruptive behavior disorders (attention-deficit/hyperactivity disorder, conduct disorder, intermittent explosive disorder, oppositional-defiant disorder), and two substance use disorders (alcohol and drug abuse with or without dependence).

Except for PTSD, the CIDI assessed lifetime prevalence of the disorder and then obtained retrospective data about age-of-onset (AOO). As noted above, PTSD was unique among these disorders in that lifetime prevalence was assessed twice – once for PTSD associated with the worst lifetime trauma and a second time for one random lifetime trauma. AOO of each disorder other than PTSD was assessed using probing techniques shown experimentally to improve recall accuracy (Knäuper et al., 1999), allowing us to determine whether respondents had a history of each disorder prior to exposure to the random trauma. This dating information is used in Chapter 11 to investigate the associations of history of psychopathology with PTSD associated with the random trauma.

Recency of disorders was assessed by asking respondents if they continued to have symptoms of each lifetime disorder at any time in the past 12 months and, if so, in the past 30 days. In the case of PTSD, respondents who had these recent symptoms were both asked about the traumas associated with those symptoms and were referred back to the lifetime trauma list they were administered at the beginning of the section. At the time this list was originally reviewed, respondents were asked to circle the number of the trauma in their Respondent Booklet (RB) with a pen provided by the interviewer each time they reported the lifetime occurrence of that trauma type. Respondents who reported recent symptoms were then asked to review this circled list and report on which traumas on the list were associated with their recent symptoms. This allowed us to determine how often cases of current PTSD in the population are complex in the sense of being associated with more than one trauma. The results of that analysis are reported in Chapter 21.

Methodological Challenges in Assessing Mental Disorders

As detailed elsewhere (Haro et al., 2006), a good concordance was found between diagnoses based on the CIDI and blinded clinical diagnoses based on SCID reappraisal interviews (First et al., 1994). In the case of PTSD, clinical reappraisal interviewers were instructed to focus on the same trauma as the one assessed in the CIDI in order to guarantee valid comparison of diagnoses, but were blinded to diagnoses based on the CIDI. Moderate CIDI–SCID concordance (Landis & Koch, 1977) of AUC = 0.69 was found between DSM-IV diagnoses of PTSD based on the CIDI and SCID in these clinical reappraisal interviews. Sensitivity and specificity were 38.3% and 99.1%, respectively, resulting in a likelihood ratio positive (sensitivity/[1 − specificity]) of 42.0 that is well above the 10.0 typically considered definitive for a positive screen (Gardner & Altman, 2000). Based on these operating characteristics, a very high proportion of CIDI cases (86.1%) were confirmed by the SCID.

As retrospective reports of lifetime occurrence of mental disorders prior to the occurrence of the random trauma play a central part in the analyses presented in this volume, it is important to recognize that previous research suggests that these reports can be inaccurate due to recall error (Giuffra & Risch, 1994; Simon & VonKorff, 1995; Patten, 2003; Moffitt et al., 2010). This problem is not unique to interviews about mental disorders, but has been recognized for years in many other areas of investigation by survey methodologists. And a considerable amount of research has been carried out by survey methodologists to address the problem (e.g., Turner & Martin, 1985; Tanur, 1992; Sudman et al., 1996) that has advanced considerably as cognitive psychologists have become increasingly interested in the survey interview as a natural laboratory for studying cognitive processes (Schwarz & Sudman, 1994; Schwarz & Sudman, 1996; Sirken et al., 1999). Several of the important tools that have emerged from these studies about how to improve the accuracy of retrospective reports were used in the modified version of the CIDI developed for the WMH surveys (Kessler & Üstün, 2004; Kessler & Üstün, 2008). We also used the results of survey methodologist research to address two other challenges in evaluating mental disorders: that mental disorders are embarrassing and thus tend to be under-reported (Tourangeau & Yan, 2007); and that some of the survey questions used to assess symptoms of mental disorders are necessarily rather complex, leading to the risk of comprehension errors (Schober et al., 2004).

Before reviewing the interview modifications that we made to address these methodological challenges, we note that analyses of the WMH data provide compelling evidence for the success of these improvements for two reasons. First, a 10-year follow-up survey of the respondents in the WMH survey carried out in the United States did not find the problem that plagued previous longitudinal psychiatric epidemiological surveys where a large number of respondents in the follow-up reported pre-baseline lifetime disorders that were not reported in the baseline interview (Borges et al., 2008). This is an important finding because it indicates that the approach we used for assessment was successful in reducing the most extreme problems of long-term recall failure. Second, the problem found in previous psychiatric epidemiological surveys of AOO reports being substantially overrepresented in the 5 years before interview do not occur in the WMH surveys (Kessler et al., 2007; Kessler et al., 2008), as shown by the fact that the distributions of AOO reports are much more substantively plausible. Again, this finding suggests that our approach to assessment addressed the problem of long-term recall failure.

These improvements were achieved by beginning with evaluations of problems in earlier versions of the CIDI made by survey methodologists in preparation for an earlier US survey that was the foundation for the WMH surveys (Kessler et al., 1998, 1999, 2000). Four main methodological challenges highlighted in those evaluations became the focus of CIDI 3.0 revision efforts: (1) that respondents might not understand some of the CIDI questions about lifetime prevalence, a number of which include multiple clauses and vaguely defined terms; (2) that some respondents might not understand the task implied by the lifetime prevalence questions, which requires a careful memory search that is unlikely to be carried out unless respondents are clearly instructed to do so; (3) that respondents might not be motivated to put in the hard work required to think back over their entire lives and answer lifetime recall questions accurately, especially in light of the fact that many CIDI questions deal with potentially embarrassing and stigmatizing experiences; and (4) that respondents might not be able to answer some CIDI questions accurately, especially those that ask about characteristics of mental disorders that are difficult to remember. AOO constitutes an especially important part of this fourth challenge, as previous research has shown that AOO is often difficult to recall accurately, even when respondents are motivated to do so (Belli, 1998; Prohaska et al., 1998). The strategies used in the CIDI 3.0 to address these four challenges are discussed in detail elsewhere (Kessler & Üstün, 2004, 2008) and will be reviewed only briefly here.

Question Comprehension

It is obvious that ambiguous questions are likely to be misconstrued, but it is somewhat less obvious just how ambiguous most structured survey questions are and how often respondents must "read between the lines" to make sense of questions. Debriefing studies of earlier versions of the CIDI found that many respondents misunderstood important aspects of key diagnostic questions. One reason for this is that many terms in surveys are vaguely defined. Another is that the survey interview situation is a special kind of interaction in which the standard rules of conversation – rules that help fill in the gaps in meaning – do not apply. Unlike someone in a normal conversation, the respondent in the survey interview often has only a vague notion of both the identity of the person to whom he/she is talking and the purpose of the conversation (Cannell et al., 1968). The person who asks the questions (the interviewer) is not the person who formulated the questions (the researcher), and the questioner is often unable to clarify the respondent's uncertainties about the intent of the questions. Furthermore, the flow of questions in the survey interview is established prior to the beginning of the conversation, which means that normal conversational rules of give-and-take in question and answer sequences do not apply. This leads to more misreading than in a normal conversation, even when questions are seemingly straightforward (Clark & Schober, 1992); this problem is compounded when the topic of the interview involves emotionally charged experiences that are often difficult to describe with clarity.

In an effort to investigate this problem, debriefing interviews were carried out with respondents administered sections of the CIDI, who were asked to explain what they thought the questions meant and why they answered them in the way that they did (Kessler et al., 1998; Kessler, 1999). Four discriminating features were found among questions that had high – as opposed to low – levels of misunderstanding. First, some questions were too complex. Second, some questions used vaguely defined terms. Third, some questions asked about odd experiences that could plausibly be interpreted in more than one way, such as those about seeing and hearing things that others do not. Many respondents were found to normalize these questions and to respond positively when the correct answer was actually negative. Fourth, some questions were misunderstood because of a contextual misunderstanding, which derived more from the question's position in the flow of the interview than from its lack of clarity.

Based on these results, we carried out detailed CIDI debriefing interviews with volunteer respondents in methodological studies to support the development of CIDI 3.0 by pinpointing questions with all four types of comprehension problems. Misunderstandings based on complex questions were addressed by breaking down the original CIDI questions into less complex subquestions. Especially complex questions were presented in a RB that provided a visual aid to respondents as the questions were being read by the interviewer. Misunderstandings based on the vagueness of terms were addressed by introducing clarifications and examples. Misunderstandings based on normalization of questions about odd experiences were addressed by prefacing the questions with the clarification that we were actually asking about odd experiences and informing respondents that it was important for us to learn how often these experiences occur. Contextual misunderstandings were resolved by reordering questions to remove the contextual effects and by adding clarifying clauses to certain questions. The number of modifications was so large that each one cannot be reviewed here.

Task Comprehension

Respondents also sometimes misunderstand the fundamental task that they are being asked to carry out. Debriefing studies showed this was especially common with the diagnostic stem questions in the CIDI (Kessler et al., 2000). The first questions asked in each diagnostic section, stem questions are used to determine whether a lifetime syndrome of a particular sort might have occurred. These questions provide brief vignettes and ask the respondent whether they ever had an experience of this sort. If a diagnostic stem question is endorsed, additional questions are asked to assess the specifics of the syndrome. If all diagnostic stem questions for a particular disorder are denied, the remaining questions about this syndrome are skipped.

Our methodological studies found that respondents often fail to understand the purpose of diagnostic stem questions. In particular, only about half of pilot respondents in our studies of the earlier version of CIDI interpreted these questions as they were intended – namely, as a request to engage in active memory search and to report the lifetime occurrence of episodes of the sort in the question. The other respondents interpreted the question as a request to report whether a memory of such an episode was readily accessible. These latter respondents did not believe that they were being asked to engage in active memory search and did not do so. Not surprisingly, the latter respondents were much less likely than those who understood the intent of the question to remember lifetime episodes.

Why did so many respondents misinterpret the intent of these lifetime recall questions? As Marquis and Cannell (1969) discovered in their early research on standard interview practice, respondents are generally both ill-informed about the purposes of the research and poorly motivated to participate actively. Furthermore, cues from interviewers often reinforce the inclination of respondents to participate in a half-hearted way. For example, when an interviewer asks a question that requires considerable thought, the respondent is likely to assume in the absence of instructions to the contrary that the interviewer is operating under normal conversational rules and is really asking for an immediate and appropriate answer. Cannell et al. (1981) showed that this conversational artifact can be minimized by explicitly instructing respondents to answer completely and accurately and that the use of such instruction can substantially improve the quality of data obtained in surveys. Based on this result, we built in clarifying statements throughout CIDI 3.0 aimed at informing respondents that accuracy was important.

Motivation

One drawback with emphasizing to respondents the need to work hard at a series of demanding and potentially embarrassing recall tasks is that it may cause them to refuse to engage in the tasks at all. Recognition of this problem among survey methodologists has led to the development of motivational techniques intended to increase the chances that respondents will accept the job of answering completely and accurately. Two techniques that have proven to be particularly useful were used in CIDI 3.0. The first consists of adding motivational components in the instructions; that is, introductory remarks at the beginning of a survey that clarify the research aims in order to motivate respondents to provide a more complete and accurate report than they might otherwise. Respondents are known to be willing to undertake laborious and possibly painful memory searches if they recognize some altruistic benefit of doing so (Cannell et al., 1981). Based on this evidence, we developed and presented a statement containing a clear rationale for administering the interview and emphasized the importance of the survey for social policy purposes.

The second technique features contingent reinforcement embedded in the interviewer feedback probes. Consistent with research on behavioral modification of verbal productions through reinforcement (e.g., Centers, 1963), several survey researchers have demonstrated that verbal reinforcers such as "thanks" and "that's useful" can significantly affect the behavior of survey respondents (Marquis & Cannell, 1969). Based on this observation, Cannell and his associates developed a method for training interviewers to use systematic feedback – both positive and negative – to reinforce respondent effort in reporting (Oksenberg et al., 1979). This method uses structured feedback statements coordinated with the content and timing of instructions aimed at reinforcing respondent performance. It is important to recognize that performance is being reinforced rather than any particular answer. For example, a difficult recall question may be prefaced with the instruction, "*This next question may be difficult, so please take your time before answering.*" In contingent feedback instruction, interviewers issue some expression of gratitude whenever the respondent seems to consider his or her answer carefully, whether they remember anything or not. Alternatively, the interviewer might instruct the precipitous respondent: "*You answered that awfully quickly. Was there anything (else), even something small?*" Such invitations to reconsider would occur whenever the respondent gives an immediate answer – whether or not anything was reported. Experiments document clearly that the combined use of these contingent reinforcement probes along with instructions explaining the importance of careful and accurate reporting leads to substantial improvement in recall of health-related events in general population surveys, including validated dates of medical events (Miller & Cannell, 1977; Vinokur et al., 1979). Importantly, these results also showed that self-enhancing response biases are reduced when these strategies are used, as indicated by both a decreased tendency to underreport potentially embarrassing conditions and behaviors (e.g., gynecologic problems, seeing an X-rated movie) and a decreased tendency to over-report self-enhancing behaviors (e.g., number of books read in the last three months, having read the editorial page of the newspaper the previous day). Based on these results, the contingent feedback approach was included as a fundamental part of the interviewer training materials developed for CIDI 3.0.

The Ability to Answer Accurately

Research on basic cognitive processes has shown that memories are organized and stored in structured sets of information packages commonly called schemas (Markus & Zajonc, 1985). When the respondent has a history of many instances of the same experience that cannot be discriminated, the separate instances tend to blend together to form a special kind of memory schema called a "semantic memory," a general memory for a prototypical experience (Jobe et al., 1990; Means & Loftus, 1991). For example, the person may have a semantic memory of what panic attacks are like but, due to the fact that he has had many such attacks in his lifetime, cannot specify details of any particular panic attack. In comparison, when a respondent has had only a small number of lifetime experiences of a certain sort or when one instance stands out as much different from the others, a memory can likely be recovered for that particular episode. This is called an "episodic memory."

In the case of memories of illness experiences, memory schemas tend to include not only semantic memories of prototypical symptoms, but also personal theories about causes, course, and cure (Leventhal et al., 1984; Skelton & Croyle, 1991). Some of these theories will conceptualize the experience in illness terms, while other theories will conceptualize the experience as a moral failing, a punishment from God, or a normal reaction to stress (Gilman, 1988). These interpretations can influence the extent to which different memory cues are capable of triggering the schemas. The effects of memory schemas and the difference between semantic and episodic memories are central themes in research on autobiographical memory. In survey research, a critical issue is whether the respondent is able to recover episodic memories or if the respondent is answering the question by drawing inferences of what the past must have been like on the basis of semantic memories.

Research shows that individuals are more likely to recover episodic memories for experiences that are recent, distinctive, and unique, while they are more likely to rely on semantic memories for experiences that are frequent, typical, and regular (Brewer, 1986; Belli, 1988; Menon, 1994). When a survey question is designed to ask about a particular instance of an experience, it must be posed in such a way that the respondent knows he is being asked to recover an episodic memory. Furthermore, the researcher must have some basis for assuming that an episodic memory can be recovered for this experience. If it cannot, a question that asks for such a memory implicitly invites the respondent to guess rather than to remember and this can have adverse effects on the quality of reporting later in the interview (Pearson et al., 1992). In comparison, when a question is designed to recover a semantic memory or to use semantic memories to arrive at an answer by estimation, that should be made clear.

One difficulty with these injunctions in the case of retrospective recall questions about lifetime mental disorders is uncertainty about what level of recall accuracy to expect. Therefore, as part of the CIDI pilot work in preparation for the WMH surveys, we debriefed pilot respondents in order to pinpoint questions that were difficult to answer on the basis of episodic memory. When questions of this sort were discovered, an attempt was made to revise the questions by allowing explicitly for estimation (e.g., explicitly asking respondents to provide a rough estimate), by providing categorical responses that reduce the complexity of the task, or by decomposing the question into subquestions that mimic effective memory search processes.

Regarding AOO questions, our pilot data showed that some individuals had a vivid memory of their first (and often only) episode of a mental disorder, especially when the disorder had a rapid onset, as in the case of panic attacks, whereas other individuals had only a vague memory of their first episode. The latter cases tended to involve accretion disorders (i.e., disorders that come on slowly) that occurred to individuals who subsequently had a great many other episodes. Based on extensive pilot work, we finally developed an approach to this problem that proved to be simple and effective: to ask respondents at the beginning of the AOO sequence if they had a clear memory of their first episode. As it turned out, the vast majority of respondents are able to answer this meta-question with no difficulty. We then varied subsequent questions, depending on the answer to that first question. Respondents who reported having a clear memory were asked a follow-up question that asked only about their age when that first episode occurred. In contrast, respondents who reported not having a clear memory were asked a more complex set of questions about the earliest age at which they could clearly remember a particular episode and their best estimate of about how old they were when they had their first episode. We carried out an experimental study to evaluate the effects of these questions by randomly assigning a group of community respondents to receive either a standard AOO question or our more complex series of AOO probes. Our new AOO probes resulted in much more plausible AOO reports than those obtained in response to standard AOO questions (Knäuper et al., 1999). In particular, the implausible pattern found in earlier studies of AOO in which answers were clustered in the five years before interview was not found in response to our AOO questions.

Combining Strategies

We also used some additional strategies that can address two or more of these memory problems at once. For example, in an effort both to motivate and to facilitate active memory search in answering diagnostic stem questions, we added a life review section at the beginning of the CIDI. This section starts out with an introduction that explains to respondents that the next questions might be difficult to answer because they require respondents to review their entire lives and then goes on to say that despite this difficulty, it is very important for the research that these questions are answered accurately. The introduction ends with the injunction to "*please take your time and think carefully before answering*."

The diagnostic stem questions for all core CIDI diagnoses are then administered directly following this commitment question. The questions are all included in the RB with a written instruction to "*take your time and think carefully before answering*." Interviewers are instructed to read the diagnostic stem questions slowly in an effort to emphasize their importance and to use motivational probes to encourage active memory search. Our intent in developing this section was both to explain the serious and difficult nature of the task and to motivate respondents to engage in active memory search by combining all the stem questions after a fairly detailed motivational introduction. Based on our debriefing studies, we recognized that CIDI respondents learn the logic of the stem-branch structure after a few sections at which point they realize that they can shorten the interview considerably by saying no to the stem questions. This problem is removed by asking all the stem questions near the beginning of the interview before the logic of the stem-branch structure becomes clear. Another important reason for including the section near the beginning of the interview is that pilot study respondents told us in debriefing interviews that their energy flagged as the interview progressed, making it much more difficult for them to carry out a serious memory search later in the interview.

We conducted an experiment to evaluate the effects of using this lifetime review section in conjunction with motivational probes. A random sample of 200 community respondents was randomized either to an earlier version of CIDI or to a version that was identical, except that it included the life review section at the beginning of the interview. As reported in detail elsewhere (Kessler et al., 1998), this experiment documented that the life review section led to a significant increase in the proportion of respondents who endorsed diagnostic stem questions. For example, while 26.7% of respondents in the standard CIDI condition endorsed a diagnostic stem question for major depression, 40.6% of respondents did so in the life review condition. Importantly, a clinical validity study documented that this increased prevalence of stem endorsement was not accompanied by a reduction in sensitivity with regard to clinical diagnoses, documenting that additional true cases were discovered by the use of the life review section and the accompanying commitment and motivation probes. These results provided the rationale for adopting the lifetime review section in CIDI 3.0.

Other Measures

We consider a number of other types of measures in this volume, including socio-demographic variables, childhood adversities, role impairments, and treatment. As these measures are the focus of specific chapters, we discuss them at the beginning of those chapters rather than here.

Translation

CIDI 3.0 was developed initially in English. One of the fundamental challenges in an undertaking such as the WMH Survey Initiative is to achieve both equivalence in meaning and consistency in measurement across surveys in multiple languages. Since the symptoms of mental disorders are described and interpreted differently in different cultures (Prince & Tcheng-Laroche, 1987; Cheng, 2001), it is often necessary to use substantially different terms or questions in different countries to assess these symptoms. Another complexity is that the CIDI source language, English, has a larger lexicon (stock of vocabulary) than any other language. This can mean that distinctions made in English cannot be matched in one or more target languages. The opposite can also be true with respect to certain areas of lexical or grammatical distinctions, in which the source language may not specify enough detail necessary for translation into a given target language.

WMH collaborators were given guidelines for translation and adaptation of the CIDI aimed at achieving both equivalence in meaning and consistency in measurement across surveys. These guidelines, which are discussed in detail by Harkness et al. (2008), are modifications of longstanding WHO guidelines for translation, back-translations, and harmonization that were updated by the staff of the WHO Data Collection Coordination Centre under the direction of Beth-Ellen Pennell in collaboration with the WMH Co-Principal Investigators.

Countries were instructed that the central aim of the translation process was to achieve target language versions of the English questionnaire that were conceptually equivalent in each of the countries/cultures rather than literally equivalent (i.e., word-for-word translations). It was emphasized that the translation should sound natural in each language (as far as that is possible in standardized instruments) and should perform in comparable fashion across the populations and languages. Independent assessors, who were experts on cross-national translation, reviewed the CIDI translations and found that these aims were generally achieved, but that some translations were at times too close to the English questionnaire language formulation and structure to sound "natural."

To achieve these aims, countries were required to follow a six-step process, which included: (1) forward translation; (2) expert panel review; (3) independent back-translation; (4) harmonization of vocabulary and formulation across different country versions of a shared language (if appropriate); (5) pretesting and cognitive interviewing; and (6) final revision, creation, and documentation of a final version of the translated questionnaire. A detailed description of these six steps is presented elsewhere (Harkness et al., 2008).

Pretesting

Consistent with best-practices recommendations (Sheatsley, 1983; Converse & Presser, 1986; Groves et al., 2004; Harkness et al., 2004; Smith, 2004), pretests of the instrument and procedures were carried out in each WMH survey prior to main study implementation. This should not be confused with the pretesting phase of translation described in the last subsection, as the latter focused only on translation, whereas the larger subsequent pretesting phase evaluated not only the instrument but all survey procedures. The pretests were designed to mirror the main study, except in those cases where they used experienced interviewer supervisors for pretest data collection rather than the interviewers who carried out the main survey. Pretest interviews were evaluated by debriefing interviewers to identify potential problem areas with the instrument and survey procedures, checking the distributions of items for high rates of missing data and out-of-range values, and using behavior coding of audio-taped pretest interviews to pinpoint questions that were often misread or often elicited respondent requests for clarification.

Pretesting is especially important in cross-national studies because of the challenges associated with working in many different languages and social contexts (Smith, 2004). A separate series of pretests was consequently required in each WMH country. Initial pretests focused on evaluating the translations. Later pretests evaluated the interview schedule and field procedures. The number of the latter pretest rounds varied from one to three, with approximately two-thirds of the countries conducting just one round of pretests and most other countries two rounds. The pretest debriefing sessions identified country-specific difficulties with questionnaire wording and response categories that were modified prior to the beginning of production interviewing. These sessions, along with quantitative analyses of responses, also detected skip pattern errors in the PAPI version and programming errors in the CAPI version that were corrected prior to the beginning of production interviewing. The pretests also allowed the investigators to evaluate the adequacy of survey procedures and sample management systems.

Interviewer Training

Although large-scale cross-national surveys have been undertaken for decades (Heath et al., 2005), there is surprisingly little research on the practical aspects of training and supervising interviewers to achieve high-quality survey data. While cultural adaptation of survey methods is widely recognized as necessary to achieve equivalence in measurement across countries (Bulmer, 1998; Jowell, 1998; Kuechler, 1998; Lynn, 2001), the literature contains few recommendations for how to achieve this equivalence across the many phases of a project's development. In the absence of standards of practice, many cross-national projects have accepted the research traditions of individual countries, which vary widely in methodological rigor. An approach at the other extreme is to implement a "one-size-fits-all" methodology, which naively imposes the same procedure and protocols across all countries and cultures, based on the assumption that good practice in one culture will invariably be good practice in other cultures (Harkness et al., 2002).

The WMH Survey Initiative sought to implement an approach between these two extremes by establishing guidelines that set minimum standards for each phase of project implementation, but allowed for country-specific adaptations. We saw this earlier in the chapter in the discussion of probability sampling methods that allowed for country-specific variations. The difficulty for the staff of the WMH Data Collection Coordination Centre was determining when variations in approach were necessary and appropriate rather than simply expedient. With regard to sampling, survey organizations in some parts of the world have a tradition of quota sampling and respondent substitution that violates the WMH requirement of probability sampling. This kind of potential conflict between local practice and best practices was found in every phase of the WMH survey implementation.

A detailed description of the WMH data quality control standards established by the WMH Data Collection Coordination Centre and the ways in which these standards were implemented in individual countries is presented elsewhere (Pennell et al., 2008). These standards were subsequently used by the senior members of the WMH Data Collection Coordination Centre to take the lead in developing internationally recognized guidelines for best practices in cross-national comparative survey research more generally (www.ccsg.isr.umich.edu). Issues of interviewer recruitment and training, research ethics, field structure, data collection procedures and quality control, and data preparation are all included in these guidelines. We will not discuss here the main practical decisions made in establishing WMH field procedures, such as the decisions to have interviews carried out face-to-face rather than by telephone and to use both paper and pencil and computer-assisted versions of the survey so as to enable individual countries to choose their preferred mode, but refer the reader to a detailed discussion of these decisions elsewhere (Pennell et al., 2008).

As noted above, CIDI 3.0 is a complex instrument. Successful implementation of such an instrument requires interviewers to be highly trained. We consequently placed high importance on careful interviewer training and quality assurance monitoring. In some countries, the research team was responsible for interviewer recruitment and management, while in other countries, the interviewing component was subcontracted to an external survey organization. Before starting the interviewer recruitment and training process, each country sent at least two interviewer supervisors to a "train-the-trainer" session presented by the WMH Data Collection Coordination Centre at the University of Michigan in the United States. These sessions, which lasted for an average of 6 days, were designed to prepare the interviewer supervisors to train and monitor interviewer performance, as well as to manage data collection and data processing in their country. Through these sessions, research teams obtained all the information and materials necessary to train their own interviewing staff using consistent procedures. These trainers, who in almost all countries came from a pool of experienced interviewers, then trained a team of supervisors to help in interviewer recruitment, training, and field quality control monitoring. Many countries were required to recruit and hire new interviewers for the WMH survey, while others were able to use field staff from ongoing survey organizations. In most countries where new interviewers were recruited, recruitment was carried out in the general population. In a few countries, though, interviewers were recruited exclusively from among college students. Careful centralized screening procedures were used in this hiring process.

Interviewer training was divided into two parts: general interviewing training (GIT) and CIDI-specific training. GIT was designed to introduce interviewers to the basic components of standardized questionnaire administration (e.g., question reading, appropriate techniques for probing and seeking clarification, providing feedback, accurate data recording). GIT sessions lasted two to three days in most countries. In addition, countries that used computer-assisted interviewing had a GIT component focused on computer hardware and software use. Some countries added other country-specific topics in their GIT sessions, such as New Zealand's inclusion of cultural empathy to Maori and Pacific Islander households and Colombia's special training on interacting with governmental authorities and armed guerrilla and paramilitary groups. All interviewers were required to demonstrate competence with GIT concepts and procedures through a variety of tests before moving on to study-specific training.

Study-specific training averaged 30 hours across countries. The content was presented as a mix of lecture and round-robin practice sessions focused on general project background and importance, rules for obtaining informed consent, definitions of eligibility and respondent selection procedures, specifics of the precise interview procedures, and discussion of production requirements. Hands-on practice was stressed throughout. Trainers assessed the skill level of each interviewer in small group exercises and often held tailored "after-hours" special sessions to address areas where interviewers needed additional assistance and practice. Most countries included in the training team a clinical consultant, typically a psychiatric social worker or a clinical psychologist, who provided interviewers with background information about the kinds of psychiatric symptoms that they would encounter during production interviewing. This clinical contact person (CCP) was also a resource person for both interviewers and respondents during data collection to address the needs of respondents who might require a referral for follow-up and interviewers who might need to debrief after a particularly difficult interview. In most cases, the CCP was available to interviewers 24 hours a day, 7 days a week. Many countries developed protocols that allowed interviewers to contact their CCP privately, without first going through a supervisor to provide interviewers a unique opportunity to speak freely about their own and their respondents' experiences.

Quality Control Monitoring

All countries required interviewers to pass a certification test before being approved for production work. Interviewers who did not pass the certification test were either terminated from the project or received additional retraining and another opportunity to obtain certification. Interviewer training often continued during the production phase of the project through periodic in-person seminars, telephone conference calls, and bulletins or newsletters.

Special procedures were also developed to monitor interviewer performance during production. Systematic monitoring is critical to survey data quality assurance (Billiet & Loosveldt, 1988; Fowler & Mangione, 1990). Consistent with best-practices guidelines for survey implementation (Biemer & Lyberg, 2003), four areas of performance were the main targets of quality assurance monitoring: detection and prevention of falsified information, compliance with the interviewing rules and guidelines set forth in the training manual, performance of non-interview tasks, and identification of interviewer–questionnaire interface problems.

These areas were evaluated by a number of methods, including supervisor re-interview of selected cases, supervisor verification of key survey elements through spot re-contact of respondents, direct observation of interviews, audio-recording, questionnaire review, analysis of performance and production measures, keystroke/trace file analysis (files that record keystrokes and movement of the interviewer through the computerized instrument), and mock interviews/tests of knowledge and practice. Interviewers were terminated from production interviewing if they were deemed unable to perform up to required standards. The recommended supervisor-to-interviewer ratio of one supervisor for every 8 to 10 interviewers was used in the majority of countries that used paper and pencil data collection, while lower ratios were used in countries with computer administration, based on the greater control over the data collection process afforded by computerized interviewing (Williams, 1986; Lavrakas, 1993).

Statistical Analysis Methods

Prevalence of Trauma Exposure and PTSD

The main focus of this volume is on the prevalence and basic descriptive predictors of trauma exposure and PTSD. Lifetime prevalence represents the proportion of people in the population who, as of the time of interview, ever were exposed to a trauma or ever met criteria for PTSD. It is important to recognize that some unknown number of respondents will be exposed to trauma and develop PTSD in the future, which means that lifetime risk (referred to in the epidemiological literature as morbid risk) is generally higher than lifetime prevalence. It is possible to estimate morbid risk by making assumptions about the stability of AOO distributions across birth cohorts. We do not emphasize morbid risk in this volume due to concerns about the implausibility of this assumption. Instead, we focus on lifetime prevalence as a conservative estimate of the proportion of the population ever affected by PTSD. However, it is important for the reader to recognize that estimates of lifetime prevalence represent lower bound estimates of the proportions of the population who will ever experience PTSD.

We also report trauma-level prevalence of PTSD; that is, the proportion of all lifetime traumas reported by all respondents that result in PTSD. The lifetime number of PTSD episodes in the population is the product of lifetime prevalence at the respondent level times the mean number of lifetime traumas experienced by individuals with lifetime PTSD times trauma-specific

PTSD risk. In addition, we report mean duration of PTSD episodes as retrospectively reported by respondents with lifetime PTSD. The societal burden of PTSD is the product of the number of lifetime episodes in the population times mean duration of these episodes. This estimate has more policy implications than either an estimate of the proportion of the population that has ever had PTSD or the number of PTSD episodes in the population.

The predictors of societal burden of PTSD represent joint associations of these predictors with probability of trauma exposures of various types, of PTSD risk given these exposures, and of PTSD duration given onset. We present information on these different components in an effort to disaggregate our estimates of overall societal burden. This disaggregated information is important because it has implications both for theory development and for intervention targeting.

Predictors of Lifetime Trauma Exposure

We think of the predictor variables examined in this volume as descriptive correlates, not causes. As a result, we use information about a number of time-invariant variables assessed in the interview (e.g., childhood adversities, respondent sex) as well as time-varying variables (e.g., education, marital status, history of other mental disorders) as predictors of exposure to traumas and subsequent onset-course of PTSD. We also control for the survey country in predicting trauma exposure and PTSD. We do this by including a series of dummy predictor variables in each equation to represent individual surveys. When all 26 surveys are included in the analysis, we use 25 dummy control variables in this way. It is important to appreciate our rationale for doing this: we are explicitly focusing on pooled within-survey associations and consciously deciding not to examine between-survey variation in risk of trauma exposure and PTSD. It would have been possible to use information about between-survey differences in central tendencies and/or distributions of predictors to predict between-survey variation in prevalence of these outcomes. Indeed, some other researchers have done exactly that by putting together published WMH country-level results (Duckers et al., 2016).

We chose not to examine cross-national differences in prevalence because the WMH surveys were optimized to search for patterns of central tendency and to highlight the most stable patterns across countries rather than to optimize examination of the reasons for cross-national differences. A serious effort to study cross-national differences would have led us to modify the sample designs of the WMH surveys to make them representative not only of countries but also of major regions within countries to increase the sample of spatial units. We would also have collected extensive data on both contemporary and short-term historical contextual factors for each country as well as regions within countries that might explain the time–space variation in prevalence. Indeed, this examination of time–space variation was the approach we took on the rare occasions when we studied cross-national differences in other parts of the WMH data (Seedat et al., 2009). And even there, we carried out the analyses to study variation in associations (i.e., sex differences in lifetime prevalence of individual disorders as of age 25) rather than prevalence in order to capitalize on the fact that these associations are less sensitive to the influence of relatively arbitrary diagnostic thresholds on estimates of cross-national differences than are prevalence estimates.

In contrast, more general comparisons of cross-national differences in predictors of prevalence are faced with the daunting task of making sense of differences across only about two dozen data points (i.e., surveys) by selecting from the literally hundreds of potentially causal variables that might account for this variation. With such a small sample, it is virtually impossible to draw unequivocal conclusions about important predictors. For example, an association of country-level economic development with prevalence might actually be due to between-country differences in methodological variables (e.g., response rate, which, as noted in Table 2.1, is considerably lower for surveys in high-income than in low-and lower-middle-income countries).

As we focus on pooled within-survey associations, a question can be raised about whether we should weight our data by population size or survey sample size. We chose the latter due to the fact that the countries included in WMH survey are not representative of all countries in the world, making it impossible to estimate worldwide prevalence or correlates of mental disorders from our pooled data. Instead, we consider each survey as having a level of importance equivalent to its sample size in generating estimates of central tendency, leading us to use weights that represent sample size rather than population size.

Discrete-time survival analysis with person-year as the unit of analysis (Efron, 1988) was used to study the predictors of first exposure to traumas. The discrete-time approach was chosen over the more traditional Cox proportional hazards analysis approach because our information about timing of onsets is available only for discrete intervals of time (i.e., years of age). The discrete-time models were operationalized as logistic regression models with person-year as the unit of analysis and first onset of the focal trauma as the outcome. This approach treats each year of each respondent's life as a separate observational record, building a data set containing n x t person-year records for a sample of n respondents with an average of t years of life at the time of interview. Each record is coded for the year of life it represents and is assigned a score of either 0 or 1 on the outcome (i.e., first lifetime occurrence of the focal trauma), depending on whether the trauma had a first onset in that year. Years of life after first exposure to the trauma are excluded from analysis. By pooling years in this way and controlling for person-year, we estimate a series of within-year models for the predictors of first exposure to the trauma in year t among respondents who never experienced the trauma as of year $t - 1$ that are combined to obtain a single parameter estimate for each predictor across all years.

Survival coefficients and their standard errors were exponentiated and are reported here as odds-ratios (ORs) with 95% confidence intervals. Confidence intervals were estimated using the design-based Taylor series linearization method (Wolter, 2007) implemented in the SAS software system (SAS Institute Inc., 2011) to adjust for the weighting and clustering of the WMH data. Multivariate significance tests for sets of dummy variables to characterize a single socio-demographic characteristic (e.g., a second degree of freedom test for the three categories of marital status) were carried out using Wald χ^2 tests based on Taylor series coefficient variance-covariance matrices. Statistical significance was consistently evaluated using 0.05-level two-sided tests.

An issue of note in discussing the person-year models is that the tens of thousands of respondents in the pooled Part II sample across all surveys considered here generated well over 2 million person-years in the data set to study predictors of each trauma type. This made it computationally intensive to estimate these models. This problem was addressed by using case-control sampling to reduce the number of observations made in estimating the models. In this approach, 100% of the person-years with first onsets of the outcome were compared to a probability sample of 10 times as many control person-years selected with stratification from the full set of person-years prior to first occurrence of the trauma and weighted to have a sum of weights equal to the sum of weights in the full set of control person-years in the pooled cross-national sample. As the logistic link function is used in these models, the coefficients are not biased by selecting a subsample of controls (Schlesselman, 1982). Furthermore, the ratio of 10 controls for every 1 case is large enough that any increase in statistical power achieved by adding more controls would be trivial.

The initial models included predictors for sex, age-at-interview (i.e., cohort), and survey. These ORs can be interpreted as the relative-odds of lifetime exposure to a given trauma for women versus men or for respondents of certain ages at interview versus those of other ages, compared to other respondents in the same survey averaged over all person-years of risk and across surveys, with these averages taking into consideration time–space variation in number of new exposures to the trauma in the cross-national data set. The latter means that any existing variation in ORs associated with a given predictor is weighted in favor of observations in the age ranges and in the surveys with highest concentrations of trauma occurrences. Subsequent models added additional predictors, the ORs of which can be interpreted as the relative-odds of lifetime exposure to the trauma among respondents with given values on the time-varying predictor as of the time of interview, compared to other individuals of the same age at interview and sex averaged over all person-years of risk and across surveys.

Decomposing Correlates of PTSD Burden

As noted above, we are especially interested in number of years with PTSD in the population because this is our most direct estimate of the burden of the disorder (i.e., an estimate of the proportion of the population having an episode of the disorder at a given point in time). When we looked at correlates, we consequently began with a consideration of associations with this outcome and then we decomposed this association into its component parts: associations with lifetime exposure to traumas in the total population (based on the survival model described in the previous subsection), associations with PTSD among individuals exposed to a random occurrence of that trauma, and association with PTSD duration among lifetime cases.

It sometimes occurs that a predictor is significantly associated with population burden of the disorder due to only one of those component associations being significant. The distinction among these components is important for policy purposes, as the primary preventive interventions designed to reduce high lifetime risk of PTSD in a particular segment of the population would be quite different from the secondary interventions designed to reduce persistence of the disorder or clinical interventions to treat active episodes.

Unlike the person-year models used to predict lifetime trauma exposure, the models to predict PTSD among respondents exposed to random traumas were person-level models estimated in the random trauma-level subsample with a logistic link function using the same design-based Taylor series linearization method as in the person-year survival models. Survival models were then used in the model for persistence among lifetime cases with person-month as the unit of analysis (as respondent reports about duration were recorded in months).

Dealing with Item-Missing Data

Item-level missing data were uncommon in the WMH surveys due to the fact that skip errors were minimized by our use of computer-assisted interviewing for most surveys and implementation of a rigorous post-interview data checking protocol that used paper and pencil administration so that missing data could be filled in quickly in brief phone calls to respondents shortly after their interview was completed. However, in some cases, there were structural problems involving a skip error in early surveys that was fixed in later surveys or the use of only a screening assessment in the main survey that was validated only later in clinical reappraisal interviews, requiring us to use regression-based imputation to estimate individual scores. In the vast majority of cases, where a variable had a very small amount of missing data, we imputed the missing values using a single regression-based imputation with an error term. The PROC MI procedure with a single imputation in SAS 9.3 (SAS Institute Inc., 2011) was used for this purpose. The method of multiple imputation (MI; Rubin, 1987) was used for more complex imputations, in which case we generated 10 imputations for each missing value and used standard procedures to adjust estimates of standard errors of parameter estimates to take into consideration the fact that many (or all) values were imputed rather than observed. These methods are discussed in more detail in the chapters in which they were used.

Acknowledgments

Portions of this chapter originally appeared in Heeringa, S. G., Wells, J. E., Hubbard, F., et al. (2008). Sample designs and sampling procedures. In R. C. Kessler & T. B. Üstün, eds., *The WHO World Mental Health Surveys: Global Perspectives on the Epidemiology of Mental Disorders*. New York, NY: Cambridge University Press, pp. 14–32; Kessler, R. C., & Üstün, T. B. (2008). The World Health Organization Composite International Diagnostic Interview. In R. C. Kessler, & T. B. Üstün, eds., *The WHO World Mental Health Surveys: Global Perspectives on the Epidemiology of Mental Disorders*. New York, NY: Cambridge University Press, pp. 58–90; Pennell, B.-E., Mneimneh, Z., Bowers, A., et al. (2008). Implementation of the World Mental Health surveys. In R. C. Kessler, & T. B. Üstün, eds., *The WHO World Mental Health Surveys: Global Perspectives on the Epidemiology of Mental Disorders*. New York, NY: Cambridge University Press, pp. 33–57; Harkness, J., Pennell, B. E., Villar, A., et al. (2008). Translation procedures and translation assessment in the World Mental Health Survey Initiative. In R. C. Kessler, & T. B. Üstün, eds., *The WHO World Mental Health Surveys: Global Perspectives on the Epidemiology of Mental Disorders*. New York, NY: Cambridge University Press, pp. 91–113; Haro, J. M., Arbabzadeh-Bouchez, S., Brugha, et al. (2008). Concordance of the Composite International Diagnostic Interview Version 3.0 (CIDI 3.0) with standardized clinical assessments in the WHO World Mental Health surveys. In R. C. Kessler, & T. B. Üstün, eds., *The WHO World Mental Health Surveys: Global Perspectives on the Epidemiology of Mental Disorders*. New York, NY: Cambridge University Press, pp. 114–30; Kessler, R. C., Heeringa, S. G., Pennell, B.-E., et al. (In press). World Mental Health Survey Methods. In K. M. Scott, P. De Jonge, D. J. Stein, & R. C. Kessler., eds., *Mental Disorders Around the World: Facts and Figures from the World Mental Health Surveys*. New York, NY: Cambridge University Press. All © World Health Organization. Used with permission.

References

Alonso, J., Angermeyer, M. C., Bernert, S., et al. (2004). Sampling and methods of the European Study of the Epidemiology of Mental Disorders (ESEMeD) project. *Acta Psychiatrica Scandinavica*, Suppl. 109, 8–20.

American Association for Public Opinion Research (2000). Standard definitions: final dispositions of case codes and outcome rates for surveys (online). Available at www.aapor.org/Standards-Ethics/Standard-Definitions-(1).aspx (Accessed April 17, 2011).

American Psychiatric Association (1994). *Diagnostic and Statistical Manual of Mental Disorders, Fourth Edition. DSM-IV*. Washington, DC: American Psychiatric Association.

Belli, R. F. (1988). Color blend retrievals: compromise memories or deliberate compromise responses? *Memory and Cognition*, 16, 314–26.

(1998). The structure of autobiographical memory and the event history calendar: potential improvements in the quality of retrospective reports in surveys. *Memory*, 6, 383–406.

Biemer, P., & Lyberg, L. (2003). *Introduction to Survey Quality*. New York, NY: John Wiley & Sons.

Billiet, J., & Loosveldt, G. (1988). Interviewer training and quality of responses. *Public Opinion Quarterly*, 52, 190–211.

Borges, G., Angst, J., Nock, M. K., Ruscio, A. M., & Kessler, R. C. (2008). Risk factors for the incidence and persistence of suicide-related outcomes: a 10-year follow-up study using the National Comorbidity Surveys. *Journal of Affective Disorders*, 105, 25–33.

Breslau, N. (2002). Epidemiologic studies of trauma, posttraumatic stress disorder, and other psychiatric disorders. *The Canadian Journal of Psychiatry. La Revue Canadienne de Psychiatrie*, 47, 923–9.

Brewer, W. F. (1986). What is autobiographical memory? In D. C. Rubin, ed., *Autobiographical Memory*. New York, NY: Cambridge University Press, pp. 25–49.

Bulmer, M. (1998). The problem of exporting social survey research. *American Behavioral Scientist*, 42, 153–67.

Cannell, C. F., Fowler, F. J., & Marquis, K. H. (1968). The influence of interviewer and respondent psychological and behavioral variables on the reporting in household interviews. *Vital and Health Statistics*, 2, 1–65.

Cannell, C. F., Miller, P. V., & Oksenberg, L. (1981). Research on interviewing techniques. In S. Leinhardt, ed., *Sociological Methodology*. San Francisco, CA: Jossey-Bass Publishers, pp. 389–487.

Centers, R. (1963). A laboratory adaptation of the conversational procedure for the conditioning of verbal operants. *Journal of Abnormal Psychology*, 67, 334–9.

Cheng, A. T. (2001). Case definition and culture: are people all the same? *British Journal of Psychiatry*, 179, 1–3.

Clark, H. H., & Schober, M. F. (1992). Asking questions and influencing answers. In J. M. Tanur, ed., *Questions about Questions: Inquiries Into the Cognitive Bases of Surveys*. New York, NY: Russell Sage Foundation, pp. 15–48.

Cochran, W. G. (1977). *Sampling Techniques*. New York, NY: John Wiley & Sons.

Converse, J., & Presser, S. (1986). *Survey Questions: Handcrafting the Standardized Questionnaire*, Sage Series No. 63. Thousand Oaks, CA: Sage Publications.

Couper, M. P., & de Leeuw, E. D. (2003). Nonresponse in cross-cultural and cross-national surveys. In J. A. Harkness, F. J. R. Van de Vijver, & P. P. Mohler, eds., *Cross-Cultural Survey Methods*. Hoboken, NJ: John Wiley & Sons, pp. 155–77.

Duckers, M. L., Alisic, E., & Brewin, C. R. (2016). A vulnerability paradox in the cross-national prevalence of post-traumatic stress disorder. *British Journal of Psychiatry*, 209, 300–5.

Efron, B. (1988). Logistic regression, survival analysis, and the Kaplan-Meier curve. *Journal of the American Statistical Association*, 83, 414–25.

First, M. B., Spitzer, R. L., Gibbon, M., & Williams, B. J. (1994). *Structured Clinical Interview for Axis I DSM-IV Disorders*. New York, NY: New York State Psychiatric Institute, Biometrics Research Department.

Fowler, F., & Mangione, T. (1990). *Standardized Survey Interviewing: Minimizing Interviewer-Related Error*. Newbury Park, CA: Sage Publications, Inc.

Galea, S., Nandi, A., & Vlahov, D. (2005). The epidemiology of post-traumatic stress disorder after disasters. *Epidemiologic Reviews*, 27, 78–91.

Gardner, M., & Altman, D. (2000). *Statistics with Confidence: Confidence Intervals and Statistical Guidelines*. London, England: BMJ Books.

Gilman, S. (1988). *Disease and Representation: Images of Illness from Madness to AIDS*. Ithaca, NY: Cornell University Press.

Giuffra, L. A., & Risch, N. (1994). Diminished recall and the cohort effect of major depression: a simulation study. *Psychological Medicine*, 24, 375–83.

Groves, R. M., Fowler, F. J., Couper, M. P., et al. (2004). *Survey Methodology*. Hoboken, NJ: John Wiley & Sons.

Harkness, J., Pennell, B. E., Villar, A., et al. (2008). Translation procedures and translation assessment in the World Mental Health Survey Initiative. In R. C. Kessler, & T. B. Üstün, eds., *The WHO World Mental Health Surveys: Global Perspectives on the Epidemiology of Mental Disorders*. New York, NY: Cambridge University Press, pp. 91–113.

Harkness, J. A., Pennell, B. E., & Schoua-Glusberg, A. (2004). Survey questionnaire translation and assessment. In S. Presser, J. Rothgeb, M. P. Couper, et al., eds., *Methods for Testing and Evaluating Survey Questionnaires*. Hoboken, NJ: John Wiley & Sons, pp. 453–74.

Harkness, J. A., Van de Vijver, J. R., & Mohler, P. P. (2002). *Cross-Cultural Survey Methods*. New York, NY: John Wiley & Sons.

Haro, J. M., Arbabzadeh-Bouchez, S., Brugha, T. S., et al. (2006). Concordance of the Composite International Diagnostic Interview Version 3.0 (CIDI 3.0) with standardized clinical assessments in the WHO World Mental Health surveys. *International Journal of Methods in Psychiatric Research*, 15, 167–80.

Heath, A., Fisher, S., & Smith, S. (2005). The globalization of public opinion research. *Annual Review of Political Science*, 8, 297–333.

Jobe, J. B., White, A. A., Kelley, C. L., et al. (1990). Recall strategies and memory for health-care visits. *Milbank Quarterly*, 68, 171–89.

Jowell, R. (1998). How comparative is comparative research? *American Behavioral Scientist*, 42, 168–77.

Kazantzis, N., Kennedy-Moffat, J., Flett, R. A., et al. (2012). Predictors of chronic trauma-related symptoms in a community sample of New Zealand motor vehicle accident survivors. *Culture, Medicine and Psychiatry*, 36, 442–64.

Kessler, R. C. (1999). The World Health Organization International Consortium in Psychiatric Epidemiology (ICPE): initial work and future directions – the NAPE Lecture 1998. *Acta Psychiatrica Scandinavica*, 99, 2–9.

Kessler, R. C., Aguilar-Gaxiola, S., Alonso, J., et al. (2008). Lifetime prevalence and age of onset distributions of mental disorders in the World Mental Health Survey Initiative. In R. C. Kessler, & T. B. Üstün, eds., *The WHO World Mental Health Surveys: Global Perspectives on the Epidemiology of Mental Disorders*. New York, NY: Cambridge University Press, pp. 511–21.

Kessler, R. C., Akiskal, H. S., Angst, J., et al. (2006). Validity of the assessment of bipolar spectrum disorders in the WHO CIDI 3.0. *Journal of Affective Disorders*, 96, 259–69.

Kessler, R. C., Angermeyer, M., Anthony, J. C., et al. (2007). Lifetime prevalence and age-of-onset distributions of mental disorders in the World Health Organization's World Mental Health Survey Initiative. *World Psychiatry*, 6, 168–76.

Kessler, R. C., Berglund, P., Chiu, W. T., et al. (2004). The US National Comorbidity Survey Replication (NCS-R): design and field procedures. *International Journal of Methods in Psychiatric Research*, 13, 69–92.

Kessler, R. C., Mroczek, D. K., & Belli, R. F. (1999). Retrospective adult assessment of childhood psychopathology. In D. Shaffer, C. P. Lucas, & J. E. Richters, eds., *Diagnostic Assessment in Child and Adolescent Psychopathology*. New York, NY: Guilford Press, pp. 256–84.

Kessler, R. C., Sonnega, A., Bromet, E., Hughes, M., & Nelson, C. B. (1995). Posttraumatic stress disorder in the National Comorbidity Survey. *Archives of General Psychiatry*, 52, 1048–60.

Kessler, R. C., & Üstün, T. B. (2004). The World Mental Health (WMH) Survey Initiative version of the World Health Organization (WHO) Composite International Diagnostic Interview (CIDI). *International Journal of Methods in Psychiatric Research*, 13, 93–121.

(2008). The World Health Organization Composite International Diagnostic Interview. In R. C. Kessler, & T. B. Üstün, eds., *The WHO World Mental Health Surveys: Global Perspectives on the Epidemiology of Mental Disorders*. New York, NY: Cambridge University Press, pp. 58–90.

Kessler, R. C., Wittchen, H. U., Abelson, J. M., et al. (1998). Methodological studies of the Composite International Diagnostic Interview (CIDI) in the US National Comorbidity Survey. *International Journal of Methods in Psychiatric Research*, 7, 33–55.

Kessler, R. C., Wittchen, H. U., Abelson, J. M., & Zhao, S. (2000). Methodological issues in assessing psychiatric disorder with self-reports. In A. A. Stone, J. S. Turrkan, C. A. Bachrach, et al., eds., *The Science of Self-Report: Implications for Research and Practice*. Mahwah, NJ: Lawrence Erlbaum Associates, pp. 229–55.

Kish, L. (1949). A procedure for objective respondent selection within the household. *Journal of the American Statistical Association*, 44, 380–7.

Kish, L. (1965). *Survey Sampling*. New York, NY: John Wiley & Sons.

Knäuper, B., Cannell, C. F., Schwarz, N., Bruce, M. L., & Kessler, R. C. (1999). Improving accuracy of major depression age-of-onset reports in the US National Comorbidity Survey. *International Journal of Methods in Psychiatric Research*, 8, 39–48.

Kuechler, M. (1998). The survey method: an indispensable tool for social science research everywhere? *American Behavioral Scientist*, 42, 178–200.

Landis, J. R., & Koch, G. G. (1977). The measurement of observer agreement for categorical data. *Biometrics*, 33, 159–74.

Lavrakas, P. J. (1993). *Telephone Survey Methods: Sampling, Selection, and Supervision*. Thousand Oaks, CA: Sage Publications.

Leventhal, H., Nerenz, D., & Steele, D. J. (1984). Illness representations and coping with health threats. In A. Baum, S. E. Taylor, & J. E. Singer, eds., *Handbook of Psychology and Health*. Hillsdale, NJ: Erlbaum Associates, pp. 219–52.

Little, R. J. A., & Rubin, D. B. (2002). *Statistical Analysis with Missing Data*, 2nd ed. New York, NY: John Wiley & Sons.

Lynn, P. (2001). Developing quality standards for cross-national survey research: five approaches. *International Journal of Social Research Methodology*, 6, 323–36.

Markus, H., & Zajonc, R. B. (1985). The cognitive perspective in social psychology. In G. Lindzey, & E. Aronson, eds., *The Handbook of Social Psychology*. New York, NY: Random House, pp. 137–230.

Marquis, K. H., & Cannell, C. F. (1969). *A Study of Interviewer–Respondent Interaction in the Urban Employment*. Ann Arbor, MI: University of Michigan, Survey Research Center.

Means, B., & Loftus, E. F. (1991). When personal history repeats itself: decomposing memories for recurring events. *Applied Cognitive Psychology*, 5, 297–318.

Menon, A. (1994). Judgements of behavioral frequencies: memory search and retrieval strategies. In N. Schwartz, & S. Sudman, eds., *Autobiographical Memory and the Validity of Retrospective Reports*. New York, NY: Springer-Verlag, pp. 161–72.

Miller, P. V., & Cannell, C. F. (1977). Communicating measurement objectives in the survey interview. In D. M. Hirsch, P. V. Miller, & F. G. Kline, eds., *Strategies for Communication Research*. Beverly Hills, CA: Sage Publications, pp. 127–51.

Moffitt, T. E., Caspi, A., Taylor, A., et al. (2010). How common are common mental disorders? Evidence that lifetime prevalence rates are doubled by prospective versus retrospective ascertainment. *Psychological Medicine*, 40, 899–909.

Nickerson, A., Aderka, I. M., Bryant, R. A., & Hofmann, S. G. (2013). The role of attribution of trauma responsibility in posttraumatic stress disorder following motor vehicle accidents. *Depression and Anxiety*, 30, 483–8.

Oksenberg, L., Vinokur, A., & Cannell, C. F. (1979). The effects of instructions, commitment and feedback on reporting in personal interviews. In C. F. Cannell, L. Oksenberg, & J. M. Converse, eds., *Experiments in Interviewing Techniques*, DHEW Publication No. (HRA) 78-3204. Washington, DC: Department of Health, Education, and Welfare, pp. 133–99.

Patten, S. B. (2003). Recall bias and major depression lifetime prevalence. *Social Psychiatry and Psychiatric Epidemiology*, 38, 290–6.

Pearson, R. W., Ross, M., & Dawes, R. M. (1992). Personal recall and the limits of retrospective questions in surveys. In J. M. Tanur, ed., *Questions about Questions: Inquiries Into the Cognitive Bases of Surveys*. New York, NY: Russell Sage Foundation, pp. 65–94.

Pennell, B. E., Mneimneh, Z., Bowers, A., et al. (2008). Implementation of the World Mental Health Surveys. In R. C. Kessler, & T. B. Üstün, eds., *The WHO World Mental Health Surveys: Global Perspectives on the Epidemiology of Mental Disorders*. New York, NY: Cambridge University Press, pp. 33–57.

Prince, R., & Tcheng-Laroche, F. (1987). Culture-bound syndromes and international disease classifications. *Cultural Medical Psychiatry*, 11, 3–52.

Prohaska, V., Brown, N. R., & Belli, R. F. (1998). Forward telescoping: the question matters. *Memory*, 6, 455–65.

Research Triangle Institute (2002). *SUDAAN: Professional Software for Survey Data Analysis, Version 8.0.1*. Research Triangle Park, NC: Research Triangle Institute.

Rosenbaum, P. R., & Rubin, D. B. (1983). The central role of the propensity score in observational studies for causal effects. *Biometrika*, 70, 41–55.

Rubin, D. B. (1987). *Multiple Imputation for Nonresponse in Surveys*. New York, NY: Wiley.

Rust, K. (1985). Variance estimation for complex estimators in sample surveys. *Journal of Official Statistics*, 1, 381–97.

SAS Institute Inc. (2011). *SAS/STAT® Software, Version 9.3 for Windows*. Cary, NC: SAS Institute Inc.

Schlesselman, J. J. (1982). *Case-Control Studies: Design, Conduct, Analysis*. New York, NY: Oxford University Press.

Schober, M. F., Conrad, F. G., & Fricker, S. S. (2004). Misunderstanding standardized language in research interviews. *Applied Cognitive Psychology*, 18, 169–88.

Schwarz, N., & Sudman, S., eds. (1994). *Autobiographical Memory and the Validity of Retrospective Reports*. New York, NY: Springer-Verlag.

Schwarz, N., & Sudman, S., eds. (1996). *Answering Questions: Methodology for Determining Cognitive and Communicative Processes in Survey Research*. San Francisco, CA: Jossey-Bass Publishers.

Seedat, S., Scott, K., Angermeyer, M. C., et al. (2009). Cross-national associations between gender and mental disorders in the World Health Organization World Mental Health Surveys. *Archives of General Psychiatry*, 66, 785–95.

Sheatsley, P. B. (1983). Questionnaire construction and item writing. In P. H. Rossi, J. D. Wright, & A. B. Anderson, eds., *Handbook of Survey Research: Quantitative Studies in Social Relations*. New York, NY: Academy Press, pp. 195–230.

Simon, G. E., & VonKorff, M. (1995). Recall of psychiatric history in cross-sectional surveys: implications for epidemiologic research. *Epidemiologic Reviews*, 17, 221–7.

Sirken, M. G., Herrmann, D. J., Schechter, S., et al., eds. (1999). *Cognition and Survey Research*. New York, NY: John Wiley & Sons.

Skelton, J. A., & Croyle, R. T. (1991). *Mental Representation in Health and Illness*. New York, NY: Springer-Verlag.

Smith, T. W. (2004). Developing and evaluating cross-national survey instruments. In S. Presser, J. M. Rothgeb, M. P. Couper, et al., eds., *Methods for Testing and Evaluating Survey Questionnaires*. New York, NY: John Wiley & Sons, pp. 431–52.

Sudman, S., Bradburn, N., & Schwarz, N. (1996). *Thinking about Answers: The Application of Cognitive Processes to Survey Methodology*. San Francisco, CA: Jossey-Bass Publishers.

Tanur, J. M. (1992). *Questions about Questions: Inquiries into the Cognitive Bases of Surveys*. New York, NY: Russell Sage Foundation.

Tiihonen Moller, A., Backstrom, T., Sondergaard, H. P., & Helstrom, L. (2014). Identifying risk factors for PTSD in women seeking medical help after rape. *PloS One*, 9, e111136.

Tourangeau, R., & Yan, T. (2007). Sensitive questions in surveys. *Psychological Bulletin*, 133, 859–83.

Turner, C., & Martin, E. (1985). *Surveying Subjective Phenomena*. New York, NY: Russell Sage Foundation.

Verma, V., Scott, C., & O'Muircheartaigh, C. (1980). Sample designs and sampling errors for the World Fertility Survey. *Journal of the Royal Statistical Society*, 143, 431–73.

Vinokur, A., Oksenberg, L., & Cannell, C. F. (1979). Effects of feedback and reinforcement on the report of health information. In C. F. Cannell, L. Oksenberg, & J. M. Converse, eds., *Experiments in Interviewing Techniques*. Ann Arbor, MI: University of Michigan, Survey Research Center.

Williams, B. J. (1986). Suggestions for the application of advanced technology in Canadian collection operations. *Journal of Official Statistics*, 2, 555–60.

Wolter, K. M. (2007). *Introduction to Variance Estimation*. New York, NY: Springer.

Chapter 3

Cross-National Prevalence, Distributions, and Clusters of Trauma Exposure

Corina Benjet, Jean-Pierre Lépine, Marina Piazza, Victoria Shahly, Arieh Shalev, and Dan J. Stein

A necessary precursor to the development of PTSD, trauma is associated with a wide range of adverse mental and physical health consequences (e.g., Turner & Lloyd, 1995; Norman et al., 2006; Galea et al., 2007; Spitzer et al., 2009; Scott et al., 2013). Research on trauma has focused mainly on the *consequences* of exposure, whereas little is known about the *distribution* of trauma exposure worldwide or about who is most vulnerable to exposure. General population studies have shown that a large proportion of individuals (estimated to be 28% to 90%) in developed countries have been exposed to at least one trauma in their lifetime, with the most common traumas being the unexpected death of a loved one, motor vehicle collisions, and being mugged (e.g., Norris, 1992; Breslau et al., 1998; Hepp et al., 2006; Storr et al., 2009; Roberts et al., 2011; Ogle et al., 2014). While more limited evidence from developing countries is available, research suggests that fatalities due to injuries and accidents are more common in low- and middle-income countries (LMICs) than in high-income countries (Herbert et al., 2011); for example, road injuries are the 10th leading cause of lost years of life in developed countries and the 8th leading cause in developing countries (GBD 2013 Mortality and Causes of Death Collaborators, 2015). However, systematic data on the cross-national prevalence of exposure to a wide range of traumas was unknown before the World Mental Health (WMH) surveys were carried out. And no study has yet examined the full range of traumas in population-based samples using the same methods across a wide range of countries that differ in level of economic development.

We are aware of only one review of the determinants of trauma exposure prior to the WMH studies (Hatch & Dohrenwend, 2007). That study considered basic socio-demographic predictors (sex, socio-economic status, race/ethnicity, and age) and focused entirely on developed countries (primarily the United States). The authors found, not surprisingly, that men and women differ in the types of traumas they experience, with men reporting more injuries, accidents, and physical assaults and women reporting more sexual assaults. They also found that low socio-economic status, racial/ethnic minority status, and being a young adult were associated with increased prevalence of trauma exposure. There is good reason to think, though, that socio-demographic predictors might vary in magnitude and by type of trauma, as some traumas such as natural disasters are more randomly distributed in the population than others. We would also expect to find significant associations of geographic location and cohort with exposure to some types of traumas due to time-space variation in the occurrence of historical events (e.g., wars, natural and human-made disasters).

Another important issue is that many individuals with a history of trauma have been exposed to multiple traumas over the course of their lives. Sledjeski et al. (2008), for example, reported that individuals reporting lifetime exposure to trauma in an epidemiological survey of the US household population experienced an average of 3.3 lifetime traumas. It is unclear, though, whether lifetime traumas are related to each other and, if so, if there are any causal associations between exposure to initial traumas and risk of subsequent exposure to the same or different types of trauma. The literature suggests that such associations exist, most notably in the discussion of the concept of an "accident-prone" personality (Visser et al., 2007). Another example is re-victimization, whereby childhood abuse is associated with subsequent exposure to interpersonal partner violence and sexual assault (Coid et al., 2001; Testa et al., 2007; Daigneault et al., 2009). However, the time-lagged associations among the full range of traumas have not been examined. Questions remain as to whether all types of trauma exposure are associated with increased risk of subsequent exposure, whether there is specificity within types, and whether specific types of trauma histories are important predictors of subsequent exposure to other types of trauma.

The current chapter reviews results of WMH analyses to address these questions by both estimating the prevalence and age-of-exposure distributions for various traumas and examining socio-demographic correlates of a wide range of traumas in the 26 WMH surveys, which are the focus of this volume. We first conducted a factor analysis to examine whether traumas cluster into interpretable factors. We then estimated lifetime prevalence of each trauma type and the proportions of all traumas due to each type both within and across countries. We then generated age-of-exposure distributions for each trauma type and examined associations of socio-demographics and prior traumas as predictors of subsequent traumas, providing a panorama of trauma exposure across the WMH countries.

Methods

Lifetime prevalence of each trauma type at the respondent level and the proportions of all traumas due to each type were calculated both within and across countries. The actuarial method was used to generate an age-of-exposure distribution for each trauma type (Halli & Rao, 1992). A matrix of tetrachoric correlations among trauma types was created and exploratory factor analysis carried out with promax rotation to determine if bivariate associations among traumas clustered into interpretable factors. Time-lagged associations of temporally primary traumas predicting the subsequent first onset of each other trauma type were then examined using discrete-time survival analysis with person-year the unit of analysis and a logistic link function (Willet & Singer, 1993). Socio-demographic predictors were also included in those models. Models were pooled across countries.

The survival models were initially estimated separately for each trauma type across all countries combined, with dummy variables to control for between-country differences in prevalence. The implicit assumption was that the odds-ratios (ORs) of predictors with outcomes were constant across countries. The person-year data files for the 29 trauma types were then pooled into more highly aggregated data files, one for the set of traumas in each factor uncovered in the exploratory factor analysis. Inspection of coefficients in the 29 trauma-specific models was used to confirm the validity of this pooling. Interaction tests subsequently were used to evaluate the assumptions of constant ORs across countries and trauma types within each factor. Logistic regression coefficients and their standard errors were exponentiated to create ORs and 95% confidence intervals (CIs). As in other analyses reported in this volume, the Taylor series linearization method (Wolter, 1985) was implemented in SAS 9.3 (SAS Institute Inc., 2011) to adjust for the weighting, including non-response and post-stratification weighting, and geographic clustering of the WMH sample. Multivariate significance was evaluated using design-based Wald χ^2 tests. Statistical significance was evaluated with 0.05-level two-sided tests.

Results

Exploratory Factor Analysis

Exploratory factor analysis found five meaningful factors underlying the matrix of tetrachoric correlations among the trauma types (see Table 3.1). The first promax rotated factor represented traumas associated with exposure to collective violence (e.g., being a civilian in a war zone, a relief worker in a war zone, a refugee). The second factor encompassed traumas associated with causing or witnessing serious bodily harm to others (e.g., purposely injuring, torturing, or killing someone; combat experience). The third factor represented traumas associated with exposure to interpersonal violence (e.g., beaten up by a caregiver as a child, witnessed physical fights at home as a child, beaten up by someone other than a romantic partner). The fourth factor represented traumas associated with exposure to intimate partner or sexual violence (e.g., physically assaulted by a romantic partner, raped, sexually assaulted). Interestingly, *other* traumas and *private* traumas both had their highest standardized partial regression coefficients (the equivalents of factor loadings) on this factor, suggesting that these highly personal traumas were more similar to intimate partner or sexual violence than to other types of trauma. The fifth factor encompassed traumas associated with accidents and injuries (e.g., natural disasters, automobile accidents). Three trauma types – unexpected death of a loved one, being mugged or threatened with a weapon, and human-made disaster – cross-loaded on more than one factor, capturing the mixture of contexts in which these events occurred. Consequently, these three traumas were examined individually in subsequent analyses.

Prevalence and Distribution of Individual Trauma Types

Pooled across all countries, 70.4% of respondents experienced at least one lifetime trauma (see Figure 3.1).

Table 3.1 Factor analysis[a] of person-year level exposure across countries (n = 68,894)

	I	II	III	IV	V
I Exposure to Organized Violence					
Relief worker in war zone	0.41	0.22	0.16	−0.33	0.28
Civilian in war zone	0.88	−0.17	−0.14	0.02	0.06
Civilian in region of terror	0.78	−0.07	0.13	−0.01	0.02
Refugee	0.80	0.05	−0.29	0.10	−0.10
Kidnapped	0.61	0.13	0.25	0.23	−0.20
II Participation in Organized Violence					
Witnessed death/dead body/serious injury	0.17	0.53	0.09	0.10	0.16
Accidentally caused serious injury/death	−0.14	0.73	0.08	0.17	−0.07
Combat experience	0.13	0.82	−0.10	−0.20	0.03
Purposely injured/tortured/killed someone	−0.21	0.97	−0.02	0.09	−0.04
Witnessed atrocities	0.36	0.58	−0.04	0.01	0.06
III Physical Violence Victimization					
Beaten by caregiver	−0.01	−0.02	0.76	0.09	0.02
Beaten by someone else	0.07	0.37	0.43	0.09	0.00
Witnessed physical fight at home	−0.14	−0.01	0.75	0.16	0.00
IV Sexual Violence Victimization					
Raped	0.00	−0.14	0.29	0.74	−0.05
Sexually assaulted	−0.07	0.00	0.17	0.69	0.02
Stalked	0.08	0.22	0.02	0.59	0.02
Beaten by spouse/romantic partner	0.04	−0.25	0.15	0.64	0.17
Trauma to loved one	0.16	0.18	0.08	0.52	−0.01
Some other trauma	0.09	0.31	−0.18	0.43	0.09
Private trauma[b]	−0.03	0.29	−0.06	0.47	0.05
V Accident/Injuries					
Natural disaster	0.11	−0.14	0.18	−0.03	0.61
Toxic chemical exposure	−0.04	0.26	0.04	−0.04	0.57
Automobile accident	−0.12	0.21	0.19	0.02	0.49
Life-threatening illness	−0.04	0.03	−0.20	0.24	0.58
Child with serious illness	−0.02	−0.17	−0.18	0.31	0.65
Other life-threatening accident	−0.04	0.18	0.16	−0.09	0.57
VI Other					
Mugged or threatened with a weapon	0.14	0.31	0.32	0.17	0.12
Human-made disaster	0.35	0.08	0.07	0.04	0.36
UD of a loved one	−0.01	0.18	−0.12	0.39	0.37

[a]Factor loadings based on a tetrachoric factor analysis with promax rotation.
[b]A *private* event is a trauma that some individuals reported in response to a question asked at the very end of the trauma section that asked if they ever had some other very upsetting experience they did not tell us about already (and this includes in response to a prior open-ended question about "any other" trauma) because they were too embarrassed or upset to talk about it. Respondents were told, before they answered, that if they reported such a trauma we would not ask them anything about what it was, only about their age when the trauma happened.

The range was quite wide across countries, from a low of 28.6% in Bulgaria to a high of 84.6% in Ukraine, although the inter-quartile range (IQR; 25th–75th percentiles) of 60.7% to 76.2% was relatively narrow across countries (see Table 3.2 and Appendix Table 3.A1). 18.2% (SE = 0.2) of the respondents had been exposed to exactly one trauma type, 12.7% (SE = 0.2) two trauma types, 9.1% (SE = 0.2) three trauma types, and 30.5% (SE = 0.3) four or more different trauma types. Because many people experienced more than one trauma type, the rate of exposure to any trauma was 321.5 per 100 respondents (see Table 3.3). Overall, the most common trauma factor was accidents/injuries (36.3%) and the least common collective violence (9.4%). The most commonly reported individual trauma type was unexpected death of a loved one, which was experienced by 31.4% of all respondents (IQR 23.3–36.9% across countries) and represented nearly one-sixth (16.5%) of all instances of trauma exposure reported in the total sample.

The second most commonly reported trauma type was direct exposure to injury or death, as indicated by either witnessing death or serious injury or discovering

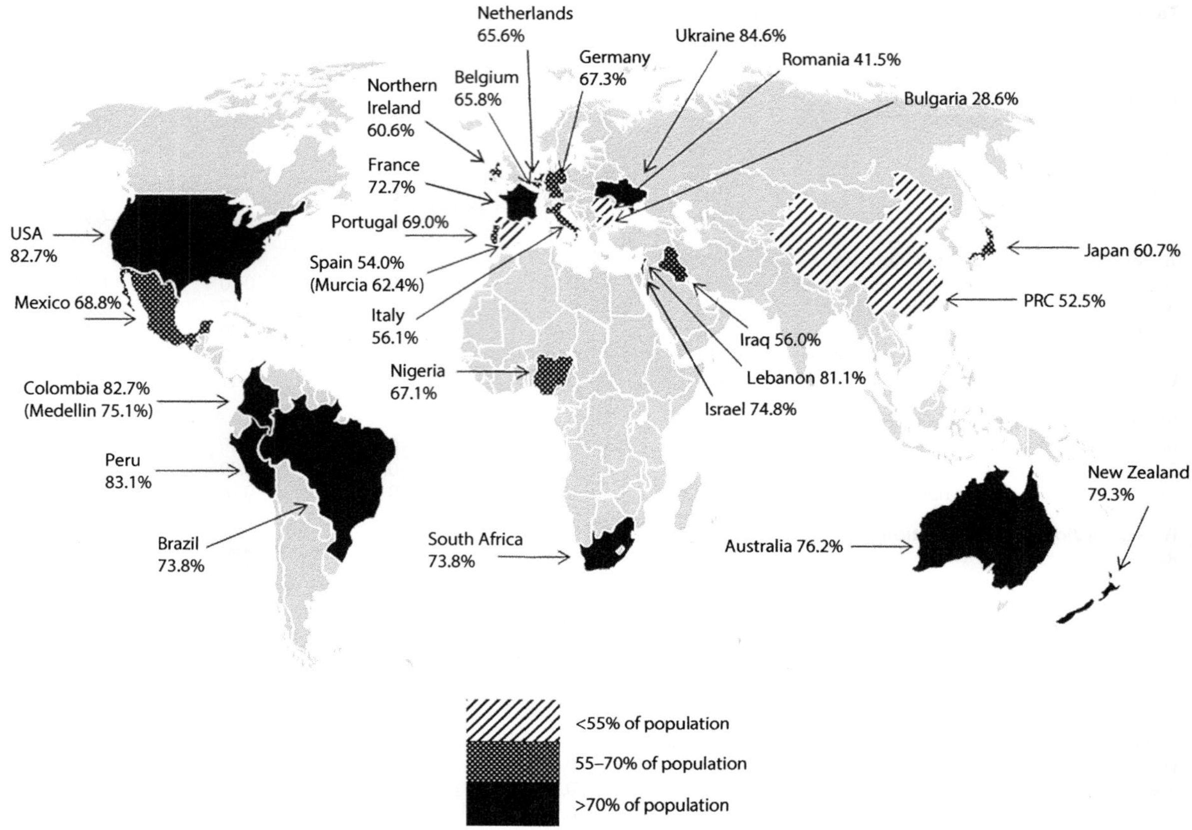

Figure 3.1 Prevalence of at least one lifetime traumatic event

a dead body (23.7%; IQR 18.0–27.3%) and represented 16.8% of all instances of trauma exposure. It should be noted that the calculation of the proportion of all trauma exposures took into consideration not only the proportion of respondents who ever experienced each trauma type, but also how many times each type occurred. This explains why witnessing death, which occurred to fewer individuals than unexpected death of a loved one (23.7% vs. 31.4%), nonetheless accounted for a similar proportion of all instances of trauma exposure (16.8% vs. 16.5%).

The next most common trauma types were being mugged (14.5%, IQR 6.5–18.3%) and life-threatening automobile accidents (14.0%, IQR 9.3–16.3%), which accounted for 7.4% and 6.1%, respectively, of all instances of trauma exposure. Only one other trauma type, life-threatening illness or injury, accounted for as much as 5% of all instances of trauma exposure. These five most common trauma types accounted for 51.9% of all instances of trauma exposure across countries.

Country-Specific Findings for Individual Trauma Types

The mean number of exposures to each trauma type per 100 respondents in each country was calculated by taking into account the percentage of respondents with the trauma and the mean number of occurrences among respondents with that trauma (see Table 3.3). Below we describe the particular trauma types that most strongly influenced the overall rates for the five trauma factors shown in the table. Prevalence of exposure to each trauma type is expressed by the number of lifetime exposures per 100 people in the population.

Exposure to Collective Violence

Exposure to collective violence was highest in Lebanon (107.6; that is, 107.6 occurrences per 100 population). This high rate was due to 55.2% of respondents reporting that they had been a civilian in a war zone

Table 3.2 Prevalence of traumas and each event as a percentage of all traumas

	Prevalence					Percentage of all traumas[a]			
				IQR of countries				IQR of countries	
	(n)	%	(SE)	25th percentile	75th percentile	%	(SE)	25th percentile	75th percentile
I Exposure to Organized Violence									
Relief worker in war zone[b]	(635)	1.1	(0.1)	0.5	1.6	0.3	(0.0)	0.2	0.7
Civilian in war zone[b]	(3,201)	5.0	(0.2)	2.4	6.8	1.4	(0.0)	0.9	3.2
Civilian in region of terror[b]	(2,501)	3.9	(0.1)	1.3	5.6	1.1	(0.0)	0.5	1.6
Refugee[c]	(1,656)	2.3	(0.1)	0.6	2.6	0.7	(0.0)	0.2	0.9
Kidnapped	(886)	1.1	(0.1)	0.5	1.4	0.4	(0.0)	0.2	0.5
Any	(6,868)	9.4	(0.2)	6.1	13.9	3.8	(0.1)	2.5	5.7
II Participation in Organized Violence									
Witnessed death/dead body/serious injury	(17,161)	23.7	(0.3)	18.0	27.3	16.8	(0.2)	14.0	19.1
Accidentally caused serious injury/death	(1,060)	1.4	(0.1)	0.6	1.6	0.7	(0.0)	0.4	0.9
Combat experience[c]	(2,038)	3.2	(0.1)	1.2	4.5	1.0	(0.0)	0.5	1.2
Purposely injured/tortured/killed someone[d]	(670)	1.0	(0.1)	0.3	1.0	0.7	(0.0)	0.3	0.6
Witnessed atrocities	(2,634)	3.7	(0.1)	1.2	3.9	2.4	(0.1)	0.5	2.5
Any	(18,965)	26.3	(0.3)	20.4	31.4	21.4	(0.2)	17.6	23.3
III Physical Violence Victimization									
Beaten by caregiver	(7,019)	7.9	(0.1)	3.1	10.2	2.5	(0.0)	1.2	3.8
Beaten by someone else	(4,558)	5.9	(0.1)	3.5	7.3	3.6	(0.1)	2.2	3.9
Witnessed physical fight at home[e]	(6,808)	12.9	(0.2)	10.4	18.2	2.5	(0.0)	2.8	5.0
Any	(13,882)	17.0	(0.2)	6.3	21.0	8.5	(0.1)	4.3	11.3
IV Sexual Violence Victimization									
Raped	(3,342)	3.2	(0.1)	0.6	3.4	1.8	(0.1)	0.5	1.9
Sexually assaulted	(5,261)	5.8	(0.1)	1.7	6.2	3.6	(0.1)	1.0	3.1
Stalked	(4,646)	5.4	(0.1)	2.8	6.0	3.0	(0.1)	2.0	3.5
Beaten by spouse/romantic partner	(4,602)	4.5	(0.1)	2.4	6.0	1.4	(0.0)	1.0	1.9
Trauma to loved one	(4,527)	5.6	(0.1)	1.7	6.2	2.7	(0.1)	1.3	2.8
Some other trauma	(3,297)	4.2	(0.1)	2.0	5.1	1.3	(0.0)	0.6	1.8
Private trauma[f]	(4,171)	4.9	(0.1)	3.5	5.8	1.5	(0.0)	1.2	2.1
Any	(19,058)	22.8	(0.3)	15.7	25.1	15.3	(0.2)	11.3	15.4

(*cont.*)

Table 3.2 *(cont.)*

	Prevalence					Percentage of all traumas[a]			
				IQR of countries				IQR of countries	
	(n)	%	(SE)	25th percentile	75th percentile	%	(SE)	25th percentile	75th percentile
V Accidents/Injuries									
Natural disaster[c]	(5,603)	7.7	(0.2)	3.9	9.6	4.1	(0.1)	1.9	6.2
Toxic chemical exposure	(3,005)	4.2	(0.1)	1.9	4.1	3.6	(0.1)	2.2	3.9
Automobile accident	(10,131)	14.0	(0.2)	9.3	16.3	6.1	(0.1)	4.8	7.3
Life-threatening illness	(9,377)	11.8	(0.2)	8.0	13.2	5.1	(0.1)	4.4	6.8
Child with serious illness	(6,370)	7.9	(0.1)	5.2	9.2	3.1	(0.1)	2.6	3.7
Other life-threatening accident	(4,537)	6.2	(0.1)	4.1	7.3	2.9	(0.1)	2.3	3.4
Any	(26,972)	36.3	(0.3)	28.5	39.4	24.9	(0.2)	21.7	28.9
VI Other									
Mugged/threatened with a weapon	(10,562)	14.5	(0.2)	6.5	18.3	7.4	(0.1)	3.6	9.8
Human-made disaster	(3,001)	4.0	(0.1)	2.4	5.3	2.1	(0.1)	1.3	3.8
UD of a loved one	(23,792)	31.4	(0.3)	23.3	36.9	16.5	(0.2)	14.2	18.3
Any	(30,218)	40.8	(0.3)	33.5	48.7	26.1	(0.2)	23.1	29.2
VII Any Event	**(50,855)**	**70.4**	**(0.3)**	**60.7**	**76.2**	**100.0**	**(0.0)**	**1.4**	**4.4**

[a]Includes information on repeat exposures.
[b]Brazil – São Paulo and Israel did not ask about this trauma.
[c]Brazil – São Paulo did not ask about this trauma.
[d]Spain – Murcia and New Zealand did not ask about this trauma.
[e]Belgium, Bulgaria, PRC – Beijing/Shanghai, France, Germany, Israel, Italy, Lebanon, Netherlands, Nigeria, South Africa, Spain, and Ukraine did not ask about this trauma.
[f]A *private* event is a trauma that some individuals reported in response to a question asked at the very end of the trauma section that asked if they ever had some other very upsetting experience they did not tell us about already (and this includes in response to a prior open-ended question about "any other" trauma) because they were too embarrassed or upset to talk about it. Respondents were told, before they answered, that if they reported such a trauma we would not ask them anything about what it was, only about their age when the trauma happened.

Table 3.3 Country-specific frequency of exposure to each type of trauma and any event per 100 respondents (n = 68,894)

	Exposure to organized violence		Participation in organized violence		Physical violence victimization		Sexual violence victimization		Accidents/ injuries		UD of a loved one		Other traumas		Any event	
	Mean per 100	(SE) per 100	Mean per 100	(SE) per 100	Mean per 100	(SE) per 100	Mean per 100	(SE) per 100	Mean per 100	(SE) per 100	Mean per 100	(SE) per 100	Mean per 100	(SE) per 100	Mean per 100	(SE) per 100
I High-Income Countries																
Australia	10.9	(0.7)	83.2	(3.6)	29.7	(1.3)	73.0	(2.8)	88.4	(2.6)	64.9	(2.2)	31.4	(1.6)	381.6	(8.9)
Belgium	21.0	(2.9)	47.3	(5.4)	11.0	(2.4)	35.6	(4.7)	56.6	(5.0)	36.1	(4.9)	23.2	(3.3)	230.7	(16.3)
France	18.5	(2.4)	77.8	(7.7)	6.7	(1.1)	40.9	(3.9)	74.5	(8.6)	41.9	(3.9)	25.4	(2.7)	285.8	(16.6)
Germany	19.3	(2.1)	63.4	(4.4)	16.2	(2.4)	40.1	(4.4)	63.7	(6.2)	43.2	(4.1)	25.9	(3.6)	271.6	(16.4)
Israel	6.5	(0.3)	104.4	(3.1)	11.8	(0.9)	46.3	(1.7)	73.7	(2.1)	65.2	(1.6)	19.6	(1.0)	327.5	(5.8)
Italy	8.3	(0.8)	102.2	(11.9)	5.9	(1.0)	16.7	(1.7)	52.8	(4.6)	29.8	(1.8)	9.1	(1.3)	224.8	(16.4)
Japan	6.5	(0.8)	42.0	(4.3)	36.7	(2.6)	33.0	(3.1)	44.9	(4.0)	37.8	(3.4)	6.2	(1.4)	207.2	(12.5)
Netherlands	16.4	(2.8)	41.8	(5.0)	9.8	(1.7)	45.7	(6.7)	47.0	(3.4)	41.6	(4.6)	35.3	(5.4)	237.6	(17.5)
New Zealand	11.8	(0.9)	70.7	(3.3)	32.9	(1.4)	83.7	(3.3)	120.0	(4.6)	67.6	(2.2)	28.1	(1.5)	414.8	(9.5)
Northern Ireland	29.1	(1.7)	47.3	(3.6)	20.3	(1.8)	39.6	(3.1)	43.5	(2.9)	42.3	(2.6)	28.6	(1.9)	250.6	(10.5)
Portugal	10.1	(1.1)	50.7	(3.3)	31.0	(1.8)	33.6	(2.9)	75.7	(3.8)	34.5	(2.4)	25.6	(2.1)	261.1	(9.4)
Spain	8.5	(0.9)	14.9	(2.1)	6.4	(1.5)	13.0	(2.2)	51.4	(3.9)	28.1	(2.2)	26.3	(3.2)	148.6	(8.9)
Spain – Murcia	3.3	(1.1)	7.4	(1.8)	15.2	(0.9)	23.1	(4.6)	51.8	(5.2)	37.6	(3.0)	18.1	(2.4)	156.6	(12.5)
United States	8.2	(0.6)	84.1	(3.3)	35.7	(1.9)	96.2	(3.1)	138.8	(4.9)	84.7	(3.4)	41.7	(1.5)	489.4	(12.9)
II Upper-Middle-Income Countries																
Brazil – São Paulo	4.1	(0.9)	101.8	(6.8)	35.4	(1.8)	30.2	(1.7)	51.6	(3.1)	47.2	(2.1)	62.5	(3.6)	332.9	(11.7)
Bulgaria	0.4	(0.2)	13.8	(1.7)	1.9	(0.7)	10.2	(1.1)	28.6	(2.2)	15.6	(2.3)	3.4	(0.9)	74.0	(4.6)
Colombia – Medellin	16.2	(2.0)	76.5	(5.7)	45.8	(3.3)	57.0	(7.3)	67.7	(6.2)	66.9	(6.6)	75.6	(4.9)	405.7	(25.9)
Lebanon	107.6	(6.9)	100.4	(8.0)	10.9	(1.8)	44.5	(4.5)	48.4	(5.2)	59.6	(4.2)	14.2	(2.0)	385.5	(22.7)
Mexico	3.3	(0.4)	39.1	(3.9)	50.1	(2.5)	36.8	(2.5)	76.9	(5.3)	34.7	(3.1)	45.6	(2.6)	286.5	(11.5)
Romania	3.7	(0.5)	25.2	(3.1)	9.7	(1.1)	13.5	(1.8)	57.2	(2.9)	15.1	(1.1)	6.2	(0.9)	130.5	(6.8)
South Africa	15.6	(1.6)	72.7	(4.6)	30.7	(1.5)	36.5	(1.4)	69.2	(2.5)	62.1	(2.6)	30.5	(1.4)	317.2	(9.6)
III Low- and Lower-Middle-Income Countries																
Colombia	13.5	(1.3)	101.1	(6.1)	53.9	(2.4)	55.1	(3.2)	91.9	(5.8)	70.2	(4.2)	72.3	(3.3)	458.0	(16.3)
Nigeria	18.5	(1.7)	100.1	(6.4)	20.5	(2.4)	22.7	(1.9)	88.6	(5.5)	62.8	(2.8)	13.8	(1.3)	327.0	(12.2)
PRC – Beijing/ Shanghai	7.7	(1.1)	34.8	(3.9)	14.8	(1.7)	15.8	(2.6)	57.7	(4.6)	12.7	(1.5)	8.6	(1.6)	152.2	(10.9)
Peru	9.4	(0.8)	54.0	(4.8)	66.4	(2.5)	41.4	(2.8)	97.3	(2.7)	44.0	(2.5)	54.8	(3.5)	367.3	(7.8)
Ukraine	18.1	(1.6)	69.6	(6.7)	43.1	(5.0)	48.8	(3.8)	105.9	(4.7)	57.9	(3.8)	30.2	(3.8)	373.6	(16.6)
IV Total	**12.2**	**(0.3)**	**68.9**	**(1.0)**	**27.3**	**(0.4)**	**49.2**	**(0.7)**	**80.2**	**(1.0)**	**53.2**	**(0.7)**	**30.6**	**(0.5)**	**321.5**	**(2.9)**

and 37.7% having been a refugee. Northern Ireland's high rate of 29.1 was due primarily to 20.8% of the respondents having been a civilian in a region of terror. The surprisingly low rate in Israel (6.5) was due to not asking about being a civilian in a war zone or region of terror, as the researchers who designed the WMH survey in Israel considered the total Israeli population to have been exposed to this type of trauma. The pattern for kidnapping differed from the aggregate results for collective violence, with the highest rates reported in Brazil (4.1), Lebanon (3.1), Medellin-Colombia (2.5), and Mexico (2.2).

Causing/Witnessing Bodily Harm

Causing or witnessing bodily harm had a high rate (above 100) in countries that have experienced war, sectarian violence, or armed conflict such as Israel, Colombia, Nigeria, and Lebanon. While witnessing death, a dead body, or serious injury was the most frequent event of this group for all countries, there was a particularly high rate of witnessing atrocities in Lebanon (20.7), Israel (20.3), and Nigeria (15.9) and of combat experience in Israel (10.8) and Lebanon (9.5). For Lebanon, a country invaded five times in the past 35 years, exposure to collective violence and causing or witnessing bodily harm accounted for 53.9% of all traumas.

Interpersonal Violence

Latin American countries had the highest rates of interpersonal violence, with overall rates in Peru (66.4), Colombia (53.9), and Mexico (50.1) explained primarily by the high prevalence of witnessing physical fights at home (20.3% to 31.5%) and having been beaten up by a caregiver (18.2% to 20.4%). These figures were difficult to compare across countries as many other countries did not ask about witnessing physical fights at home.

Intimate Partner/Sexual Violence

Rates of sexual violence were highest in the United States (96.2), New Zealand (83.7), and Australia (73.0), and represented 19% to 20% of all traumas in these countries. All of the individual traumas in this group had elevated rates in these three countries. However, one specific trauma – being beaten up by a spouse or romantic partner – had similar or even higher rates in Colombia, Medellin-Colombia, and Peru (7.2–7.8).

Accidents and Injuries

The highest rates of accidents and injuries were reported in the United States (138.8), New Zealand (120.0), and Ukraine (105.9), representing 28% of all traumas in these countries. These high rates were due primarily to automobile accidents (in all three countries), personal life-threatening illness (in the United States and Ukraine), serious illness of a child (in Ukraine), and natural disasters (in the United States).

Unexpected Death of a Loved One

Rates of the unexpected death of a loved one, defined as someone very close dying unexpectedly by being killed in an accident, homicide, suicide, or a fatal heart attack at a young age, were consistently high across countries, with a pooled rate of 53.2. China had a remarkably low rate (12.7) compared to other countries, presumably due to the one child policy, although this still represented 8.1% of all traumas in China.

Other Traumas

Rates of exposure to human-made disaster in Ukraine (16.7), where the Chernobyl disaster occurred, were more than double the pooled average across countries (6.9). Northern Ireland, a country with frequent car bombings during the troubles, had the second highest rate of human-made disaster (14.2). The rate of having been mugged or threatened with a weapon was highest in the five Latin American surveys, ranging from 42.9 in Mexico to 71.2 in Medellin-Colombia.

Predictors of Trauma Exposure

In the aggregate, age-of-exposure curves showed that interpersonal violence had the earliest ages of exposure (see Figure 3.2a), generally in childhood, followed by collective violence (see Figure 3.2b) and causing/witnessing bodily harm (see Figure 3.2c), generally in early adulthood. Intimate partner/sexual violence (see Figure 3.2d) had varying age-of-exposure distributions: rape and sexual assault centered narrowly in early adolescence whereas the other sexual violence events had shallower slopes and later median ages-of-exposure ranging from 25 to 48. Later still, accidents and injuries (see Figure 3.2e) showed two distinct sets of slopes: toxic chemical exposure, automobile accidents, other life-threatening accidents, and natural disasters occurred earlier with median ages-of-exposure

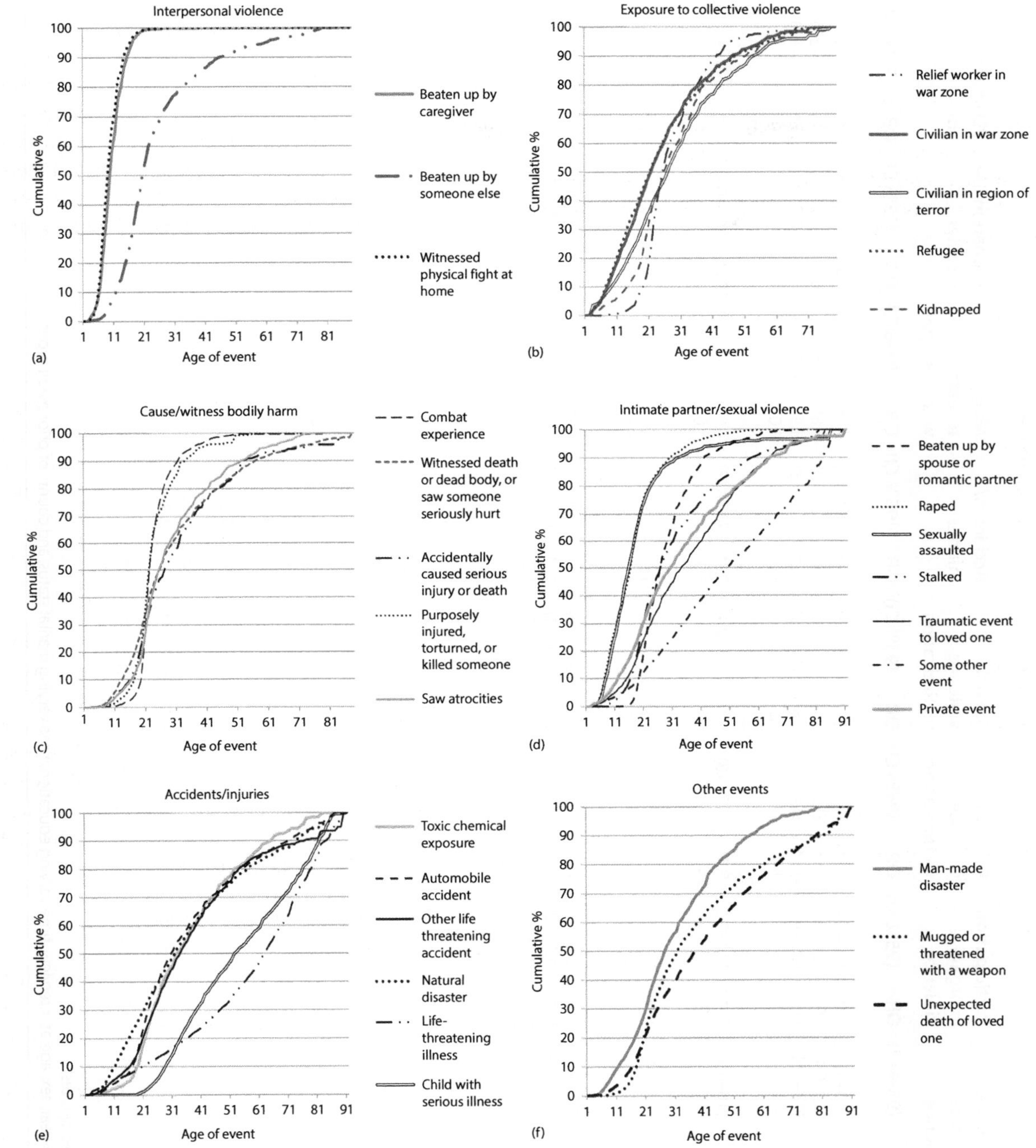

Figure 3.2 Age-of-onset curves for trauma exposure in countries with the event

between 29 and 32, whereas having a life-threatening illness or a child with a serious illness occurred later with median age-of-exposure of 61 and 51, respectively. The other traumas (see Figure 3.2f) – exposure to human-made disasters, being mugged, and the unexpected death of a loved one – had median onsets spanning ages 26 to 37.

We examined predictors of trauma exposure for each of the 29 trauma types both separately and pooled across the factors. Only the pooled models plus models for the three individual cross-loading traumas are shown in Table 3.4, although we comment briefly below on trauma-specific deviations from these aggregate results. Females were more likely than males to

Table 3.4 Associations of socio-demographic variables and prior traumas predicting event categories in 26 WMH surveys from 24 countries[a]

	Exposure to organized violence		Participation in organized violence		Physical violence victimization		Sexual violence victimization		Accidents/ injuries		Mugged/ threatened with a weapon		Human-made disaster		UD of a loved one	
	OR	(95% CI)	OR	(95% CI)	OR	(95% CI)	OR	(95% CI)	OR	(95% CI)	OR	(95% CI)	OR	(95% CI)	OR	(95% CI)
I Age at Interview																
18–34 years old	0.3*	(0.3–0.3)	1.3*	(1.2–1.4)	1.8*	(1.6–1.9)	3.3*	(3.0–3.5)	1.8*	(1.7–1.9)	5.2*	(4.6–6.0)	0.9	(0.8–1.1)	3.8*	(3.5–4.1)
35–49 years old	0.4*	(0.3–0.4)	1.0	(0.9–1.1)	1.8*	(1.6–2.0)	2.3*	(2.1–2.5)	1.3*	(1.3–1.4)	2.8*	(2.5–3.2)	0.9	(0.7–1.0)	2.1*	(2.0–2.3)
50–64 years old	0.4*	(0.4–0.5)	1.0	(0.9–1.0)	1.5*	(1.4–1.7)	1.8*	(1.6–1.9)	1.2*	(1.2–1.3)	1.9*	(1.7–2.2)	0.8*	(0.7–0.9)	1.6*	(1.5–1.7)
65+ years old	1.0	–	1.0	–	1.0	–	1.0	–	1.0	–	1.0	–	1.0	–	1.0	–
II Sex																
Female	0.8*	(0.8–0.9)	0.4*	(0.4–0.4)	0.8*	(0.7–0.8)	2.3*	(2.2–2.4)	0.7*	(0.7–0.7)	0.5*	(0.4–0.5)	0.7*	(0.6–0.7)	1.1*	(1.1–1.2)
Male	1.0	–	1.0	–	1.0	–	1.0	–	1.0	–	1.0	–	1.0	–	1.0	–
III Student																
Student	0.8*	(0.7–0.9)	1.3*	(1.2–1.5)	1.4*	(1.3–1.6)	1.2*	(1.2–1.3)	1.0	(0.9–1.1)	1.6*	(1.4–1.8)	1.1	(0.9–1.3)	1.7*	(1.6–1.9)
Non-student	1.0	–	1.0	–	1.0	–	1.0	–	1.0	–	1.0	–	1.0	–	1.0	–
IV Time Varying Education																
Low education	0.6*	(0.5–0.7)	1.0	(0.9–1.1)	1.4*	(1.2–1.6)	0.9	(0.9–1.0)	1.0	(0.9–1.1)	0.8*	(0.8–0.9)	0.9	(0.8–1.1)	1.2*	(1.1–1.3)
Low-average	0.6*	(0.6–0.7)	1.2*	(1.1–1.3)	1.3*	(1.2–1.6)	1.0	(1.0–1.1)	1.1*	(1.0–1.2)	1.0	(0.9–1.1)	0.9	(0.8–1.1)	1.3*	(1.3–1.4)
High-average	0.8*	(0.7–0.9)	1.2*	(1.1–1.3)	1.1	(1.0–1.3)	1.0	(1.0–1.1)	1.2*	(1.1–1.2)	1.1	(1.0–1.2)	1.0	(0.8–1.2)	1.3*	(1.2–1.4)
High	1.0	–	1.0	–	1.0	–	1.0	–	1.0	–	1.0	–	1.0	–	1.0	–
V Time Varying Marital Status																
Currently married	0.8*	(0.7–0.9)	0.7*	(0.7–0.8)	0.5*	(0.5–0.6)	0.9*	(0.8–0.9)	1.0	(0.9–1.0)	0.6*	(0.6–0.7)	0.8*	(0.7–0.9)	0.8*	(0.8–0.9)
Previously married	0.8*	(0.7–1.0)	0.9*	(0.8–1.0)	1.4*	(1.2–1.8)	1.3*	(1.2–1.4)	1.0	(0.9–1.0)	1.0	(0.9–1.1)	0.9	(0.8–1.2)	1.2*	(1.1–1.3)
Never married	1.0	–	1.0	–	1.0	–	1.0	–	1.0	–	1.0	–	1.0	–	1.0	–
VI Prior Trauma-Type Count																
Exposure to organized violence	1.8*	(1.6–2.1)	1.6*	(1.5–1.8)	1.4*	(1.2–1.6)	1.3*	(1.2–1.4)	1.3*	(1.2–1.3)	1.4*	(1.3–1.6)	2.1*	(1.8–2.5)	1.1*	(1.0–1.2)
Participation in organized violence	1.7*	(1.6–1.9)	1.7*	(1.6–1.8)	1.4*	(1.3–1.6)	1.5*	(1.4–1.6)	1.4*	(1.3–1.5)	1.8*	(1.7–1.9)	1.9*	(1.6–2.2)	1.3*	(1.3–1.4)
Physical violence victimization	1.5*	(1.4–1.7)	1.6*	(1.6–1.7)	2.6*	(2.4–2.8)	2.2*	(2.1–2.3)	1.4*	(1.4–1.5)	1.6*	(1.5–1.7)	1.3*	(1.2–1.5)	1.4*	(1.4–1.5)
Sexual violence victimization	1.3*	(1.2–1.5)	1.4*	(1.3–1.5)	1.5*	(1.4–1.7)	1.7*	(1.6–1.8)	1.4*	(1.3–1.4)	1.5*	(1.4–1.6)	1.4*	(1.2–1.7)	1.3*	(1.2–1.4)
Accident/injuries	1.4*	(1.2–1.5)	1.4*	(1.4–1.5)	1.4*	(1.3–1.5)	1.4*	(1.4–1.5)	1.5*	(1.4–1.5)	1.5*	(1.4–1.6)	1.9*	(1.6–2.2)	1.4*	(1.3–1.5)
Mugged/threatened with a weapon	1.7*	(1.5–2.0)	1.4*	(1.3–1.5)	0.9	(0.8–1.1)	1.3*	(1.2–1.4)	1.3*	(1.2–1.4)			1.5*	(1.2–1.8)	1.2*	(1.1–1.3)
Human-made disaster	1.4*	(1.2–1.8)	1.4*	(1.3–1.6)	1.4*	(1.2–1.6)	1.3*	(1.2–1.4)	1.2*	(1.2–1.3)	1.4*	(1.2–1.6)			1.2*	(1.1–1.4)
UD of a loved one	1.1*	(1.0–1.3)	1.3*	(1.3–1.4)	1.1*	(1.0–1.2)	1.3*	(1.2–1.4)	1.2*	(1.2–1.3)	1.3*	(1.3–1.5)	1.4*	(1.2–1.6)	1.2*	(1.1–1.3)

*Significant at the 0.05 level, two-sided test.
[a]Model includes country, person-year, sex, age at interview, time varying education, time varying marital status, and counts of prior event types.

be exposed to intimate partner/sexual violence (OR = 2.3) and to the unexpected death of a loved one (OR = 1.1), with the latter a small but statistically reliable effect. On the other hand, females were less likely than males to be exposed to traumas from the other four factors (ORs = 0.4–0.8). Two specific traumas deviated from these aggregate results: females had greater odds of being a refugee and of having a child with a serious illness. Being a civilian in a war zone, having a life-threatening illness, and experiencing a self-nominated *other* trauma had no association with sex. Clearly, if a child is seriously ill and the child has both a mother and a father, men and women should have the same rates of exposure to their child being seriously ill. That this was not the case suggests that the traumas reported in the WMH surveys are to some extent self-selected by the respondents based on salience, which was presumably higher for women than men in the case of child illnesses. This finding is consistent with long-standing evidence that women are more emotionally affected than men by stressful life events that occur to individuals in their social networks (Kessler & McLeod, 1984).

Married respondents had reduced odds, compared to the never married, of all trauma factors (ORs = 0.5–0.9) except accidents/injuries (OR = 1.0). Two specific trauma types deviated from these aggregate results: married respondents had greater odds than the unmarried of being beaten up by a spouse or romantic partner (OR = 1.7) and of having a child with a serious illness (OR = 2.4). Previously married respondents, in comparison to those never married, had lower odds of exposure to collective violence and causing/witnessing bodily harm (OR = 0.8–0.9), but elevated odds of unexpected death of a loved one (OR = 1.2), interpersonal violence (OR = 1.4), and sexual violence (OR = 1.3). Importantly, these associations were based on models that adjusted for age of exposure, such that the high odds of exposure among the never married were not due to age effects.

Regarding cohort effects, compared to respondents aged 65 or older, all three younger cohorts had lower odds of exposure to collective violence but higher odds of exposure to interpersonal violence, sexual violence, accidents/injuries, unexpected death of a loved one, and being mugged. Only the youngest cohort had increased odds of causing/witnessing bodily harm. These odd-ratios were on the order of 1.3 to 5.2 and generally decreased with increasing age. The odds for each individual trauma type were very consistent with the aggregate results. Only natural disasters, being beaten up by a caregiver, and having purposefully injured or killed were unrelated to cohort.

Being a student was associated with low odds of exposure to traumas associated with collective violence (OR = 0.8), but elevated odds of exposure to traumas in each of the other factors (ORs = 1.2–1.7). Two specific trauma types deviated from these aggregate results: students had reduced odds of a life-threatening illness (OR = 0.9) and having a child with a serious illness (OR = 0.3). Student status was not associated with 15 of the 29 trauma types.

In general, education was inversely associated with exposure to traumas related to causing/witnessing bodily harm, experiencing interpersonal violence, having accidents/injuries, and the unexpected death of a loved one, but positively associated with exposure to collective violence and being mugged. Automobile accidents deviated from the aggregate results for injuries/accidents, in that education was positively associated with automobile accidents (OR = 1.1). Sexual violence was not associated with education in the aggregate, as the individual events within this factor had opposing odds (i.e., education was inversely associated with being raped, beaten up by a spouse or romantic partner, or stalked [ORs = 0.4–0.8], but positively associated with sexual assault, a private or other trauma, or a trauma that occurred to a loved one [ORs = 1.2–1.7]).

Prior Trauma Exposure

The mean number of lifetime trauma exposures was 3.2 in the total sample (IQR = 2.2–3.7) and 4.6 among those with any trauma exposure (IQR = 3.5–4.7). At the aggregate level, temporally primary traumas in all five factors as well as the three separate traumas were positively associated with subsequent exposure to traumas in all five factors and the other three separate traumas, the only exception being a nonsignificant association between being mugged and subsequent interpersonal violence. The strength of these associations varied across trauma types. The strongest associations in the aggregate were temporally primary exposure to traumas related to collective violence predicting subsequent human-made disasters (OR = 2.1), and temporally primary traumas related to interpersonal violence with predicting subsequent exposure to other traumas in the same group (OR = 2.6) as well as traumas in the sexual violence group (OR = 2.2). For individual traumas, there were significant associations for traumas within the same factor as well as across factors, though the associations across factors were weaker.

Discussion

The use of retrospective reports may have led to the underestimation of traumas, especially for those encountered early in life. Consistent with this possibility, a review of the literature on the validity of retrospective reports of childhood abuse indicates that false negatives are common and false positives are rare (Hardt & Rutter, 2004). One would expect this to be true for other traumas as well. Furthermore, there may be cultural differences in the willingness to disclose sensitive information. We attempted to minimize the under-reporting of sensitive information by including an option to report an unspecified private event. The private event accounted for 1.2% to 2.1% of all traumas worldwide, with an interquartile range between countries of 3.5% to 5.8%. The narrowness of this range provided indirect evidence that cultural differences in disclosing stigmatizing traumas were not substantial. However, the possibility of cross-cultural differences in the willingness to acknowledge even a private event cannot be excluded. Bulgaria, in particular, had low rates of all traumas and yet the private event in Bulgaria accounted for a greater proportion of all events (3.3%) than in any other country (except Japan), suggesting that under-reporting of stigmatizing traumas may have been implicated in the low rates in that country.

Notwithstanding these likely limitations involving under-estimation, our results are noteworthy in several respects. First, we found that trauma exposure is a common experience worldwide, with over two-thirds of individuals reporting a lifetime trauma and the biases noted in the prior paragraph suggesting that this estimate is conservative. Second, a small number of trauma types account for a large proportion of all trauma exposure. Five trauma types are especially common: witnessing death or serious injury, experiencing the unexpected death of loved one, being mugged, being in a life-threatening automobile accident, and experiencing a life-threatening illness or injury. Together, these five trauma types account for over half of all instances of trauma exposure in the population, a pattern that is rather consistent across countries. Third, trauma exposure does not occur randomly in the population. The types of traumas to which people are exposed and the frequencies of these exposures vary according to the country of residence, socio-demographic characteristics, and history of prior trauma exposure. Rather than identifying a particular group of vulnerable individuals, though, a more nuanced portrait emerges from the analysis showing that the vast majority of individuals experience traumas that differ in type and frequency, depending on individual differences in life circumstances. Fourth, trauma exposure increases risk of subsequent exposure, although the strength of this association varies by type of trauma. Fifth, most traumas are first experienced in childhood, adolescence, or early adulthood.

Our finding that trauma exposure is common is consistent with previous reports from developed countries (Breslau et al., 1998; Ogle et al., 2014). However, the WMH data addressed an important limitation of previous studies: the lack of even basic descriptive data on trauma exposure in developing countries. Our findings did not support the prevailing assumption that individuals in lower-income countries are much more likely to be exposed to trauma than those in higher-income countries. One reason for this is that a substantial proportion of residents in high-income countries are immigrants from war-torn countries. In 2005, developed countries had 60% of the world's immigrants, with the United States alone having 20% of the world's immigrants (representing almost 13% of the US population), and Australia 2% (representing 20% of Australian population) (United Nations, Department of Economic and Social Affairs, Population Division, 2009). The wars and conflicts to which high-income countries have sent soldiers, peacekeepers, and relief workers also add to the proportion of the population in high-income countries exposed to collective violence.

It is noteworthy that the United States and New Zealand have the highest rates of accidents and injuries among the countries considered here, especially given that low-income countries have the highest fatality rates due to accidents and injuries (World Health Organization, 2009; Herbert et al., 2011). It has been estimated that there are 20 severe road traffic accidents for every fatality (Abrahams et al., 2014). Taking into consideration access to and quality of emergency medical services, however, it is likely that more individuals who have experienced accidents and injuries in high-income countries survive – and consequently are more likely to be interviewed – than those in low-income countries.

Our findings were strengthened by the uniform measurement across countries. This is particularly relevant for sexual violence where question wording and operationalization is known to impact estimates (Fisher, 2009). Varying prevalence rates across countries are likely due to a combination of true differences, cultural willingness to disclose, and cultural differences in labeling an experience as "rape" or "unwanted/

inappropriate sexual contact" due to differences in perceptions of autonomy over one's body or right to deny sexual advances. Our finding that sexual violence is reported most often in Australia, New Zealand, and the United States, which is consistent with two recent publications (Stoltenborgh et al., 2011; Abrahams et al., 2014), may very well be due to this latter explanation.

We found that the identification of vulnerable groups is more complex than previously reported in the literature. In contrast to Hatch and Dohrenwend (2007), who reported greater trauma exposure among disadvantaged groups in general and the less educated in particular in the United States, we found that the association between education and trauma exposure varies by trauma type. Those with less education have increased risk of causing/witnessing bodily harm (perhaps because they are more likely to enlist in military service), experiencing interpersonal violence, and having accidents and injuries, but reduced risk of exposure to collective violence. Those with high education have elevated risk of automobile accidents and sexual assaults, but reduced risk of being raped.

The most consistent finding involving correlates is that being married is associated with low risk of many traumas. Given that our classification of being married did not include cohabitating couples, our estimates are likely to be conservative. Married people may spend less time outside the home, at later hours, unaccompanied, and in potentially vulnerable situations (such as parties or bars) than the unmarried. Consistent with this explanation, a survey conducted in 17 industrialized countries found that single individuals had double the risk of contact crime, and those who went out more frequently were 20% more likely than others to become crime victims (van Kesteren et al., 2000). Additionally, married individuals may have more resources and consequently face fewer stressors such as living in unsafe communities than unmarried individuals. The main exceptions to this general pattern are that being married is associated with elevated odds of being beaten up by a spouse/romantic partner and of having a child with a serious illness.

No obvious single vulnerable group emerged from this analysis as being at especially elevated risk of trauma exposure other than the unmarried. However, preventive interventions for trauma exposure might more reasonably be focused on the segments of the population most likely to be exposed to multiple types of trauma. The fact that risk of trauma exposure is correlated over time is of particular interest in this regard, as this presumably reflects individual differences in predispositions, coping resources, and lifestyles that influence the risk of trauma exposure. The WMH surveys were not designed to facilitate a search for modifiable risk factors that might be targeted to prevent future trauma exposure, but the strong patterning of inter-temporal associations among traumas suggests that such an investigation might make sense in future studies by focusing on individuals exposed to initial traumas. Preventive interventions with this focus already exist for recurrence of drunk driving (Miller et al., 2015), intimate partner violence (Ramsay et al., 2009), and sexual violence (Marques et al., 2005), but our results raise the possibility of developing risk models to target broader types of secondary preventive interventions as well.

Acknowledgment

Portions of this chapter are based on Benjet, C., Bromet, E., Karam, E. G., et al. (2016). The epidemiology of traumatic event exposure worldwide: results from the World Mental Health Consortium. *Psychological Medicine*, **46**, 327–43, by permission of Cambridge University Press.

References

Abrahams, N., Devries, K., Watts, C., et al. (2014). Worldwide prevalence of non-partner sexual violence: a systematic review. *Lancet*, 383, 1648–54.

Breslau, N., Kessler, R. C., Chilcoat, H. D., et al. (1998). Trauma and posttraumatic stress disorder in the community: the 1996 Detroit area survey of trauma. *Archives of General Psychiatry*, 55, 626–32.

Coid, J., Petruckevitch, A., Feder, G., et al. (2001). Relation between childhood sexual and physical abuse and risk of revictimisation in women: a cross-sectional survey. *Lancet*, 358, 450–4.

Daigneault, I., Herbert, M., & McDuff, P. (2009). Men's and women's childhood sexual abuse and victimization in adult partner relationships: a study of risk factors. *Child Abuse & Neglect*, 33, 638–47.

Fisher, B. S. (2009). The effects of survey question wording on rape estimates: evidence from a quasi-experimental design. *Violence Against Women*, 15, 133–47.

GBD 2013 Mortality and Causes of Death Collaborators (2015). Global, regional, and national age-sex specific all-cause and cause-specific mortality for 240 causes of death, 1990–2013: a systematic analysis for the Global Burden of Disease Study 2013. *Lancet*, 385, 117–71.

Galea, S., Brewin, C. R., Gruber, M., et al. (2007). Exposure to hurricane-related stressors and mental illness after Hurricane Katrina. *Archives of General Psychiatry*, 64, 1427–34.

Halli, S. S., & Rao, K. V. (1992). *Advanced Techniques of Population Analysis*. New York, NY: Plenum.

Hardt, J., & Rutter, M. (2004). Validity of adult retrospective reports of adverse childhood experiences: review of the evidence. *Journal of Child Psychology and Psychiatry*, 45, 260–73.

Hatch, S. L., & Dohrenwend, B. P. (2007). Distribution of traumatic and other stressful life events by race/ethnicity, gender, SES and age: a review of the research. *American Journal of Community Psychology*, 40, 313–32.

Hepp, U., Gamma, A., Milos, G., et al. (2006). Prevalence of exposure to potentially traumatic events and PTSD: the Zurich Cohort Study. *European Archives of Psychiatry and Clinical Neuroscience*, 256, 151–8.

Herbert, H. K., Hyder, A. A., Butchart, A., & Norton, R. (2011). Global health: injuries and violence. *Infectious Disease Clinics of North America*, 25, 653–68.

Kessler, R. C., & McLeod, J. D. (1984). Sex differences in vulnerability to undesirable life events. *American Sociological Review*, 49, 620–31.

Marques, J. K., Wiederanders, M., Day, D. M., Nelson, C., & van Ommeren, A. (2005). Effects of a relapse prevention program on sexual recidivism: final results from California's sex offender treatment and evaluation project (SOTEP). *Sexual Abuse*, 17, 79–107.

Miller, P. G., Curtis, A., Sonderlund, A., Day, A., & Droste, N. (2015). Effectiveness of interventions for convicted DUI offenders in reducing recidivism: a systematic review of the peer-reviewed scientific literature. *American Journal of Drug and Alcohol Abuse*, 41, 16–29.

Norman, S. B., Means-Christensen, A. J., Craske, M. G., et al. (2006). Associations between psychological trauma and physical illness in primary care. *Journal of Traumatic Stress*, 19, 461–70.

Norris, F. H. (1992). Epidemiology of trauma: frequency and impact of different potentially traumatic events on different demographic groups. *Journal of Consulting and Clinical Psychology*, 60, 409–18.

Ogle, C. M., Rubin, D. C., & Siegler, I. C. (2014). Cumulative exposure to traumatic events in older adults. *Aging and Mental Health*, 18, 316–25.

Ramsay, J., Carter, Y., Davidson, L., et al. (2009). Advocacy interventions to reduce or eliminate violence and promote the physical and psychosocial well-being of women who experience intimate partner abuse. *The Cochrane Database of Systematic Reviews*, Issue 3, Cd005043.

Roberts, A. L., Gilman, S. E., Breslau, J., Breslau, N., & Koenen, K. C. (2011). Race/ethnic differences in exposure to traumatic events, development of post-traumatic stress disorder, and treatment-seeking for post-traumatic stress disorder in the United States. *Psychological Medicine*, 41, 71–83.

SAS Institute Inc. (2011). *SAS/STAT® Software, Version 9.3 for Windows*. Cary, NC: SAS Institute Inc.

Scott, K. M., Koenen, K. C., Aguilar-Gaxiola, S., et al. (2013). Associations between lifetime traumatic events and subsequent chronic physical conditions: a cross-national, cross-sectional study. *PLoS One*, 8, e80573.

Sledjeski, E. M., Speisman, B., & Dierker, L. C. (2008). Does number of lifetime traumas explain the relationship between PTSD and chronic medical conditions? Answers from the National Comorbidity Survey-Replication (NCS-R). *Journal of Behavioral Medicine*, 31, 341–9.

Spitzer, C., Barnow, S., Volzke, H., et al. (2009). Trauma, posttraumatic stress disorder, and physical illness: findings from the general population. *Psychosomatic Medicine*, 71, 1012–17.

Stoltenborgh, M., van Ijzendoorn, M. H., Euser, E. M., & Bakermans-Kranenburg, M. J. (2011). A global perspective on child sexual abuse: meta-analysis of prevalence around the world. *Child Maltreatment*, 16, 79–101.

Storr, C. L., Schaeffer, C. M., Petras, H., Ialongo, N. S., & Breslau, N. (2009). Early childhood behavior trajectories and the likelihood of experiencing a traumatic event and PTSD by young adulthood. *Social Psychiatry and Psychiatric Epidemiology*, 44, 398–406.

Testa, M., VanZile-Tamsen, C., & Livingston, J. A. (2007). Prospective prediction of women's sexual victimization by intimate and nonintimate male perpetrators. *Journal of Consulting and Clinical Psychology*, 75, 52–60.

Turner, R. J., & Lloyd, D. A. (1995). Lifetime traumas and mental health: the significance of cumulative adversity. *Journal of Health and Social Behavior*, 36, 360–76.

United Nations, Department of Economic and Social Affairs, Population Division (2009). International migration report 2006: a global assessment (online). Available at: www.un.org/esa/population/publications/2006_MigrationRep/exec_sum.pdf (Accessed January 1, 2017).

van Kesteren, J., Mayhew, P., & Nieuwbeerta, P. (2000). *Criminal Victimization in Seventeen Industrialized Countries: Key Findings from the 2000 International Crime Victims Survey*. Den Haag, Netherlands: WODC.

Visser, E., Pijl, Y. J., Stolk, R. P., Neeleman, J., & Rosmalen, J. G. M. (2007). Accident proneness, does it exist? A review and meta-analysis. *Accident Analysis and Prevention*, 39, 556–64.

Willett, J. B., & Singer, J. D. (1993). Investigating onset, cessation, relapse, and recovery: why you should, and how you can, use discrete-time survival analysis to examine event occurrence. *Journal of Consulting and Clinical Psychology*, 61, 952–65.

Wolter, K. M. (1985). *Introduction to Variance Estimation*. New York, NY: Springer-Verlag.

World Health Organization (2009). Global status report on road safety: time for action (online). Available at: www.who.int/violence_injury_prevention/road_safety_status/2009 (Accessed January 1, 2016).

Appendix

Table 3.A1 Prevalence of traumas and each trauma as a percentage of all traumas by country in decreasing order of percentage for any trauma

	Ukraine				Peru				Colombia				United States			
	Prevalence of trauma		Trauma as a percentage of all trauma		Prevalence of trauma		Trauma as a percentage of all trauma		Prevalence of trauma		Trauma as a percentage of all trauma		Prevalence of trauma		Trauma as a percentage of all trauma	
	%	(SE)	%	(SE)	%	(SE)	%	(SE)	%	(SE)	%	(SE)	%	(SE)	%	(SE)
I Exposure to Organized Violence																
Relief worker in war zone	1.8	(0.5)	0.5	(0.1)	0.5	(0.2)	0.1	(0.1)	1.1	(0.2)	0.2	(0.1)	1.4	(0.2)	0.3	(0.1)
Civilian in war zone	11.9	(1.4)	3.2	(0.4)	1.7	(0.4)	0.5	(0.1)	3.4	(0.4)	0.7	(0.1)	2.1	(0.3)	0.4	(0.1)
Civilian in region of terror	1.6	(0.4)	0.4	(0.1)	5.8	(0.6)	1.6	(0.2)	6.4	(0.6)	1.4	(0.1)	2.4	(0.2)	0.5	(0.1)
Refugee	1.8	(0.4)	0.5	(0.1)	0.1	(0.0)	0.0	(0.0)	0.7	(0.2)	0.2	(0.0)	0.8	(0.3)	0.2	(0.1)
Kidnapped	0.9	(0.3)	0.3	(0.1)	1.3	(0.3)	0.3	(0.1)	1.9	(0.5)	0.4	(0.1)	1.4	(0.2)	0.3	(0.0)
Any	15.0	(1.3)	4.8	(0.4)	8.1	(0.6)	2.5	(0.2)	10.5	(0.8)	3.0	(0.3)	6.8	(0.4)	1.7	(0.1)
II Participation in Organized Violence																
Witnessed death/dead body/serious injury	23.8	(1.9)	14.3	(1.2)	22.9	(1.1)	13.1	(1.1)	36.2	(1.6)	19.9	(0.9)	28.2	(0.8)	12.4	(0.5)
Accidentally caused serious injury/death	1.1	(0.4)	0.5	(0.1)	1.0	(0.1)	0.4	(0.1)	1.3	(0.2)	0.4	(0.1)	1.4	(0.1)	0.5	(0.1)
Combat experience	4.5	(0.6)	1.2	(0.2)	1.8	(0.4)	0.5	(0.1)	2.4	(0.6)	0.5	(0.1)	4.9	(0.4)	1.0	(0.1)
Purposely injured/tortured/killed someone	1.3	(0.4)	0.7	(0.2)	0.3	(0.1)	0.1	(0.1)	0.9	(0.3)	0.3	(0.1)	1.9	(0.3)	1.0	(0.1)
Witnessed atrocities	3.9	(0.5)	2.0	(0.5)	1.2	(0.3)	0.5	(0.1)	2.5	(0.5)	0.9	(0.1)	5.5	(0.5)	2.3	(0.2)
Any	28.8	(1.9)	18.6	(1.4)	24.8	(1.3)	14.7	(1.2)	37.3	(1.6)	22.1	(0.8)	31.3	(0.8)	17.2	(0.6)
III Physical Violence Victimization																
Beaten by caregiver	8.7	(1.0)	2.3	(0.2)	20.4	(0.8)	5.5	(0.2)	22.9	(1.5)	5.0	(0.3)	6.6	(0.3)	1.3	(0.1)
Beaten by someone else	14.0	(1.5)	9.2	(1.1)	8.4	(0.9)	3.9	(0.4)	5.6	(0.6)	2.2	(0.4)	7.1	(0.5)	3.0	(0.2)
Witnessed physical fight at home					31.5	(1.1)	8.6	(0.3)	21.0	(1.9)	4.6	(0.3)	14.3	(0.7)	2.9	(0.1)
Any	20.6	(1.8)	11.5	(1.2)	43.0	(1.1)	18.1	(0.6)	37.6	(2.4)	11.8	(0.7)	21.4	(0.9)	7.3	(0.3)
IV Sexual Violence Victimization																
Raped	2.2	(0.4)	0.8	(0.2)	3.0	(0.3)	1.4	(0.2)	4.5	(0.6)	1.7	(0.3)	8.9	(0.6)	3.4	(0.2)
Sexually assaulted	4.4	(0.6)	1.9	(0.3)	6.2	(0.9)	2.7	(0.4)	6.9	(0.5)	2.4	(0.2)	12.2	(0.5)	5.4	(0.3)
Stalked	4.9	(0.6)	1.9	(0.3)	3.7	(0.5)	1.5	(0.2)	6.0	(0.9)	2.1	(0.3)	9.6	(0.5)	3.4	(0.2)
Beaten by spouse/romantic partner	7.9	(0.9)	2.1	(0.2)	7.2	(0.6)	1.9	(0.2)	7.7	(0.6)	1.7	(0.1)	7.8	(0.7)	1.6	(0.1)
Trauma to loved one	4.0	(0.5)	1.3	(0.2)	5.1	(0.6)	1.5	(0.2)	8.9	(0.8)	2.8	(0.2)	9.7	(0.5)	3.1	(0.2)
Some other trauma	9.7	(1.1)	2.6	(0.3)	1.9	(0.5)	0.5	(0.1)	2.4	(0.5)	0.5	(0.1)	7.0	(0.4)	1.4	(0.1)
Private trauma[a]	9.3	(0.9)	2.5	(0.2)	6.2	(0.5)	1.7	(0.1)	4.2	(0.5)	0.9	(0.1)	6.8	(0.4)	1.4	(0.1)
Any	29.9	(1.8)	13.1	(0.8)	25.0	(1.4)	11.3	(0.7)	27.7	(1.7)	12.0	(0.5)	36.9	(1.4)	19.6	(0.4)

(cont.)

Table 3.A1 *(cont.)*

	Ukraine				Peru				Colombia				United States			
	Prevalence of trauma		Trauma as a percentage of all trauma		Prevalence of trauma		Trauma as a percentage of all trauma		Prevalence of trauma		Trauma as a percentage of all trauma		Prevalence of trauma		Trauma as a percentage of all trauma	
	%	(SE)	%	(SE)	%	(SE)	%	(SE)	%	(SE)	%	(SE)	%	(SE)	%	(SE)
V Accidents/Injuries																
Natural disaster	3.0	(0.7)	1.2	(0.4)	16.4	(0.9)	6.9	(0.6)	9.9	(1.2)	3.8	(0.5)	17.4	(1.0)	7.2	(0.4)
Toxic chemical exposure	5.4	(0.7)	2.5	(0.4)	3.3	(0.4)	1.9	(0.3)	4.9	(0.8)	2.0	(0.3)	7.1	(0.4)	4.3	(0.3)
Automobile accident	21.1	(1.3)	7.3	(0.6)	20.1	(1.2)	7.4	(0.4)	19.2	(1.1)	6.6	(0.4)	19.2	(0.9)	6.0	(0.2)
Life-threatening illness	21.7	(1.4)	7.9	(0.5)	12.1	(0.8)	4.2	(0.4)	10.5	(1.1)	3.0	(0.3)	16.0	(0.6)	4.6	(0.2)
Child with serious illness	18.0	(1.3)	6.1	(0.5)	8.3	(0.6)	2.7	(0.2)	9.7	(1.0)	2.5	(0.2)	11.5	(0.7)	3.0	(0.1)
Other life-threatening accident	9.6	(1.1)	3.4	(0.4)	8.4	(0.8)	3.4	(0.4)	7.5	(1.0)	2.3	(0.3)	9.7	(0.5)	3.3	(0.2)
Any	52.5	(1.7)	28.3	(1.3)	47.9	(1.4)	26.5	(0.8)	39.4	(1.7)	20.1	(0.9)	50.6	(1.3)	28.4	(0.6)
VI Other																
Mugged/threatened with a weapon	10.2	(1.5)	3.6	(0.5)	28.8	(1.4)	12.8	(0.7)	38.2	(1.5)	14.2	(0.5)	18.6	(0.6)	6.4	(0.2)
Human-made disaster	8.9	(1.2)	4.5	(0.5)	5.3	(0.5)	2.1	(0.3)	4.9	(0.6)	1.6	(0.2)	6.7	(0.5)	2.2	(0.2)
UD of a loved one	41.0	(2.1)	15.5	(0.9)	31.6	(1.0)	12.0	(0.8)	39.7	(1.2)	15.3	(0.7)	41.9	(1.2)	17.3	(0.5)
Any	49.5	(2.2)	23.6	(1.0)	50.4	(1.4)	26.9	(0.8)	60.4	(1.5)	31.1	(1.0)	52.1	(1.2)	25.8	(0.5)
VII Total	**84.6**	**(1.7)**	**100.0**	**(0.0)**	**83.1**	**(0.8)**	**100.0**	**(0.0)**	**82.7**	**(1.3)**	**100.0**	**(0.0)**	**82.7**	**(0.9)**	**100.0**	**(0.0)**

[a]A *private* event is a trauma that some individuals reported in response to a question asked at the very end of the trauma section that asked if they ever had some other very upsetting experience they did not tell us about already (and this includes in response to a prior open-ended question about "any other" trauma) because they were too embarrassed or upset to talk about it. Respondents were told, before they answered, that if they reported such a trauma we would not ask them anything about what it was, only about their age when the trauma happened.

Table 3.A2 Prevalence of traumas and each trauma as a percentage of all traumas by country in decreasing order of percentage for any trauma

	Lebanon				New Zealand				Australia				Colombia – Medellin			
	Prevalence of trauma		Trauma as a percentage of all trauma		Prevalence of trauma		Trauma as a percentage of all trauma		Prevalence of trauma		Trauma as a percentage of all trauma		Prevalence of trauma		Trauma as a percentage of all trauma	
	%	(SE)	%	(SE)	%	(SE)	%	(SE)	%	(SE)	%	(SE)	%	(SE)	%	(SE)
I Exposure to Organized Violence																
Relief worker in war zone	3.0	(0.9)	0.8	(0.2)	1.0	(0.2)	0.2	(0.0)	0.9	(0.1)	0.2	(0.0)	0.5	(0.3)	0.1	(0.1)
Civilian in war zone	55.2	(2.9)	14.3	(0.8)	5.1	(0.4)	1.2	(0.1)	4.2	(0.3)	1.1	(0.1)	4.6	(0.9)	1.1	(0.2)
Civilian in region of terror	8.6	(1.5)	2.2	(0.4)	3.9	(0.4)	0.9	(0.1)	3.2	(0.3)	0.8	(0.1)	7.7	(1.1)	1.9	(0.3)
Refugee	37.7	(3.6)	9.8	(0.6)	0.7	(0.2)	0.2	(0.1)	1.6	(0.2)	0.4	(0.1)	0.9	(0.2)	0.2	(0.1)
Kidnapped	3.1	(0.7)	0.8	(0.2)	1.1	(0.1)	0.3	(0.0)	1.0	(0.2)	0.3	(0.1)	2.5	(0.6)	0.6	(0.1)
Any	65.0	(3.2)	27.9	(1.1)	9.2	(0.5)	2.8	(0.2)	8.2	(0.4)	2.9	(0.2)	12.6	(1.4)	4.0	(0.4)
II Participation in Organized Violence																
Witnessed death/dead body/ serious injury	29.5	(2.3)	17.3	(1.0)	25.5	(0.7)	13.2	(0.6)	27.3	(0.8)	17.4	(0.5)	31.0	(2.1)	15.8	(0.9)
Accidentally caused serious injury/ death	0.9	(0.4)	0.3	(0.2)	1.8	(0.2)	0.7	(0.1)	1.4	(0.2)	0.7	(0.1)	2.7	(0.8)	0.7	(0.2)
Combat experience	9.5	(1.0)	2.5	(0.3)	2.4	(0.3)	0.6	(0.1)	2.0	(0.2)	0.5	(0.1)	3.6	(0.9)	0.9	(0.2)
Purposely injured/tortured/killed someone	0.9	(0.4)	0.5	(0.2)	–	–	–	–	1.1	(0.2)	0.9	(0.1)	1.5	(0.6)	0.4	(0.2)
Witnessed atrocities	11.2	(1.4)	5.4	(0.7)	4.7	(0.4)	2.5	(0.2)	3.7	(0.2)	2.4	(0.2)	2.6	(0.6)	1.0	(0.2)
Any	34.9	(2.6)	26.0	(1.4)	28.2	(0.8)	17.0	(0.7)	29.0	(0.8)	21.8	(0.7)	33.3	(2.2)	18.8	(1.1)
III Physical Violence Victimization																
Beaten by caregiver	4.1	(0.9)	1.1	(0.2)	6.4	(0.3)	1.5	(0.1)	5.1	(0.4)	1.3	(0.1)	20.7	(1.9)	5.1	(0.4)
Beaten by someone else	4.1	(0.7)	1.8	(0.3)	7.8	(0.5)	3.8	(0.3)	6.5	(0.4)	3.7	(0.3)	4.6	(0.7)	1.7	(0.3)
Witnessed physical fight at home	–	–	–	–	10.9	(0.4)	2.6	(0.1)	10.4	(0.5)	2.7	(0.1)	18.2	(1.7)	4.5	(0.4)
Any	7.4	(1.2)	2.8	(0.4)	19.0	(0.7)	7.9	(0.3)	16.8	(0.6)	7.8	(0.3)	32.9	(2.2)	11.3	(0.7)
IV Sexual Violence Victimization																
Raped	0.3	(0.1)	0.1	(0.1)	6.5	(0.4)	2.7	(0.2)	5.4	(0.4)	2.8	(0.2)	4.1	(0.5)	1.9	(0.3)
Sexually assaulted	1.9	(0.4)	0.8	(0.2)	11.6	(0.5)	5.8	(0.3)	10.0	(0.5)	5.8	(0.3)	7.2	(0.8)	3.0	(0.4)
Stalked	4.5	(1.0)	2.8	(0.6)	7.5	(0.5)	3.2	(0.2)	7.0	(0.4)	3.5	(0.2)	5.3	(1.0)	1.9	(0.3)
Beaten by spouse/romantic partner	1.6	(0.3)	0.4	(0.1)	5.5	(0.3)	1.3	(0.1)	4.9	(0.3)	1.3	(0.1)	7.8	(0.9)	1.9	(0.2)
Trauma to loved one	13.2	(1.1)	5.4	(0.6)	10.4	(0.5)	4.1	(0.3)	7.9	(0.4)	3.3	(0.2)	8.5	(1.2)	3.8	(1.2)
Some other trauma	2.0	(0.6)	0.5	(0.1)	7.6	(0.5)	1.8	(0.1)	5.0	(0.3)	1.3	(0.1)	2.4	(0.6)	0.6	(0.1)
Private trauma[a]	5.8	(1.2)	1.5	(0.3)	5.1	(0.3)	1.2	(0.1)	4.7	(0.3)	1.2	(0.1)	4.1	(0.9)	1.0	(0.2)
Any	21.9	(1.8)	11.5	(0.8)	33.3	(0.9)	20.2	(0.7)	28.5	(0.8)	19.1	(0.6)	26.9	(1.9)	14.1	(1.2)

(cont.)

Table 3.A2 *(cont.)*

	Lebanon				New Zealand				Australia				Colombia – Medellin			
	Prevalence of trauma		Trauma as a percentage of all trauma		Prevalence of trauma		Trauma as a percentage of all trauma		Prevalence of trauma		Trauma as a percentage of all trauma		Prevalence of trauma		Trauma as a percentage of all trauma	
	%	(SE)	%	(SE)	%	(SE)	%	(SE)	%	(SE)	%	(SE)	%	(SE)	%	(SE)
V Accidents/Injuries																
Natural disaster	5.9	(1.3)	2.0	(0.4)	9.6	(0.6)	4.9	(0.5)	8.8	(0.4)	4.7	(0.3)	5.1	(0.8)	1.7	(0.3)
Toxic chemical exposure	0.7	(0.3)	0.3	(0.1)	7.9	(0.5)	6.3	(0.5)	5.3	(0.3)	3.9	(0.2)	3.5	(0.7)	1.8	(0.5)
Automobile accident	12.8	(1.4)	4.4	(0.5)	16.3	(0.6)	6.3	(0.3)	13.2	(0.6)	4.8	(0.2)	18.4	(1.7)	6.5	(0.6)
Life-threatening illness	5.2	(0.9)	1.7	(0.3)	14.3	(0.6)	5.0	(0.2)	12.1	(0.4)	4.4	(0.2)	8.5	(1.3)	3.1	(0.6)
Child with serious illness	4.4	(0.9)	1.3	(0.2)	9.2	(0.4)	3.1	(0.2)	8.4	(0.4)	2.7	(0.1)	5.1	(0.6)	1.5	(0.2)
Other life-threatening accident	7.3	(1.6)	2.9	(0.7)	8.2	(0.5)	3.4	(0.2)	6.1	(0.4)	2.5	(0.2)	6.4	(1.1)	2.0	(0.4)
Any	28.7	(2.6)	12.6	(1.0)	43.3	(0.9)	28.9	(0.8)	37.7	(0.8)	23.2	(0.6)	33.4	(2.4)	16.7	(1.0)
VI Other																
Mugged/threatened with a weapon	5.1	(0.9)	2.0	(0.4)	13.0	(0.6)	5.0	(0.3)	12.3	(0.5)	5.5	(0.2)	37.4	(2.1)	17.5	(0.9)
Human-made disaster	5.5	(0.9)	1.7	(0.2)	4.2	(0.3)	1.7	(0.2)	5.0	(0.4)	2.8	(0.3)	2.7	(0.5)	1.1	(0.3)
UD of a loved one	36.6	(2.5)	15.4	(0.9)	36.9	(0.9)	16.3	(0.5)	35.0	(0.8)	17.0	(0.4)	33.0	(2.3)	16.5	(1.0)
Any	41.0	(2.6)	19.1	(1.1)	44.4	(1.0)	23.1	(0.6)	42.9	(0.8)	25.2	(0.5)	53.2	(2.5)	35.1	(1.1)
VII Total	**81.1**	**(2.7)**	**100.0**	**(0.0)**	**79.3**	**(0.8)**	**100.0**	**(0.0)**	**76.2**	**(0.7)**	**100.0**	**(0.0)**	**75.1**	**(2.6)**	**100.0**	**(0.0)**

[a]A *private* event is a trauma that some individuals reported in response to a question asked at the very end of the trauma section that asked if they ever had some other very upsetting experience they did not tell us about already (and this includes in response to a prior open-ended question about "any other" trauma) because they were too embarrassed or upset to talk about it. Respondents were told, before they answered, that if they reported such a trauma we would not ask them anything about what it was, only about their age when the trauma happened.

Table 3.A3 Prevalence of traumas and each trauma as a percentage of all trauma by country in decreasing order of percentage for any trauma

	Israel				South Africa				Brazil– São Paulo				France			
	Prevalence of trauma		Trauma as a percentage of all trauma		Prevalence of trauma		Trauma as a percentage of all trauma		Prevalence of trauma		Trauma as a percentage of all trauma		Prevalence of trauma		Trauma as a percentage of all trauma	
	%	(SE)	%	(SE)	%	(SE)	%	(SE)	%	(SE)	%	(SE)	%	(SE)	%	(SE)
I Exposure to Organized Violence																
Relief worker in war zone	–	–	–	–	2.1	(0.3)	0.7	(0.1)	–	–	–	–	1.5	(0.5)	0.5	(0.2)
Civilian in war zone	–	–	–	–	3.6	(0.7)	1.1	(0.2)	–	–	–	–	9.7	(1.4)	3.4	(0.4)
Civilian in region of terror	–	–	–	–	7.1	(0.7)	2.2	(0.2)	–	–	–	–	4.1	(1.0)	1.4	(0.4)
Refugee	6.1	(0.4)	1.9	(0.1)	1.6	(0.3)	0.5	(0.1)	–	–	–	–	2.6	(0.5)	0.9	(0.2)
Kidnapped	0.5	(0.1)	0.1	(0.0)	1.2	(0.2)	0.4	(0.1)	1.9	(0.4)	1.2	(0.3)	0.6	(0.3)	0.2	(0.1)
Any	6.4	(0.4)	2.0	(0.1)	11.5	(0.9)	4.9	(0.5)	1.9	(0.4)	1.2	(0.3)	14.8	(1.9)	6.5	(0.6)
II Participation in Organized Violence																
Witnessed death/dead body/ serious injury	26.8	(0.5)	19.1	(0.4)	28.5	(1.3)	18.2	(0.9)	35.7	(1.0)	26.5	(1.2)	24.0	(1.5)	19.1	(1.2)
Accidentally caused serious injury/death	1.3	(0.2)	0.5	(0.1)	1.9	(0.3)	1.0	(0.2)	2.5	(0.4)	1.4	(0.5)	2.7	(0.6)	2.1	(0.8)
Combat experience	10.8	(0.5)	3.3	(0.1)	2.6	(0.4)	0.8	(0.1)					6.1	(0.8)	2.1	(0.3)
Purposely injured/tortured/killed someone	3.2	(0.2)	2.7	(0.2)	0.9	(0.2)	0.5	(0.1)	1.0	(0.3)	0.6	(0.2)	0.5	(0.2)	0.4	(0.3)
Witnessed atrocities	9.6	(0.5)	6.2	(0.3)	3.9	(0.5)	2.5	(0.4)	3.5	(0.4)	2.1	(0.4)	4.9	(1.1)	3.5	(0.7)
Any	34.2	(0.6)	31.9	(0.7)	31.8	(1.4)	22.9	(1.0)	36.8	(1.1)	30.6	(1.3)	29.3	(1.8)	27.2	(1.6)
III Physical Violence Victimization																
Beaten by caregiver	3.4	(0.3)	1.0	(0.1)	12.0	(0.8)	3.8	(0.3)	15.4	(1.1)	4.6	(0.3)	2.8	(0.5)	1.0	(0.2)
Beaten by someone else	3.5	(0.3)	2.6	(0.2)	12.4	(0.6)	5.9	(0.3)	3.9	(0.5)	2.2	(0.3)	1.9	(0.4)	1.4	(0.3)
Witnessed physical fight at home	–	–	–	–	–	–	–	–	12.6	(0.7)	3.8	(0.2)	–	–	–	–
Any	6.3	(0.4)	3.6	(0.2)	21.0	(0.9)	9.7	(0.5)	25.2	(1.0)	10.6	(0.4)	4.6	(0.6)	2.4	(0.4)
IV Sexual Violence Victimization																
Raped	0.8	(0.1)	0.3	(0.1)	2.1	(0.3)	0.9	(0.1)	1.0	(0.2)	0.4	(0.1)	1.3	(0.3)	0.7	(0.2)
Sexually assaulted	6.1	(0.4)	3.6	(0.2)	1.6	(0.2)	0.9	(0.2)	1.7	(0.2)	1.0	(0.2)	4.5	(0.8)	3.1	(0.9)
Stalked	6.6	(0.4)	3.7	(0.3)	4.5	(0.4)	2.6	(0.2)	5.5	(0.5)	2.9	(0.3)	7.4	(0.8)	4.1	(0.7)
Beaten by spouse/romantic partner	1.6	(0.2)	0.5	(0.1)	7.9	(0.5)	2.5	(0.1)	3.7	(0.4)	1.1	(0.1)	2.5	(0.6)	0.9	(0.2)
Trauma to loved one	3.8	(0.3)	1.8	(0.2)	5.8	(0.4)	2.5	(0.3)	5.2	(0.5)	2.2	(0.3)	3.7	(0.5)	1.6	(0.2)
Some other trauma	5.2	(0.3)	1.6	(0.1)	3.0	(0.4)	0.9	(0.1)	2.1	(0.3)	0.6	(0.1)	5.8	(1.1)	2.0	(0.4)
Private trauma[a]	8.7	(0.4)	2.7	(0.1)	3.9	(0.4)	1.2	(0.1)	2.5	(0.3)	0.8	(0.1)	5.2	(0.8)	1.8	(0.3)
Any	23.8	(0.6)	14.1	(0.5)	22.5	(0.7)	11.5	(0.4)	16.7	(0.8)	9.1	(0.5)	22.0	(1.4)	14.3	(1.7)

(*cont.*)

Table 3.A3 *(cont.)*

	Israel				South Africa				Brazil– São Paulo				France			
	Prevalence of trauma		Trauma as a percentage of all trauma		Prevalence of trauma		Trauma as a percentage of all trauma		Prevalence of trauma		Trauma as a percentage of all trauma		Prevalence of trauma		Trauma as a percentage of all trauma	
	%	(SE)	%	(SE)	%	(SE)	%	(SE)	%	(SE)	%	(SE)	%	(SE)	%	(SE)
V Accidents/Injuries																
Natural disaster	1.6	(0.2)	1.0	(0.1)	4.1	(0.5)	1.7	(0.2)	–	–	–	–	7.8	(1.3)	6.2	(2.8)
Toxic chemical exposure	5.6	(0.3)	4.6	(0.3)	3.2	(0.4)	2.2	(0.3)	3.4	(0.5)	2.5	(0.4)	4.1	(0.9)	3.3	(0.8)
Automobile accident	11.6	(0.4)	4.7	(0.2)	13.2	(0.6)	5.1	(0.3)	15.4	(0.8)	6.2	(0.3)	15.4	(1.2)	7.2	(0.7)
Life-threatening illness	10.6	(0.4)	4.7	(0.2)	13.2	(0.8)	6.8	(0.4)	6.4	(0.6)	2.4	(0.2)	9.2	(1.0)	4.4	(0.5)
Child with serious illness	9.4	(0.5)	4.0	(0.2)	8.1	(0.5)	3.5	(0.3)	6.7	(0.9)	2.4	(0.3)	6.4	(0.7)	2.4	(0.2)
Other life-threatening accident	7.5	(0.4)	3.6	(0.2)	5.6	(0.4)	2.6	(0.3)	5.0	(0.5)	2.1	(0.3)	4.3	(0.9)	2.6	(0.9)
Any	34.4	(0.7)	22.5	(0.6)	35.0	(1.1)	21.8	(0.5)	28.9	(1.3)	15.5	(0.7)	36.0	(2.0)	26.1	(2.3)
VI Other																
Mugged/threatened with a weapon	9.3	(0.4)	4.7	(0.3)	18.3	(0.8)	8.4	(0.4)	34.0	(1.5)	18.2	(1.1)	11.7	(1.0)	6.5	(0.6)
Human-made disaster	2.7	(0.2)	1.3	(0.1)	2.8	(0.3)	1.2	(0.1)	1.4	(0.2)	0.6	(0.1)	4.6	(0.8)	2.4	(0.5)
UD of a loved one	38.3	(0.8)	19.9	(0.5)	39.2	(1.2)	19.6	(0.6)	31.0	(1.1)	14.2	(0.6)	28.2	(1.9)	14.7	(1.3)
Any	44.6	(0.7)	25.9	(0.5)	48.7	(1.2)	29.2	(0.7)	52.3	(1.8)	33.0	(1.4)	38.3	(1.8)	23.5	(1.2)
VII Total	**74.8**	**(0.6)**	**100.0**	**(0.0)**	**73.8**	**(1.2)**	**100.0**	**(0.0)**	**73.8**	**(1.5)**	**100.0**	**(0.0)**	**72.7**	**(2.3)**	**100.0**	**(0.0)**

[a]A *private* event is a trauma that some individuals reported in response to a question asked at the very end of the trauma section that asked if they ever had some other very upsetting experience they did not tell us about already (and this includes in response to a prior open-ended question about "any other" trauma) because they were too embarrassed or upset to talk about it. Respondents were told, before they answered, that if they reported such a trauma we would not ask them anything about what it was, only about their age when the trauma happened.

Table 3.A4 Prevalence of trauma and each trauma as a percentage of all traumas by country in decreasing order of percentage for any trauma

	Portugal				Mexico				Germany				Nigeria			
	Prevalence of trauma		Trauma as a percentage of all trauma		Prevalence of trauma		Trauma as a percentage of all trauma		Prevalence of trauma		Trauma as a percentage of all trauma		Prevalence of trauma		Trauma as a percentage of all trauma	
	%	(SE)	%	(SE)	%	(SE)	%	(SE)	%	(SE)	%	(SE)	%	(SE)	%	(SE)
I Exposure to Organized Violence																
Relief worker in war zone	1.7	(0.5)	0.7	(0.2)	0.2	(0.1)	0.1	(0.0)	1.1	(0.3)	0.4	(0.1)	2.3	(0.8)	0.7	(0.2)
Civilian in war zone	4.3	(0.5)	1.6	(0.2)	0.1	(0.1)	0.0	(0.0)	9.9	(1.1)	3.6	(0.4)	3.7	(0.6)	1.1	(0.2)
Civilian in region of terror	2.0	(0.4)	0.8	(0.1)	0.8	(0.2)	0.3	(0.1)	2.3	(0.7)	0.9	(0.2)	5.3	(0.6)	1.6	(0.2)
Refugee	1.9	(0.4)	0.7	(0.2)	0.0	(0.0)	0.0	(0.0)	5.6	(0.9)	2.0	(0.3)	6.1	(0.7)	1.9	(0.2)
Kidnapped	0.2	(0.1)	0.1	(0.0)	2.2	(0.3)	0.8	(0.1)	0.3	(0.1)	0.1	(0.1)	1.0	(0.3)	0.3	(0.1)
Any	7.5	(0.8)	3.9	(0.4)	3.0	(0.4)	1.1	(0.1)	14.7	(1.3)	7.1	(0.6)	13.9	(1.2)	5.7	(0.5)
II Participation in Organized Violence																
Witnessed death/dead body/ serious injury	20.5	(1.3)	14.7	(0.9)	16.3	(1.1)	12.1	(0.9)	22.4	(1.4)	17.8	(1.1)	27.3	(1.3)	24.3	(1.3)
Accidentally caused serious injury/death	1.6	(0.3)	0.7	(0.2)	1.3	(0.2)	1.1	(0.3)	1.4	(0.4)	0.9	(0.4)	1.4	(0.4)	0.6	(0.2)
Combat experience	4.6	(0.8)	1.8	(0.3)	0.0	(0.0)	0.0	(0.0)	5.1	(0.7)	1.9	(0.3)	1.8	(0.3)	0.5	(0.1)
Purposely injured/tortured/killed someone	0.3	(0.1)	0.5	(0.2)	0.4	(0.1)	0.2	(0.1)	0.6	(0.2)	0.6	(0.2)	0.5	(0.3)	0.3	(0.1)
Witnessed atrocities	2.2	(0.3)	1.8	(0.4)	0.5	(0.2)	0.2	(0.1)	2.9	(0.5)	2.2	(0.5)	7.5	(0.6)	4.9	(0.4)
Any	23.9	(1.3)	19.4	(0.9)	17.2	(1.1)	13.6	(1.0)	25.1	(1.3)	23.3	(1.2)	30.5	(1.4)	30.6	(1.5)
III Physical Violence Victimization																
Beaten by caregiver	9.3	(1.0)	3.6	(0.4)	18.3	(1.0)	6.4	(0.3)	5.5	(0.9)	2.0	(0.3)	10.2	(0.8)	3.1	(0.2)
Beaten by someone else	3.6	(0.4)	3.3	(0.5)	7.4	(0.8)	4.0	(0.4)	4.8	(0.8)	3.9	(0.7)	5.4	(0.7)	3.2	(0.6)
Witnessed physical fight at home	13.0	(0.8)	5.0	(0.3)	20.3	(1.2)	7.1	(0.3)	–	–	–	–	–	–	–	–
Any	20.0	(1.3)	11.9	(0.7)	33.4	(1.4)	17.5	(0.7)	9.3	(1.0)	5.9	(0.7)	13.8	(1.0)	6.3	(0.7)
IV Sexual Violence Victimization																
Raped	1.1	(0.2)	0.8	(0.3)	3.9	(0.5)	2.4	(0.5)	2.6	(0.5)	1.8	(0.6)	0.6	(0.3)	0.3	(0.2)
Sexually assaulted	3.4	(0.5)	3.0	(0.5)	5.4	(0.7)	3.1	(0.4)	5.9	(0.8)	4.3	(0.8)	1.3	(0.3)	0.6	(0.1)
Stalked	5.8	(0.6)	4.6	(0.6)	3.7	(0.6)	2.0	(0.3)	6.5	(0.8)	3.3	(0.4)	2.0	(0.3)	1.1	(0.2)
Beaten by spouse/romantic partner	2.7	(0.4)	1.0	(0.2)	6.0	(0.5)	2.1	(0.2)	2.8	(0.8)	1.0	(0.3)	4.2	(0.6)	1.3	(0.2)
Trauma to loved one	2.3	(0.4)	1.3	(0.2)	3.5	(0.4)	1.4	(0.2)	4.0	(0.7)	1.9	(0.3)	4.4	(0.6)	1.8	(0.4)
Some other trauma	2.7	(0.4)	1.0	(0.2)	1.4	(0.3)	0.5	(0.1)	3.3	(0.6)	1.2	(0.2)	2.3	(0.4)	0.7	(0.1)
Private trauma[a]	3.0	(0.5)	1.2	(0.2)	3.8	(0.4)	1.3	(0.1)	3.5	(0.6)	1.3	(0.2)	4.2	(0.5)	1.2	(0.2)
Any	15.8	(1.2)	12.9	(1.0)	19.3	(1.1)	12.8	(0.9)	20.7	(1.5)	14.7	(1.4)	15.7	(1.2)	6.9	(0.6)

(cont.)

Table 3.A4 *(cont.)*

	Portugal				Mexico				Germany				Nigeria			
	Prevalence of trauma		Trauma as a percentage of all trauma		Prevalence of trauma		Trauma as a percentage of all trauma		Prevalence of trauma		Trauma as a percentage of all trauma		Prevalence of trauma		Trauma as a percentage of all trauma	
	%	(SE)	%	(SE)	%	(SE)	%	(SE)	%	(SE)	%	(SE)	%	(SE)	%	(SE)
V Accidents/Injuries																
Natural disaster	4.2	(0.6)	1.9	(0.2)	12.2	(1.3)	6.7	(1.0)	5.5	(0.7)	3.5	(1.2)	2.4	(0.4)	1.5	(0.4)
Toxic chemical exposure	1.5	(0.3)	1.2	(0.2)	4.1	(0.6)	3.4	(0.7)	3.4	(0.6)	4.0	(0.9)	3.1	(1.2)	2.8	(1.5)
Automobile accident	21.3	(1.3)	11.8	(0.8)	15.3	(1.2)	6.8	(0.5)	9.1	(1.1)	3.8	(0.6)	12.3	(0.9)	5.2	(0.5)
Life-threatening illness	14.2	(1.1)	6.9	(0.6)	10.0	(0.9)	4.5	(0.5)	14.1	(1.3)	6.7	(0.5)	24.3	(1.3)	10.8	(0.6)
Child with serious illness	7.3	(0.8)	3.7	(0.5)	7.2	(0.8)	3.0	(0.4)	6.7	(1.0)	2.8	(0.5)	10.5	(0.7)	4.6	(0.4)
Other life-threatening accident	6.8	(0.8)	3.4	(0.4)	5.1	(0.5)	2.5	(0.3)	4.5	(0.6)	2.5	(0.4)	5.2	(0.5)	2.1	(0.3)
Any	41.2	(1.5)	29.0	(1.1)	37.4	(1.5)	26.8	(1.3)	32.2	(1.8)	23.4	(1.9)	39.6	(1.5)	27.1	(1.2)
VI Other																
Mugged/threatened with a weapon	9.9	(0.8)	5.7	(0.5)	24.6	(1.2)	15.0	(0.8)	6.5	(0.8)	4.1	(0.8)	8.1	(0.8)	3.6	(0.3)
Human-made disaster	6.0	(0.9)	4.1	(0.6)	2.3	(0.4)	0.9	(0.1)	6.7	(1.1)	5.4	(0.8)	1.1	(0.3)	0.6	(0.2)
UD of a loved one	23.3	(1.2)	13.2	(0.7)	22.7	(1.4)	12.1	(1.0)	27.2	(2.0)	15.9	(1.3)	38.6	(1.2)	19.2	(0.8)
Any	33.5	(1.5)	23.0	(1.1)	40.1	(1.7)	28.0	(1.4)	34.1	(2.2)	25.5	(1.4)	42.1	(1.3)	23.4	(0.8)
VII Total	**69.0**	**(1.7)**	**100.0**	**(0.0)**	**68.8**	**(1.8)**	**100.0**	**(0.0)**	**67.3**	**(2.2)**	**100.0**	**(0.0)**	**67.1**	**(1.3)**	**100.0**	**(0.0)**

[a]A *private* event is a trauma that some individuals reported in response to a question asked at the very end of the trauma section that asked if they ever had some other very upsetting experience they did not tell us about already (and this includes in response to a prior open-ended question about "any other" trauma) because they were too embarrassed or upset to talk about it. Respondents were told, before they answered, that if they reported such a trauma we would not ask them anything about what it was, only about their age when the trauma happened.

Table 3.A5 Prevalence of traumas and each trauma as a percentage of all traumas by country in decreasing order of percentage for any trauma

	Belgium				Netherlands				Spain – Murcia				Japan			
	Prevalence of trauma		Trauma as a percentage of all trauma		Prevalence of trauma		Trauma as a percentage of all trauma		Prevalence of trauma		Trauma as a percentage of all trauma		Prevalence of trauma		Trauma as a percentage of all trauma	
	%	(SE)	%	(SE)	%	(SE)	%	(SE)	%	(SE)	%	(SE)	%	(SE)	%	(SE)
I Exposure to Organized Violence																
Relief worker in war zone	1.4	(0.4)	0.6	(0.2)	0.6	(0.4)	0.3	(0.2)	1.2	(0.4)	0.8	(0.3)	0.1	(0.1)	0.0	(0.0)
Civilian in war zone	11.8	(2.0)	5.1	(0.8)	8.3	(1.3)	3.5	(0.5)	1.2	(0.5)	0.8	(0.3)	5.2	(0.6)	2.5	(0.3)
Civilian in region of terror	2.6	(0.6)	1.1	(0.2)	3.0	(0.7)	1.3	(0.3)	0.5	(0.3)	0.3	(0.2)	0.2	(0.1)	0.1	(0.1)
Refugee	4.1	(1.2)	1.8	(0.5)	3.0	(0.9)	1.3	(0.4)	0.1	(0.1)	0.0	(0.0)	0.5	(0.1)	0.2	(0.1)
Kidnapped	1.1	(0.5)	0.5	(0.2)	1.3	(0.4)	0.6	(0.1)	0.4	(0.3)	0.2	(0.2)	0.7	(0.2)	0.3	(0.1)
Any	15.3	(2.0)	9.1	(1.1)	12.6	(1.8)	6.9	(1.0)	3.0	(1.0)	2.1	(0.7)	5.9	(0.7)	3.2	(0.4)
II Participation in Organized Violence																
Witnessed death/dead body/ serious injury	18.0	(1.8)	15.5	(1.5)	19.1	(1.5)	14.8	(1.7)	5.4	(1.3)	3.9	(0.6)	18.0	(1.1)	16.8	(1.2)
Accidentally caused serious injury/death	1.4	(0.4)	0.7	(0.2)	2.2	(0.8)	1.0	(0.3)	0.5	(0.3)	0.6	(0.3)	1.4	(0.3)	1.0	(0.3)
Combat experience	2.5	(0.6)	1.1	(0.3)	1.7	(0.6)	0.7	(0.2)	0.4	(0.2)	0.3	(0.2)	2.0	(0.6)	1.0	(0.3)
Purposely injured/tortured/killed someone	0.6	(0.2)	0.6	(0.2)	0.2	(0.1)	0.1	(0.1)					0.4	(0.2)	0.6	(0.4)
Witnessed atrocities	2.8	(0.6)	2.5	(0.6)	1.7	(0.8)	0.9	(0.4)	0.1	(0.1)	0.1	(0.0)	1.2	(0.3)	0.9	(0.3)
Any	20.6	(2.0)	20.5	(1.6)	21.7	(1.6)	17.6	(2.0)	6.0	(1.4)	4.7	(0.8)	20.4	(1.2)	20.3	(1.5)
III Physical Violence Victimization																
Beaten by caregiver	2.0	(0.5)	0.9	(0.2)	3.2	(0.6)	1.3	(0.3)	5.3	(0.7)	3.4	(0.4)	6.9	(0.8)	3.3	(0.3)
Beaten by someone else	4.5	(0.7)	3.9	(0.9)	4.1	(0.7)	2.8	(0.5)	2.9	(0.4)	2.4	(0.3)	7.3	(0.7)	9.3	(0.7)
Witnessed physical fight at home	–	–	–	–	–	–	–	–	6.0	(0.9)	3.9	(0.8)	10.6	(1.0)	5.1	(0.5)
Any	6.2	(0.9)	4.8	(1.0)	6.1	(0.9)	4.1	(0.6)	12.2	(0.8)	9.7	(1.0)	19.7	(1.1)	17.7	(0.9)
IV Sexual Violence Victimization																
Raped	1.7	(0.8)	1.5	(0.6)	3.4	(0.5)	3.2	(0.6)	1.0	(0.4)	1.7	(0.7)	0.6	(0.2)	0.5	(0.1)
Sexually assaulted	2.9	(0.8)	2.6	(0.7)	3.2	(0.6)	2.6	(0.6)	2.0	(0.4)	2.7	(0.7)	1.7	(0.4)	2.0	(0.5)
Stalked	5.1	(0.8)	3.6	(0.7)	3.6	(0.6)	3.4	(0.7)	5.2	(0.9)	6.0	(1.4)	2.7	(0.5)	2.9	(0.6)
Beaten by spouse/romantic partner	2.7	(0.7)	1.2	(0.3)	2.5	(0.7)	1.1	(0.3)	2.4	(0.5)	1.5	(0.3)	4.4	(0.5)	2.1	(0.2)
Trauma to loved one	3.0	(0.5)	1.9	(0.4)	6.2	(1.3)	5.0	(1.1)	1.7	(0.7)	1.4	(0.4)	1.1	(0.3)	1.1	(0.5)
Some other trauma	4.5	(0.8)	1.9	(0.3)	5.4	(0.8)	2.3	(0.3)	0.9	(0.4)	0.6	(0.2)	4.7	(0.8)	2.3	(0.4)
Private trauma[a]	6.2	(1.9)	2.7	(0.9)	3.9	(0.6)	1.6	(0.3)	1.5	(0.3)	0.9	(0.2)	10.3	(1.1)	5.0	(0.6)
Any	20.5	(2.3)	15.4	(1.7)	20.3	(1.9)	19.2	(2.2)	11.9	(1.6)	14.8	(2.3)	19.9	(1.3)	15.9	(1.3)

(cont.)

Table 3.A5 *(cont.)*

	Belgium				Netherlands				Spain – Murcia				Japan			
	Prevalence of trauma		Trauma as a percentage of all trauma		Prevalence of trauma		Trauma as a percentage of all trauma		Prevalence of trauma		Trauma as a percentage of all trauma		Prevalence of trauma		Trauma as a percentage of all trauma	
	%	(SE)	%	(SE)	%	(SE)	%	(SE)	%	(SE)	%	(SE)	%	(SE)	%	(SE)
V Accidents/Injuries																
Natural disaster	4.4	(1.3)	2.2	(0.5)	3.9	(1.1)	2.0	(0.5)	12.1	(2.3)	9.0	(1.7)	5.4	(0.7)	3.6	(0.6)
Toxic chemical exposure	3.5	(0.7)	4.4	(1.0)	2.3	(0.5)	2.8	(0.9)	1.3	(0.7)	2.3	(1.2)	0.8	(0.3)	0.7	(0.2)
Automobile accident	11.2	(1.8)	6.0	(0.9)	7.1	(1.1)	3.5	(0.5)	11.9	(0.7)	9.6	(1.2)	6.5	(0.8)	4.3	(0.5)
Life-threatening illness	9.4	(1.4)	5.6	(0.9)	10.8	(1.0)	6.5	(0.9)	7.7	(0.9)	6.4	(1.0)	10.3	(1.1)	6.6	(0.8)
Child with serious illness	9.3	(0.9)	4.7	(0.5)	6.0	(1.4)	3.1	(0.6)	5.2	(0.7)	3.6	(0.4)	6.1	(0.9)	3.4	(0.6)
Other life-threatening accident	3.3	(1.1)	1.6	(0.5)	3.9	(1.0)	1.8	(0.4)	2.9	(0.7)	2.3	(0.6)	4.1	(0.7)	3.0	(0.5)
Any	32.2	(2.6)	24.5	(1.7)	28.2	(1.9)	19.8	(1.2)	32.9	(2.3)	33.1	(2.2)	25.2	(1.7)	21.7	(1.3)
VI Other																
Mugged/threatened with a weapon	10.4	(1.5)	6.9	(1.3)	15.1	(2.1)	9.8	(1.2)	9.6	(1.2)	7.8	(1.1)	2.1	(0.4)	2.0	(0.5)
Human-made disaster	3.8	(1.0)	3.1	(0.8)	4.9	(1.0)	5.1	(1.7)	3.2	(0.5)	3.8	(1.1)	1.7	(0.4)	1.0	(0.3)
UD of a loved one	24.4	(2.2)	15.7	(1.7)	25.4	(2.1)	17.5	(1.5)	29.6	(2.3)	24.0	(1.3)	23.7	(1.4)	18.3	(1.3)
Any	34.5	(2.6)	25.7	(1.9)	38.6	(2.8)	32.4	(2.2)	36.7	(2.2)	35.6	(1.9)	25.8	(1.5)	21.3	(1.3)
VII Total	**65.8**	**(3.1)**	**100.0**	**(0.0)**	**65.6**	**(2.8)**	**100.0**	**(0.0)**	**62.4**	**(1.9)**	**100.0**	**(0.0)**	**60.7**	**(1.7)**	**100.0**	**(0.0)**

[a]A *private* event is a trauma that some individuals reported in response to a question asked at the very end of the trauma section that asked if they ever had some other very upsetting experience they did not tell us about already (and this includes in response to a prior open-ended question about "any other" trauma) because they were too embarrassed or upset to talk about it. Respondents were told, before they answered, that if they reported such a trauma we would not ask them anything about what it was, only about their age when the trauma happened.

Table 3.A6 Prevalence of traumas and each trauma as a percentage of all traumas by country in decreasing order of percentage for any trauma

	Northern Ireland				Italy				Spain				PRC – Beijing/Shanghai			
	Prevalence of trauma		Trauma as a percentage of all trauma		Prevalence of trauma		Trauma as a percentage of all trauma		Prevalence of trauma		Trauma as a percentage of all trauma		Prevalence of trauma		Trauma as a percentage of all trauma	
	%	(SE)	%	(SE)	%	(SE)	%	(SE)	%	(SE)	%	(SE)	%	(SE)	%	(SE)
I Exposure to Organized Violence																
Relief worker in war zone	1.8	(0.4)	0.7	(0.2)	0.8	(0.3)	0.3	(0.1)	1.0	(0.3)	0.6	(0.2)	0.2	(0.1)	0.1	(0.1)
Civilian in war zone	3.5	(0.6)	1.4	(0.2)	4.6	(0.7)	2.1	(0.3)	4.6	(0.5)	3.1	(0.3)	2.6	(0.6)	1.7	(0.4)
Civilian in region of terror	20.8	(1.3)	8.3	(0.5)	1.1	(0.3)	0.5	(0.1)	1.6	(0.4)	1.1	(0.3)	3.8	(0.7)	2.5	(0.4)
Refugee	1.6	(0.5)	0.6	(0.2)	0.5	(0.2)	0.2	(0.1)	0.6	(0.3)	0.4	(0.2)	0.7	(0.2)	0.5	(0.2)
Kidnapped	1.4	(0.3)	0.5	(0.1)	1.3	(0.4)	0.6	(0.2)	0.8	(0.3)	0.5	(0.2)	0.3	(0.2)	0.2	(0.2)
Any	24.3	(1.3)	11.6	(0.6)	6.9	(0.7)	3.7	(0.4)	7.0	(0.7)	5.7	(0.6)	6.1	(0.9)	5.0	(0.7)
II Participation in Organized Violence																
Witnessed death/dead body/ serious injury	19.1	(1.2)	14.0	(0.7)	25.4	(2.2)	44.0	(2.9)	7.3	(1.0)	8.5	(1.1)	16.0	(1.8)	21.8	(1.7)
Accidentally caused serious injury/death	0.5	(0.1)	0.5	(0.2)	0.6	(0.2)	0.3	(0.1)	0.5	(0.1)	0.4	(0.1)	0.3	(0.1)	0.3	(0.1)
Combat experience	3.1	(0.5)	1.3	(0.2)	1.0	(0.3)	0.4	(0.2)	1.1	(0.2)	0.8	(0.1)	0.7	(0.3)	0.4	(0.2)
Purposely injured/tortured/ killed someone	0.3	(0.1)	0.3	(0.1)	0.2	(0.1)	0.2	(0.2)	0.0	(0.0)	0.0	(0.0)	0.1	(0.1)	0.1	(0.0)
Witnessed atrocities	3.6	(0.5)	2.8	(0.5)	0.5	(0.2)	0.5	(0.2)	0.4	(0.2)	0.4	(0.2)	0.4	(0.1)	0.3	(0.1)
Any	21.7	(1.2)	18.9	(1.0)	25.8	(2.2)	45.5	(2.8)	8.7	(1.0)	10.1	(1.2)	16.8	(1.8)	22.9	(1.7)
III Physical Violence Victimization																
Beaten by caregiver	2.9	(0.5)	1.1	(0.2)	2.8	(0.6)	1.2	(0.2)	2.5	(0.5)	1.7	(0.3)	7.8	(0.9)	5.2	(0.5)
Beaten by someone else	7.3	(0.8)	4.9	(0.4)	1.5	(0.3)	1.4	(0.3)	1.6	(0.5)	2.6	(0.9)	3.9	(0.9)	4.6	(0.8)
Witnessed physical fight at home	5.2	(0.7)	2.1	(0.3)	–	–	–	–	–	–	–	–	–	—	–	–
Any	12.6	(1.1)	8.1	(0.6)	4.1	(0.6)	2.6	(0.4)	3.8	(0.6)	4.3	(0.9)	10.5	(1.2)	9.7	(1.0)
IV Sexual Violence Victimization																
Raped	2.8	(0.4)	2.4	(0.4)	0.7	(0.2)	0.6	(0.1)	0.4	(0.1)	0.5	(0.2)	0.1	(0.1)	0.0	(0.0)
Sexually assaulted	4.8	(0.4)	3.8	(0.5)	1.1	(0.3)	1.1	(0.3)	0.7	(0.2)	0.8	(0.2)	1.8	(0.4)	3.1	(0.9)
Stalked	2.8	(0.4)	2.1	(0.4)	2.2	(0.4)	1.8	(0.3)	1.8	(0.3)	2.1	(0.6)	2.8	(0.6)	3.5	(0.8)
Beaten by spouse/romantic partner	2.6	(0.4)	1.0	(0.2)	1.1	(0.3)	0.5	(0.1)	0.7	(0.2)	0.5	(0.2)	0.8	(0.2)	0.5	(0.1)
Trauma to loved one	4.9	(0.4)	2.8	(0.3)	0.7	(0.2)	0.3	(0.1)	1.3	(0.3)	1.9	(1.0)	1.2	(0.3)	0.9	(0.2)
Some other trauma	4.4	(0.5)	1.7	(0.2)	2.5	(0.5)	1.1	(0.2)	0.6	(0.2)	0.4	(0.1)	1.2	(0.3)	0.8	(0.2)
Private trauma[a]	4.6	(0.6)	1.8	(0.2)	4.8	(0.6)	2.1	(0.3)	3.7	(0.6)	2.5	(0.4)	2.2	(0.4)	1.4	(0.3)
Any	18.3	(0.9)	15.8	(1.1)	11.3	(0.9)	7.4	(0.6)	7.7	(0.7)	8.8	(1.3)	8.4	(1.0)	10.4	(1.4)

(cont.)

Table 3.A6 *(cont.)*

	Northern Ireland				Italy				Spain				PRC – Beijing/Shanghai			
	Prevalence of trauma		Trauma as a percentage of all trauma		Prevalence of trauma		Trauma as a percentage of all trauma		Prevalence of trauma		Trauma as a percentage of all trauma		Prevalence of trauma		Trauma as a percentage of all trauma	
	%	(SE)	%	(SE)	%	(SE)	%	(SE)	%	(SE)	%	(SE)	%	(SE)	%	(SE)
V Accidents/Injuries																
Natural disaster	1.4	(0.6)	0.7	(0.2)	7.8	(1.3)	4.9	(0.8)	2.9	(0.5)	2.5	(0.6)	18.9	(1.6)	15.4	(1.1)
Toxic chemical exposure	2.1	(0.4)	2.8	(0.5)	1.8	(0.4)	3.0	(0.7)	1.9	(0.4)	3.0	(0.8)	2.8	(0.6)	3.9	(0.7)
Automobile accident	8.5	(0.9)	4.7	(0.4)	11.7	(1.2)	6.6	(0.7)	14.1	(1.2)	12.3	(1.1)	6.9	(0.7)	6.2	(0.8)
Life-threatening illness	7.8	(0.7)	4.2	(0.4)	8.0	(0.8)	4.4	(0.6)	8.9	(0.9)	9.4	(1.2)	7.3	(0.9)	5.6	(0.7)
Child with serious illness	5.8	(0.6)	2.6	(0.3)	5.4	(0.7)	2.8	(0.4)	4.3	(0.5)	3.4	(0.3)	3.2	(0.5)	2.4	(0.5)
Other life-threatening accident	4.0	(0.4)	2.3	(0.3)	2.9	(0.5)	1.8	(0.4)	5.1	(0.9)	3.9	(0.7)	4.9	(0.7)	4.4	(0.6)
Any	22.8	(1.3)	17.3	(1.0)	27.9	(1.9)	23.5	(1.7)	28.5	(1.4)	34.6	(1.7)	33.7	(1.9)	37.9	(1.9)
VI Other																
Mugged/threatened with a weapon	9.8	(0.8)	5.7	(0.5)	4.7	(0.7)	2.7	(0.5)	13.1	(1.4)	12.8	(1.5)	3.4	(0.6)	3.3	(0.6)
Human-made disaster	7.0	(0.6)	5.7	(0.5)	2.3	(0.4)	1.4	(0.3)	4.3	(0.7)	4.9	(1.3)	2.8	(0.9)	2.4	(0.6)
UD of a loved one	26.7	(1.2)	16.9	(0.9)	20.4	(1.2)	13.3	(0.9)	20.6	(1.4)	18.9	(1.3)	11.1	(1.1)	8.4	(1.0)
Any	34.9	(1.3)	28.3	(0.7)	24.3	(1.4)	17.3	(1.1)	32.0	(1.6)	36.6	(2.0)	15.3	(1.5)	14.0	(1.3)
VII Total	**60.6**	**(1.7)**	**100.0**	**(0.0)**	**56.1**	**(2.2)**	**100.0**	**(0.0)**	**54.0**	**(1.7)**	**100.0**	**(0.0)**	**52.5**	**(2.6)**	**100.0**	**(0.0)**

[a]A *private* event is a trauma that some individuals reported in response to a question asked at the very end of the trauma section that asked if they ever had some other very upsetting experience they did not tell us about already (and this includes in response to a prior open-ended question about "any other" trauma) because they were too embarrassed or upset to talk about it. Respondents were told, before they answered, that if they reported such a trauma we would not ask them anything about what it was, only about their age when the trauma happened.

Table 3.A7 Prevalence of traumas and each trauma as a percentage of all traumas by country in decreasing order of percentage for any trauma

	Romania				Bulgaria			
	Prevalence of trauma		Trauma as a percentage of all trauma		Prevalence of trauma		Trauma as a percentage of all trauma	
	%	(SE)	%	(SE)	%	(SE)	%	(SE)
I Exposure to Organized Violence								
Relief worker in war zone	0.3	(0.2)	0.2	(0.1)	0.1	(0.0)	0.1	(0.1)
Civilian in war zone	1.7	(0.2)	1.3	(0.2)	0.0	(0.0)	0.1	(0.0)
Civilian in region of terror	0.5	(0.1)	0.4	(0.1)	0.0	(0.0)	0.1	(0.0)
Refugee	0.8	(0.2)	0.6	(0.1)	0.1	(0.1)	0.2	(0.1)
Kidnapped	0.4	(0.2)	0.3	(0.1)	0.2	(0.1)	0.2	(0.2)
Any	3.1	(0.4)	2.9	(0.4)	0.4	(0.2)	0.6	(0.2)
II Participation in Organized Violence								
Witnessed death/dead body/serious injury	10.7	(0.7)	15.7	(1.5)	6.7	(0.7)	17.2	(1.8)
Accidentally caused serious injury/death	0.6	(0.2)	0.5	(0.2)	0.1	(0.0)	0.1	(0.1)
Combat experience	1.2	(0.3)	0.9	(0.2)	0.5	(0.2)	0.7	(0.3)
Purposely injured/tortured/killed someone	0.3	(0.2)	0.5	(0.3)	0.2	(0.1)	0.3	(0.2)
Witnessed atrocities	1.3	(0.2)	1.7	(0.4)	0.2	(0.1)	0.3	(0.1)
Any	12.0	(0.8)	19.3	(1.7)	7.1	(0.7)	18.7	(1.9)
III Physical Violence Victimization								
Beaten by caregiver	3.1	(0.5)	2.4	(0.3)	0.7	(0.2)	0.9	(0.3)
Beaten by someone else	2.0	(0.3)	2.2	(0.5)	0.5	(0.2)	1.6	(0.8)
Witnessed physical fight at home	3.7	(0.4)	2.8	(0.3)				
Any	7.5	(0.7)	7.4	(0.7)	1.2	(0.3)	2.6	(0.9)
IV Sexual Violence Victimization								
Raped	0.6	(0.3)	0.5	(0.2)	0.2	(0.0)	0.3	(0.1)
Sexually assaulted	0.7	(0.2)	1.0	(0.4)	0.3	(0.2)	0.5	(0.3)
Stalked	1.9	(0.4)	3.6	(0.9)	0.5	(0.2)	1.1	(0.3)
Beaten by spouse/romantic partner	3.1	(0.4)	2.4	(0.4)	1.4	(0.2)	1.9	(0.3)
Trauma to loved one	0.3	(0.1)	0.3	(0.1)	0.6	(0.2)	1.3	(0.6)
Some other trauma	1.1	(0.2)	0.9	(0.2)	3.1	(0.5)	5.5	(0.9)
Private trauma[a]	2.2	(0.4)	1.7	(0.3)	2.5	(0.4)	3.3	(0.5)
Any	8.1	(0.8)	10.3	(1.2)	6.6	(0.6)	13.8	(1.1)

(cont.)

Table 3.A7 *(cont.)*

	Romania				Bulgaria			
	Prevalence of trauma		Trauma as a percentage of all trauma		Prevalence of trauma		Trauma as a percentage of all trauma	
	%	(SE)	%	(SE)	%	(SE)	%	(SE)
V Accidents/Injuries								
Natural disaster	5.2	(0.5)	7.9	(1.0)	1.3	(0.3)	2.8	(0.7)
Toxic chemical exposure	2.4	(0.4)	3.8	(0.8)	0.8	(0.2)	2.4	(0.5)
Automobile accident	9.3	(0.6)	10.2	(0.8)	6.9	(0.9)	12.8	(1.4)
Life-threatening illness	10.0	(0.8)	11.9	(1.3)	5.1	(0.8)	9.4	(1.1)
Child with serious illness	4.7	(0.6)	4.3	(0.7)	3.7	(0.6)	6.2	(1.0)
Other life-threatening accident	5.5	(0.6)	5.6	(0.7)	2.7	(0.4)	4.9	(1.1)
Any	26.4	(0.9)	43.8	(2.1)	16.1	(1.2)	38.7	(2.3)
VI Other								
Mugged/threatened with a weapon	3.5	(0.7)	3.4	(0.5)	1.2	(0.3)	3.2	(1.2)
Human-made disaster	1.4	(0.3)	1.4	(0.3)	0.9	(0.2)	1.4	(0.3)
UD of a loved one	10.5	(0.7)	11.5	(0.8)	11.0	(1.0)	21.1	(2.9)
Any	13.9	(1.0)	16.3	(1.0)	12.6	(1.1)	25.7	(2.8)
VII Total	**41.5**	**(1.1)**	**100.0**	**(0.0)**	**28.6**	**(1.3)**	**100.0**	**(0.0)**

[a]A *private* event is a trauma that some individuals reported in response to a question asked at the very end of the trauma section that asked if they ever had some other very upsetting experience they did not tell us about already (and this includes in response to a prior open-ended question about "any other" trauma) because they were too embarrassed or upset to talk about it. Respondents were told, before they answered, that if they reported such a trauma we would not ask them anything about what it was, only about their age when the trauma happened.

Table 3.A8 Country-specific frequency of exposure to each type of trauma and any event per 100 respondents (n = 68,894)

	Exposure to organized violence		Participation in organized violence		Physical violence victimization		Sexual violence victimization		Accidents/ injuries		UD of a loved one		Other traumas		Any event	
	Mean per 100	(SE) per 100	Mean per 100	(SE) per 100	Mean per 100	(SE) per 100	Mean per 100	(SE) per 100	Mean per 100	(SE) per 100	Mean per 100	(SE) per 100	Mean per 100	(SE) per 100	Mean per 100	(SE) per 100
I High-Income Countries																
Australia	10.9	(0.7)	83.2	(3.6)	29.7	(1.3)	73.0	(2.8)	88.4	(2.6)	64.9	(2.2)	31.4	(1.6)	381.6	(8.9)
Belgium	21.0	(2.9)	47.3	(5.4)	11.0	(2.4)	35.6	(4.7)	56.6	(5.0)	36.1	(4.9)	23.2	(3.3)	230.7	(16.3)
France	18.5	(2.4)	77.8	(7.7)	6.7	(1.1)	40.9	(3.9)	74.5	(8.6)	41.9	(3.9)	25.4	(2.7)	285.8	(16.6)
Germany	19.3	(2.1)	63.4	(4.4)	16.2	(2.4)	40.1	(4.4)	63.7	(6.2)	43.2	(4.1)	25.9	(3.6)	271.6	(16.4)
Israel	6.5	(0.3)	104.4	(3.1)	11.8	(0.9)	46.3	(1.7)	73.7	(2.1)	65.2	(1.6)	19.6	(1.0)	327.5	(5.8)
Italy	8.3	(0.8)	102.2	(11.9)	5.9	(1.0)	16.7	(1.7)	52.8	(4.6)	29.8	(1.8)	9.1	(1.3)	224.8	(16.4)
Japan	6.5	(0.8)	42.0	(4.3)	36.7	(2.6)	33.0	(3.1)	44.9	(4.0)	37.8	(3.4)	6.2	(1.4)	207.2	(12.5)
Netherlands	16.4	(2.8)	41.8	(5.0)	9.8	(1.7)	45.7	(6.7)	47.0	(3.4)	41.6	(4.6)	35.3	(5.4)	237.6	(17.5)
New Zealand	11.8	(0.9)	70.7	(3.3)	32.9	(1.4)	83.7	(3.3)	120.0	(4.6)	67.6	(2.2)	28.1	(1.5)	414.8	(9.5)
Northern Ireland	29.1	(1.7)	47.3	(3.6)	20.3	(1.8)	39.6	(3.1)	43.5	(2.9)	42.3	(2.6)	28.6	(1.9)	250.6	(10.5)
Portugal	10.1	(1.1)	50.7	(3.3)	31.0	(1.8)	33.6	(2.9)	75.7	(3.8)	34.5	(2.4)	25.6	(2.1)	261.1	(9.4)
Spain	8.5	(0.9)	14.9	(2.1)	6.4	(1.5)	13.0	(2.2)	51.4	(3.9)	28.1	(2.2)	26.3	(3.2)	148.6	(8.9)
Spain – Murcia	3.3	(1.1)	7.4	(1.8)	15.2	(0.9)	23.1	(4.6)	51.8	(5.2)	37.6	(3.0)	18.1	(2.4)	156.6	(12.5)
United States	8.2	(0.6)	84.1	(3.3)	35.7	(1.9)	96.2	(3.1)	138.8	(4.9)	84.7	(3.4)	41.7	(1.5)	489.4	(12.9)
II Upper-Middle-Income Countries																
Brazil – São Paulo	4.1	(0.9)	101.8	(6.8)	35.4	(1.8)	30.2	(1.7)	51.6	(3.1)	47.2	(2.1)	62.5	(3.6)	332.9	(11.7)
Bulgaria	0.4	(0.2)	13.8	(1.7)	1.9	(0.7)	10.2	(1.1)	28.6	(2.2)	15.6	(2.3)	3.4	(0.9)	74.0	(4.6)
Lebanon	107.6	(6.9)	100.4	(8.0)	10.9	(1.8)	44.5	(4.5)	48.4	(5.2)	59.6	(4.2)	14.2	(2.0)	385.5	(22.7)
Colombia – Medellin	16.2	(2.0)	76.5	(5.7)	45.8	(3.3)	57.0	(7.3)	67.7	(6.2)	66.9	(6.6)	75.6	(4.9)	405.7	(25.9)
Mexico	3.3	(0.4)	39.1	(3.9)	50.1	(2.5)	36.8	(2.5)	76.9	(5.3)	34.7	(3.1)	45.6	(2.6)	286.5	(11.5)
Romania	3.7	(0.5)	25.2	(3.1)	9.7	(1.1)	13.5	(1.8)	57.2	(2.9)	15.1	(1.1)	6.2	(0.9)	130.5	(6.8)
South Africa	15.6	(1.6)	72.7	(4.6)	30.7	(1.5)	36.5	(1.4)	69.2	(2.5)	62.1	(2.6)	30.5	(1.4)	317.2	(9.6)
III Low- and Lower-Middle-Income Countries																
Colombia	13.5	(1.3)	101.1	(6.1)	53.9	(2.4)	55.1	(3.2)	91.9	(5.8)	70.2	(4.2)	72.3	(3.3)	458.0	(16.3)
Nigeria	18.5	(1.7)	100.1	(6.4)	20.5	(2.4)	22.7	(1.9)	88.6	(5.5)	62.8	(2.8)	13.8	(1.3)	327.0	(12.2)
PRC – Beijing/ Shanghai	7.7	(1.1)	34.8	(3.9)	14.8	(1.7)	15.8	(2.6)	57.7	(4.6)	12.7	(1.5)	8.6	(1.6)	152.2	(10.9)
Peru	9.4	(0.8)	54.0	(4.8)	66.4	(2.5)	41.4	(2.8)	97.3	(2.7)	44.0	(2.5)	54.8	(3.5)	367.3	(7.8)
Ukraine	18.1	(1.6)	69.6	(6.7)	43.1	(5.0)	48.8	(3.8)	105.9	(4.7)	57.9	(3.8)	30.2	(3.8)	373.6	(16.6)
IV Total	**12.2**	**(0.3)**	**68.9**	**(1.0)**	**27.3**	**(0.4)**	**49.2**	**(0.7)**	**80.2**	**(1.0)**	**53.2**	**(0.7)**	**30.6**	**(0.5)**	**321.5**	**(2.9)**

Chapter 4

Childhood Adversities and Preexisting Psychopathology as Predictors of Trauma

Victoria Shahly, Corina Benjet, Graça Cardoso, Louisa Degenhardt, and Elie G. Karam

Epidemiological research has begun unraveling the risk pathways leading from trauma exposures to pathological stress reactions and beyond to syndromic PTSD, focusing heavily on trauma-related features (e.g., type or severity) and differential reactivity of respondents during and following exposures. However, to date, studies have rarely examined differential liability to trauma exposure, even though this information may be both methodologically and clinically relevant (Jang et al., 2003; Briggs-Gowan et al., 2010; Amstadter et al., 2013; Brown et al., 2014; Overstreet et al., 2017).

We saw in Chapter 3 that traumas are highly prevalent, non-randomly distributed, begin early in life, and tend to pile up over time. Socio-demographic predictors of traumas vary substantially across trauma types, but generally include sex, age, economic status, and marital status. Because of variation in both the sign and strength of these predictors – with women having higher risk than men of sexual assault victimization, but men having higher risk of other traumas – no single high-risk trauma vulnerability profile emerged from our descriptive analyses in Chapter 3 apart from an apparently protective effect of being married.

We also showed in Chapter 3 that traumas are correlated over time; that the prior occurrence of one trauma is associated with increased risk of exposure to subsequent traumas. This is an important finding because it suggests that stable individual differences affect the risk of trauma exposure. If identified, the determinants of these individual differences might point to novel cross-cutting prevention targets that could help reduce future exposure (Howlett & Stein, 2016). Unfortunately, we were unaware of any of these subtle patterns when launching the WMH Initiative. As a result, survey questions were not developed to optimize study of the links across traumas. Many of the significant predictors of such links considered in previous research, most notably those of "event proneness" (Stein et al., 2002b), have involved intrinsic factors such as intelligence (Macklin et al., 1998; Breslau et al., 2006) or core personality dimensions such as dispositional negativity (Shackman et al., 2016), negative emotionality (Eisenberg et al., 2002; Wolff & Baglivio, 2016), irritable/fearful temperament (Schmeck & Poustka, 2001; Helzer et al., 2009; Taskesen et al., 2017), neuroticism (Kendler et al., 2002, 2003; Jaksic et al., 2012), and impulsivity/extraversion (Netto et al., 2016; Moore et al., 2017). However, despite their considerable explanatory value, such constitutional factors are highly resistant to modification and thus have limited clinical utility at present.

As a result, we conducted post hoc analyses of WMH data to explore two other types of pre-trauma vulnerability that offer promising inroads to behavioral change. First, we investigated the possibility that childhood adversities (CAs) are associated with elevated risk of subsequent adult traumas. In the case of intergenerational transmission of family violence, prior research has shown that childhood physical or sexual abuse predicts greatly enhanced odds of adult intimate partner victimization (IPV) (Ehrensaft et al., 2003; Noll et al., 2003; Barnes et al., 2009; Black et al., 2010; Cui et al., 2010) and perpetration (Stith et al., 2004; Millett et al., 2013). Numerous evidence-based primary interventions for these kinds of CAs have already been developed (McClennen et al., 2016), which employ a rich variety of psychosocial and cognitive-behavioral techniques suitable for ethnically and culturally diverse populations in various settings (Silverman et al., 2008; Dorsey et al., 2017). It is conceivable that these kinds of interventions could be expanded based on evidence we uncover of other kinds of inter-temporal trauma clustering.

Second, we investigated the possibility that temporally primary lifetime mental disorders are associated with elevated risk of exposures to a wide range of subsequent adult traumas. Such associations have been documented in previous studies. Prior research has shown, for example, that bipolar disorder predicts greatly increased odds of both future violence-related traumas – violent crime victimization, crime perpetration (Fazel et al., 2010), and sexual assault (Darves-Bornoz et al., 1995) – and accident-related traumas (Hiroeh et al., 2001). The risk reduction programs that already screen for and treat emerging behavioral disorders before they progress to serious criminal or accident-related sequelae of this sort (Lam et al., 2005) might accommodate prevention arms for potential downstream traumas. However, a clearer characterization of the extent to which DSM-IV disorders predict subsequent trauma exposure is needed for optimal targeting of pre-trauma risk factors.

Methods

Using the same sample and analytical framework as in Chapter 3, we expanded the models developed in that chapter to include predictors for CAs and temporally prior (to index traumas) lifetime mental disorders. As discussed in detail in Chapter 10, the WMH surveys assessed 12 dichotomously measured CAs. These included three types of interpersonal loss (parent death, parent divorce, and other loss of contact with parents or caregivers), four types of parent maladjustment (psychopathology, substance abuse, criminality, and family violence), three types of respondent maltreatment (physical abuse, sexual abuse, and neglect), respondent serious physical illness, and family economic adversity. Parent death and divorce were assessed only for biological parents, but other loss of contact with caregivers included any disruption of a caregiving relationship for six months or longer. Respondents born to an unwed mother or who were adopted at birth were not coded as experiencing the loss of their fathers or biological parents, respectively.

Physical abuse of the respondent by caregivers was assessed with a modified version of the Conflict Tactics Scale (CTS) (Straus, 1979) and with an item from the trauma section of the Composite International Diagnostic Interview (CIDI) (Kessler & Üstün, 2004). Sexual abuse of the respondent by caregivers or other family members was assessed with questions from the CIDI regarding sexual assault, attempted rape, and rape, which asked whether these traumas were one-time vs. recurrent experiences. Neglect was assessed with questions used in studies of child welfare that assessed the frequency of having inadequate food, clothing, medical care, or supervision, and being required to do age-inappropriate chores (Courtney et al., 1998).

Parent criminality was assessed with questions about whether a parent engaged in criminal activities or was ever arrested or sent to prison. Parent psychopathology (major depression, generalized anxiety disorder, panic disorder, or suicide attempt) and parent substance abuse were assessed with a revised version of the Family History Research Diagnostic Criteria Interview (Endicott et al., 1978; Kendler et al., 1991). Family violence was assessed with the modified CTS and a question in the trauma section of the CIDI about parent violence. Economic adversity was assessed with questions about whether the respondent's family received welfare or other government assistance or had insufficient money for necessities. Physical illness was assessed with a standard chronic conditions checklist.

It should be noted that since several of the CAs considered here were either themselves listed among the individual trauma types assessed in Chapter 3 (e.g., childhood physical abuse, witnessing family violence during childhood, childhood physical illness) or included as components of these trauma types (e.g., sexual assault victimization, unexpected death of a loved one), certain of the analyses planned here naturally echoed those in Chapter 3 that traced prior traumas to subsequent ones. In cases of direct overlap, we removed the CA questions from the CA battery, treating them as traumas rather than childhood adversities. Although this resulted in the complete elimination of the CA sexual abuse category and the narrowing of the CA physical abuse category in some cases, most of the study CAs were unaffected.

Consistent with final models generated for Chapter 10, the CA models predicted trauma exposure controlling for socio-demographics and prior trauma measures along with methodological controls for survey and person-year. We began with a series of models examining each CA separately along with these controls and then estimated models that included a separate predictor variable for each of the CAs followed by multivariate models that evaluated the joint predictive effects of all CAs. We distinguished between CAs in a highly inter-correlated set that we referred to in previous reports as indicators of maladaptive family functioning (MFF) CAs (Kessler et al., 2010). The logic of these models is described in Chapter 10. The MFF CAs included parent mental illness, parent substance abuse, parent criminality, family violence, physical and sexual abuse of the respondent, and neglect of the respondent.

The final CA models were then expanded to include information about lifetime occurrence of 14 DSM-IV Axis I disorders that had initial onsets prior to the respondent's history of criminality, family violence, physical and sexual abuse, these disorders were assessed with the CIDI. The disorders included two mood disorders (major depressive disorder/dysthymic disorder and broadly defined bipolar disorder [bipolar I and II and sub-threshold bipolar disorder, defined using criteria described elsewhere]) (Kessler et al., 2006), six anxiety disorders (generalized anxiety disorder, panic disorder and/or agoraphobia, post-traumatic stress disorder, separation anxiety disorder, social phobia, and specific phobia), four disruptive behavior disorders (attention-deficit/hyperactivity disorder, conduct disorder, intermittent explosive disorder, and oppositional-defiant disorder), and two substance disorders (alcohol and drug abuse with or without dependence). As noted in Chapter 2, age-of-onset of each disorder was assessed using probing techniques shown experimentally to improve recall accuracy (Knäuper et al., 1999), enabling us to determine whether respondents had a history of each disorder prior to exposure to the index trauma.

Associations of Childhood Adversities with Subsequent Traumas

We examined predictors of trauma exposure for each of the 29 trauma types both separately and pooled across the trauma factors described in Chapter 3. As in that chapter, we also focus here primarily on the pooled models as well as on models for each of the three individual cross-loading traumas. However, trauma-specific models are briefly mentioned and are presented in the appendix tables. We began with inspection of bivariate associations in which only one CA was considered at a time to predict the subsequent occurrence of each of the 29 trauma types controlling for respondent sex, person-year, and age at interview along with dummy controls for survey. About two-thirds (68%) of these 319 (11 CAs predicting each of 29 traumas) ORs were greater than 1.0 and significant at the 0.05 level (two-sided tests). However, given that the CAs were strongly inter-correlated, much smaller proportions of ORs remained significant in multivariate models. The 11 CAs were significant as a set in predicting subsequent exposures to traumas in all five broad trauma groups as well as the three cross-loading traumas ($\chi^2_{11} = 166.9$–$2{,}043.7$, $p < 0.001$) (see Table 4.1). MFF CAs consistently were stronger predictors ($\chi^2_6 = 122.7$–$1{,}546.7$, $p < 0.001$) than other CAs ($\chi^2_5 = 20.0$–181.3, $p = 0.001$ to <0.001).

Inspection of ORs in the aggregated models showed that the most consistent predictors, significant in all models, were parent mental illness (OR = 1.4–2.0), parent criminality (OR = 1.2–1.7), and other parent loss (OR = 1.1–1.6). The extent to which controls for exogenous associations among predictors influenced these estimates is indicated by the fact that the bivariate associations of these three predictors with the outcomes were in the range OR = 1.6–2.7 for parent mental illness, OR = 1.4–3.1 for parent criminality, and OR = 1.2–2.1 for other parent loss. The multivariate ORs were more strongly elevated and consistently significant for MFF CAs (81% of ORs significant, with a median of 1.8 and inter-quartile range [IQR] of 1.5–2.3) than other CAs (52% of ORs significant, with a median of 1.3 and IQR of 1.1–1.5). Similar patterns held in bivariate models, where median (IQR) ORs predicting each of the 29 traumas was highest for parent mental illness [OR = 2.2 (1.6–2.5)] followed by neglect [OR = 2.0 (1.7–2.8)] and parent criminality [OR = 2.0 (1.6–2.5)]. The other MFF CAs and other parent loss had lower bivariate ORs [other MFF CAs OR = 1.5 (1.4–2.1); other parent loss OR = 1.7 (1.4–1.9)], whereas the remaining CAs (parent death, parent divorce, serious physical illness, economic adversity) had much lower bivariate ORs [OR = 1.2 (1.1–1.5)].

As expected, the CAs most strongly predicted trauma exposures in the domains of physical and sexual violence victimization. Parent neglect (OR = 1.7–2.6) and parent mental illness (OR = 1.8–1.9) consistently had the highest ORs in those models followed by parent substance abuse (OR = 1.8 predicting physical violence victimization but only OR = 1.1 predicting sexual violence victimization) and other parent loss (OR = 1.7–1.5). Disaggregation showed that the traumas within the broad groups involving physical and sexual violence victimization most strongly predicted by the above CAs were being raped (OR = 2.4–3.9) and witnessing physical fights between parents at home (OR = 1.8–4.8) in bivariate models. These CAs also strongly predicted subsequently being beaten by a spouse or romantic partner (OR = 1.9–3.2 in bivariate models), beaten up by someone else (OR = 1.9–3.0), mugged (OR = 1.3–1.6), and all other traumas in the sexual assault victimization group (OR = 1.3–2.6). Childhood neglect typically had the highest OR in predicting these outcomes, followed by parent mental illness and parent criminality.

Table 4.1 Multivariate associations of CAs with the subsequent onset of traumas aggregated into categories in 26 WMH surveys[a]

	Exposure to organized violence		Participation in organized violence		Physical violence victimization		Sexual violence victimization		Accidents/ injuries		Mugged/ threatened with a weapon		Human-made disaster		UD of a loved one	
	OR	(95% CI)	OR	(95% CI)	OR	(95% CI)	OR	(95% CI)	OR	(95% CI)	OR	(95% CI)	OR	(95% CI)	OR	(95% CI)
I MFF CAs																
Parent psychopathology	1.7*	(1.5–1.9)	1.6*	(1.5–1.8)	1.8*	(1.7–2.0)	1.9*	(1.8–2.1)	1.5*	(1.5–1.6)	1.4*	(1.3–1.6)	2.0*	(1.6–2.4)	1.5*	(1.4–1.6)
Parent substance misuse	1.0	(0.8–1.2)	1.1	(1.0–1.3)	1.8*	(1.6–2.0)	1.1*	(1.0–1.2)	1.1*	(1.1–1.2)	1.2*	(1.1–1.4)	1.0	(0.8–1.4)	1.2*	(1.1–1.3)
Parent criminality	1.5*	(1.3–1.8)	1.5*	(1.4–1.8)	1.7*	(1.5–1.9)	1.5*	(1.3–1.7)	1.2*	(1.1–1.4)	1.3*	(1.2–1.5)	1.6*	(1.2–2.1)	1.3*	(1.2–1.5)
Family violence	1.2	(0.8–1.7)	1.0	(0.8–1.2)	1.1	(0.9–1.3)	1.3*	(1.1–1.6)	1.1	(0.9–1.2)	0.9	(0.6–1.3)	1.0	(0.6–1.6)	1.0	(0.8–1.2)
Physical abuse	1.4	(1.0–1.9)	1.3*	(1.0–1.5)	1.0	(0.8–1.3)	1.1	(1.0–1.3)	1.3*	(1.1–1.5)	1.5*	(1.2–1.9)	1.0	(0.7–1.6)	1.4*	(1.2–1.6)
Neglect	1.5*	(1.2–1.8)	1.4*	(1.3–1.6)	2.6*	(2.3–2.8)	1.7*	(1.6–1.9)	1.3*	(1.2–1.4)	1.2*	(1.1–1.3)	1.4*	(1.1–1.8)	1.1	(1.0–1.2)
$\chi^{2\,b}_{6}$	178.2*		354.4*		1546.7*		718.8*		375.7*		169.6*		122.7*		271.3*	
II Other CAs																
Parent death	1.2*	(1.0–1.3)	1.1	(1.0–1.2)	1.1	(1.0–1.1)	1.1*	(1.1–1.2)	1.1*	(1.1–1.2)	1.0	(0.9–1.1)	0.9	(0.8–1.1)	1.5*	(1.4–1.5)
Parent divorce	1.3*	(1.1–1.5)	1.3*	(1.1–1.4)	1.4*	(1.3–1.6)	1.3*	(1.2–1.5)	1.2*	(1.1–1.3)	1.3*	(1.1–1.4)	1.2	(0.9–1.4)	1.1	(1.0–1.2)
Other parent loss	1.5*	(1.3–1.7)	1.4*	(1.2–1.5)	1.7*	(1.5–1.8)	1.5*	(1.4–1.6)	1.3*	(1.2–1.4)	1.2*	(1.1–1.3)	1.6*	(1.3–2.0)	1.1*	(1.0–1.2)
Serious physical illness	0.7	(0.4–1.2)	1.1	(0.8–1.4)	1.2	(0.9–1.6)	1.3*	(1.0–1.6)	1.2*	(1.0–1.5)	1.8*	(1.3–2.5)	1.0	(0.5–2.0)	1.2	(0.9–1.5)
Economic adversity	0.9	(0.7–1.1)	0.9*	(0.8–1.0)	1.2*	(1.0–1.3)	1.1	(1.0–1.2)	1.0	(0.9–1.1)	1.1	(0.9–1.3)	1.1	(0.9–1.4)	1.0	(0.9–1.1)
$\chi^{2\,b}_{5}$	44.0*		72.9*		181.3*		172.2*		121.9*		42.5*		20.0*		152.7*	
$\chi^{2\,c}_{11}$	262.0*		451.3*		2043.7*		1015.7*		584.0*		245.7*		166.9*		460.1*	

*Significant at the 0.05 level, two-sided test.
[a]Based on a series of multivariate survival models with person-year the unit of analysis and a logistic link function in which information about prior CAs was used to predict the subsequent first onset of traumas. Controls were included for person-year, sex, age-at-interview, and survey.
[b]The joint significance of the set of ORs for CAs in the group.
[c]The joint significance of all CAs in the model.

Associations of Temporally Prior DSM-IV/CIDI Disorders with Subsequent Traumas

We next considered associations of temporally primary lifetime mental disorders with subsequent first onset of traumas. We used the same modeling approach as in the analysis of CAs. We began with bivariate models for the association of each temporally primary lifetime mental disorders predicting subsequent first onset of each trauma, controlling for type and number of CAs, respondent sex, person-year, age at interview, and dummy controls for survey. The vast majority (96.3%) of these 406 (14 mental disorders predicting each of 29 traumas) ORs were greater than 1.0% and 78.5% were both greater than 1.0 and statistically significant at the 0.05 level (two-sided tests). This number did not decrease greatly in multivariate models, where 74.1% of ORs were greater than 1.0 and were also statistically significant.

In multivariate models, the 14 disorders were significant as a set in predicting subsequent exposures to traumas in all five broad trauma groups as well as in the three cross-loading traumas (χ^2_{14} = 224.1–1,710.8, $p < 0.001$) (see Table 4.2). Mood disorders were significant in seven of eight models (χ^2_2 = 6.4–223.8, p = 0.040–<0.001), and each other class of disorders was significant in all eight models (anxiety disorders χ^2_6 = 40.1–598.9, $p < 0.001$; disruptive behavior disorders χ^2_4 =15.0–158.5, p = 0.005–<0.001; substance disorders χ^2_2 = 34.1–191.6, $p < 0.001$).

Within the mood disorders, major depression was more consistently significant than bipolar spectrum disorder (in seven vs. two models, with ORs = 1.1–1.6 vs. in two models with OR = 1.3–1.4). However, this difference reflected the stronger comorbidities of BP spectrum disorder than major depression with the other disorders in the set. This can be seen in the bivariate models wherein we considered only one mental disorder at a time, the median (IQR) ORs across all 29 traumas was higher for BP spectrum disorder [OR = 2.2 (1.6–2.9)] than major depression [OR = 1.7 (1.4–2.6)]. The traumas predicted most strongly by BP spectrum disorder in bivariate models included being kidnapped (OR = 5.1), stalked (OR = 4.6), beaten by a romantic partner (OR = 4.0), and beaten up by someone else (OR = 3.5). ORs for all these outcomes were also elevated but lower for major depression. The only case where major depression had a substantially higher OR than BP spectrum disorders in bivariate models was in predicting purposefully injuring, torturing, or killing someone (OR = 3.9 for major depression, OR = 2.7 for BP spectrum disorder).

Within the anxiety disorders, social phobia and specific phobia were the most consistently significant predictors in multivariate models, as they were significant in all models. They had ORs in the range OR = 1.1–1.3 for specific phobia and OR = 1.2–1.8 for social phobia. As with mood disorders, though, these results reflect differences in comorbidities among the disorders. The bivariate models tell a somewhat different story, showing that separation anxiety disorder (SAD) had the strongest median (IQR) OR across the 29 traumas [OR = 2.1 (2.0–2.9)] followed by panic/agoraphobia [OR = 1.9 (1.6–2.3)], generalized anxiety disorder [OR = 1.8 (1.4–2.4)], social phobia [OR = 1.8 (1.4–2.4)], and specific phobia [OR = 1.8 (1.6–2.2). Interestingly, PTSD had the lowest median OR of all anxiety disorders [OR = 1.2 (1.0–1.4)]. The traumas predicted most strongly by SAD in bivariate models included purposefully injured/killed someone (OR = 7.9), accidentally caused serious injury/death (OR = 3.8), and stalked (OR = 3.8). The traumas predicted most strongly by all anxiety disorders other than PTSD were those involving sexual assault victimization (OR = 2.2–3.3). PTSD, in comparison, consistently had the weakest predictive associations of all anxiety disorders across the traumas [OR = 1.2 (1.0–1.4)].

All disruptive behavior disorders other than ADHD were consistently significant predictors in multivariate models (OR = 1.2–1.8). ADHD, in comparison, was significant in half the multivariate models with significant ORs of 1.2–1.7. Bivariate models show, in comparison, conduct disorder (CD) and oppositional-defiant disorder (ODD) had the highest median (IQR) ORs [CD OR = 3.1 (2.6–4.0); ODD OR = 3.1 (2.5–3.6)] followed by ADHD [OR = 2.7 (2.3–3.2)] and IED [OR = 2.2 (1.7–2.7)]. The traumas most strongly predicted by CD and ODD were in the domains of participation in organized violence (accidentally and purposefully causing serious injury or death OR = 7.2–9.9), physical violence victimization (beaten up by someone else OR = 4.4–6.5), and especially sexual assault victimization (raped OR = 4.5–4.7, stalked OR = 4.1–3.6, beaten up by romantic partner OR = 6.9–4.9). The traumas most strongly predicted by ADHD and IED were similar, but with lower ORs than those for CD and ODD. It is noteworthy, given prominent discussions to the contrary in the clinical ADHD literature (Garner et al., 2014; Chang et al., 2017), that the OR of ADHD predicting automobile accidents (OR = 2.3) was in line with ORs for other

Table 4.2 Multivariate associations of lifetime DSM-IV/CIDI disorders with the subsequent onset of traumas aggregated into categories in 26 WMH surveys[a]

	Exposure to organized violence		Participation in organized violence		Physical violence victimization		Sexual violence victimization		Accidents/ injuries		Mugged/ threatened with a weapon		Human-made disaster		UD of a loved one	
	OR	(95% CI)	OR	(95% CI)	OR	(95% CI)	OR	(95% CI)	OR	(95% CI)	OR	(95% CI)	OR	(95% CI)	OR	(95% CI)
I Mood Disorders																
MDD or dysthymic disorder	1.2*	(1.0–1.4)	1.2*	(1.1–1.4)	1.3*	(1.2–1.5)	1.6*	(1.5–1.7)	1.2*	(1.1–1.3)	1.4*	(1.3–1.6)	1.1	(0.9–1.4)	1.1*	(1.1–1.2)
BPD (broad definition)	1.1	(0.8–1.5)	1.1	(0.9–1.4)	1.2	(0.9–1.6)	1.4*	(1.2–1.6)	1.0	(0.9–1.2)	1.1	(0.9–1.5)	1.3	(0.8–2.1)	1.3*	(1.1–1.5)
$\chi^{2\,b}_{2}$	6.4*		21.9*		21.5*		223.8*		53.0*		47.4*		2.8		27.8*	
II Anxiety Disorders																
Panic disorder or agoraphobia	1.1	(0.9–1.4)	1.3*	(1.2–1.5)	1.4*	(1.2–1.6)	1.4*	(1.3–1.6)	1.2*	(1.1–1.3)	1.2*	(1.0–1.4)	1.1	(0.7–1.6)	1.2*	(1.1–1.4)
GAD	0.9	(0.7–1.1)	0.9	(0.8–1.1)	1.0	(0.8–1.2)	1.2*	(1.1–1.4)	1.2*	(1.1–1.3)	0.9	(0.8–1.1)	1.3	(0.9–1.9)	1.1	(1.0–1.2)
PTSD	1.0	(0.9–1.1)	1.0	(1.0–1.1)	1.0	(0.9–1.0)	1.2*	(1.1–1.2)	0.9*	(0.9-1.0)	1.1	(1.0–1.2)	1.1	(1.0–1.3)	0.9*	(0.9–1.0)
Social phobia	1.2*	(1.0–1.4)	1.1*	(1.0–1.3)	1.2*	(1.0–1.4)	1.3*	(1.2–1.4)	1.1*	(1.0–1.2)	1.3*	(1.1–1.5)	1.3*	(1.0–1.7)	1.1*	(1.0–1.2)
Specific phobia	1.2*	(1.1–1.4)	1.5*	(1.4–1.6)	1.8*	(1.7–2.0)	1.6*	(1.5–1.7)	1.3*	(1.3–1.4)	1.4*	(1.3–1.6)	1.4*	(1.2–1.7)	1.4*	(1.3–1.5)
Separation anxiety disorder	1.7*	(1.3–2.4)	1.4*	(1.2–1.6)	1.2	(1.0–1.3)	1.5*	(1.3–1.6)	1.3*	(1.2–1.5)	1.5*	(1.3–1.7)	1.3	(0.9–1.8)	1.5*	(1.4–1.7)
$\chi^{2\,b}_{6}$	40.1*		149.5*		319.5*		598.9*		253.1*		166.1*		44.2*		269.7*	
III Disruptive Behavioral Disorders																
ADHD	1.2	(0.9–1.7)	1.4*	(1.2–1.7)	1.7*	(1.4–2.2)	1.2*	(1.1–1.5)	1.4*	(1.2–1.6)	1.0	(0.8–1.3)	1.5	(0.9–2.7)	1.2	(1.0–1.3)
CD	1.8*	(1.3–2.7)	1.7*	(1.4–2.1)	1.8*	(1.4–2.2)	1.5*	(1.3–1.8)	1.4*	(1.3–1.6)	1.7*	(1.3–2.2)	1.7*	(1.1–2.6)	1.3*	(1.1–1.6)
IED	1.3*	(1.0–1.7)	1.6*	(1.4–1.9)	1.4*	(1.2–1.7)	1.3*	(1.1–1.4)	1.3*	(1.1–1.4)	1.5*	(1.3–1.8)	1.3	(0.9–1.9)	1.3*	(1.1–1.5)
ODD	1.7*	(1.2–2.3)	1.4*	(1.2–1.7)	1.4*	(1.1–1.8)	1.3*	(1.1–1.6)	1.2*	(1.1–1.4)	1.4*	(1.1–1.8)	1.3	(0.9–2.0)	1.5*	(1.3–1.8)
$\chi^{2\,b}_{4}$	63.4*		125.5*		158.5*		123.2*		175.9*		68.6*		15.0*		93.7*	
IV Substance Use Disorders																
Alcohol abuse or dependence	1.4*	(1.1–1.8)	1.3*	(1.2–1.5)	1.8*	(1.6–2.1)	1.4*	(1.3–1.5)	1.5*	(1.4–1.6)	1.3*	(1.2–1.5)	2.1*	(1.6–2.7)	1.4*	(1.3–1.6)
Drug abuse or dependence	1.6*	(1.2–2.2)	1.6*	(1.3–1.9)	1.3*	(1.0–1.6)	1.5*	(1.3–1.7)	1.2*	(1.1–1.4)	1.8*	(1.5–2.2)	0.9	(0.7–1.3)	1.2*	(1.0–1.3)
$\chi^{2\,b}_{2}$	39.6*		81.4*		97.3*		149.5*		191.6*		92.0*		34.1*		109.4*	
$\chi^{2\,c}_{14}$	281.3*		661.6*		988.6*		1710.8*		1215.7*		629.8*		224.1*		892.7*	

*Significant at the 0.05 level, two-sided test.
[a]Based on a series of multivariate survival models with person-year the unit of analysis and a logistic link function in which information about prior lifetime mental disorders was used to predict the subsequent first onset of traumas. Controls were included for person-year, sex, age-at-interview, survey, and CAs.
[b]The joint significance of the set of ORs for mental disorders in the group.
[c]The joint significance of all mental disorders in the model.

disruptive behavior disorders (OR = 2.1–2.7). With the exceptions of BP spectrum disorder and substance use disorder (OR = 1.8–2.2), disruptive behavior disorders had higher bivariate ORs predicting automobile accidents than did any other mental disorders (OR = 1.0–1.6).

Both substance use disorders were consistently significant predictors of traumas in multivariate models (OR = 1.2–2.1). Both alcohol and drug use disorders also had significant elevated ORs with 86.2%–82.8% of the 29 individual traumas in bivariate models, with median (IQR) values somewhat higher for drug use disorders [OR = 2.4 (1.8–2.9)] than alcohol use disorders [OR = 1.7 (1.6–2.5)]. The highest bivariate ORs are with accidentally and purposefully injuring or killing someone (OR = 2.9–6.5), being kidnapped (OR = 3.6–4.7), being beaten by a romantic partner (OR = 5.1–7.0), and being stalked (OR = 2.7–4.0), in each case with drug use disorder having a higher OR than alcohol use disorder.

The traumas most strongly predicted by temporally primary mental disorders were those involving sexual assault victimization, both in bivariate models [OR = 2.6 (2.3–2.9)] and in multivariate models (OR = 1.2–1.6). Traumas involving physical violence victimization were next most strongly predicted [OR = 2.3 (1.9–2.7) in bivariate models; OR = 1.2–1.8 in multivariate models]. The traumas least strongly predicted by prior mental disorders were unexpected death of a loved one [OR = 1.7 (1.5–2.9) in bivariate models; OR = 1.1–1.5 in multivariate models] and accidents/injuries [OR = 1.8 (1.7–1.9) in bivariate models; 1.1–1.5 in multivariate models].

Discussion

In this chapter, we evaluated two potentially important classes of predictors of trauma exposure, childhood adversities and prior mental disorders, both of which are highly prevalent, heavily paired with particular trauma trajectories in the clinical literature, and associated with evidence-based treatment protocols that might be leveraged for prevention of subsequent trauma exposure (Howlett & Stein, 2016). Our finding that CAs most strongly predict traumas in the domains of physical and sexual violence victimization is consistent with a large observational literature linking child maltreatment to heightened risk of subsequent adult relationship violence (Coid et al., 2001; Ehrensaft et al., 2003; Noll et al., 2003; Gover et al., 2008; Barnes et al., 2009; Black et al., 2010; Cui et al., 2010; Conley et al., 2017; Lang & Gartstein, 2017) and with similar findings in studies of child maltreatment among representative U.S. samples (Finkelhor et al., 2007; Cuevas et al., 2009).

Our finding that childhood neglect is the strongest predictor of trauma risk is surprising, given the strong focus on child *maltreatment* in contemporary epidemiological research relative to neglect (Kanai et al., 2016; Cohen et al., 2017; Naughton et al., 2017). Although we were unable to find other population-based comparators, the notion that early neglect may lead to subsequent trauma is indirectly consistent with strong neurobiological evidence linking deprivation to aberrant neurodevelopment (Calem et al., 2017) associated with a cascade of persistent cognitive deficits (Center on the Developing Child at Harvard University, 2012; McLaughlin et al., 2017) and incident psychopathology (Busso et al., 2017; Walsh et al., 2017).

Somewhat unexpected as well was the comparatively weak association of childhood physical abuse with overall trauma liability (with only 55.2% of its bivariate associations with traumas significant positives) vs. those for neglect (with 96.6% of bivariate associations with traumas significant positives) and parent maladjustment (with 86.2%–93.1% significant positives). Altogether, such findings hint that trauma proneness is mediated both by early neglect, which may reflect environmental influences on brain hardwiring during sensitive developmental periods and by parent maladjustment, which may reflect heritable influences on self-selection into hazardous situations (Jang et al., 2003; Ogle et al., 2014) and/or the durable effects of vicissitudes in early attachment (Ogden, 2016). Our robust finding from Chapter 3 of lower trauma exposure among married respondents perhaps assumes better definition in this context; although we initially attributed the result to marriage-related benefits of an instrumental or material sort (e.g., home during evenings, fewer bar fights, greater income), the more qualitative, relational aspects of marriage may be more pertinent (e.g., caring, companionship, belonging). Conversely, being unmarried may serve less as an index of chronic exposures to situational hazards and more as a potent marker of disturbed early attachment and entrenched psychopathology (Breslau et al., 2011).

Psychopathology is generally considered an outcome of trauma exposure instead of a predictor, limiting comparators for our results in the prior literature. Nonetheless, our finding that preexisting behavior disorders are associated with elevated risk of most traumas is consistent with data from several longitudinal cohort studies (Koenen et al., 2002, 2007; Breslau et al., 2006; Storr et al., 2007). Our finding that preexisting conduct disorder in particular confers strongest risk of lifetime traumatic exposure is consistent with previous findings in both U.S. civilian (Afifi et al., 2011) and military (Koenen et al., 2002, 2005) samples. Preexisting ADHD, in contrast, confers the least overall trauma liability relative to other disruptive disorders. Its modest relative risk for auto accidents was especially unexpected, given the vast public health literature devoted to ADHD-related road accidents (Barkley et al., 1993). However, a recent meta-analysis isolated such excess risk to ADHD-related drivers to cases with comorbid ODD, CD, and/or other conduct problems (Vaa, 2014). The modest risk of accidents among drivers with ADHD may also reflect higher treatment rates and/or more effective treatments for ADHD vs. other high-risk psychiatric disorders. A 58% reduction in risk of serious transport accidents was found for male Swedish Registry ADHD drivers under psychostimulants vs. untreated ADHD drivers (Chang et al., 2014).

Our finding that preexisting PTSD confers least overall risk for subsequent exposure to trauma seems at odds with the central role that trauma is hypothesized to play in the etiology and maintenance of the disorder. One possible interpretation of this finding is that trauma-exposed individuals become reactively risk averse, systematically selecting themselves *out* of future hazardous situations and settings. Slight support for this is seen in the minimally decreased but significant odds of accidents and injuries (OR = 0.9) and unexpected death of a loved one (OR = 0.9) among multivariate analyses. However, there is no corresponding decrease in relative risk for highly threatening traumas such as exposure to organized violence, participation in organized violence, or physical violence victimization (all OR = 1.0). Bivariate analyses show insignificantly reduced odds of being a civilian in a war zone and witnessing a physical fight at home, but significantly reduced odds of combat experience (OR = 0.8).

Another possibility is that traumatized individuals might defensively *disavow* danger as well as actively avoid it. Memory encoding and retrieval deficits are paradigmatic of PTSD phenomenology, and are characterized by overgeneral, fragmented, or biased recall (Klein et al., 2003; Brewin, 2011, 2016); and inaccurate self-report of discrete autobiographical memories in particular (Brennen et al., 2010). A limitation to interpretation here is that history of both prior psychiatric symptoms and traumas was assessed by self-report contemporaneously and retrospectively, after the onset of PTSD, and this may have impacted recall of the traumas. A final noteworthy possibility is that the low relative-risk of trauma exposure following PTSD diagnosis may reflect a beneficial treatment effect (i.e., effective treatment may have reduced the rates of recurrent exposures). However, this seems unlikely given that the survey was conducted in 29 countries across 6 continents, including numerous developing countries with poor access to mental health treatment.

An interesting corollary to PTSD's lowest overall trauma risk is separation anxiety's highest (96.6% significant positives in bivariate analyses). In the case of separation anxiety, however, disproportionately high, significant exposures to "fateful" events, such as toxic chemical exposure (OR = 2.8), human-made disaster (OR = 2.1), and natural disaster (OR = 1.6), suggest that these respondents may have higher "experienced" traumas, but not higher "actual" traumas. Something of this sort was demonstrated in a city-specific, prospective longitudinal survey that coded events with both Criterion A1 and A2 (intense fear response and helplessness) (Stein et al., 2002a). Presence of an anxiety disorder at baseline predicted increased reports of high A2 exposures at follow up. If a similar dynamic is at work in the WMH data, then the consistent association of separation anxiety disorder with high trauma exposure might be due to a reporting artifact.

Taken together, the results reported in this chapter show clearly that trauma exposure is far from random. To the extent that the associations documented here are causal, interventions either to prevent CAs or, more realistically, to provide treatment for individuals exposed to CAs might profitably include components designed to reduce the elevated risks of future trauma exposure documented here. The same could be said for psychotherapies provided to patients with the DSM-IV disorders considered here. It is relevant in this regard that the subsequent traumas linked to the CAs and disorders considered here are not only required for subsequent PTSD, but are also known to be powerful predictors of major depression (Dorsey et al., 2017), behavioral and substance use problems (Kilpatrick et al., 2003), psychosis (Read et al., 2005; Mayo et al., 2017), personality disorders (Golier et al., 2003; Bandelow et al., 2005), developmental delays

(Briggs-Gowan et al., 2010) and cognitive deficits (Karstens et al., 2017). Trauma has also been implicated in the transitions both between psychiatric disorders (Walsh et al., 2017) and from psychiatric disorders to serious physical disorders (McLaughlin et al., 2016). While an evaluation of the plausibility of developing interventions to reduce trauma exposure is beyond the scope of this chapter, the results reported here make it clear that the associations that might be the targets of such interventions are substantial.

References

Afifi, T. O., McMillan, K. A., Asmundson, G. J., Pietrzak, R. H., & Sareen, J. (2011). An examination of the relation between conduct disorder, childhood and adulthood traumatic events, and posttraumatic stress disorder in a nationally representative sample. *Journal of Psychiatric Research*, 45, 1564–72.

Amstadter, A. B., Aggen, S. H., Knudsen, G. P., Reichborn-Kjennerud, T., & Kendler, K. S. (2013). Potentially traumatic event exposure, posttraumatic stress disorder, and Axis I and II comorbidity in a population-based study of Norwegian young adults. *Social Psychiatry and Psychiatric Epidemiology*, 48, 215–23.

Bandelow, B., Krause, J., Wedekind, D., et al. (2005). Early traumatic life events, parental attitudes, family history, and birth risk factors in patients with borderline personality disorder and healthy controls. *Psychiatry Research*, 134, 169–79.

Barkley, R. A., Guevremont, D. C., Anastopoulos, A. D., DuPaul, G. J., & Shelton, T. L. (1993). Driving-related risks and outcomes of attention deficit hyperactivity disorder in adolescents and young adults: a 3- to 5-year follow-up survey. *Pediatrics*, 92, 212–18.

Barnes, J. E., Noll, J. G., Putnam, F. W., & Trickett, P. K. (2009). Sexual and physical revictimization among victims of severe childhood sexual abuse. *Child Abuse and Neglect*, 33, 412–20.

Black, D. S., Sussman, S., & Unger, J. B. (2010). A further look at the intergenerational transmission of violence: witnessing interparental violence in emerging adulthood. *Journal of Interpersonal Violence*, 25, 1022–42.

Brennen, T., Hasanovic, M., Zotovic, M., et al. (2010). Trauma exposure in childhood impairs the ability to recall specific autobiographical memories in late adolescence. *Journal of Traumatic Stress*, 23, 240–7.

Breslau, J., Miller, E., Jin, R., et al. (2011). A multinational study of mental disorders, marriage, and divorce. *Acta Psychiatrica Scandinavica*, 124, 474–86.

Breslau, N., Lucia, V. C., & Alvarado, G. F. (2006). Intelligence and other predisposing factors in exposure to trauma and posttraumatic stress disorder: a follow-up study at age 17 years. *Archives of General Psychiatry*, 63, 1238–45.

Brewin, C. R. (2011). The nature and significance of memory disturbance in posttraumatic stress disorder. *Annual Review of Clinical Psychology*, 7, 203–27.

(2016). Coherence, disorganization, and fragmentation in traumatic memory reconsidered: a response to Rubin et al. (2016). *Journal of Abnormal Psychology*, 125, 1011–17.

Briggs-Gowan, M. J., Carter, A. S., Clark, R., et al. (2010). Exposure to potentially traumatic events in early childhood: differential links to emergent psychopathology. *Journal of Child Psychology and Psychiatry and Allied Disciplines*, 51, 1132–40.

Brown, R. C., Berenz, E. C., Aggen, S. H., et al. (2014). Trauma exposure and Axis I psychopathology: a co-twin control analysis in Norwegian young adults. *Psychological Trauma: Theory, Research, Practice and Policy*, 6, 652–60.

Busso, D. S., McLaughlin, K. A., Brueck, S., et al. (2017). Child abuse, neural structure, and adolescent psychopathology: a longitudinal study. *Journal of the American Academy of Child and Adolescent Psychiatry*, 56, 321–8.e1.

Calem, M., Bromis, K., McGuire, P., Morgan, C., & Kempton, M. J. (2017). Meta-analysis of associations between childhood adversity and hippocampus and amygdala volume in non-clinical and general population samples. *NeuroImage: Clinical*, 14, 471–9.

Center on the Developing Child at Harvard University (2012). The science of neglect: the persistent absence of responsive care disrupts the developing brain, Working Paper No. 12 (online). Available at: www.developingchild.harvard.edu (Accessed July 1, 2017).

Chang, Z., Lichtenstein, P., D'Onofrio, B. M., Sjolander, A., & Larsson, H. (2014). Serious transport accidents in adults with attention-deficit/hyperactivity disorder and the effect of medication: a population-based study. *JAMA Psychiatry*, 71, 319–25.

Chang, Z., Quinn, P. D., Hur, K., et al. (2017). Association between medication use for attention-deficit/hyperactivity disorder and risk of motor vehicle crashes. *JAMA Psychiatry*, 74, 597–603.

Cohen, J. R., Menon, S. V., Shorey, R. C., Le, V. D., & Temple, J. R. (2017). The distal consequences of physical and emotional neglect in emerging adults: a person-centered, multi-wave, longitudinal study. *Child Abuse and Neglect*, 63, 151–61.

Coid, J., Petruckevitch, A., Feder, G., et al. (2001). Relation between childhood sexual and physical abuse and risk of revictimisation in women: a cross-sectional survey. *Lancet*, 358, 450–4.

Conley, A. H., Overstreet, C. M., Hawn, S. E., et al. (2017). Prevalence and predictors of sexual assault among a college sample. *Journal of American College Health*, 65, 41–9.

Courtney, M. E., Piliavin, I., Grogan-Kaylor, A., & Nesmith, A. (1998). *Foster Youth Transitions to Adulthood: A Longitudinal View of Youth Leaving Care*. Madison, WI: Institute for Research on Poverty.

Cuevas, C. A., Finkelhor, D., Ormrod, R., & Turner, H. (2009). Psychiatric diagnosis as a risk marker for victimization in a national sample of children. *Journal of Interpersonal Violence*, 24, 636–52.

Cui, M., Durtschi, J. A., Donnellan, M. B., Lorenz, F. O., & Conger, R. D. (2010). Intergenerational transmission of relationship aggression: a prospective longitudinal study. *Journal of Family Psychology*, 24, 688–97.

Darves-Bornoz, J. M., Lempérière, T., Degiovanni, A., & Gaillard, P. (1995). Sexual victimization in women with schizophrenia and bipolar disorder. *Social Psychiatry and Psychiatric Epidemiology*, 30, 78–84.

Dorsey, S., McLaughlin, K. A., Kerns, S. E. U., et al. (2017). Evidence base update for psychosocial treatments for children and adolescents exposed to traumatic events. *Journal of Clinical Child and Adolescent Psychology*, 46, 303–30.

Ehrensaft, M. K., Cohen, P., Brown, J., et al. (2003). Intergenerational transmission of partner violence: a 20-year prospective study. *Journal of Consulting and Clinical Psychology*, 71, 741–53.

Eisenberg, N., Fabes, R. A., Guthrie, I. K., & Reiser, M. (2002). The role of emotionality and regulation in children's social competence and adjustment. In L. Pulkkinen, & A. Caspi, eds., *Paths to Successful Development: Personality in the Life Course*. Cambridge, England: Cambridge University Press, pp. 46–72.

Endicott, J., Andreasen, N., & Spitzer, R. L. (1978). *Family History Research Diagnostic Criteria*. New York, NY: Biometrics Research, NY State Psychiatric Institute.

Fazel, S., Lichtenstein, P., Grann, M., Goodwin, G. M., & Langstrom, N. (2010). Bipolar disorder and violent crime: new evidence from population-based longitudinal studies and systematic review. *Archives of General Psychiatry*, 67, 931–8.

Finkelhor, D., Ormrod, R. K., & Turner, H. A. (2007). Poly-victimization: a neglected component in child victimization. *Child Abuse and Neglect*, 31, 7–26.

Garner, A. A., Gentry, A., Welburn, S. C., et al. (2014). Symptom dimensions of disruptive behavior disorders in adolescent drivers. *Journal of Attention Disorders*, 18, 496–503.

Golier, J. A., Yehuda, R., Bierer, L. M., et al. (2003). The relationship of borderline personality disorder to posttraumatic stress disorder and traumatic events. *American Journal of Psychiatry*, 160, 2018–24.

Gover, A. R., Kaukinen, C., & Fox, K. A. (2008). The relationship between violence in the family of origin and dating violence among college students. *Journal of Interpersonal Violence*, 23, 1667–93.

Helzer, E. G., Connor-Smith, J. K., & Reed, M. A. (2009). Traits, states, and attentional gates: temperament and threat relevance as predictors of attentional bias to social threat. *Anxiety Stress Coping*, 22, 57–76.

Hiroeh, U., Appleby, L., Mortensen, P. B., & Dunn, G. (2001). Death by homicide, suicide, and other unnatural causes in people with mental illness: a population-based study. *Lancet*, 358, 2110–12.

Howlett, J. R., & Stein, M. B. (2016). Prevention of trauma and stressor-related disorders: a review. *Neuropsychopharmacology*, 41, 357–69.

Jaksic, N., Brajkovic, L., Ivezic, E., Topic, R., & Jakovljevic, M. (2012). The role of personality traits in posttraumatic stress disorder (PTSD). *Psychiatria Danubina*, 24, 256–66.

Jang, K. L., Stein, M. B., Taylor, S., Asmundson, G. J., & Livesley, W. J. (2003). Exposure to traumatic events and experiences: aetiological relationships with personality function. *Psychiatry Research*, 120, 61–9.

Kanai, Y., Takaesu, Y., Nakai, Y., et al. (2016). The influence of childhood abuse, adult life events, and affective temperaments on the well-being of the general, nonclinical adult population. *Neuropsychiatric Disease and Treatment*, 12, 823–32.

Karstens, A. J., Rubin, L. H., Shankman, S. A., et al. (2017). Investigating the separate and interactive associations of trauma and depression on neurocognition in urban dwelling adults. *Journal of Psychiatric Research*, 89, 6–13.

Kendler, K. S., Gardner, C. O., & Prescott, C. A. (2003). Personality and the experience of environmental adversity. *Psychological Medicine*, 33, 1193–202.

Kendler, K. S., Myers, J., & Prescott, C. A. (2002). The etiology of phobias: an evaluation of the stress-diathesis model. *Archives of General Psychiatry*, 59, 242–8.

Kendler, K. S., Silberg, J. L., Neale, M. C., et al. (1991). The family history method: whose psychiatric history is measured? *American Journal of Psychiatry*, 148, 1501–4.

Kessler, R. C., Akiskal, H. S., Angst, J., et al. (2006). Validity of the assessment of bipolar spectrum disorders in the WHO CIDI 3.0. *Journal of Affective Disorders*, 96, 259–69.

Kessler, R. C., McLaughlin, K. A., Green, J. G., et al. (2010). Childhood adversities and adult psychopathology in the WHO World Mental Health Surveys. *British Journal of Psychiatry*, 197, 378–85.

Kessler, R. C., & Üstün, T. B. (2004). The World Mental Health (WMH) Survey Initiative version of the World Health Organization (WHO) Composite International Diagnostic Interview (CIDI). *International Journal of Methods in Psychiatric Research*, 13, 93–121.

Kilpatrick, D. G., Ruggiero, K. J., Acierno, R., et al. (2003). Violence and risk of PTSD, major depression, substance abuse/dependence, and comorbidity: results from the National Survey of Adolescents. *Journal of Consulting and Clinical Psychology*, 71, 692–700.

Klein, E., Caspi, Y., & Gil, S. (2003). The relation between memory of the traumatic event and PTSD: evidence from studies of traumatic brain injury. *The Canadian Journal of Psychiatry. La Revue Canadienne de Psychiatrie*, 48, 28–33.

Knäuper, B., Cannell, C. F., Schwarz, N., Bruce, M. L., & Kessler, R. C. (1999). Improving accuracy of major depression age-of-onset reports in the US National Comorbidity Survey. *International Journal of Methods in Psychiatric Research*, 8, 39–48.

Koenen, K. C., Fu, Q. J., Lyons, M. J., et al. (2005). Juvenile conduct disorder as a risk factor for trauma exposure and posttraumatic stress disorder. *Journal of Traumatic Stress*, 18, 23–32.

Koenen, K. C., Harley, R., Lyons, M. J., et al. (2002). A twin registry study of familial and individual risk factors for trauma exposure and posttraumatic stress disorder. *Journal of Nervous and Mental Disease*, 190, 209–18.

Koenen, K. C., Moffitt, T. E., Poulton, R., Martin, J., & Caspi, A. (2007). Early childhood factors associated with the development of post-traumatic stress disorder: results from a longitudinal birth cohort. *Psychological Medicine*, 37, 181–92.

Lam, D. H., Hayward, P., Watkins, E. R., Wright, K., & Sham, P. (2005). Relapse prevention in patients with bipolar disorder: cognitive therapy outcome after 2 years. *American Journal of Psychiatry*, 162, 324–9.

Lang, A. J., & Gartstein, M. A. (2017). Intergenerational transmission of traumatization: theoretical framework and implications for prevention. *Journal of Trauma & Dissociation*, 19, 162–75.

Macklin, M. L., Metzger, L. J., Litz, B. T., et al. (1998). Lower precombat intelligence is a risk factor for posttraumatic stress disorder. *Journal of Consulting and Clinical Psychology*, 66, 323–6.

Mayo, D., Corey, S., Kelly, L. H., et al. (2017). The role of trauma and stressful life events among individuals at clinical high risk for psychosis: a review. *Frontiers in Psychiatry*, 8, 55.

McClennen, J. C., Keys, A. M., & Dugan-Day, M. L. (2016). *Social Work and Family Violence: Theories, Assessment, and Intervention*, 2nd edn. New York, NY: Springer Publishing Company.

McLaughlin, K. A., Basu, A., Walsh, K., et al. (2016). Childhood exposure to violence and chronic physical conditions in a national sample of US adolescents. *Psychosomatic Medicine*, 78, 1072–83.

McLaughlin, K. A., Sheridan, M. A., & Nelson, C. A. (2017). Neglect as a violation of species-expectant experience: neurodevelopmental consequences. *Biological Psychiatry*, 82, 462–71.

Millett, L. S., Kohl, P. L., Jonson-Reid, M., Drake, B., & Petra, M. (2013). Child maltreatment victimization and subsequent perpetration of young adult intimate partner violence. *Child Maltreatment*, 18, 71–84.

Moore, A. A., Overstreet, C., Kendler, K. S., et al. (2017). Potentially traumatic events, personality, and risky sexual behavior in undergraduate college students. *Psychological Trauma: Theory, Research, Practice and Policy*, 9, 105–12.

Naughton, A. M., Cowley, L. E., Tempest, V., et al. (2017). Ask Me! self-reported features of adolescents experiencing neglect or emotional maltreatment: a rapid systematic review. *Child: Care, Health and Development*, 43, 348–60.

Netto, L. R., Pereira, J. L., Nogueira, J. F., et al. (2016). Impulsivity is relevant for trauma exposure and PTSD symptoms in a non-clinical population. *Psychiatry Research*, 239, 204–11.

Noll, J. G., Horowitz, L. A., Bonanno, G. A., Trickett, P. K., & Putnam, F. W. (2003). Revictimization and self-harm in females who experienced childhood sexual abuse: results from a prospective study. *Journal of Interpersonal Violence*, 18, 1452–71.

Ogden, T. H. (2016). Destruction reconceived: on Winnicott's 'The Use of an Object and Relating through Identifications'. *International Journal of Psycho-Analysis*, 97, 1243–62.

Ogle, C. M., Rubin, D. C., & Siegler, I. C. (2014). Cumulative exposure to traumatic events in older adults. *Aging & Mental Health*, 18, 316–25.

Overstreet, C., Berenz, E. C., Kendler, K. S., Dick, D. M., & Amstadter, A. B. (2017). Predictors and mental health outcomes of potentially traumatic event exposure. *Psychiatry Research*, 247, 296–304.

Read, J., van Os, J., Morrison, A. P., & Ross, C. A. (2005). Childhood trauma, psychosis and schizophrenia: a literature review with theoretical and clinical implications. *Acta Psychiatrica Scandinavica*, 112, 330–50.

Schmeck, K., & Poustka, F. (2001). Temperament and disruptive behavior disorders. *Psychopathology*, 34, 159–63.

Shackman, A. J., Stockbridge, M. D., Tillman, R. M., et al. (2016). The neurobiology of dispositional negativity and attentional biases to threat: implications for understanding anxiety disorders in adults and youth. *Journal of Experimental Psychopathology*, 7, 311–42.

Silverman, W. K., Ortiz, C. D., Viswesvaran, C., et al. (2008). Evidence-based psychosocial treatments for children and adolescents exposed to traumatic events. *Journal of Clinical Child and Adolescent Psychology*, 37, 156–83.

Stein, M. B., Hofler, M., Perkonigg, A., et al. (2002a). Patterns of incidence and psychiatric risk factors for traumatic events. *International Journal of Methods in Psychiatric Research*, 11, 143–53.

Stein, M. B., Jang, K. L., Taylor, S., Vernon, P. A., & Livesley, W. J. (2002b). Genetic and environmental influences on trauma exposure and posttraumatic stress disorder symptoms: a twin study. *American Journal of Psychiatry*, 159, 1675–81.

Stith, S. M., Smith, D. B., Penn, C. E., Ward, D. B., & Tritt, D. (2004). Intimate partner physical abuse perpetration and victimization risk factors: a meta-analytic review. *Aggression and Violent Behavior*, 10, 65–98.

Storr, C. L., Ialongo, N. S., Anthony, J. C., & Breslau, N. (2007). Childhood antecedents of exposure to traumatic events and posttraumatic stress disorder. *American Journal of Psychiatry*, 164, 119–25.

Straus, M. A. (1979). Measuring intrafamily conflict and violence: the Conflict Tactics (CT) Scales. *Journal of Marriage and the Family*, 41, 75–88.

Taskesen, A., Demirkale, I., Taskesen, N., Okumus, M., & Can, D. O. (2017). Irritable temperament profile prevails among patients with boxer fractures. *European Journal of Trauma and Emergency Surgery*, 43, 869–83.

Vaa, T. (2014). ADHD and relative risk of accidents in road traffic: a meta-analysis. *Accident Analysis and Prevention*, 62, 415–25.

Walsh, K., McLaughlin, K. A., Hamilton, A., & Keyes, K. M. (2017). Trauma exposure, incident psychiatric disorders, and disorder transitions in a longitudinal population representative sample. *Journal of Psychiatric Research*, 92, 212–18.

Wolff, K. T., & Baglivio, M. T. (2016). Adverse childhood experiences, negative emotionality, and pathways to juvenile recidivism. *Crime & Delinquency*, 63, 1495–521.

Appendix

Table 4.A1 Bivariate associations of MFF CAs with the subsequent onset of traumas aggregated in 26 WMH surveys[a]

	Parent psychopathology		Parent substance misuse		Parent criminality		Family violence		Physical abuse		Neglect	
	OR	(95% CI)	OR	(95% CI)	OR	(95% CI)	OR	(95% CI)	OR	(95% CI)	OR	(95% CI)
I Exposure to Organized Violence												
Relief worker in war zone	1.4	(0.9–2.2)	1.5	(0.8–2.7)	0.7	(0.3–1.6)	0.8	(0.3–2.7)	0.9	(0.4–2.1)	1.5	(0.9–2.6)
Civilian in war zone	1.4*	(1.0–1.8)	1.1	(0.8–1.5)	1.8*	(1.2–2.7)	1.2	(0.7–2.0)	1.5	(0.9–2.6)	1.7*	(1.2–2.4)
Civilian in region of terror	2.0*	(1.6–2.5)	1.7*	(1.3–2.2)	1.6*	(1.2–2.2)	2.2*	(1.3–3.7)	2.1*	(1.3–3.3)	2.0*	(1.5–2.7)
Refugee	2.7*	(1.8–4.0)	1.4	(0.8–2.3)	1.7	(0.9–3.3)	1.1	(0.5–2.4)	1.4	(0.6–3.2)	2.0*	(1.2–3.4)
Kidnapped	2.2*	(1.6–2.9)	1.9*	(1.3–2.9)	3.2*	(2.2–4.6)	1.4	(0.5–4.4)	2.1*	(1.1–4.3)	2.8*	(1.9–4.2)
Any	1.9*	(1.6–2.1)	1.4*	(1.2–1.7)	1.9*	(1.6–2.3)	1.7*	(1.2–2.4)	1.6*	(1.2–2.3)	2.0*	(1.6–2.4)
II Participation in Organized Violence												
Witnessed death/dead body/serious injury	1.8*	(1.7–1.9)	1.5*	(1.4–1.7)	1.9*	(1.7–2.1)	1.4*	(1.2–1.8)	1.4*	(1.2–1.7)	1.7*	(1.5–1.8)
Accidentally caused serious injury/death	2.3*	(1.7–3.3)	2.2*	(1.4–3.5)	2.5*	(1.5–4.1)	1.2	(0.5–3.2)	2.0	(0.9–4.8)	2.9*	(1.9–4.4)
Combat experience	1.3	(0.9–1.7)	1.2	(0.8–1.8)	1.6	(1.0–2.4)	1.1	(0.5–2.5)	2.2*	(1.1–4.4)	1.7*	(1.1–2.4)
Purposely injured/tortured/killed someone	3.9*	(2.6–5.7)	2.2*	(1.3–3.5)	2.6*	(1.6–4.2)	2.8*	(1.1–6.8)	1.0	(0.4–2.5)	3.6*	(2.1–6.2)
Witnessed atrocities	2.0*	(1.6–2.5)	1.7*	(1.3–2.3)	2.0*	(1.5–2.6)	1.5	(0.8–2.7)	2.3*	(1.6–3.5)	2.3*	(1.8–3.0)
Any	1.9*	(1.7–2.0)	1.5*	(1.4–1.7)	1.9*	(1.7–2.2)	1.5*	(1.2–1.8)	1.5*	(1.2–1.8)	1.8*	(1.6–2.0)
III Physical Violence Victimization												
Beaten by caregiver	2.9*	(2.5–3.3)	3.0*	(2.5–3.5)	2.9*	(2.5–3.5)	4.3*	(3.2–5.8)	1.3	(0.9–1.8)	5.0*	(4.3–5.8)
Beaten by someone else	2.3*	(2.0–2.6)	1.9*	(1.5–2.3)	2.2*	(1.9–2.7)	2.3*	(1.7–3.2)	1.9*	(1.3–2.7)	3.0*	(2.5–3.5)
Witnessed physical fight at home	3.2*	(2.8–3.7)	4.8*	(4.1–5.6)	3.7*	(3.0–4.6)	0.4*	(0.2–0.8)	2.7*	(2.0–3.6)	3.6*	(3.1–4.2)
Any	2.7*	(2.5–2.9)	3.1*	(2.8–3.4)	3.2*	(2.9–3.5)	2.3*	(1.9–2.8)	1.7*	(1.4–2.0)	4.0*	(3.6–4.3)
IV Sexual Violence Victimization												
Raped	2.7*	(2.2–3.2)	2.7*	(2.2–3.4)	2.9*	(2.3–3.7)	2.3*	(1.6–3.4)	2.3*	(1.5–3.5)	3.9*	(3.2–4.7)
Sexually assaulted	2.5*	(2.2–2.8)	2.0*	(1.7–2.4)	2.5*	(2.0–3.1)	2.2*	(1.5–3.1)	1.7*	(1.2–2.3)	2.3*	(1.9–2.7)
Stalked	2.5*	(2.1–2.8)	1.8*	(1.5–2.2)	2.4*	(2.0–2.9)	2.3*	(1.5–3.4)	1.5*	(1.1–2.1)	2.5*	(2.1–3.0)
Beaten by spouse/romantic partner	2.3*	(2.2–2.5)	2.0*	(1.7–2.4)	2.0*	(1.6–2.5)	2.1*	(1.5–2.8)	1.8*	(1.3–2.4)	3.2*	(2.7–3.8)
Trauma to loved one	2.4*	(2.0–2.8)	1.7*	(1.4–2.1)	2.5*	(2.0–3.2)	2.4*	(1.6–3.5)	1.5*	(1.1–2.1)	2.0*	(1.7–2.4)
Some other trauma	2.5*	(2.1–2.9)	1.3*	(1.0–1.7)	1.9*	(1.5–2.5)	1.4	(0.9–2.2)	1.3	(0.9–2.0)	2.1*	(1.7–2.7)
Private trauma[b]	2.6*	(2.2–3.0)	1.6*	(1.3–1.9)	2.2*	(1.7–2.7)	2.6*	(1.8–3.7)	1.5*	(1.0–2.1)	1.9*	(1.6–2.3)
Any	2.3*	(2.2–2.5)	1.8*	(1.6–2.0)	2.3*	(2.0–2.5)	2.1*	(1.7–2.5)	1.7*	(1.4–1.9)	2.5*	(2.3–2.8)

V Accidents/Injuries												
Natural disaster	1.6*	(1.4–1.9)	1.3*	(1.1–1.5)	1.5*	(1.3–1.8)	1.1	(0.7–1.7)	1.2	(0.9–1.7)	1.6*	(1.3–1.8)
Toxic chemical exposure	2.1*	(1.8–2.5)	1.5*	(1.1–1.9)	2.0*	(1.5–2.6)	2.3*	(1.4–3.8)	2.0*	(1.2–3.1)	2.2*	(1.7–2.9)
Automobile accident	1.6*	(1.4–1.8)	1.4*	(1.2–1.6)	1.5*	(1.3–1.8)	1.3	(1.0–1.7)	1.7*	(1.4–2.2)	1.2*	(1.1–1.4)
Life-threatening illness	1.8*	(1.6–2.0)	1.5*	(1.3–1.7)	1.5*	(1.3–1.8)	1.6*	(1.2–2.0)	1.5*	(1.1–1.9)	1.7*	(1.5–1.9)
Child with serious illness	1.6*	(1.4–1.9)	1.5*	(1.2–1.7)	1.6*	(1.3–1.9)	1.7*	(1.2–2.4)	1.5*	(1.1–2.2)	1.5*	(1.3–1.8)
Other life-threatening accident	1.8*	(1.5–2.1)	1.6*	(1.3–1.9)	1.4*	(1.1–1.8)	1.3	(0.8–1.9)	1.4	(1.0–1.8)	1.7*	(1.4–2.0)
Any	1.7*	(1.6–1.8)	1.4*	(1.3–1.6)	1.5*	(1.4–1.7)	1.4*	(1.2–1.7)	1.5*	(1.3–1.7)	1.6*	(1.4–1.7)
VI Other												
Mugged/threatened with a weapon	1.6	(1.5–1.8)	1.5*	(1.3–1.7)	1.6*	(1.4–1.9)	1.3	(0.9–1.9)	1.7*	(1.3–2.1)	1.5*	(1.3–1.6)
Human-made disaster	2.3	(1.9–2.7)	1.6*	(1.2–2.1)	2.1*	(1.7–2.7)	1.6*	(1.1–2.5)	1.4	(0.9–2.1)	1.9*	(1.5–2.5)
UD of a loved one	1.6	(1.5–1.7)	1.4*	(1.3–1.5)	1.6*	(1.4–1.7)	1.3*	(1.0–1.5)	1.5*	(1.3–1.8)	1.3*	(1.2–1.4)
VII Summary Statistics for Predictor across Traumas												
Percent positive ORs	100.0%		100.0%		96.6%		93.1%		93.1%		100.0%	
Percent positive and significant ORs	93.1%		86.2%		89.7%		55.2%		65.5%		96.6%	
Median (IQR) ORs	2.2	(1.6–2.5)	1.6	(1.5–1.9)	2.0	(1.6–2.5)	1.5	(1.3–2.3)	1.5	(1.4–2.0)	2.0	(1.7–2.8)

*Significant at the 0.05 level, two-sided test.

[a]Based on a series of multivariate survival models with person-year the unit of analysis and a logistic link function in which information about one and only one CA was used to predict the subsequent first onset of traumas. Controls were included for person-year, sex, age-at-interview, and survey.

[b]A *private* event is a trauma that some individuals reported in response to a question asked at the very end of the trauma section that asked if they ever had some other very upsetting experience they did not tell us about already (and this includes in response to a prior open-ended question about "any other" trauma) because they were too embarrassed or upset to talk about it. Respondents were told, before they answered, that if they reported such a trauma we would not ask them anything about what it was, only about their age when the trauma happened.

Table 4.A2 Bivariate associations of other CAs with the subsequent onset of individual traumas in 26 WMH surveys[a]

	Parent death		Parent divorce		Other parent loss		Serious physical illness		Economic adversity	
	OR	(95% CI)	OR	(95% CI)	OR	(95% CI)	OR	(95% CI)	OR	(95% CI)
I Exposure to Organized Violence										
Relief worker in war zone	1.2	(0.8–1.7)	1.1	(0.6–1.9)	1.2	(0.7–2.0)	0.9	(0.3–3.0)	0.5	(0.3–3.0)
Civilian in war zone	1.0	(0.9–1.3)	1.2	(0.9–1.7)	1.5*	(1.0–2.1)	0.4	(0.1–1.2)	0.8	(0.6–1.2)
Civilian in region of terror	1.2	(1.0–1.4)	1.1	(0.8–1.5)	1.5*	(1.1–1.9)	0.5*	(0.2–1.0)	1.3	(1.0–1.7)
Refugee	1.2	(0.9–1.6)	1.0	(0.6–1.6)	2.2*	(1.6–3.1)	1.1	(0.4–3.4)	1.5	(1.0–2.2)
Kidnapped	1.7*	(1.3–2.3)	2.2*	(1.5–3.2)	2.5*	(1.7–3.5)	2.5	(0.8–7.4)	1.5	(0.9–2.3)
Any	1.2*	(1.0–1.3)	1.4*	(1.2–1.6)	1.6*	(1.4–1.9)	0.7	(0.4–1.2)	1.0	(0.9–1.2)
II Participation in Organized Violence										
Witnessed death/dead body/serious injury	1.1	(1.0–1.1)	1.4*	(1.3–1.5)	1.4*	(1.3–1.5)	1.2	(0.9–1.5)	1.0	(0.9–1.1)
Accidentally caused serious injury/death	1.3	(0.9–1.8)	1.3	(0.9–1.9)	2.2*	(1.5–3.2)	2.9*	(1.1–7.4)	1.2	(0.7–1.9)
Combat experience	1.1	(0.9–1.3)	1.0	(0.7–1.4)	1.2	(0.9–1.6)	1.2	(0.5–2.8)	0.8	(0.6–1.2)
Purposely injured/tortured/killed someone	1.4*	(1.0–2.1)	1.6*	(1.0–2.5)	2.4*	(1.6–3.6)	1.6	(0.4–5.6)	1.8*	(1.2–2.9)
Witnessed atrocities	0.9	(0.8–1.1)	1.3*	(1.0–1.6)	1.7*	(1.4–2.2)	1.2	(0.6–2.6)	1.0	(0.7–1.3)
Any	1.1	(1.0–1.2)	1.3*	(1.2–1.5)	1.5*	(1.3–1.6)	1.1	(0.8–1.5)	1.0	(0.9–1.1)
III Physical Violence Victimization										
Beaten by caregiver	1.1*	(1.0–1.3)	1.6*	(1.3–1.8)	2.3*	(2.0–2.6)	1.4	(0.9–2.1)	1.5*	(1.3–1.9)
Beaten by someone else	1.2*	(1.0–1.4)	1.6*	(1.3–1.9)	2.2*	(1.8–2.6)	1.0	(0.6–1.8)	1.5*	(1.2–1.8)
Witnessed physical fight at home	0.9	(0.7–1.0)	2.2*	(1.9–2.6)	1.8*	(1.5–2.1)	1.2	(0.8–1.8)	1.8*	(1.5–2.3)
Any	1.1*	(1.0–1.2)	1.7*	(1.5–1.8)	2.1*	(1.9–2.3)	1.2	(0.9–1.6)	1.5*	(1.4–1.7)
IV Sexual Violence Victimization										
Raped	1.4*	(1.1–1.7)	1.6*	(1.3–2.0)	2.4*	(2.0–3.0)	2.0*	(1.2–3.5)	1.9*	(1.5–2.3)
Sexually assaulted	1.2*	(1.0–1.4)	1.6*	(1.4–1.9)	1.6*	(1.4–1.9)	1.1	(0.6–2.1)	1.6*	(1.3–1.9)
Stalked	1.1	(1.0–1.3)	1.5*	(1.3–1.8)	1.7*	(1.4–2.0)	1.3	(0.8–2.2)	1.2	(1.0–1.5)
Beaten by spouse/romantic partner	1.4*	(1.2–1.6)	1.5*	(1.2–1.9)	1.9*	(1.6–2.3)	1.5	(0.9–2.3)	1.4*	(1.1–1.7)
Trauma to loved one	1.1	(0.9–1.3)	1.5*	(1.3–1.8)	1.6*	(1.4–1.9)	1.3	(0.8–1.9)	1.6*	(1.3–1.9)
Some other trauma	1.0	(0.8–1.2)	1.2	(0.9–1.5)	1.7*	(1.4–2.2)	1.5	(0.9–2.6)	1.1	(0.8–1.4)
Private trauma[b]	1.1	(0.9–1.2)	1.5*	(1.2–1.8)	1.7*	(1.4–2.0)	1.3	(0.8–2.2)	1.3*	(1.1–1.6)
Any	1.2*	(1.1–1.2)	1.5*	(1.4–1.6)	1.8*	(1.7–2.0)	1.3*	(1.0–1.7)	1.4*	(1.3–1.5)

V Accidents/Injuries										
Natural disaster	1.2*	(1.0–1.4)	1.1	(0.9–1.4)	1.4*	(1.3–1.7)	1.2	(0.8–1.8)	0.9	(0.8–1.1)
Toxic chemical exposure	1.0	(0.9–1.2)	1.5*	(1.2–1.9)	1.4*	(1.1–1.8)	0.5*	(0.3–1.0)	1.2	(0.9–1.6)
Automobile accident	1.1	(1.0–1.2)	1.2*	(1.1–1.4)	1.3*	(1.2–1.5)	1.7*	(1.2–2.3)	1.0	(0.9–1.2)
Life-threatening illness	1.1*	(1.0–1.2)	1.3*	(1.1-1.4)	1.5*	(1.3–1.7)	1.1	(0.8–1.6)	1.2*	(1.1–1.4)
Child with serious illness	1.2*	(1.0–1.3)	1.3*	(1.1–1.6)	1.4*	(1.2–1.6)	1.1	(0.7–1.9)	1.2	(0.9–1.6)
Other life-threatening accident	1.0	(0.9–1.2)	1.5*	(1.2–1.8)	1.7*	(1.4–2.0)	1.5	(0.9–2.5)	1.1	(0.9–1.4)
Any	1.1*	(1.1–1.2)	1.3*	(1.2–1.4)	1.4*	(1.3–1.5)	1.3*	(1.1–1.5)	1.1*	(1.0–1.2)
VI Other										
Mugged/threatened with a weapon	1.0	(0.9–1.1)	1.4*	(1.2–1.5)	1.3*	(1.2–1.5)	1.8*	(1.3–2.5)	1.2*	(1.0–1.4)
Human-made disaster	1.0	(0.8–1.2)	1.3*	(1.1–1.6)	1.8*	(1.5–2.3)	1.0	(0.6–2.0)	1.3*	(1.0–1.6)
UD of a loved one	1.5*	(1.4–1.6)	1.1	(1.0–1.2)	1.2*	(1.1–1.3)	1.2	(0.9–1.5)	1.2*	(1.1–1.3)
VII Summary Statistics for Predictor across Traumas										
Percent positive ORs	89.7%		96.6%		100.0%		86.2%		79.3%	
Percent positive and significant ORs	37.9%		69.0%		93.1%		13.8%		44.8%	
Median (IQR) ORs	1.1	(1.0–1.2)	1.4	(1.2–1.5)	1.7	(1.4–1.9)	1.2	(1.1–1.5)	1.2	(1.1–1.5)

*Significant at the 0.05 level, two-sided test.

[a]Based on a series of multivariate survival models with person-year the unit of analysis and a logistic link function in which information about one and only one CA was used to predict the subsequent first onset of traumas. Controls were included for person-year, sex, age-at-interview, and survey.

[b]A *private* event is a trauma that some individuals reported in response to a question asked at the very end of the trauma section that asked if they ever had some other very upsetting experience they did not tell us about already (and this includes in response to a prior open-ended question about "any other" trauma) because they were too embarrassed or upset to talk about it. Respondents were told, before they answered, that if they reported such a trauma we would not ask them anything about what it was, only about their age when the trauma happened.

Table 4.A3 Bivariate associations of lifetime DSM-IV/CIDI mood and substance use disorders with the subsequent onset of individual traumas in 26 WMH surveys[a]

	Mood disorders				Substance use disorders			
	MDD or dysthymic disorder		BPD (broad definition)		Alcohol abuse or dependence		Drug abuse or dependence	
	OR	(95% CI)	OR	(95% CI)	OR	(95% CI)	OR	(95% CI)
I Exposure to Organized Violence								
Relief worker in war zone	1.1	(0.7–1.7)	1.0	(0.5–2.1)	2.0*	(1.4–3.0)	1.5	(0.8–2.8)
Civilian in war zone	1.2	(0.9–1.5)	1.7*	(1.1–2.7)	1.7*	(1.2–2.4)	2.9*	(1.8–4.6)
Civilian in region of terror	1.1	(0.9–1.4)	1.4	(0.9–2.3)	1.4*	(1.0–1.9)	1.9*	(1.3–2.7)
Refugee	1.9*	(1.3–2.6)	0.8	(0.3–2.1)	1.1	(0.6–2.1)	1.7	(0.8–3.6)
Kidnapped	2.5*	(1.9–3.4)	5.1*	(3.1–8.5)	3.6*	(2.4–5.2)	4.7*	(2.9–7.4)
Any	1.5*	(1.3–1.7)	2.2*	(1.7–2.8)	1.8*	(1.5–2.2)	2.6*	(2.0–3.3)
II Participation in Organized Violence								
Witnessed death/dead body/serious injury	1.6*	(1.5–1.7)	2.0*	(1.7–2.4)	1.7*	(1.5–1.9)	2.4*	(2.0–2.8)
Accidentally caused serious injury/death	2.6*	(1.9–3.5)	2.7*	(1.5–5.1)	2.9*	(2.1–3.9)	4.9*	(3.3–7.4)
Combat experience	1.0	(0.7–1.3)	1.4	(0.8–2.7)	1.2	(0.9–1.6)	1.4	(0.9–2.2)
Purposely injured/tortured/killed someone	3.9*	(2.5–6.1)	2.7*	(1.1–6.6)	3.8*	(2.5–5.7)	6.5*	(3.8–11.0)
Witnessed atrocities	1.5*	(1.2–1.9)	2.0*	(1.3–3.0)	1.5*	(1.2–1.8)	2.0*	(1.4–2.8)
Any	1.7*	(1.5–1.8)	2.2*	(1.9–2.6)	1.8*	(1.6–2.0)	2.5*	(2.2–2.9)
III Physical Violence Victimization								
Beaten by caregiver	1.2	(0.9–1.5)	1.5	(0.7–3.0)	0.3*	(0.1–0.6)	0.3*	(0.1–0.7)
Beaten by someone else	2.8*	(2.4–3.2)	3.5*	(2.6–4.6)	3.0*	(2.5–3.5)	3.5*	(2.8–4.4)
Witnessed physical fight at home	1.1	(0.8–1.5)	1.4	(0.7–2.8)	0.4*	(0.2–0.6)	0.4*	(0.2–0.7)
Any	2.0*	(1.8–2.3)	2.5*	(2.0–3.2)	2.4*	(2.2–2.8)	2.7*	(2.2–3.2)
IV Sexual Violence Victimization								
Raped	3.2*	(2.6–4.0)	3.5*	(2.3–5.4)	2.7*	(1.9–3.6)	2.9*	(2.0–4.4)
Sexually assaulted	2.6*	(2.2–3.0)	2.9*	(2.1–4.1)	1.7*	(1.3–2.1)	2.4*	(1.7–3.3)
Stalked	3.2*	(2.8–3.6)	4.6*	(3.7–5.8)	2.7*	(2.3–3.2)	4.0*	(3.3–4.9)
Beaten by spouse/romantic partner	2.6*	(2.3–2.9)	4.0*	(3.1–5.1)	5.1*	(4.2–6.1)	7.0*	(5.5–8.8)
Trauma to loved one	2.2*	(1.9–2.5)	2.7*	(2.1–3.5)	1.8*	(1.5–2.1)	2.4*	(1.9–2.9)
Some other trauma	2.6*	(2.3–3.0)	2.6*	(1.9–3.5)	1.6*	(1.4–1.9)	2.5*	(1.9–3.2)
Private trauma[b]	2.3*	(2.0–2.7)	2.9*	(2.1–3.9)	1.7*	(1.4–2.0)	2.5*	(1.8–3.3)
Any	2.5*	(2.4–2.7)	3.3*	(2.9–3.7)	2.2*	(2.0–2.4)	2.9*	(2.7–3.3)

V Accidents/Injuries								
Natural disaster	1.3*	(1.2–1.5)	1.8*	(1.4–2.4)	1.4*	(1.2–1.7)	1.4*	(1.0–1.8)
Toxic chemical exposure	1.6*	(1.3–1.9)	1.9*	(1.4–2.6)	2.4*	(2.0–2.8)	3.2*	(2.5–4.1)
Automobile accident	1.5*	(1.3–1.6)	2.2*	(1.8–2.7)	1.9*	(1.7–2.1)	2.0*	(1.7–2.3)
Life-threatening illness	1.6*	(1.4–1.7)	1.6*	(1.2–2.0)	1.7*	(1.5–1.9)	1.9*	(1.5–2.3)
Child with serious illness	1.6*	(1.4–1.8)	1.3	(1.0–1.6)	1.6*	(1.4–1.8)	1.8*	(1.4–2.3)
Other life-threatening accident	1.7*	(1.5–2.0)	2.2*	(1.7–2.9)	2.0*	(1.7–2.3)	2.3*	(1.8–2.8)
Any	1.5*	(1.4–1.6)	1.8*	(1.6–2.0)	1.7*	(1.6–1.8)	2.0*	(1.8–2.2)
VI Other								
Mugged/threatened with a weapon	2.0*	(1.8–2.1)	2.4*	(2.0–2.9)	1.9*	(1.7–2.1)	2.9*	(2.5–3.4)
Human-made disaster	1.7*	(1.5–2.1)	2.9*	(2.0–4.1)	2.5*	(2.0–3.2)	2.1*	(1.6–2.7)
UD of a loved one	1.4*	(1.3–1.5)	2.0*	(1.8–2.3)	1.7*	(1.5–1.8)	1.7*	(1.5–1.9)
VII Summary Statistics for Predictor across Traumas								
Percent positive ORs	96.6%		96.6%		93.1%		93.1%	
Percent positive and significant ORs	79.3%		75.9%		86.2%		82.8%	
Median (IQR) ORs	1.7	(1.4–2.6)	2.2	(1.6–2.9)	1.7	(1.6–2.5)	2.4	(1.8–2.9)

*Significant at the 0.05 level, two-sided test.

[a]Based on a series of multivariate survival models with person-year the unit of analysis and a logistic link function in which information about one and only one temporally primary disorder was used to predict the subsequent first onset of traumas. Controls were included for person-year, sex, age-at-interview, and survey.

[b]A *private* event is a trauma that some individuals reported in response to a question asked at the very end of the trauma section that asked if they ever had some other very upsetting experience they did not tell us about already (and this includes in response to a prior open-ended question about "any other" trauma) because they were too embarrassed or upset to talk about it. Respondents were told, before they answered, that if they reported such a trauma we would not ask them anything about what it was, only about their age when the trauma happened.

Table 4.A4 Bivariate associations of lifetime DSM-IV/CIDI anxiety disorders with the subsequent onset of individual traumas in 26 WMH surveys[a]

	Anxiety disorders											
	Panic disorder or agoraphobia		GAD		PTSD		Social phobia		Specific phobia		Separation anxiety disorder	
	OR	(95% CI)	OR	(95% CI)	OR	(95% CI)	OR	(95% CI)	OR	(95% CI)	OR	(95% CI)
I Exposure to Organized Violence												
Relief worker in war zone	1.2	(0.7–2.1)	0.4*	(0.2–0.9)	1.3	(0.9–1.8)	1.0	(0.6–1.6)	1.5	(1.0–2.4)	1.8	(0.9–3.7)
Civilian in war zone	1.5*	(1.0–2.2)	1.1	(0.7–1.6)	0.9	(0.8–1.1)	1.3	(1.0–1.7)	1.3*	(1.0–1.7)	2.7*	(1.6–4.6)
Civilian in region of terror	1.6*	(1.2–2.2)	1.3	(0.9–1.9)	1.0	(0.8–1.2)	1.3*	(1.0–1.7)	1.3*	(1.1–1.6)	2.0*	(1.3–3.0)
Refugee	0.9	(0.5–1.6)	1.1	(0.6–2.0)	1.6*	(1.2–2.1)	1.2	(0.8–1.8)	1.5	(0.9–2.4)	3.2 *	(1.6–6.3)
Kidnapped	3.0*	(2.1–4.4)	3.2*	(2.1–4.7)	1.6*	(1.3–2.1)	2.5*	(1.8–3.5)	2.0*	(1.5–2.7)	2.9 *	(1.9–4.6)
Any	1.6*	(1.3–1.9)	1.3*	(1.0–1.6)	1.1	(1.0–1.2)	1.6*	(1.4–1.9)	1.5*	(1.3–1.7)	2.4*	(1.8–3.1)
II Participation in Organized Violence												
Witnessed death/dead body/serious injury	2.0*	(1.8–2.2)	1.6*	(1.4–1.8)	1.2*	(1.1–1.2)	1.7*	(1.5–1.8)	1.9*	(1.7–2.0)	2.1*	(1.8–2.4)
Accidentally caused serious injury/death	2.1*	(1.3–3.4)	2.0*	(1.3–3.1)	1.4*	(1.1–1.8)	1.9*	(1.4–2.7)	2.1*	(1.5–3.0)	3.8*	(2.3–6.2)
Combat experience	1.6*	(1.1–2.5)	0.9	(0.5–1.5)	0.8*	(0.6–1.0)	1.4*	(1.0–2.0)	1.3	(1.0–1.9)	2.0*	(1.1–3.8)
Purposely injured/tortured/killed someone	3.3*	(1.9–5.8)	3.8*	(1.9–7.6)	2.0*	(1.5–2.8)	3.5*	(2.2–5.7)	1.8*	(1.2–2.7)	7.9*	(4.0—15.7)
Witnessed atrocities	1.7*	(1.3–2.4)	1.3	(0.9–1.8)	1.2	(1.0–1.3)	1.4*	(1.1–1.8)	1.8*	(1.5–2.2)	2.7*	(2.1–3.6)
Any	2.0*	(1.8–2.3)	1.5*	(1.4–1.8)	1.1*	(1.1–1.2)	1.7*	(1.6–1.9)	1.8*	(1.7–2.0)	2.1*	(1.8–2.4)
III Physical Violence Victimization												
Beaten by caregiver	2.3*	(1.7–3.1)	1.3	(0.8–1.9)	1.0	(0.9–1.2)	1.8*	(1.4–2.3)	2.5*	(2.2–2.9)	1.5*	(1.1–2.0)
Beaten by someone else	2.6*	(2.1–3.3)	2.4*	(1.9–2.9)	1.3*	(1.2–1.5)	2.5*	(2.1–2.9)	2.6*	(2.3–3.0)	3.0*	(2.3–3.7)
Witnessed physical fight at home	2.1*	(1.6–2.8)	1.5*	(1.1–2.2)	0.9	(0.8–1.1)	1.6*	(1.3–2.0)	2.2*	(1.9–2.5)	1.9*	(1.4–2.5)
Any	2.3*	(2.0–2.6)	1.9*	(1.6–2.2)	1.1*	(1.0–1.2)	1.8*	(1.6–2.0)	2.2*	(2.0–2.3)	1.8*	(1.6–2.1)
IV Sexual Violence Victimization												
Raped	4.6*	(3.5–6.0)	3.3*	(2.6–4.2)	1.4*	(1.2–1.7)	3.0*	(2.5–3.6)	2.8*	(2.4–3.3)	2.6*	(2.0–3.5)
Sexually assaulted	3.1*	(2.5–3.9)	2.2*	(1.8–2.7)	1.3*	(1.1–1.5)	2.9*	(2.5–3.3)	2.3*	(2.0–2.6)	2.7*	(2.2–3.4)
Stalked	2.9*	(2.4–3.5)	2.9*	(2.4–3.4)	1.7*	(1.6–1.9)	2.6*	(2.2–3.0)	2.5*	(2.2–2.8)	3.8*	(3.2–4.6)
Beaten by spouse/romantic partner	3.3*	(2.8–3.9)	2.5*	(2.1–3.1)	1.5*	(1.4–1.7)	2.6*	(2.2–3.1)	2.3*	(2.0–2.6)	3.0*	(2.6–3.6)
Trauma to loved one	2.3*	(1.9–2.8)	2.3*	(2.0–2.8)	1.4*	(1.3–1.6)	2.1*	(1.8–2.4)	2.1*	(1.8–2.3)	2.0*	(1.6–2.5)
Some other trauma	1.9*	(1.5–2.5)	2.6*	(2.2–3.1)	1.3*	(1.1–1.4)	1.8*	(1.5–2.1)	1.9*	(1.6–2.2)	2.2*	(1.6–2.9)
Private trauma[b]	2.3*	(1.9–2.9)	2.4*	(1.9–2.9)	1.2*	(1.1–1.3)	2.4*	(2.1–2.8)	2.2*	(1.9–2.6)	2.9*	(2.2–3.6)
Any	2.6*	(2.4–2.9)	2.5*	(2.3–2.7)	1.4*	(1.3–1.4)	2.3*	(2.1–2.4)	2.2*	(2.0–2.3)	2.6*	(2.4–2.9)

V Accidents/Injuries												
Natural disaster	1.9*	(1.5–2.4)	1.4*	(1.1–1.7)	1.1	(1.0–1.2)	1.1	(1.0–1.3)	1.8*	(1.5–2.0)	1.6*	(1.3–2.0)
Toxic chemical exposure	1.8*	(1.4–2.3)	2.1*	(1.7–2.7)	1.2*	(1.1–1.4)	2.1*	(1.8–2.5)	2.0*	(1.6–2.5)	2.8*	(2.1–3.9)
Automobile accident	1.5*	(1.3–1.8)	1.4*	(1.2–1.6)	1.0	(1.0–1.1)	1.6*	(1.4–1.8)	1.6*	(1.4–1.7)	1.8*	(1.5–2.1)
Life-threatening illness	1.5*	(1.3–1.8)	1.7*	(1.5–2.0)	0.9*	(0.9–1.0)	1.4*	(1.3–1.6)	1.5*	(1.4–1.7)	1.9*	(1.6–2.3)
Child with serious illness	1.7*	(1.5–2.0)	1.9*	(1.6–2.2)	1.0	(0.9–1.1)	1.6*	(1.4–1.8)	1.6*	(1.5–1.8)	1.7*	(1.4–2.1)
Other life-threatening accident	2.0*	(1.7–2.5)	1.8*	(1.4–2.2)	1.2*	(1.1–1.3)	1.4*	(1.2–1.7)	1.6*	(1.4–1.9)	2.1*	(1.7–2.6)
Any	1.7*	(1.5–1.8)	1.6*	(1.5–1.8)	1.0	(1.0–1.1)	1.5*	(1.4–1.6)	1.6*	(1.5–1.7)	1.8*	(1.6–2.0)
VI Other												
Mugged/threatened with a weapon	1.9*	(1.7–2.2)	1.7*	(1.5–2.0)	1.2*	(1.1–1.3)	1.9*	(1.8–2.2)	1.8*	(1.7–2.0)	2.1*	(1.9–2.4)
Human-made disaster	1.9*	(1.4–2.7)	2.0*	(1.4–2.7)	1.3*	(1.1–1.5)	1.9*	(1.6–2.3)	1.8*	(1.5–2.1)	2.1*	(1.6–2.8)
UD of a loved one	1.6*	(1.5–1.8)	1.5*	(1.3–1.6)	1.0	(0.9–1.0)	1.5*	(1.4–1.6)	1.7*	(1.6–1.8)	2.1*	(1.8–2.3)
VII Summary Statistics for Predictor across Traumas												
Percent positive ORs	96.6%		93.1%		79.3%		100.0%		100.0%		100.0%	
Percent positive and significant ORs	93.1%		75.9%		58.6%		86.2%		89.7%		96.6%	
Median (IQR) ORs	1.9	(1.6–2.3)	1.8	(1.4–2.4)	1.2	(1.0–1.4)	1.8	(1.4–2.4)	1.8	(1.6–2.2)	2.1	(2.0–2.9)

*Significant at the 0.05 level, two-sided test.

[a]Based on a series of multivariate survival models with person-year the unit of analysis and a logistic link function in which information about one and only one temporally primary disorder was used to predict the subsequent first onset of traumas. Controls were included for person-year, sex, age-at-interview, and survey.

[b]A *private* event is a trauma that some individuals reported in response to a question asked at the very end of the trauma section that asked if they ever had some other very upsetting experience they did not tell us about already (and this includes in response to a prior open-ended question about "any other" trauma) because they were too embarrassed or upset to talk about it. Respondents were told, before they answered, that if they reported such a trauma we would not ask them anything about what it was, only about their age when the trauma happened.

Table 4.A5 Bivariate associations of lifetime DSM-IV/CIDI disruptive behavior disorders with the subsequent onset of individual traumas in 26 WMH surveys[a]

	Disruptive behavioral disorders							
	ADHD		CD		IED		ODD	
	OR	(95% CI)	OR	(95% CI)	OR	(95% CI)	OR	(95% CI)
I Exposure to Organized Violence								
Relief worker in war zone	2.6*	(1.0–6.6)	2.5*	(1.1–5.8)	2.0	(0.8–4.8)	4.2*	(1.8–10.1)
Civilian in war zone	1.6	(0.9–2.8)	2.8*	(1.5–4.9)	1.2	(0.8–1.9)	3.5*	(2.2–5.8)
Civilian in region of terror	2.5*	(1.6–3.8)	3.3*	(2.0–5.4)	1.7*	(1.1–2.6)	3.3*	(2.1–5.0)
Refugee	2.4*	(1.2–4.5)	4.0*	(2.1–7.5)	1.7	(0.9–3.2)	2.1*	(1.0–4.4)
Kidnapped	2.8*	(1.5–5.3)	5.4*	(3.0–9.5)	2.5*	(1.5–4.1)	2.9*	(1.6–5.0)
Any	2.7*	(2.1–3.4)	3.9*	(2.9–5.2)	2.0*	(1.6–2.6)	3.5*	(2.7–4.4)
II Participation in Organized Violence								
Witnessed death/dead body/serious injury	2.7*	(2.3–3.2)	3.3*	(2.8–3.8)	2.2*	(2.0–2.6)	2.6*	(2.2–3.1)
Accidentally caused serious injury/death	4.9*	(2.8–8.9)	7.2*	(4.1–12.6)	7.0*	(4.1–12.1)	9.9*	(5.5–17.9)
Combat experience	2.3*	(1.4–3.8)	2.7*	(1.7–4.3)	2.4*	(1.6–3.7)	3.5*	(2.1–5.7)
Purposely injured/tortured/killed someone	5.8*	(3.2–10.8)	8.4*	(4.5–15.7)	7.3*	(4.5–11.7)	7.6*	(4.2–13.7)
Witnessed atrocities	3.3*	(2.2–5.1)	3.9*	(2.6–5.9)	2.8*	(1.9–4.1)	3.5*	(2.3–5.2)
Any	2.6*	(2.2–3.1)	3.4*	(2.8–4.2)	2.6*	(2.2–3.0)	3.1*	(2.6–3.7)
III Physical Violence Victimization								
Beaten by caregiver	3.6*	(2.6–4.9)	3.1*	(2.1–4.6)	1.2	(0.8–1.7)	3.7*	(2.6–5.3)
Beaten by someone else	3.6*	(2.5–5.0)	6.5*	(4.9–8.5)	4.0*	(3.0–5.1)	4.4*	(3.4–5.6)
Witnessed physical fight at home	2.6*	(1.8–3.7)	1.0	(0.6–1.8)	1.4	(0.9–2.1)	2.5*	(1.7–3.6)
Any	3.1*	(2.6–3.7)	3.8*	(3.2–4.4)	2.4*	(2.0–2.8)	3.2*	(2.7–3.8)
IV Sexual Violence Victimization								
Raped	4.5*	(3.0–6.8)	4.5*	(3.0–6.7)	2.5*	(1.9–3.2)	4.7*	(3.5–6.4)
Sexually assaulted	3.0*	(2.4–3.9)	3.5*	(2.4–4.9)	2.8*	(2.2–3.6)	3.4*	(2.6–4.4)
Stalked	3.3*	(2.6–4.2)	4.1*	(2.9–5.6)	3.2*	(2.6–4.0)	3.6*	(2.8–4.5)
Beaten by spouse/romantic partner	3.2*	(2.3–4.3)	6.9*	(5.0–9.6)	3.4*	(2.8–4.1)	4.9*	(3.8–6.3)
Trauma to loved one	3.2*	(2.4–4.4)	2.6*	(1.9–3.4)	2.3*	(1.7–3.0)	3.1*	(2.4–3.9)
Some other trauma	2.3*	(1.6–3.2)	2.8*	(2.0–4.0)	1.8*	(1.3–2.4)	2.9*	(2.2–3.9)
Private trauma[b]	3.1*	(2.2–4.3)	3.1*	(2.3–4.2)	2.7*	(2.0–3.6)	2.9*	(2.1–4.0)
Any	2.9*	(2.6–3.3)	3.6*	(3.2–4.0)	2.5*	(2.3–2.8)	3.2*	(2.9–3.6)

V Accidents/Injuries								
Natural disaster	2.4*	(1.9–3.0)	1.9*	(1.4–2.6)	1.6*	(1.2–2.0)	2.0*	(1.6–2.5)
Toxic chemical exposure	3.1*	(2.2–4.3)	2.7*	(1.9–3.8)	2.1*	(1.6–2.8)	2.8*	(1.9–4.1)
Automobile accident	2.3*	(1.9–2.8)	2.7*	(2.2–3.2)	2.1*	(1.7–2.5)	2.3*	(1.9–2.7)
Life-threatening illness	1.9*	(1.4–2.6)	2.0*	(1.4–2.8)	1.5*	(1.2–1.8)	2.1*	(1.6–2.7)
Child with serious illness	1.5*	(1.1–2.1)	1.9*	(1.4–2.5)	1.8*	(1.5–2.2)	1.9*	(1.5–2.6)
Other life-threatening accident	2.1*	(1.6–2.9)	2.4*	(1.7–3.4)	1.6*	(1.2–2.2)	2.1*	(1.6–2.9)
Any	2.2*	(1.9–2.5)	2.4*	(2.1–2.7)	1.8*	(1.6–2.0)	2.3*	(2.0–2.5)
VI Other								
Mugged/threatened with a weapon	2.1*	(1.7–2.4)	3.3*	(2.8–4.0)	2.5*	(2.1–2.8)	2.9*	(2.5–3.5)
Human-made disaster	2.9*	(1.8–4.7)	3.6*	(2.4–5.4)	2.4*	(1.8–3.3)	3.3*	(2.4–4.5)
UD of a loved one	2.0*	(1.7–2.2)	2.2*	(1.9–2.6)	1.7*	(1.5–2.0)	2.5*	(2.2–2.8)
VII Summary Statistics for Predictor across Traumas								
Percent positive ORs	100.0%		100.0%		100.0%		100.0%	
Percent positive and significant ORs	96.6%		96.6%		82.8%		100.0%	
Median (IQR) ORs	2.7	(2.3–3.2)	3.1	(2.6–4.0)	2.2	(1.7–2.7)	3.1	(2.5–3.6)

*Significant at the 0.05 level, two-sided test.

[a]Based on a series of multivariate survival models with person-year the unit of analysis and a logistic link function in which information about one and only one temporally primary disorder was used to predict the subsequent first onset of traumas. Controls were included for person-year, sex, age-at-interview, and survey.

[b]A *private* event is a trauma that some individuals reported in response to a question asked at the very end of the trauma section that asked if they ever had some other very upsetting experience they did not tell us about already (and this includes in response to a prior open-ended question about "any other" trauma) because they were too embarrassed or upset to talk about it. Respondents were told, before they answered, that if they reported such a trauma we would not ask them anything about what it was, only about their age when the trauma happened.

Chapter 5

Population Prevalence of Posttraumatic Stress Disorder

Karestan C. Koenen, Andrew Ratanatharathorn, Evelyn J. Bromet, Elie G. Karam, and Dan J. Stein

We saw in Chapter 3 that trauma is very common globally. Although the majority of trauma-exposed individuals respond with resilience, a substantial minority go on to develop posttraumatic stress disorder (PTSD), the cardinal trauma-related mental disorder. Previous studies have shown that lifetime prevalence of PTSD varies widely across countries (Breslau, 2009). Surveys that ask about the worst trauma (as identified by respondents) generally find higher rates of PTSD, ranging from 1.7% in South Korea (Jeon et al., 2007) to 9.2% in Canada (Van Ameringen et al., 2008), than surveys that assess PTSD in relation to a random trauma. Examples of the lower PTSD prevalence rates found in surveys based on random traumas are 2.3% in South Africa (Atwoli et al., 2013), 2.5% in Iraq (Alhasnawi et al., 2009), and 3.4% in Lebanon (Karam et al., 2008). The wide variation in the national prevalence estimates suggests that an accurate picture of the worldwide prevalence of PTSD requires surveying countries across the globe using a consistent instrument, sampling procedures, and analytic approach.

No previous study brought together estimates of lifetime, 12-month, and 30-day PTSD prevalence across the range of countries available in the WMH surveys. While the proportion of 12-month cases among lifetime cases is an indicator of PTSD persistence, the 30-day prevalence estimate gives the most direct estimate of the population burden of PTSD at a point in time. We report country-specific estimates of PTSD prevalence for all these time frames in the current chapter.

Reviews and meta-analyses examining the correlates of PTSD have consistently found that socio-demographic indicators of social disadvantage are associated with high prevalence of the disorder (Brewin et al., 2000; Tolin & Foa, 2006; Ozer et al., 2008). These include younger age at the time of trauma, low socio-economic status, and being female. However, these associations between demographic correlates and PTSD have been found to vary by study design (e.g., prospective vs. retrospective), study population (e.g., civilian vs. military) (Brewin et al., 2000), and country income level (Atwoli et al., 2015).

Few studies have examined socio-demographic correlates of PTSD persistence. Research on other mental disorders has shown differing associations of socio-demographic factors with disorder onset and course. For example, in the United States, racial/ethnic minority status is associated with decreased risk of developing a substance-abuse-related disorder, but increased risk of the disorder becoming chronic (Breslau et al., 2005). Also in the United States, major depressive disorder is less prevalent, but more likely to be chronic, among minority groups (Williams et al., 2007). Likewise, women are at higher risk than men of lifetime depression, even though they typically have a similar course of depression to men (Kessler, 2003).

The current chapter fills in the above gaps by presenting country-specific data on PTSD prevalence. Specifically, we address three limitations of previous research. First, no previous report has brought together trauma exposure and PTSD prevalence rates across all the WMH survey countries for summary and comparison. Second, the WMH surveys addressed issues of study heterogeneity affecting cross-national prevalence estimates by using standardized methods for sample selection and assessment across all countries. Third, this report examines whether socio-demographic correlates, extensively documented in United States and European samples, are evident across country income levels.

Methods

The set of low- and lower-middle-income countries considered here is different in two ways from the core set described in Chapter 2 and used in the analyses in Chapters 3 and 4. First, the national WMH survey in Iraq is included here, as that survey assessed PTSD. The Iraq survey is not included in the core set of WMH surveys used in most other chapters, though, because information was not collected about type of trauma exposure. Second, the regional WMH survey in Nigeria is not included here because of the extremely low prevalence of PTSD. The revised sample included 26 surveys in 24 countries, 18 of which are based on nationally representative samples, and the other eight on regional samples. A total of 123,298 respondents in these surveys completed Part I of the interview, and 71,083 completed Part II, with a weighted mean response rate of 70.6%.

As detailed in Chapter 2, the Composite International Diagnostic Interview (CIDI) was used to assess PTSD according to DSM-IV criteria. Six measures of PTSD prevalence are reported in this chapter: lifetime prevalence in the total sample; lifetime prevalence among respondents who were exposed to at least one lifetime trauma; 12-month prevalence among the lifetime-exposed; 30-day prevalence among the lifetime-exposed; 12-month prevalence among lifetime cases; and 30-day prevalence among 12-month cases. The last two estimates provide indirect data on persistence. We also look at socio-demographic correlates, including age, sex, employment status (employed, student, homemaker, retired, unemployed), marital status (never married, divorced/separated/widowed, currently married), education level (no education, some primary, finished primary, some secondary, finished secondary, some college, finished college), and household income relative to national standards (low, low-average, high-average, high).

Cross-tabulations were used to calculate prevalence. The actuarial method implemented in SAS 9.4 was used to generate age-of-onset (AOO) and projected lifetime risk of PTSD (Wolter, 2007). Survival models were used to estimate the associations of correlates with lifetime PTSD controlling for country. Associations between socio-demographic correlates and 12-month PTSD among lifetime cases were estimated using logistic regression controlling for time since PTSD onset, age of PTSD onset, sex, and country. Age of PTSD onset was defined separately within each country with the 25% of PTSD cases (25th percentile) having earliest onsets defined as early-onset cases followed by early-average (50th percentile), late-average (75th percentile), and late onset. Significance was calculated using Wald and McNemar's Chi-square tests. Because the data were weighted and clustered, the Taylor series linearization method implemented in the SUDAAN software package was used to estimate design-based standard errors. Statistical significance was evaluated using two-sided tests, with $p < 0.05$ considered significant.

Results

Prevalence

Lifetime prevalence of PTSD in the total sample was 3.9%, but with significant variation across countries. Prevalence in high-income countries (5.0%) was more than twice the rate found in both upper-middle-income countries (2.3%) and low- and lower-middle-income countries (2.1%) (see Table 5.1). Among respondents who experienced a trauma, lifetime PTSD prevalence was 5.6% and varied significantly across countries, income groups, and World Health Organization (WHO) regions, with lifetime prevalence of PTSD higher among trauma-exposed individuals in high-income countries (6.9%) than in both upper-middle-income countries (3.9%) and low- and lower-middle-income countries (3.0%). A similar pattern was observed for 12-month and 30-day prevalence among the trauma-exposed. The 12-month prevalence among the exposed was 2.8% and varied significantly by country income level, with the prevalence in high-income countries (3.6%) more than twice that in upper-middle income countries (1.6%) and low- and lower-middle-income (1.5%). The 30-day prevalence among the exposed was 1.4% and varied significantly by country income level, with the prevalence in high-income countries (1.9%) about three times that in upper-middle income countries (0.7%) and low- and lower-middle-income (0.6%). Twelve-month prevalence among the exposed also varied across WHO regions, with the Western Pacific region reporting a prevalence (4.3%) more than four times that in the Africa region (1.0%). Thirty-day prevalence among the exposed also varied across WHO regions, with the Western Pacific region reporting a 30-day prevalence among the exposed (2.4%), which was 12 times the prevalence in the Africa region (0.2%).

Symptom Persistence and Reduction

The 12-month prevalence estimates among lifetime cases and 30-day prevalence estimates among 12-month cases are presented in Table 5.2. Twelve-month prevalence among lifetime cases, which is one indicator of symptom persistence, varied by country, country income group, and WHO region. The proportion of cases with persistent PTSD varied widely

Table 5.1 Prevalence of DSM-IV/CIDI PTSD in the WMH surveys (n = 71,083)

	Lifetime prevalence of PTSD in total sample			Trauma exposure			Lifetime prevalence of PTSD among exposed			12-month prevalence of PTSD among exposed			30-day prevalence of PTSD among exposed			Sample size used
	%	(SE)	(n)	%	(SE)	(n)	%	(SE)	(n)	%	(SE)	(n)	%	(SE)	(n)	(n)
I High-Income Countries	5.0	(0.1)	(3,107)	72.4	(0.4)	(32,001)	6.9	(0.2)	(3,107)	3.6	(0.1)	(1,615)	1.9	(0.1)	(817)	(42,308)
Australia	7.3	(0.4)	(640)	76.2	(0.7)	(6,519)	9.6	(0.5)	(640)	5.8	(0.3)	(382)	3.3	(0.3)	(216)	(8,463)
Belgium	2.7	(0.5)	(51)	65.8	(3.1)	(710)	4.1	(0.8)	(51)	1.2	(0.2)	(22)	0.3	(0.1)	(9)	(1,043)
France	3.9	(0.6)	(98)	72.7	(2.3)	(1,071)	5.4	(0.7)	(98)	3.2	(0.6)	(58)	1.4	(0.4)	(23)	(1,436)
Germany	1.7	(0.3)	(54)	67.3	(2.2)	(928)	2.5	(0.5)	(54)	1.0	(0.2)	(25)	0.4	(0.2)	(11)	(1,323)
Israel	1.6	(0.2)	(73)	74.8	(0.7)	(3,679)	2.1	(0.3)	(73)	0.8	(0.2)	(25)	0.3	(0.1)	(10)	(4,859)
Italy	2.4	(0.6)	(65)	56.1	(2.2)	(1,064)	4.3	(1.0)	(65)	1.3	(0.4)	(25)	0.6	(0.2)	(11)	(1,779)
Japan	1.3	(0.2)	(38)	60.7	(1.7)	(1,138)	2.1	(0.4)	(38)	1.2	(0.3)	(19)	0.4	(0.2)	(6)	(1,682)
Netherlands	4.4	(0.8)	(90)	65.6	(2.8)	(788)	6.7	(1.2)	(90)	4.1	(1.1)	(50)	1.6	(0.5)	(27)	(1,093)
New Zealand	6.1	(0.3)	(828)	79.3	(0.8)	(6,089)	7.6	(0.4)	(828)	3.8	(0.3)	(416)	2.1	(0.2)	(218)	(7,312)
Northern Ireland	8.8	(0.7)	(238)	60.6	(1.7)	(1,287)	14.5	(1.1)	(238)	8.4	(0.9)	(129)	4.0	(0.7)	(61)	(1,986)
Portugal	5.3	(0.5)	(180)	69.0	(1.7)	(1,548)	7.7	(0.7)	(180)	3.3	(0.5)	(77)	1.4	(0.3)	(32)	(2,060)
Spain	2.2	(0.4)	(85)	54.0	(1.7)	(1,284)	4.0	(0.8)	(85)	1.0	(0.2)	(35)	0.3	(0.1)	(16)	(2,121)
Spain – Murcia	2.8	(0.5)	(65)	62.4	(1.9)	(942)	4.5	(0.7)	(65)	1.4	(0.4)	(26)	0.7	(0.1)	(16)	(1,459)
United States	6.9	(0.4)	(602)	82.7	(0.9)	(4,954)	8.3	(0.5)	(602)	4.3	(0.3)	(326)	2.1	(0.2)	(161)	(5,692)
II Upper-Middle-Income Countries	2.3	(0.1)	(602)	63.2	(0.6)	(11,266)	3.6	(0.2)	(602)	1.6	(0.1)	(273)	0.7	(0.1)	(116)	(16,913)
Brazil – São Paulo	3.2	(0.2)	(160)	73.8	(1.5)	(2,330)	4.3	(0.3)	(160)	2.1	(0.3)	(81)	0.9	(0.2)	(35)	(2,942)
Bulgaria	1.9	(0.3)	(73)	28.6	(1.3)	(776)	6.5	(1.1)	(73)	4.0	(0.6)	(45)	2.8	(0.6)	(27)	(2,233)
Colombia – Medellin	3.7	(0.6)	(109)	75.1	(2.6)	(1,387)	4.9	(0.8)	(109)	1.3	(0.3)	(39)	0.3	(0.1)	(9)	(1,673)
Lebanon	3.4	(0.6)	(70)	81.1	(2.7)	(873)	4.2	(0.7)	(70)	2.4	(0.8)	(30)	1.5	(0.7)	(16)	(1,031)
Mexico	1.5	(0.3)	(68)	68.8	(1.8)	(1,818)	2.1	(0.4)	(68)	0.8	(0.2)	(29)	0.3	(0.1)	(15)	(2,362)
Romania	1.2	(0.3)	(31)	41.5	(1.1)	(997)	2.8	(0.7)	(31)	1.8	(0.6)	(16)	0.9	(0.4)	(6)	(2,357)
South Africa	2.3	(0.3)	(91)	73.8	(1.2)	(3,085)	3.0	(0.4)	(91)	1.0	(0.2)	(33)	0.2	(0.1)	(8)	(4,315)
III Low- and Lower-Middle-Income Countries	2.1	(0.2)	(394)	69.1	(0.7)	(8,530)	3.0	(0.2)	(394)	1.5	(0.2)	(198)	0.6	(0.1)	(95)	(11,862)
Colombia	1.8	(0.4)	(58)	82.7	(1.4)	(2,068)	2.2	(0.5)	(58)	0.7	(0.2)	(25)	0.2	(0.1)	(6)	(2,381)
Iraq	2.5	(0.2)	(140)	56.0	(0.8)	(2,458)	4.4	(0.4)	(140)	2.0	(0.3)	(61)	0.7	(0.2)	(23)	(4,332)
PRC – Beijing/Shanghai	0.3	(0.1)	(11)	52.5	(2.6)	(929)	0.5	(0.2)	(11)	0.4	(0.2)	(8)	0.1	(0.1)	(2)	(1,628)
Peru	0.7	(0.1)	(22)	83.1	(0.8)	(1,530)	0.8	(0.2)	(22)	0.2	(0.1)	(7)	0.1	(0.1)	(2)	(1,801)
Ukraine	4.8	(0.6)	(163)	84.6	(1.7)	(1,545)	5.7	(0.7)	(163)	3.4	(0.6)	(97)	2.0	(0.4)	(62)	(1,720)

(cont.)

Table 5.1 *(cont.)*

	Lifetime prevalence of PTSD in total sample			Trauma exposure			Lifetime prevalence of PTSD among exposed			12-month prevalence of PTSD among exposed			30-day prevalence of PTSD among exposed			Sample size used
	%	(SE)	(n)	%	(SE)	(n)	%	(SE)	(n)	%	(SE)	(n)	%	(SE)	(n)	(n)
IV WHO Regions[a]																
Region of the Americas	3.8	(0.2)	(1,019)	78.5	(0.6)	(14,087)	4.8	(0.2)	(1,019)	2.2	(0.1)	(507)	1.0	(0.1)	(228)	(16,851)
African region	2.3	(0.3)	(91)	73.8	(1.2)	(3,085)	3.0	(0.4)	(91)	1.0	(0.2)	(33)	0.2	(0.1)	(8)	(4,315)
Western Pacific region	5.7	(0.2)	(1,517)	74.0	(0.5)	(14,675)	7.7	(0.3)	(1,517)	4.3	(0.2)	(825)	2.4	(0.2)	(442)	(19,085)
Eastern Mediterranean region	2.1	(0.1)	(283)	67.5	(0.6)	(7,010)	3.2	(0.2)	(283)	1.4	(0.2)	(116)	0.6	(0.1)	(49)	(10,222)
Western European region	4.0	(0.2)	(926)	63.0	(0.7)	(9,622)	6.3	(0.3)	(926)	2.9	(0.2)	(447)	1.3	(0.1)	(206)	(14,300)
Eastern European region	2.4	(0.2)	(267)	48.7	(1.0)	(3,318)	4.9	(0.5)	(267)	3.0	(0.4)	(158)	1.8	(0.3)	(95)	(6,310)
V Total	3.9	(0.1)	(4,103)	69.7	(0.3)	(51,797)	5.6	(0.1)	(4,103)	2.8	(0.1)	(2,086)	1.4	(0.1)	(1,028)	(71,083)
χ^2_{25} [b]	33.7*			81.8*			32.7*			25.4*			13.2*			
χ^2_2 [c]	135.8*			74.5*			115.3*			87.0*			50.5*			
χ^2_5 [d]	46.3*			148.2*			40.7*			36.7*			38.1*			

*Significant at the 0.05 level, two-sided test.

[a]Region of the Americas (Brazil – São Paulo, Colombia, Mexico, Peru, United States, Colombia – Medellin); African region (South Africa); Western Pacific region (Australia, Japan, New Zealand, PRC – Beijing/Shanghai); Eastern Mediterranean region (Lebanon, Iraq, Israel); Western European region (Belgium, France, Germany, Italy, Netherlands, Northern Ireland, Portugal, Spain, Spain – Murcia); Eastern European region (Bulgaria, Romania, Ukraine).

[b]The significance of the differences in prevalence between all countries.

[c]The significance of the differences in prevalence by country income.

[d]The significance of the differences in prevalence by WHO regions.

Table 5.2 Prevalence of persistent DSM-IV/CIDI PTSD in the WMH surveys (n = 71,083)

	12-month prevalence of PTSD among lifetime cases			30-day prevalence of PTSD among 12-month cases			Sample size used
	%	(SE)	(n)	%	(SE)	(n)	(n)
I High-Income Countries	**52.1**	**(1.2)**	**(1,615)**	**51.3**	**(1.8)**	**(817)**	**(42,308)**
Australia	60.0	(2.2)	(382)	56.6	(3.3)	(216)	(8,463)
Belgium	28.0	(6.2)	(22)	29.7	(9.5)	(9)	(1,043)
France	59.5	(6.8)	(58)	44.8	(8.0)	(23)	(1,436)
Germany	40.9	(8.3)	(25)	36.9	(11.5)	(11)	(1,323)
Israel	37.3	(5.9)	(25)	44.1	(10.3)	(10)	(4,859)
Italy	30.0	(7.6)	(25)	48.8	(13.1)	(11)	(1,779)
Japan	55.4	(7.1)	(19)	35.0	(14.0)	(6)	(1,682)
Netherlands	62.0	(8.3)	(50)	39.3	(10.8)	(27)	(1,093)
New Zealand	50.0	(2.5)	(416)	54.9	(3.8)	(218)	(7,312)
Northern Ireland	57.5	(3.8)	(129)	48.0	(6.4)	(61)	(1,986)
Portugal	42.6	(4.5)	(77)	42.3	(6.5)	(32)	(2,060)
Spain	26.1	(6.7)	(35)	33.5	(9.0)	(16)	(2,121)
Spain – Murcia	32.1	(8.5)	(26)	47.4	(9.5)	(16)	(1,459)
United States	52.4	(2.9)	(326)	49.3	(4.1)	(161)	(5,692)
II Upper-Middle-Income Countries	**43.5**	**(2.7)**	**(273)**	**44.3**	**(4.5)**	**(116)**	**(16,913)**
Brazil – São Paulo	48.8	(4.9)	(81)	44.8	(8.4)	(35)	(2,942)
Bulgaria	61.9	(4.9)	(45)	69.3	(10.4)	(27)	(2,233)
Colombia – Medellin	26.4	(5.3)	(39)	26.9	(9.2)	(9)	(1,673)
Lebanon	58.2	(11.2)	(30)	62.3	(12.6)	(16)	(1,031)
Mexico	39.2	(8.6)	(29)	40.3	(11.9)	(15)	(2,362)
Romania	64.6	(8.7)	(16)	47.7	(14.1)	(6)	(2,357)
South Africa	31.7	(5.5)	(33)	20.0	(7.4)	(8)	(4,315)
III Low- and Lower-Middle-Income Countries	**47.8**	**(3.9)**	**(198)**	**43.2**	**(5.4)**	**(95)**	**(11,862)**
Colombia	34.2	(9.6)	(25)	29.2	(13.7)	(6)	(2,381)
Iraq	46.1	(6.2)	(61)	33.7	(9.4)	(23)	(4,332)
PRC – Beijing/Shanghai	82.1	(11.5)	(8)	17.9	(14.0)	(2)	(1,628)
Peru	23.1	(8.9)	(7)	37.5	(26.1)	(2)	(1,801)
Ukraine	58.9	(5.3)	(97)	59.2	(7.5)	(62)	(1,720)
VI WHO Regions[a]							
Region of the Americas	46.9	(2.2)	(507)	45.9	(3.3)	(228)	(16,851)
African region	31.7	(5.5)	(33)	20.0	(7.4)	(8)	(4,315)
Western Pacific region	56.0	(1.6)	(825)	55.3	(2.5)	(442)	(19,085)
Eastern Mediterranean region	44.9	(4.2)	(116)	42.6	(6.7)	(49)	(10,222)
Western European region	46.7	(2.3)	(447)	44.1	(3.3)	(206)	(14,300)
Eastern European region	60.7	(3.6)	(158)	59.8	(5.7)	(95)	(6,310)
V Total	**50.5**	**(1.0)**	**(2,086)**	**49.8**	**(1.6)**	**(1,028)**	**(71,083)**
$\chi^{2\,b}_{25}$	4.0*			1.7*			
$\chi^{2\,c}_{2}$	4.3*			1.8			
$\chi^{2\,d}_{5}$	7.1*			4.1*			

*Significant at the 0.05 level, two-sided test.
[a]Region of the Americas (Brazil – São Paulo, Colombia, Mexico, Peru, United States, Colombia – Medellin); African region (South Africa); Western Pacific region (Australia, Japan, New Zealand, PRC – Beijing/Shanghai); Eastern Mediterranean region (Lebanon, Iraq, Israel); Western European region (Belgium, France, Germany, Italy, Netherlands, Northern Ireland, Portugal, Spain, Spain – Murcia); Eastern European region (Bulgaria, Romania, Ukraine).
[b]The significance of the differences in prevalence between all countries.
[c]The significance of the differences in prevalence by country income.
[d]The significance of the differences in prevalence by WHO region.

across countries, even countries with similar lifetime prevalence. For example, Belgium and Lebanon had a similar lifetime prevalence of PTSD among the exposed (4.1–4.2%), but 12-month prevalence among the exposed was twice as high in Lebanon (2.4%) as in Belgium (1.2%). Lebanon's 12-month prevalence of PTSD among lifetime cases (58.2%) was consequently roughly twice as high as that of Belgium's (28.0%).

The results regarding 30-day prevalence among 12-month cases provide insight into how the duration of PTSD varies across countries. Of note, this ratio varied significantly by country and WHO region, but not by country income. Again using the example of Lebanon and Belgium, Lebanon's 30-day prevalence of PTSD among the exposed (1.5%) was five times that of Belgium's (0.3%), even though lifetime prevalence of PTSD among the exposed was similar in the two countries.

Age-of-Onset

Cumulative distributions for the age of PTSD onset stratified by country income group are presented in Figure 5.1. Onset of PTSD was earlier on average in high-income countries than in low- and lower-middle-income countries and in upper-middle-income countries, with half of lifetime cases in high-income countries reporting onset before age 30 compared to age 43 for lifetime cases in low- and lower-middle-income countries. In high-income countries, 30% of respondents reported PTSD onset before age 18 compared to fewer than 16% in upper-middle income and 10% in low- and lower-middle-income countries. Across all groups, the vast majority of respondents reported symptoms beginning immediately after the trauma.

Socio-Demographic Correlates

Table 5.3 presents associations of socio-demographics with trauma exposure, lifetime PTSD among the exposed, and 12-month PTSD among lifetime cases in all countries combined. Socio-demographic correlates of trauma exposure are presented for reference to the other outcomes, even though they were already reported in Chapter 3 for a slightly different sample. All socio-demographic correlates were significantly associated with lifetime PTSD among the trauma-exposed. Respondents who were younger, female, not employed, not currently married, less educated, and had a lower household income were more likely than others to develop PTSD after trauma exposure. However, female sex, marital status, and education level were not significantly associated with persistence as defined by 12-month PTSD among lifetime cases controlling for number of years since onset. In addition, all household

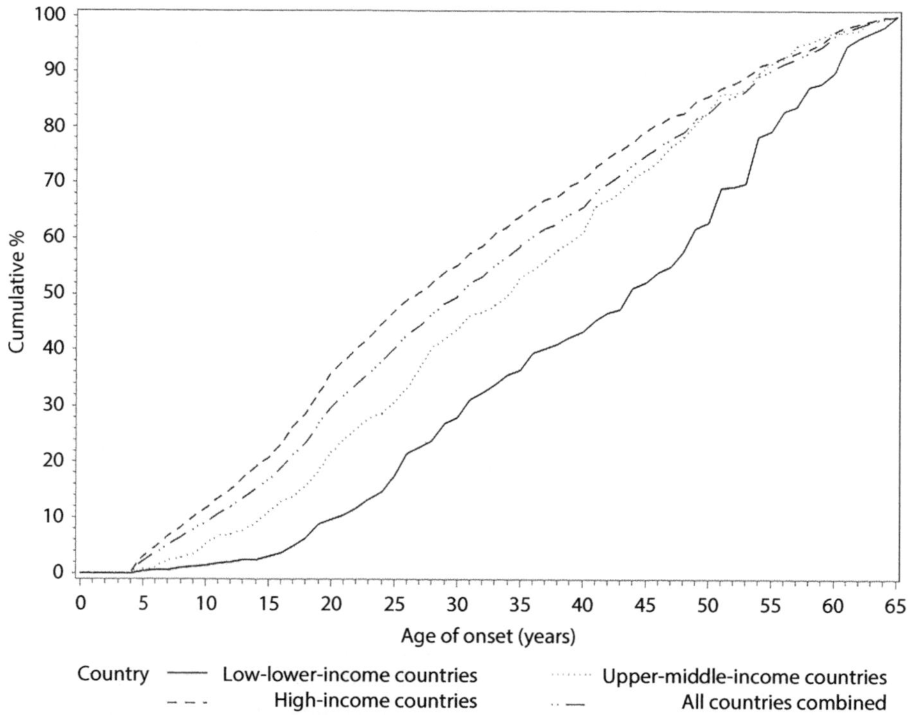

Figure 5.1 Age of onset distributions of DSM-IV PTSD by income-group countries

Table 5.3 Bivariate associations between socio-demographic correlates and DSM-IV PTSD among trauma-exposed (all countries combined n = 71,083)

	Exposure to trauma[a,b]		Lifetime PTSD among exposed[a,b]		12-month PTSD among lifetime cases[c]	
	OR	(95% CI)	OR	(95% CI)	OR	(95% CI)
I Age						
18–29	2.0*	(1.9–2.1)	2.5*	(2.1–3.0)		
30–44	1.6*	(1.5–1.6)	2.1*	(1.8–2.4)		
45–59	1.3*	(1.2–1.3)	1.8*	(1.6–2.1)		
60+	1.0	–	1.0	–		
χ^2_3	1,063.8*		122.1*			
II Sex						
Female	0.9*	(0.8–0.9)	2.6*	(2.4–2.9)	1.1	(0.9–1.3)
Male	1.0	–	1.0	–	1.0	–
III Education						
No education	0.7*	(0.6–0.8)	1.5	(0.9–2.7)	0.6	(0.3–1.2)
Some primary	0.9*	(0.8–0.9)	1.4*	(1.2–1.8)	1.0	(0.7–1.5)
Finished primary	0.9*	(0.8–0.9)	1.7*	(1.3–2.1)	1.2	(0.8–1.8)
Some secondary	1.0	(0.9–1.0)	1.4*	(1.2–1.6)	0.9	(0.7–1.2)
Finished secondary	1.0	(1.0–1.0)	1.1	(0.9–1.3)	1.1	(0.8–1.5)
Some college	1.1*	(1.0–1.1)	1.1	(0.9–1.3)	1.1	(0.8–1.5)
Finished college	1.0	–	1.0	–	1.0	–
χ^2_6	85.7		36.9*		5.8	
IV Marital Status						
Currently married	1.0	–	1.0	–	1.0	–
Previously married	1.2*	(1.1–1.2)	1.7*	(1.5–1.9)	1.2	(1.0–1.5)
Never married	1.0	(1.0–1.0)	1.3*	(1.1–1.5)	1.1	(0.8–1.4)
χ^2_2	67.2*		70.8*		3.8	
V Employment Status						
Student	1.0	(0.9–1.1)	1.0	(0.7–1.3)	1.7	(1.0–3.0)
Homemaker	0.9*	(0.8–0.9)	1.2*	(1.0–1.4)	1.2	(0.9–1.6)
Retired	1.0	(0.9–1.1)	1.3*	(1.1–1.6)	1.1	(0.8–1.5)
Other	1.1*	(1.0–1.1)	1.7*	(1.5–2.0)	1.5*	(1.2–1.9)
Employed	1.0	–	1.0	–	1.0	–
χ^2_4	39.2*		77.7*		12.3*	
VI Household Income						
Low	0.9*	(0.9–1.0)	1.7*	(1.5–1.9)	1.5*	(1.2–1.9)
Low-average	1.0	(0.9–1.0)	1.5*	(1.3–1.7)	1.3	(1.0–1.7)
High-average	1.0	(1.0–1.0)	1.4*	(1.3–1.7)	1.0	(0.8–1.3)
High	1.0	–	1.0	–	1.0	–
χ^2_3	13.3*		55.2*		15.8*	
VII Age-of-Onset[d]						
Early					1.1	(0.9–1.5)
Early-average					0.8*	(0.6–1.0)
Late-average					0.7*	(0.5–0.9)
Late					1.0	–
χ^2_3					21.7*	
VIII Years Since Onset (continuous)					**0.97***	**(0.97–0.98)**
(n)[e]	(1,646,308)		(1,310,008)		(4,103)	

*Significant at the 0.05 level, two-sided test.
[a]These estimates are based on survival models adjusted for age-cohorts, sex, person-years, and country.
[b]Iraq is not included in the analysis related to exposure to traumas because the age of first exposure to traumas is not available in Iraq. Excluding Iraq, there were 49,339 people exposed to traumas and 3,963 people with PTSD.
[c]These estimates are based on logistic regression models adjusted for time since PTSD onset, age of PTSD onset, sex, and country.
[d]Defined in terms of within-survey quartiles of the AOO distribution.
[e]Denominator n: 71,083 = total sample; 1,646,308, 1,310,008, and 3,067,607 = number of person-years in the survival models; 4,103 = number of lifetime cases of PTSD.

income categories (where income was defined for the year before interview, which means that income in most cases was assessed after onset of PTSD) below the highest income level were associated with lifetime PTSD, but only the lowest income category was associated with persistent PTSD. Being a homemaker, retired, or "other" employment status was associated with an increased risk of lifetime PTSD compared to being employed, but only an employment status of "other" was associated with persistent PTSD.

Parallel analyses of socio-demographic correlates by country income level, which are presented in Appendix Tables 5.A2–5.A4, showed that patterns were largely consistent for lifetime PTSD among the exposed across income level. However, there were three major exceptions. First, lower education was not associated with PTSD prevalence in upper-middle-income countries, but was in other countries. Second, younger respondents were not more likely to develop PTSD in low- and lower-middle-income countries, but were in high-income countries. Third, there was no significant association between employment status and PTSD prevalence in low- and lower-middle-income countries. For 12-month PTSD among lifetime cases, socio-demographic results differed markedly between the high-income countries and low- and lower-middle-income countries. No socio-demographic variables were associated with persistent PTSD in the low- and lower-middle-income countries, while lower household income, "other" employment status, and being divorced, separated, or widowed was associated with more persistent PTSD in high-income countries.

Discussion

The WMH surveys have four limitations with particular relevance for interpreting the results in this chapter. First, substantial variation in the response rate across countries might have biased estimates of prevalence and correlates. We post-stratified the data to the extent possible to reduce this problem, but there is no guarantee that this improved estimates. Second, trauma exposure and PTSD were assessed retrospectively, which may have led to underreporting of lifetime prevalence or bias in estimation of AOO. Third, while the WMH surveys used the same assessment in all countries, cultural differences may have affected respondents' willingness to discuss sensitive issues, especially stigmatizing traumas. We attempted to mitigate underreporting by including an open-ended question about traumas that respondents did not want to describe. As noted in Chapter 2, this question was endorsed by 6.1% of the total sample, but there is no guarantee that all respondents who were reluctant to report stigmatizing traumas endorsed this question. Fourth, the WMH surveys did not include many countries with recent mass violence and armed conflicts. Nor did the surveys include individuals who were not residing in the household population, which means that the millions displaced by sectarian violence (most notably in Iraq) were excluded from the surveys. The limited data available about these excluded populations suggests that PTSD prevalence is much higher than in the household population (de Jong et al., 2001).

Despite these limitations, the WMH surveys have several strengths. First, they assessed a large sample within each country, two-thirds of which were nationally representative. These samples were sufficiently large to permit estimates of 30-day prevalence in addition to 12-month and lifetime prevalence of PTSD. For many countries, these were the first published prevalence estimates of PTSD, and thus provided important information on the burden of PTSD. An additional strength was the use of standardized measures to assess trauma and PTSD across all countries, which facilitated cross-national comparisons and pooling of data. In addition, we collected detailed, standardized socio-demographic information for all respondents, enabling us to examine the associations of individual- and social-level factors with PTSD prevalence and persistence.

Three notable findings merit discussion. First, we found that 5.6% of respondents who were exposed to traumas at some time in their lives had a lifetime diagnosis of PTSD. This prevalence estimate varied from 0.5% to 14.5% across countries, which may stem from variation in trauma types across countries. We show elsewhere (see Chapter 9) that PTSD prevalence was associated with type of trauma and that interpersonal traumas (e.g., sexual violence) were associated with highest risk of PTSD. Half of respondents with lifetime PTSD had symptoms in the 12 months before interview, and almost half of 12-month cases reported symptoms in the 30 days before interview. These results suggest that PTSD is a highly persistent disorder. It is likely that at least some participants with 12-month but without 30-day PTSD experienced relapsing and remitting symptoms over the year, a pattern that has been documented in several longitudinal studies (Osenbach et al., 2014; Bryant et al., 2015). The DSM system, however, does not distinguish between those who fully remit and those whose symptoms are sensitive to flaring up again with reminders. Consequently, the 30-day prevalence of PTSD, which represents the burden of PTSD at the specific time the survey was conducted, may underestimate the current burden of PTSD. Similarly, the burden of PTSD may be overestimated if symptoms were waxing at the time of interview, leading to more individuals meeting formal diagnostic criteria.

Second, our results confirm earlier reports that PTSD onset often occurs later in life than some other DSM-IV anxiety disorders, especially the phobias (Kessler et al., 2005, 2007). However, we found wide variation in AOO across countries and income groups, with PTSD developing significantly earlier in high-income countries (median age 25–28) compared to low- and lower-middle- (median age 43) and upper-middle- (median age 30) income countries. Interestingly, the relatively late AOO of PTSD contrasts with the finding in Chapter 3 that incident trauma exposure is more common among children, adolescents, and young adults than among older individuals (Benjet et al., 2016). While this may imply that conditional risk of developing PTSD is higher in older adults exposed to trauma, results presented in Table 5.A4 show that younger respondents were at greater risk of developing PTSD. One possible reason for this discrepancy may be that younger individuals are more likely to be exposed to the types of traumas that have greater risk for the development of PTSD. Exploring this issue is beyond the scope of this chapter, but we plan to address it in future analyses of WMH data.

Third, we examined socio-demographic correlates of PTSD prevalence and persistence. We found that lifetime PTSD among those exposed to trauma was associated with being younger, female, not employed, not currently married, having a lower education level, and having a lower household income. These results were mostly consistent across country income groups. Moreover, our results for female sex are consistent with a large literature on sex differences in risk for PTSD (Tolin & Foa, 2006). Only income level and employment status were associated with persistent PTSD in the overall sample. When countries were stratified by country income, no socio-demographic variables were correlated with persistent PTSD in low- and lower-middle-income countries, whereas lower socio-economic status was associated with persistent PTSD in high-income countries. Given the lack of information on the temporal ordering of socio-demographic factors and PTSD onset, we cannot determine whether factors such as marital status or socio-economic status are risk factors for, or consequences of, the disorder.

Acknowledgment

Portions of this chapter are based on Koenen, K. C., Ratanatharathorn, A., Ng, L. C., et al. (2017). Posttraumatic stress disorder in the World Mental Health Surveys. *Psychological Medicine*, **47**, 2260–74. Reproduced with permission of Cambridge University Press.

References

Alhasnawi, S., Sadik, S., Rasheed, M., et al. (2009). The prevalence and correlates of DSM-IV disorders in the Iraq Mental Health Survey (IMHS). *World Psychiatry*, 8, 97–109.

Atwoli, L., Stein, D. J., Koenen, K. C., & Mclaughlin, K. A. (2015). Epidemiology of posttraumatic stress disorder: prevalence, correlates and consequences. *Current Opinion in Psychiatry*, 28, 307–11.

Atwoli, L., Stein, D. J., Williams, D. R., et al. (2013). Trauma and posttraumatic stress disorder in South Africa: analysis from the South African Stress and Health Study. *BMC Psychiatry*, 13, 182.

Benjet, C., Bromet, E., Karam, E. G., et al. (2016). The epidemiology of traumatic event exposure worldwide: results from the World Mental Health Survey Consortium. *Psychological Medicine*, 46, 327–43.

Breslau, J., Kendler, K. S., Su, M., Gaxiola-Aguilar, S., & Kessler, R. C. (2005). Lifetime risk and persistence of psychiatric disorders across ethnic groups in the United States. *Psychological Medicine*, 35, 317–27.

Breslau, N. (2009). The epidemiology of trauma, PTSD, and other posttrauma disorders. *Trauma, Violence, & Abuse*, 10, 198–210.

Brewin, C. R., Andrews, B., & Valentine, J. D. (2000). Meta-analysis of risk factors for posttraumatic stress disorder in trauma-exposed adults. *Journal of Consulting and Clinical Psychology*, 68, 748–66.

Bryant, R. A., Nickerson, A., Creamer, M., et al. (2015). Trajectory of post-traumatic stress following traumatic injury: 6-year follow-up. *The British Journal of Psychiatry*, 206, 417–23.

de Jong, J. T., Komproe, I. H., Van Ommeren, M., et al. (2001). Lifetime events and posttraumatic stress disorder in 4 postconflict settings. *JAMA*, 286, 555–62.

Jeon, H. J., Suh, T., Lee, H. J., et al. (2007). Partial versus full PTSD in the Korean community: prevalence, duration, correlates, comorbidity, and dysfunctions. *Depression and Anxiety*, 24, 577–85.

Karam, E. G., Mneimneh, Z. N., Dimassi, H., et al. (2008). Lifetime prevalence of mental disorders in

Lebanon: first onset, treatment, and exposure to war. *PLoS Medicine*, 5, e61.

Kessler, R. C. (2003). Epidemiology of women and depression. *Journal of Affective Disorders*, 74, 5–13.

Kessler, R. C., Amminger, G. P., Aguilar-Gaxiola, S., et al. (2007). Age of onset of mental disorders: a review of recent literature. *Current Opinion in Psychiatry*, 20, 359–64.

Kessler, R. C., Berglund, P., Demler, O., et al. (2005). Lifetime prevalence and age-of-onset distributions of DSM-IV disorders in the National Comorbidity Survey Replication. *Archives of General Psychiatry*, 62, 593–602.

Osenbach, J. E., Lewis, C., Rosenfeld, B., et al. (2014). Exploring the longitudinal trajectories of posttraumatic stress disorder in injured trauma survivors. *Psychiatry*, 77, 386–97.

Ozer, E. J., Best, S. R., Lipsey, T. L., & Weiss, D. S. (2008, August). Predictors of posttraumatic stress disorder and symptoms in adults: a meta-analysis. In *Annual Meeting of the International Society for Traumatic Stress Studies*, Washington, DC. This article is based on a paper presented at the aforementioned meeting. Educational Publishing Foundation.

Tolin, D. F., & Foa, E. B. (2006). Sex differences in trauma and posttraumatic stress disorder: a quantitative review of 25 years of research. *Psychological Bulletin*, 132, 959–92.

Van Ameringen, M., Mancini, C., Patterson, B., & Boyle, M. H. (2008). Post-traumatic stress disorder in Canada. *CNS Neuroscience & Therapeutics*, 14, 171–81.

Williams, D. R., Gonzalez, H. M., Neighbors, H., et al. (2007). Prevalence and distribution of major depressive disorder in African Americans, Caribbean blacks, and non-Hispanic whites: results from the National Survey of American Life. *Archives of General Psychiatry*, 64, 305–15.

Wolter, K. M. (2007). *Introduction to Variance Estimation*. New York, NY: Springer.

Appendix

Table 5.A1 WMH sample characteristics by World Bank income categories[a]

Country by income category	Survey[b]	Sample characteristics[c]	Field dates	Age range	Sample size		Response rate[d]
					Part I	Part II	
I Low- and Lower-Middle-Income Countries							
Colombia	NSMH	All urban areas of the country (approximately 73% of the total national population)	2003	18–65	4,426	2,381	87.7
Iraq	IMHS	Nationally representative	2006–7	18–96	4,332	4,332	95.2
PRC – Beijing/Shanghai	B-WMH/S-WMH	Beijing and Shanghai metropolitan areas.	2002–3	18–70	5,201	1,628	74.7
Peru	EMSMP	Five urban areas of the country (approximately 38% of the total national population)	2004–5	18–65	3,930	1,801	90.2
Ukraine	CMDPSD	Nationally representative	2002	18–91	4,724	1,719	78.3
(Total)					(22,613)	(11,861)	83.9
II Upper-Middle-Income Countries							
Brazil – São Paulo	São Paulo Megacity	São Paulo metropolitan area	2005–7	18–93	5,037	2,942	81.3
Bulgaria	NSHS	Nationally representative	2003–7	18–98	5,318	2,233	72.0
Colombia – Medellin[e]	MMHHS	Medellin metropolitan area	2011–12	19–65	3,261	1,673	97.2
Lebanon	LEBANON	Nationally representative	2002–3	18–94	2,857	1,031	70.0
Mexico	M-NCS	All urban areas of the country (approximately 75% of the total national population)	2001–2	18–65	5,782	2,362	76.6
Romania	RMHS	Nationally representative	2005–6	18–96	2,357	2,357	70.9
South Africa[f]	SASH	Nationally representative	2003–4	18–92	4,315	4,315	87.1
(Total)					(28,927)	(16,913)	78.5
III High-Income Countries							
Australia[f]	NSMHWB	Nationally representative	2007	18–85	8,463	8,463	60.0
Belgium	ESEMeD	Nationally representative – The sample was selected from a national register of Belgium residents.	2001–2	18–95	2,419	1,043	50.6
France	ESEMeD	Nationally representative – The sample was selected from a national list of households with listed telephone numbers.	2001–2	18–97	2,894	1,436	45.9
Germany	ESEMeD	Nationally representative	2002–3	19–95	3,555	1,323	57.8
Israel	NHS	Nationally representative	2002–4	21–98	4,859	4,859	72.6
Italy	ESEMeD	Nationally representative – The sample was selected from municipality resident registries	2001–2	18–100	4,712	1,779	71.3
Japan	WMHJ 2002–2006	Eleven metropolitan areas	2002–6	20–98	4,129	1,682	55.1
Netherlands	ESEMeD	Nationally representative – The sample was selected from municipal postal registries.	2002–3	18–95	2,372	1,094	56.4
New Zealand[f]	NZMHS	Nationally representative	2003–4	18–98	12,790	7,312	73.3
Northern Ireland	NISHS	Nationally representative	2004–7	18–97	4,340	1,986	68.4
Portugal	NMHS	Nationally representative	2008–9	18–81	3,849	2,060	57.3

(cont.)

Table 5.A1 *(cont.)*

Country by income category	Survey[b]	Sample characteristics[c]	Field dates	Age range	Sample size		Response rate[d]
					Part I	Part II	
Spain	ESEMeD	Nationally representative	2001–2	18–98	5,473	2,121	78.6
Spain – Murcia	PEGASUS – Murcia	Murcia region	2010–12	18–96	2,621	1,459	67.4
United States	NCS-R	Nationally representative	2002–3	18–99	9,282	5,692	70.9
(Total)					(71,758)	(42,309)	64.4
IV Total					**(123,298)**	**(71,083)**	**70.6**

[a]The World Bank (2012) Data. Accessed May 12, 2012 at: http://data.worldbank.org/country. Some of the WMH countries have moved into new income categories since the surveys were conducted. The income groupings above reflect the status of each country at the time of data collection. The current income category of each country is available at the preceding URL.

[b]NSMH (The Colombian National Study of Mental Health); IMHS (Iraq Mental Health Survey); B-WMH (The Beijing World Mental Health Survey); S-WMH (The Shanghai World Mental Health Survey); EMSMP (La Encuesta Mundial de Salud Mental en el Peru); CMDPSD (Comorbid Mental Disorders during Periods of Social Disruption); NSHS (Bulgaria National Survey of Health and Stress); MMHHS (Medellín Mental Health Household Study); LEBANON (Lebanese Evaluation of the Burden of Ailments and Needs of the Nation); M-NCS (The Mexico National Comorbidity Survey); RMHS (Romania Mental Health Survey); SASH (South Africa Health Survey); NSMHWB (National Survey of Mental Health and Wellbeing); ESEMeD (The European Study Of The Epidemiology Of Mental Disorders); NHS (Israel National Health Survey); WMHJ 2002-2006 (World Mental Health Japan Survey); NZMHS (New Zealand Mental Health Survey); NISHS (Northern Ireland Study of Health and Stress); NMHS (Portugal National Mental Health Survey); PEGASUS-Murcia (Psychiatric Enquiry to General Population in Southeast Spain-Murcia); NCS-R (The US National Comorbidity Survey Replication).

[c]Most WMH surveys are based on stratified multistage clustered area probability household samples in which samples of areas equivalent to counties or municipalities in the United States were selected in the first stage followed by one or more subsequent stages of geographic sampling (e.g., towns within counties, blocks within towns, households within blocks) to arrive at a sample of households, in each of which a listing of household members was created and one or two people were selected from this listing to be interviewed. No substitution was allowed when the originally sampled household resident could not be interviewed. These household samples were selected from census area data in all countries other than France (where telephone directories were used to select households) and the Netherlands (where postal registries were used to select households). Several WMH surveys (Belgium, Germany, Italy, Spain – Murcia) used municipal resident or universal health-care registries to select respondents without listing households. The Japanese sample is the only totally un-clustered sample, with households randomly selected in each of the 11 metropolitan areas and one random respondent selected in each sample household. Eighteen of the 26 surveys are based on nationally representative household samples.

[d]The response rate is calculated as the ratio of the number of households in which an interview was completed to the number of households originally sampled, excluding from the denominator households known not to be eligible either because of being vacant at the time of initial contact or because the residents were unable to speak the designated languages of the survey. The weighted average response rate is 70.6%.

[e]Colombia moved from the "lower- and lower-middle-income" to the "upper-middle-income" category between 2003 (when the Colombian National Study of Mental Health was conducted) and 2010 (when the Medellin Mental Health Household Study was conducted), hence Colombia's appearance in both income categories. For more information, please see footnote a.

[f]For the purposes of cross-national comparisons we limit the sample to those 18+.

Table 5.A2 Bivariate associations between socio-demographics correlates and DSM-IV PTSD (low- and lower-middle-income countries)

	Exposure to trauma[a,b]		Lifetime PTSD among exposed[a,b]		12-month PTSD among lifetime cases[c]	
	OR	(95% CI)	OR	(95% CI)	OR	(95% CI)
I Age						
18–29	1.9*	(1.6–2.2)	0.8	(0.4–1.6)		
30–44	1.3*	(1.2–1.5)	0.9	(0.6–1.5)		
45–59	1.0	(0.9–1.2)	0.9	(0.5–1.7)		
60+	1.0	–	1.0	–		
χ^2_3	139.8*		0.4			
II Sex						
Female	0.9*	(0.8–0.9)	2.9*	(1.8–4.8)	1.0	(0.5–1.9)
Male	1.0	–	1.0	–	1.0	–
III Education						
No education	0.8	(0.6–1.1)			0.5	(0.2–1.6)
Some primary	1.0	(0.9–1.2)	1.9	(1.0–3.5)	1.1	(0.4–3.2)
Finished primary	1.1	(1.0–1.3)	1.8	(1.0–3.4)	0.9	(0.3–2.6)
Some secondary	1.0	(0.9–1.2)	1.1	(0.6–2.3)	0.8	(0.3–2.0)
Finished secondary	1.0	(0.9–1.1)	1.0	(0.6–1.7)	0.8	(0.3–2.4)
Some college	1.0	(0.9–1.2)	0.8	(0.5–1.5)	1.2	(0.3–3.9)
Finished college	1.0	–	1.0	–	1.0	–
χ^2_3	6.4		13.6		2.3	
IV Marital Status						
Currently married	1.0	–	1.0	–	1.0	–
Previously married	1.1*	(1.0–1.3)	1.7*	(1.1–2.6)	1.7	(0.8–3.4)
Never married	1.0	(0.9–1.1)	1.9	(0.7–5.1)	1.5	(0.6–4.2)
χ^2_2	4.3		6.7*		2.6	
V Employment Status						
Student	0.8	(0.7–1.0)				
Homemaker	0.8*	(0.7–0.9)	1.6	(0.7–3.3)	0.9	(0.3–2.1)
Retired	1.0	(0.8–1.2)	1.9	(0.9–3.7)	1.4	(0.5–4.1)
Other	1.1	(1.0–1.2)	1.4	(0.8–2.6)	0.9	(0.4–2.1)
Employed	1.0	–	1.0	–	1.0	–
χ^2_4	15.0*		8.0		4.8	
VI Household Income						
Low	0.9	(0.8–1.0)	1.9	(0.9–4.3)	1.8	(0.7–4.2)
Low-average	0.9*	(0.8–0.9)	2.5*	(1.4–4.4)	1.6	(0.7–3.4)
High-average	0.9	(0.9–1.0)	1.6	(0.9–2.8)	1.3	(0.6–2.8)
High	1.0	–	1.0	–	1.0	–
χ^2_3	10.6*		10.2*		2.1	
VII AOO						
Early					2.3	(0.7–7.8)
Early-average					0.7	(0.3–1.5)
Late-average					0.8	(0.3–1.8)
Late					1.0	–
χ^2_3					5.6	
VIII Years Since Onset (continuous)					**0.95***	**(0.93–0.98)**
(n)[d]	(153,510)		(157,483)		(394)	

*Significant at the 0.05 level, two-sided test.
[a]These estimates are based on survival models adjusted for age-cohorts, sex, person-years, and low- and lower-middle-income countries.
[b]Iraq is not included in the analysis related to exposure to traumas because the age of first exposure to traumas is not available in Iraq.
[c]These estimates are based on logistic regression models adjusted for time since PTSD onset, age of PTSD onset, sex, and low- and lower-middle-income countries.
[d]Denominator n: 11,862 = total sample; 153,510, 157,483, and 467,383 = number of person-years in the survival models; 394 = number of lifetime cases of PTSD; 198 = number of 12-month cases of PTSD.

Table 5.A3 Associations between socio-demographics correlates and DSM-IV/CIDI PTSD (upper-middle-income countries)

	Exposure to trauma[a]		Lifetime PTSD among exposed[a]		12-month PTSD among lifetime cases[b]	
	OR	(95% CI)	OR	(95% CI)	OR	(95% CI)
I Age						
18–29	3.3*	(2.9–3.6)	1.7*	(1.0–3.0)		
30–44	2.3*	(2.1–2.6)	1.4	(0.8–2.4)		
45–59	1.7*	(1.6–1.8)	1.4	(0.9–2.1)		
60+	1.0	–	1.0	–		
χ^2_3	524.9*		4.5			
II Sex						
Female	0.9*	(0.8–0.9)	2.7*	(1.9–3.6)	0.9	(0.6–1.5)
Male	1.0	–	1.0	–	1.0	–
III Education						
No education	0.9	(0.8–1.1)	1.4	(0.8–2.4)	0.6	(0.2–2.4)
Some primary	1.1	(1.0–1.2)	1.4	(0.9–2.3)	2.4	(0.9–6.8)
Finished primary	0.9	(0.8–1.1)	1.3	(0.7–2.3)	3.2	(0.9–11.1)
Some secondary	1.1	(1.0–1.2)	1.5	(0.9–2.4)	2.1	(0.8–5.4)
Finished secondary	1.1	(1.0–1.2)	1.4	(0.9–2.3)	1.4	(0.5–3.9)
Some college	1.2*	(1.0–1.3)	1.4	(0.9–2.3)	2.4	(0.8–7.5)
Finished college	1.0	–	1.0	–	1.0	–
χ^2_6	20.6*		3.2		9.5	
IV Marital Status						
Currently married	1.0	–	1.0	–	1.0	–
Previously married	1.2*	(1.1–1.3)	1.7*	(1.2–2.4)	0.6	(0.3–1.2)
Never married	1.0	(0.9–1.1)	0.7	(0.5–1.0)	1.1	(0.6–2.2)
χ^2_2	14.0*		13.8*		2.4	
V Employment Status						
Student	0.9	(0.8–1.1)	0.6	(0.2–1.6)	–	–
Homemaker	0.9*	(0.8–1.0)	1.1	(0.8–1.5)	1.3	(0.7–2.3)
Retired	1.0	(0.9–1.1)	1.3	(0.8–2.1)	1.1	(0.4–2.7)
Other	1.1	(1.0–1.1)	1.4*	(1.0–2.0)	1.3	(0.8–2.3)
Employed	1.0	–	1.0	–	1.0	–
χ^2_4	12.4*		7.4		4.8	
VI Household Income						
Low	0.9*	(0.8–1.0)	1.5*	(1.1–2.0)	0.9	(0.5–1.6)
Low-average	0.9	(0.9–1.0)	1.4	(0.9–2.0)	1.0	(0.5–2.2)
High-average	1.0	(0.9–1.0)	1.6*	(1.1–2.1)	0.6	(0.3–1.2)
High	1.0	–	1.0	–	1.0	–
χ^2_3	9.2*		8.2*		2.7	
VII AOO						
Early					0.7	(0.4–1.5)
Early-average					0.7	(0.4–1.2)
Late-average					0.6	(0.3–1.1)
Late					1.0	–
χ^2_3					3.3	
VIII **Years Since Onset (Continuous)**					**0.96***	**(0.93–0.98)**
(n)[c]	(461,399)		(254,602)		(602)	

*Significant at the 0.05 level, two-sided test.

[a]These estimates are based on survival models adjusted for age-cohorts, sex, person-years, and upper-middle-income countries.

[b]These estimates are based on logistic regression models adjusted for time since PTSD onset, age of PTSD onset, sex, and upper-middle-income countries.

[c]Denominator n: 16,913 = total sample; 461,399, 254,602, and 705,959 = number of person-years in the survival models; 602 = number of lifetime cases of PTSD; 273 = number of 12-month cases of PTSD.

Table 5.A4 Bivariate associations between socio-demographics correlates and DSM-IV/CIDI PTSD (high-income countries)

	Exposure to trauma[a]		Lifetime PTSD among exposed[a]		12-month PTSD among lifetime cases[b]	
	OR	(95% CI)	OR	(95% CI)	OR	(95% CI)
I Age						
18–29	1.8*	(1.7–1.9)	3.1*	(2.5–3.7)		
30–44	1.5*	(1.4–1.6)	2.4*	(2.0–2.8)		
45–59	1.2*	(1.2–1.3)	2.0*	(1.7–2.4)		
60+	1.0	–	1.0	–		
χ^2_3	621.7*		138.3*			
II Sex						
Female	0.9*	(0.8–0.9)	2.6*	(2.3–2.9)	1.1	(0.8–1.3)
Male	1.0	–	1.0	–	1.0	–
III Education						
No education	0.7*	(0.6–0.9)	1.4	(0.7–2.9)	–	–
Some primary	0.8*	(0.8–0.9)	1.7*	(1.3–2.2)	1.0	(0.5–1.7)
Finished primary	0.9*	(0.8–0.9)	2.0*	(1.5–2.7)	1.3	(0.8–2.2)
Some secondary	1.0	(0.9–1.0)	1.5*	(1.3–1.8)	0.9	(0.7–1.3)
Finished secondary	1.0	(0.9–1.0)	1.1	(0.9–1.2)	1.2	(0.9–1.7)
Some college	1.0	(1.0–1.1)	1.1	(0.9–1.3)	1.1	(0.8–1.6)
Finished college	1.0	–	1.0	–	1.0	–
χ^2_6	40.4*		47.9*		$\chi^2_5 = 5.3$	
IV Marital Status						
Currently married	1.0	–	1.0	–	1.0	–
Previously married	1.2*	(1.1–1.2)	1.6*	(1.4–1.8)	1.4*	(1.1–1.7)
Never married	1.0	(1.0–1.1)	1.4*	(1.2–1.6)	1.1	(0.8–1.4)
χ^2_2	35.1*		54.2*		5.8	
V Employment Status						
Student	1.0	(0.9–1.1)	1.0	(0.7–1.4)	1.4	(0.8–2.5)
Homemaker	0.9	(0.9–1.0)	1.3*	(1.1–1.5)	1.4	(1.0–1.9)
Retired	1.0	(0.9–1.1)	1.4*	(1.1–1.7)	1.1	(0.8–1.7)
Other	1.2*	(1.1–1.2)	2.0*	(1.8–2.4)	1.8*	(1.3–2.4)
Employed	1.0	–	1.0	–	1.0	–
χ^2_4	29.4*		98.2*		15.5*	
VI Household Income						
Low	1.0	(0.9–1.0)	1.7*	(1.5–2.0)	1.6*	(1.2–2.1)
Low-average	1.0	(0.9–1.0)	1.4*	(1.2–1.7)	1.3	(0.9–1.7)
High-average	1.0	(0.9–1.0)	1.4*	(1.2–1.6)	1.0	(0.8–1.4)
High	1.0	–	1.0	–	1.0	–
χ^2_3	2.3		48.2*		14.6*	
VII AOO						
Early					1.1	(0.8–1.5)
Early-average					0.7*	(0.6–1.0)
Late-average					0.7*	(0.5–0.9)
Late					1.0	–
χ^2_3					17.7*	
VIII Years Since Onset (Continuous)					**0.98***	**(0.97–0.98)**
(n)[c]	(1,031,399)		(89,7923)		(3,078)	

Note: En dashes were inserted for small cell counts (<5).
*Significant at the 0.05 level, two-sided test.
[a]These estimates are based on survival models adjusted for age-cohorts, sex, person-years, and upper-middle-income countries.
[b]These estimates are based on logistic regression models adjusted for time since PTSD onset, age of PTSD onset, sex, and high-income countries.
[c]Denominator n: 42,280 = total sample; 1,031,399, 897,923, and 1,897,969 = number of person-years in the survival models; 3,078 = number of lifetime cases of PTSD; 1,600 = number of 12-month cases of PTSD.

Chapter 6

The Associations of Posttraumatic Stress Disorder with Secondary Mental and Physical Health Disorders

Ronald C. Kessler, Peter de Jonge, Yueqin Huang, John J. McGrath, Elie G. Karam, and Kate Scott

Comorbidity is often seen in mental disorders (Demyttenaere et al., 2004; Kessler et al., 2005). With posttraumatic stress disorder (PTSD), more than two-thirds of cases also meet criteria for at least one other mental disorder (Alonso et al., 2004; Kessler et al., 2005). One reason for this high comorbidity could be that a history of prior mental disorders predicts the onset and persistence of PTSD, a possibility considered directly in Chapter 4. Another might be that PTSD is a risk factor for the subsequent onset and/or persistence of other mental disorders. Individuals with PTSD, for example, might be at increased risk of developing an alcohol or drug abuse problem due to a desire to relieve their anxiety by self-medicating. Alternatively, those with PTSD who already suffered from an anxiety disorder prior to the exposure to trauma might develop more persistent and severe symptoms than they might have otherwise. If so, these debilitating effects should be counted among the negative consequences of PTSD. Likewise, since there is evidence that PTSD is also associated with a wide variety of physical conditions (Pacella et al., 2013), the elevated prevalence of these disorders might also be understood as an additional adverse sequela of PTSD. Analyses of the World Mental Health (WMH) data examined both of these issues. This chapter presents an overview of those analyses.

Comorbidities with Other Mental Disorders

A number of studies have documented strong comorbidities of PTSD with other mental disorders, including major depression (Flory & Yehuda, 2015), attention-deficit/hyperactivity disorder (ADHD; Spencer et al., 2016), conduct disorder (Bernhard et al., 2016), schizophrenia (Seow et al., 2016), alcohol abuse (Petrakis & Simpson, 2017), and drug abuse (Danovitch, 2016), but little research has considered comorbidities of PTSD with the full range of these other disorders. However, a growing body of literature has examined the structure of comorbidity among all common mental disorders, and these studies can help us better understand the particular comorbidities of PTSD. Numerous researchers have documented that bivariate associations among hierarchy-free anxiety, mood, behavior, and substance disorders can be accounted for by correlated latent predispositions to internalizing and externalizing disorders – with the internalizing disorders, in turn, divided into the secondary dimensions of fear (e.g., panic, phobia) and distress (e.g., major depressive episode, generalized anxiety disorder) disorders (Krueger, 1999; Vollebergh et al., 2001; Cox & Swinson, 2002; Krueger & Markon, 2006a; Slade & Watson, 2006; Lahey et al., 2008; Beesdo-Baum et al., 2009). These results have been used to argue for a reorganization of the classification of mental disorders in both the DSM and ICD diagnostic systems (Watson, 2005; Krueger & Markon, 2006b; Andrews et al., 2009; Goldberg et al., 2009). However, additional work is needed to evaluate the empirical support for such reorganization, as the framework has only recently been expanded to include additional forms of psychopathology, such as psychotic experiences (Markon, 2010). Moreover, additional research on the stability of the structure across socio-demographic variables (e.g., age, sex, education) would be informative.

These results have also been used to investigate whether risk factors for individual disorders are better conceptualized as risk factors for the latent dimensions underlying these disorders rather than for the individual disorders per se. Kramer et al. (2008), for example, found that observed sex differences in several internalizing and externalizing disorders became statistically nonsignificant when the results were adjusted for latent internalizing and externalizing dimensions. Such evidence can be valuable in distinguishing between specific and nonspecific risk factors. This use of latent variable models is only in its infancy. One obvious application is to the development of comorbidity itself. In particular, while the cross-sectional structure of comorbidity has been examined in a number of studies, we are unaware of other attempts besides the WMH surveys to investigate the role of latent dimensions in accounting for the *development* of comorbidity.

Although several studies used longitudinal data to determine whether the structure of internalizing and externalizing disorders is stable over time (Krueger et al., 1998; Vollebergh et al., 2001; Wittchen et al., 2009), none investigated whether this structure accounts for the associations between temporally primary disorders and subsequent first onset of comorbid disorders, with PTSD being the disorder of particular interest in the current chapter. A number of other longitudinal studies examined temporal progression (Stein et al., 2001; Fergusson et al., 2007) or sequencing (Newman et al., 1996; Costello et al., 2003; Burke et al., 2005; Copeland et al., 2009) between earlier and later mental disorders, documenting strong persistence of individual disorders over time and significant predictive associations between some, but not other, temporally primary and later disorders, but none of them looked at PTSD. For example, Fergusson et al. (2007) found that childhood conduct disorder, but not ADHD, predicted subsequent substance disorders.

None of the above studies other than those described here in the WMH data investigated whether associations of earlier disorders with onset of later disorders were mediated by latent variables. Such analyses could be useful in identifying potentially modifiable risk pathways by focusing attention on subsets of disorders with especially strong predictive associations that could subsequently be examined in more focused analyses (Angold et al., 1999; Jensen, 2003). For example, clinical studies finding childhood impulse-control problems in a subset of patients with early-onset obsessive compulsive disorder (OCD; Thomsen & Jensen, 1991; Geller et al., 1996), along with those finding that impulse-control disorders figure prominently in some cases of adult OCD (Hoehn-Saric & Barksdale, 1983; Matsunaga et al., 2005), have created interest in the importance of inhibitory dyscontrol in the pathogenesis of OCD (Chamberlain et al., 2005). However, the role of putative neurobiological markers of such dyscontrol in accounting for the associations of impulse-control disorders with subsequent OCD remains unstudied. The documentation in epidemiological data of special associations between a cluster of early-onset impulse-control disorders and subsequent OCD could help spur such research by suggesting that more focused prospective neurobiological studies of this cluster beginning in childhood might yield important information about this putative OCD subtype.

Methods

At the time the WMH analyses of these issues were carried out, only 14 WMH surveys assessed the full range of hierarchy-free comorbid disorders we wanted to consider – seven in high-income countries (Belgium, France, Germany, Italy, the Netherlands, Spain, and the United States) and seven in low-and-middle-income countries (LMICs; Brazil, Colombia, India [which was at the time part of the WMH series], Lebanon, Mexico, the People's Republic of China [PRC], and Romania). The 29,410 Part II respondents in those surveys were the focus of the analyses summarized here. In an effort to shed light on the issues reviewed above, a novel approach to the study of latent variables in the development of comorbidity was carried out (Kessler et al., 2011a, 2011b). Exploratory principal axis tetrachoric factor analysis with promax rotation was used to examine bivariate associations between all logically possible pairs of hierarchy-free disorders assessed in the WMH surveys. Discrete-time survival analysis (Efron, 1988) with person-year as the unit of analysis and a logistic link function (Willett & Singer, 1993) was then used to study associations of temporally primary lifetime disorders with subsequent first onset of later disorders in order to test the hypothesis that all these associations were mediated by latent variables corresponding to the factors found in the exploratory factor analysis (EFA).

It is noteworthy that the behavioral disorders included in the EFA were disaggregated more than in other WMH analyses in order to allow for the possibility that disorder subtypes might have different associations with comorbidity. Included in the analysis were the same DSM-IV anxiety and mood disorders examined in previous chapters: anxiety disorders including agoraphobia with or without panic disorder, generalized anxiety disorder (GAD), OCD, panic disorder with or without agoraphobia, PTSD, separation anxiety disorder, social phobia, and specific phobia; and mood disorders including bipolar I-II or sub-threshold disorder and major depressive episode/dysthymia. But the assessment of ADHD distinguished between attention-deficit disorder (AD) and hyperactivity disorder (HD) allowing for the possibility that respondents could have either or both, while the assessment of conduct disorder (CD) distinguished between CD with covert symptoms (CD1; e.g., lying, shoplifting) and CD with overt symptoms (CD2; e.g., bullying, being physically cruel to people), again allowing for the possibility that individual respondents could have either or both. The other disorders included in the analyses were intermittent explosive disorder (IED), oppositional-defiant disorder (ODD), and substance use disorders (alcohol and drug abuse with or without dependence).

The initial survival models predicted first onset of each of the DSM-IV/CIDI disorders assessed in the WMH surveys from information about prior lifetime occurrence of the other disorders. We began with 18 disorders, resulting in 306 (18 × 17) pair-wise associations. Each predictor disorder was treated as a time-varying covariate, controlling for respondent age, sex, and survey. Retrospective age-of-onset (AOO) reports were used to define the predictor disorders as time-varying and to define AOO of the outcome disorders. We then estimated a latent variable model that constrained the coefficients in the observed variable models to be mediated by hypothesized continuous time-varying latent variables corresponding to the factors found in the EFA. The coefficients in the observed variable model were *constrained* in the sense that this model included 306 coefficients (see Figure 6.1), whereas the latent variable model, which assumed the existence of two patent mediating variables, used only 36 independent coefficients to reproduce these same associations (see Figure 6.2): 10 coefficients (one of which was non-independent because the 10 coefficients together perfectly predict the time *t* latent variable) for the time *t* lifetime internalizing disorders predicting the time *t* latent internalizing variable; eight coefficients (one of which was non-independent because the eight coefficients together perfectly predict the time *t* latent variable) for the time *t* lifetime externalizing disorders predicting the time *t* latent externalizing variable; four coefficients (two of which were non-independent because the pair of time *t* latent variables perfectly predict each of the two time $t+1$ latent variables) for the time *t* latent internalizing and externalizing variables predicting the time $t+1$ latent internalizing and externalizing variables; 10 coefficients for the time $t+1$ latent internalizing variable predicting first onsets of the 10 time $t+1$ internalizing disorders; and eight coefficients for the time $t+1$ latent externalizing variable predicting first onsets of the eight time $t+1$ externalizing disorders.

It is necessary to note that the latent variables were actually weighted (by ORs of disorders predicting latent variables) composites of all predictor disorders. The assumption that a single weighted composite could represent the associations of all predictor disorders is equivalent to assuming that the ratios of the ORs across predictors were constant across outcomes. These constraints were the key features of the model.

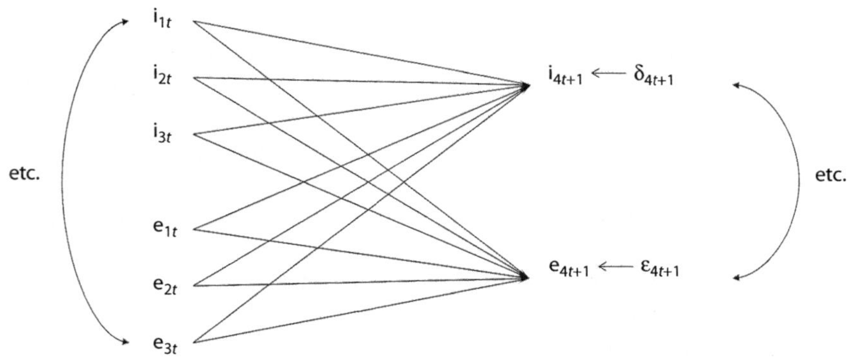

Figure 6.1 Schematic of the multivariate observed variable model[a]

[a]Only three observed lifetime time *t* internalizing disorders (e.g., i_{1t} represents internalizing disorder 1 at time *t*) and externalizing disorders along with only one observed internalizing and one observed externalizing observed at time $t+1$ are shown to simplify the presentation, but there were 10 observed lifetime internalizing and 8 observed externalizing disorders in the actual survival model at each time point. First onset of each of these 18 disorders between times *t* and $t+1$ was predicted by prior lifetime history of the other 17 disorders as of time *t*. Estimation was made in 18 separate survival equations, each with 17 predictors by prior history of the other disorders, for a total of 306 (18 × 17) pair-wise time-lagged associations between earlier and later mental disorders. The 17 predictor disorders were treated as time-varying covariates in a discrete-time (person-year) survival framework. Controls were also included for respondent age at interview, sex, person-year, and country.

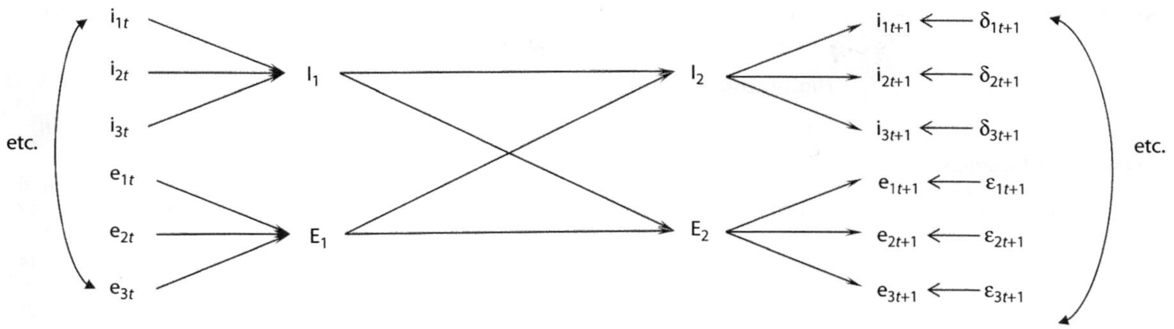

Figure 6.2 Schematic of the multivariate latent variable model[a]

[a]Only three observed lifetime time *t* internalizing disorders (e.g., i_{1t} represents internalizing disorder 1 at time *t*) and externalizing disorders and only three disorders of each set at time $t + 1$ are shown to simplify the presentation, but there were 10 observed lifetime internalizing and 8 observed externalizing disorders in the actual survival model. First onset of each of these 18 disorders between times *t* and $t + 1$ was predicted by latent internalizing or latent externalizing variables at time $t + 1$. These latent variables, in turn, were predicted by lifetime history of latent internalizing and externalizing variables as of time *t*. These time *t* latent variables, finally, were predicted by lifetime history of observed internalizing or externalizing variables as of time *t*. Estimation was carried out using a three-part iterative procedure. See the text for more details. A total of 36 independent associations were estimated, 270 fewer than in the model for associations among observed disorders. As in the earlier observed variable model, the predictor disorders were treated as time-varying covariates in a discrete-time (person-year) survival framework and controls were included for respondent age at interview, sex, person-year, and country.

The standard covariance structure analysis programs used in previous studies of the structure of comorbidity could not be used to impose these constraints, as discrete-time survival analysis is based on a person-year data array that varies in size across the outcomes. An iterative maximum-likelihood (ML) method implemented in an SAS macro was consequently written to estimate the coefficients (SAS Institute Inc., 2002). This procedure sequentially estimated the coefficients in the three parts of the model (time *t* observed variables predicting time *t* latent variables, time *t* latent variables predicting time $t + 1$ latent variables, time $t + 1$ latent variables predicting time $t + 1$ observed variables), each time holding constant the coefficients in the other two parts of the model to their values in the previous iteration, until estimates converged.

Once estimated, a likelihood ratio χ^2 test was used to compare the fit of the latent variable model and the observed variable model with 270 (306 – 36) degrees of freedom. As described below, the latent variable model provided a better fit. We also investigated whether any of the 306 pair-wise associations remained significant after controlling for the latent variables. Simple pair-wise tests were inappropriate because separate 0.05-level tests would generate more than a dozen false positives out of 306 tests. The Bonferroni method and its extensions address this problem (Shaffer, 1995), but these are low-power tests that make it difficult to detect all but the largest true associations (Perneger, 1998). We consequently used an internal sub-sampling strategy to pinpoint pair-wise associations for further investigation by estimating observed-variable survival models controlling for the latent variables in subsets of person-years. Rather than use random subsamples, which would simply have produced patterns determined by sampling theory, we focused on meaningfully different subsamples defined by four independent life course stages (childhood: ages 4–12; adolescence: ages 13–19; young adulthood: ages 20–29; middle adulthood: ages 30–44) and considered a given pair-wise association substantively significant only if it was statistically significant at the 0.05 level both in the total sample and in at least two independent sub-samples with consistent sign patterns and ORs (exponentiated survival coefficients) either greater than or equal to 2.0 or less than or equal to 0.5. As the WMH data were both clustered and weighted, the design-based method of jackknife repeated replications (JRR; Wolter, 1985) was used to calculate standard errors and assess statistical significance. A SAS macro was used for this purpose (SAS Institute Inc., 2002).

Results

Exploratory Factor Analysis (EFA)

EFA of the 18 lifetime DSM-IV disorders was carried out separately in high-income countries and LMICs. Only two meaningful factors were found, with

Table 6.1 Rotated (promax) factor pattern (standardized regression coefficients) of lifetime DSM-IV/CIDI disorders separately in WMH surveys carried out in high-income countries and LMICs[a]

	High-income countries		LMICs		Total	
	I	II	I	II	I	II
I Internalizing Disorders						
MDD or dysthymic disorder	0.72	0.07	0.69	0.09	0.71	0.09
BPD (broad definition)	0.37	0.31	0.54	0.20	0.46	0.27
Panic disorder[b]	0.65	0.10	0.51	0.17	0.60	0.17
Agoraphobia[c]	0.87	−0.11	0.74	−0.16	0.82	−0.14
GAD	0.67	0.04	0.72	−0.02	0.69	0.05
PTSD	0.57	0.18	0.43	0.18	0.52	0.21
Social phobia	0.72	0.09	0.74	−0.04	0.71	0.09
Specific phobia	0.75	−0.13	0.78	−0.16	0.79	−0.16
Separation anxiety disorder	0.54	0.20	0.47	0.14	0.50	0.15
OCD	0.51	0.12	0.71	−0.17	0.63	−0.04
II Externalizing Disorders						
Attention-deficit disorder	0.30	0.51	0.36	0.57	0.31	0.55
Hyperactivity disorder	0.19	0.58	0.32	0.60	0.22	0.61
CD (overt)[d]	−0.09	0.94	−0.03	0.90	−0.08	0.93
CD (covert)[e]	−0.04	0.90	0.05	0.84	−0.01	0.87
IED	0.15	0.61	0.48	0.30	0.29	0.47
ODD	0.10	0.80	−0.02	0.73	0.02	0.78
Alcohol abuse or dependence	0.01	0.76	−0.14	0.63	−0.06	0.73
Drug abuse or dependence	−0.06	0.79	−0.15	0.69	−0.08	0.77
(n)[f]	(7,360)		(13,869)		(21,229)	

[a]Results are based on principal axis factor analysis of tetrachoric correlation matrices estimated in person-year datasets.
[b]With or without agoraphobia.
[c]With or without panic disorder.
[d]E.g., bullying, fighting, being physically cruel to people.
[e]E.g., lying, shoplifting.
[f]The n's are for the numbers of respondents. The numbers of person-years (every year of life of the respondents beginning at age four up to and including the age at interview) are 214,738 (high-income), 376,961 (low- and middle-income), and 591,699 (total).

unrotated eigenvalues of 8.0 and 1.8 (developed) and 6.6 and 2.3 (developing). Promax rotated factor loadings (standardized partial regression coefficients) showed the factors correspond to internalizing and externalizing dimensions (see Table 6.1). PTSD along with all other anxiety and mood disorders other than bipolar disorder (BPD) loaded clearly on the internalizing factor (0.43–0.87 standardized regression coefficients). All the behavior and substance disorders other than IED loaded clearly on the externalizing factor (0.51–0.94 standardized regression coefficients). The factor loading for PTSD on the internalizing factor was 0.43–0.57 compared to 0.18–0.21 on the externalizing factor. BPD cross-loaded in LMICs (0.31–0.37) and IED in high-income countries (0.30–0.48). However, country-level analyses (results not shown) found that BPD generally loaded more strongly on the internalizing factor and IED on the externalizing factor, leading us to classify them with these dimensions in further analyses. A separate EFA of only the internalizing disorders found no reliable secondary distinction between fear and other distress disorders (unrotated eigenvalues of 4.8 and 1.0 in high-income countries and 4.3 and 1.3 in LMICs).

Bivariate and Multivariate Associations between Earlier and Later Disorders

As noted above, we estimated 306 bivariate survival equations, each with first onset of one disorder predicted by the prior occurrence of one of the other 17 disorders. Of the 306 survival coefficients, 98.0% were positive and 95.1% were significant (see Table 6.2). The median (and IQR) ORs were 3.4 (2.7–4.3). None of the ORs less than 1.0 was significant. Within-domain ORs were generally larger than between-domain ORs, with within-domain median ORs of 3.6–5.5 compared to between-domain medians of 3.0–3.2.

This largely positive pattern persisted in attenuated form in multivariate models, with 80.0% of ORs

Table 6.2 Associations of lifetime DSM-IV/CIDI disorders with subsequent first onset of other DSM-IV/CIDI disorders based on bivariate and multivariate survival models in the total sample (n = 21,229)[a]

	Distribution of ORs					
	Median	Range	IQR	Percent positive	Percent positive and significant	Number of ORs
I Internalizing Predicting Internalizing						**90**
Bivariate	3.6	1.2–10.4	3.0–4.3	100	97.8	
Multivariate	1.6	0.4–5.5	1.1–2.0	87.8	58.9	
II Externalizing Predicting Internalizing						**80**
Bivariate	3.2	1.7–7.5	2.6–3.7	100	98.8	
Multivariate	1.3	0.5–3.2	1.0–1.6	80.0	28.8	
III Internalizing Predicting Externalizing						**80**
Bivariate	3.0	0.4–10.3	2.4–3.9	96.3	90.0	
Multivariate	1.3	0.1–3.2	0.9–1.6	70.0	33.8	
IV Externalizing Predicting Externalizing						**56**
Bivariate	5.5	0.5–30.0	3.3–8.2	94.5	92.7	
Multivariate	1.6	0.2–13.4	1.2–2.9	81.8	50.9	
V Total						**306**
Bivariate	3.4	0.4–30.0	2.7–4.3	98.0	95.1	
Multivariate	1.4	0.1–13.4	1.1–1.9	80.0	43.0	

[a]First lifetime onset of each of 18 DSM-IV/CIDI disorders was predicted either by a single dummy variable for prior lifetime history of one of the other disorders (bivariate model) or 17 dummy variables for prior history of each of the 17 other disorders (multivariate model). In discrete-time (person-year) survival models, the predictor disorders and latent variables were treated as time-varying covariates. Controls were included for respondent age at interview, person-year, sex, and country.

positive and 43.0% positive and statistically significant. The median (OR = 1.4) and IQR (OR = 1.1–1.9) of ORs were considerably lower than in bivariate models due to strong inter-correlations among predictor disorders. Nine of the 306 multivariate ORs were negative and significant (GAD predicting agoraphobia and specific phobia and HD, PTSD and CD1 predicting OCD, CD2 predicting GAD and PTSD, and alcohol abuse predicting AD and HD). 50.9–58.9% of within-domain ORs were positive and significant compared to 28.8–33.8% of between-domain ORs. The median OR was higher within (OR = 1.6) than between (OR = 1.3) domains.

Multivariate Associations in the Latent Variable Model

The latent variable model fit the observed data better than the observed variable model, as indicated by both a lower Bayesian Information Criterion (BIC; Kass & Raftery, 1995) of 7,514.3 (latent) versus 7,530.0 (observed) and an insignificant improvement in likelihood ratio χ^2 of the observed variable model (χ^2_{270} = 107.8, p = 0.99). Latent variable coefficients were quite stable, as indicated by the Pearson correlations of model coefficients across four samples (the total sample and the three subsamples of all high-income countries, all LMICs, and all countries excluding the four with survey response rates less than 60% [Belgium, France, Germany, and Spain]) being 0.88–0.97.

As noted earlier, the latent variables can be interpreted as weighted (by ORs of disorders predicting latent variables) composites of all predictor disorders. The assumption that a single weighted composite represented the effects of all the predictor disorders on all outcomes would be equivalent to assuming that the ratios of the ORs across predictors were constant across outcomes. The good fit of the latent variable model showed that this assumption was generally consistent with the data, which means that the predictive effects of these disorders on each other could plausibly be assumed to be mediated by common internalizing and externalizing pathways.

The metric of the time t latent variables was set by fixing the slope of the latent variable on the strongest time t predictor to 1.0 and scaling other slopes relative to that value (see Table 6.3). Within the internalizing domain, specific phobia was by far the most powerful predictor (1.00 by definition) followed by OCD (0.62) and other phobias (0.46–0.48). GAD

Table 6.3 Parameter estimates for associations between observed disorders and latent variables in the latent variable model (n = 21,229)[a]

	Time *t* disorders predicting time *t* latent variables		Time *t* + 1 latent variables predicting time *t* + 1 first onset of disorders	
	Est	(SE)	Est	(SE)
I Internalizing				
MDD or dysthymic disorder	0.29*	(0.06)	0.68*	(0.04)
BPD (broad definition)	0.18*	(0.08)	0.85*	(0.05)
Panic disorder[b]	−0.02	(0.10)	0.82*	(0.05)
Agoraphobia[c]	0.48*	(0.09)	1.00*	(0.09)
GAD	0.02	(0.07)	0.72*	(0.05)
PTSD	0.21*	(0.08)	0.68*	(0.05)
Social phobia	0.46*	(0.05)	0.97*	(0.05)
Specific phobia	1.00*	(0.09)	0.86*	(0.10)
Separation anxiety disorder	0.44*	(0.06)	0.74*	(0.05)
OCD	0.62*	(0.07)	0.87*	(0.06)
II Externalizing				
Attention-deficit disorder	0.77*	(0.24)	1.00*	(0.31)
Hyperactivity disorder	1.00*	(0.23)	0.95*	(0.16)
CD (overt)[d]	0.43*	(0.18)	0.74*	(0.16)
CD (covert)[e]	0.57*	(0.23)	0.78*	(0.16)
IED	0.77*	(0.15)	0.52*	(0.08)
ODD	0.97*	(0.18)	0.69*	(0.15)
Alcohol abuse or dependence	−0.53	(0.35)	0.44*	(0.08)
Drug abuse or dependence	0.51	(0.31)	0.38*	(0.13)

*Significant at the 0.05 level, two-sided test.
[a]Based on an iteratively estimated pooled discrete-time (person-year) survival model with 17 dummy variables for prior history of each other disorder predicting subsequent first onset of each of the 18 disorders assuming the existence of latent internalizing and externalizing disorders that explain the direct effects of the observed predictor disorders on the outcome disorders. The predictor disorders and latent variables were treated as time-varying covariates. Controls were included for respondent age at interview, person-year, sex, and country. See the text for a discussion of estimation methods.
[b]With or without agoraphobia.
[c]With or without panic disorder.
[d]E.g., bullying, fighting, being physically cruel to people.
[e]E.g., lying, shoplifting.

and panic disorder, at the other extreme, were nonsignificant predictors. The remaining internalizing disorders had ORs of intermediate strength (0.18–0.44). Within the externalizing domain, HD (1.00) and ODD (0.97) were the most powerful predictors. Alcohol and drug abuse were nonsignificant and the remaining externalizing disorders had ORs in the range of 0.43–0.77.

The ORs for the disorders as outcomes were much more consistent than for the disorders as predictors, with ranges of 0.68–1.00 (internalizing) and 0.44–1.00 (externalizing). Agoraphobia and social phobia were the most strongly predicted internalizing disorders, while AD and HD were the most strongly predicted externalizing disorders. The relative importance of internalizing and externalizing disorders predicting each other was estimated in the set of four ORs between the latent variables at times *t* and *t* + 1 (see Table 6.4). Weighted (by relative prevalence of disorders) within-domain ORs (1.6 for internalizing; 1.4 for externalizing) were higher than between-domain ORs (1.3 for time *t* internalizing predicting time *t* + 1 externalizing; 1.1 for time *t* externalizing predicting

Table 6.4 Parameter estimates for associations among latent variables in the latent variable model (n = 21,229)

Time 1 predictor group	Time 2 dependent group			
	Internalizing		Externalizing	
	OR	(95% CI)	OR	(95% CI)
Internalizing	1.6*	(1.5–1.6)	1.3*	(1.2–1.3)
Externalizing	1.1*	(1.1–1.2)	1.4*	(1.3–1.4)

*Significant at the 0.05 level, two-sided test.

time $t + 1$ internalizing), but between-domain ORs were nonetheless statistically significant.

Residual Associations Not Explained by the Latent Variable Model

A key question in the current chapter is whether any residual associations involving PTSD could be found in further analyses of the above model. As it happened, only 13 of the 306 residual pair-wise time-lagged associations between observed disorders passed our test of statistical significance. Nine of these 13 were positive and the other 4 negative. PTSD was involved in 2 of these 13, both of them negative associations. The 9 positive associations involved 4 within-disorder reciprocal ORs between CDI and CD2 (3.2–4.8) and between AD and HD (4.0–19.4), 2 asymmetrical associations between well-known disorder pairs (panic predicting agoraphobia [2.0–2.22] and depression predicting GAD [2.0–6.0], although the latter association was limited to child-adolescent onsets), and that might have reflected diagnostic confusions [agoraphobia predicting specific phobia (2.2–4.8); and HD but, importantly, not AD, predicting BPD (1.9–3.9)], and one for IED predicting OCD (1.5–4.0). The 4 significant negative residual associations included PTSD predicting OCD (0.4–0.7), CD2 predicting both BPD (0.2–0.5) and PTSD (0.2–0.4) and IED (0.5–0.6) predicting drug abuse.

Discussion

Several limitations of the analysis of comorbidities of PTSD with other mental disorders are noteworthy. First, as noted in previous chapters, the diagnoses were based on fully structured lay interviews rather than on semi-structured clinical interviews, and these interviews typically produce more reliable (i.e., reproducible across multiple interviewers) diagnoses (Wittchen, 1994) as well as somewhat more conservative prevalence estimates (Haro et al., 2006). However, fully structured interviews, unlike semi-structured clinical interviews, are unable to clarify symptom responses or check questions across disorders to facilitate differential diagnosis, potentially leading to inflated estimates of comorbidity. Second, disorders were assessed dichotomously rather than dimensionally, presumably reducing our ability to detect for subtle aspects of structure in the data. This might help explain why we did not detect higher-order sub-factors in the two-factor exploratory factor analysis model. Third, data were combined across countries with very different cultures and across surveys with very different response rates (which could have introduced variation in sample selection bias), different rates of sample exclusion (due to cross-national differences in rates of suicide, homelessness, and institutionalization), and different languages in which interviews were administered. Even though every effort was made to make the translations as comparable as possible (Harkness et al., 2008), residual variation in meaning almost certainly contributed to cross-national variation in results. Fourth, lifetime diagnoses were based on retrospective reports rather than on prospective assessments, probably leading to recall bias that underestimated prevalence (Moffitt et al., 2010) and distorted AOO estimates (Simon & VonKorff, 1995) despite the use of special memory priming methods (Knäuper et al., 1999). Bias in model coefficients might have varied across disorders as a function of AOO and/or recency. Given the importance of this potential bias, it is noteworthy that the onset distributions based on these retrospective data were quite consistent with those based on prospective studies and studies carried out at separate life course stages (Kessler et al., 2007). In addition, model coefficients in subsamples defined by life course stage were very consistent, suggesting that variation in recall across the sample age range did not significantly influence results. Fifth, models were based on the simplifying assumptions that the time-lagged associations among mental disorders were constant across countries and sex, stable across the life course, and unrelated either to AOO or time-since-onset of the predictor disorders. Sensitivity analyses showed that these assumptions were a reasonable first approximation. Sixth, we did not take history of treatment into consideration, even though early treatment, which varies in frequency across countries (Wang et al., 2007), might interrupt the progression of comorbidity and thereby distort estimates of predictive associations.

In the context of these limitations, our finding of a two-factor internalizing-externalizing structure among WMH disorders is consistent with previous research (Vollebergh et al., 2001; Cox & Swinson, 2002; Krueger & Markon, 2006a; Slade & Watson, 2006; Lahey et al., 2008; Beesdo-Baum et al., 2009), but does not support the distinction in some previous studies between distress (e.g., depression, GAD, PTSD) and fear (i.e., panic and phobias) disorders. As noted in the introduction, other studies also failed to find a distinction between distress and fear disorders (Krueger et al.,

1998; Krueger & Finger, 2001). This less differentiated structure in the WMH data might be due to our focus on lifetime disorders, whereas 12-month disorders were the focus of most studies that distinguished distress and fear disorders. Our finding that PTSD loaded with internalizing disorders is consistent with these previous studies.

Our finding of significant time-lagged associations across virtually all pairs of the disorders considered here is broadly consistent with evidence of associations between earlier and later disorders in previous longitudinal studies (Newman et al., 1996; Stein et al., 2001; Costello et al., 2003; Burke et al., 2005; Fergusson et al., 2007; Copeland et al., 2009), although most previous studies focused on prevalent cases whereas we studied first onsets. As with previous studies, we also found stronger and more consistent time-lagged associations within than between the internalizing and externalizing domains but significant between-domain time-lagged associations (Newman et al., 1996; Costello et al., 2003).

Our analysis then went beyond previous studies to investigate the role of latent variables in the development of comorbidity. We showed that the vast majority of the 306 pair-wise time-lagged associations among the 18 disorders considered here could be explained by a model that assumed the existence of mediating latent internalizing and externalizing variables. This finding extends previous cross-cultural work on the structure of comorbidity (Krueger et al., 2003). The fact that the predictive associations across this large number of disorders was mediated by two higher-order variables makes the internalizing and externalizing spectrum dimensions compelling targets for inquiry aimed at reducing the burden of mental disorders around the world by interrupting the processes leading to the onset of comorbidity.

Our finding of 13 significant residual associations shows that the latent variables explain the vast majority of the comorbidity of PTSD with the other disorders considered here. The negative residual association of CD2 (overt CD) with subsequent PTSD might be related to the findings that *blunted* psychophysiological and emotional reactivity to fear stimuli are predictors of CD (Herpertz et al., 2005; Sterzer et al., 2005) whereas *heightened* physiological reactivity to trauma-related stress cues is a predictor of PTSD (Orr & Roth, 2000; Marshall & Garakani, 2002). These observations suggest that a more differentiated latent variable model with separate internalizing and externalizing sub-dimensions might explain the significant negative associations involving PTSD found here in the less differentiated WMH latent variable model. Reconciliation of these results with those in our earlier analyses of the associations of temporally primary comorbid disorders with the onset (Chapter 11) and course (Chapter 16) of PTSD would require analyses based on prospective data.

Even if prospective studies subsequently show our specifications to be reliable, their existence should not deflect attention from our main finding: that the consistently significant comorbidities found between PTSD and other mental disorders assessed in the WMH surveys are likely due to common underlying processes that should be a major focus of future research on the development and consequences of comorbidity. One important implication of this finding is that future research on comorbidities of PTSD with other mental disorders should guard against interpreting results as unique without first investigating, as we did here, whether or not they are specific rather than mere realizations of larger processes involving all internalizing and/or externalizing disorders. Finally, the fact that we found only two factors does not mean that only two underlying processes are at work, as multiple processes could underlie each factor, and all these diverse processes need to be studied in order to enrich our understanding of the causal influences leading to the higher-order structure found here.

Comorbidities with Physical Disorders

We turn now to a consideration of comorbidities between PTSD and physical disorders. It is well documented that PTSD is associated with an increased risk of several chronic physical conditions. Most of this research has focused on links between PTSD and cardiometabolic diseases, with the association between PTSD and incident coronary heart disease the best substantiated. Early studies of the association between PTSD and subsequent heart disease were based on male military veterans (Kubzansky et al., 2007; Boscarino, 2008) but this association has now been confirmed in a diverse range of prospective studies, including among women (Kubzansky et al., 2009; Jordan et al., 2011; Vaccarino et al., 2013; Sumner et al., 2015). A growing number of prospective studies are also finding associations of PTSD with incident stroke (Emdin et al., 2016), hypertension (Schnurr et al., 2000; Sumner et al., 2016), and type 2 diabetes (Boyko et al., 2013; Vaccarino et al., 2014), as is noted in several recent reviews of this literature (Levine et al., 2014; Edmondson & von Känel, 2017; Koenen et al., 2017).

A second cluster of physical conditions associated with PTSD are chronic pain conditions (e.g., chronic headache and backache; fibromyalgia, chronic pelvic pain). Most of this research has focused on concurrent comorbidity, based on the observation that PTSD and pain conditions often develop in close temporal proximity to one another and have mutually reinforcing links (Sharp & Harvey, 2001; Brennstuhl et al., 2015; Holley et al., 2016). The specific question in this chapter, though, is whether PTSD might increase the risk of the *subsequent* development of chronic pain conditions. Although there are not many prospective studies specifically examining this question, some researchers have taken as a starting point the finding that chronic pain in adulthood is among the most common of the medical outcomes of abuse in childhood (Davis et al., 2005; Paras et al., 2009) and have queried the role of intervening PTSD. Evidence has shown PTSD to be both a mediator (Lang et al., 2006; Campbell et al., 2008) and a moderator (Raphael & Widom, 2011) of the associations between child abuse and subsequent onset of chronic pain conditions in adulthood (Lee et al., 2016).

The mounting research linking PTSD with incident cardiometabolic and chronic pain conditions, together with recent studies linking PTSD with other diseases such as rheumatoid arthritis (Lee et al., 2016) and asthma (de la Hoz et al., 2016), suggests that PTSD may have serious and persistent ramifications for physical health. However, one important methodological issue is whether PTSD constitutes the "bad actor" in these associations with physical ill-health or whether other mental disorders with which PTSD is commonly comorbid are the true causes. Depression is the most obvious candidate both because it is highly comorbid with PTSD and because it has even better substantiated associations with cardiometabolic outcomes than PTSD (Whooley & Wong, 2013; Scott, 2014). Although several of the prospective studies on PTSD and cardiovascular diseases have controlled for depression, most studies linking PTSD with physical conditions have not. Moreover, no study prior to the WMH analyses described below has controlled for a range of mental disorders other than depression. This may be important because various anxiety disorders that often precede PTSD in onset are also associated with cardiovascular diseases (Thurston et al., 2013). We did this by using WMH retrospectively-reported data on AOO of mental disorders and AOO (or diagnosis) of physical conditions. We examined associations in these data between temporally prior PTSD and the subsequent onset/diagnosis of 11 chronic physical conditions, with and without control for lifetime comorbid mental disorders.

Methods

These analyses were based on data from WMH surveys in 19 countries, including 13 high-income countries (Belgium, Italy, France, Germany, The Netherlands, Portugal, Spain, Northern Ireland, Poland, Israel, Japan, New Zealand, and the United States) and 6 LMICs (Mexico, Colombia, Iraq, Peru, PRC, and Romania). It is noteworthy that the analysis was not carried out with a special focus on PTSD, but rather considered the multivariate associations of all the mental disorders assessed in the WMH surveys with the subsequent onset of chronic physical disorders. Not all these mental disorders were assessed in all the surveys used in the analyses. Poland and Iraq, in particular, did not assess PTSD in a way that could be used in the analyses reported below. These analyses were conducted in the pooled cross-national WMH dataset that combined data across all countries, based on the weighted Part II combined subsample of 52,095 respondents in these surveys. The initial WMH work on these analyses was reported in an earlier volume in this series (Von Korff et al., 2009) and later work in a series of journal articles cited below.

The 11 chronic physical conditions that were included in these analyses as outcome variables were selected from a slightly larger set of physical conditions assessed in the WMH surveys. Selection was based on consideration of whether there was existing research on their associations with temporally prior mental disorders, together with consideration of the frequency of the physical conditions in the WMH surveys. Assessment of the physical conditions involved a brief series of questions in Part II of the interview together with a checklist based on the US Health Interview Survey. Respondents were asked whether a health professional had ever told them they had any of a series of medical conditions (e.g., heart disease, stroke, cancer, diabetes, high blood pressure, asthma, other chronic lung disease, peptic ulcer), or whether they had a lifetime history of a chronic symptomatic condition (e.g., arthritis [primarily osteoarthritis], chronic back or neck pain, chronic or severe headaches). Respondents were asked how old they were when first diagnosed with the condition (for the medical conditions) or first experienced the condition (for the symptomatic conditions). This year is referred to herein as the AOO or diagnosis of these conditions, although it is recognized that the underlying pathology of these conditions usually develops over many years. Lifetime prevalence of these conditions among WMH respondents was reported in our earlier publications (Scott et al., 2013a, 2013b, 2016; Alonso et al., 2014; de Jonge et al., 2014; O'Neill et al., 2014; Stein et al., 2014; Bruffaerts et al., 2015; Rapsey et al., 2015; Swain et al., 2015; Aguilar-Gaxiola et al., 2016).

The associations of PTSD with subsequent chronic physical condition were studied using discrete-time survival analyses, based on retrospective reports about AOO of PTSD and of the symptomatic physical conditions, and age of diagnosis of the medical conditions. For all but 3 of the 11 physical conditions (the exceptions being chronic back pain, chronic headache, and peptic ulcer) the start of the period at risk of the physical condition was set at age 20. That is, the small number of people who reported that a given physical condition had an onset before age 21 were excluded from analysis. This was because childhood onsets of these conditions were likely to be congenital and unrelated to mental disorders.

For these analyses, a person-year data set was created with each year in the life of each respondent up to and including the AOO of the physical condition or their age at interview (whichever came first) treated as a separate observational record, with the year of physical condition onset coded 1 and earlier years coded 0 on a dichotomous outcome variable. PTSD was coded 1 from the year *after* first onset. This time lag ensured that first onsets of PTSD in the same year as the physical condition were not included in the predictor set. Only person-years up to the diagnosis/onset of the physical condition were analyzed so that only PTSD occurring prior to the onset of the physical condition was examined as a predictor. Survival coefficients were transformed into ORs. Separate models were estimated for each physical condition outcome.

The bivariate models predicted onset of each physical condition as a function of temporally prior PTSD controlling for age cohort (18–29, 30–44, 45–59, 60+), person year, sex, and country. The main analyses were then repeated controlling for smoking history and education, but few material differences emerged with control for either of these additional covariates. Multivariate models were then estimated that included dummy variables for other DSM-IV mental disorders. The latter included panic disorder, agoraphobia without panic, specific phobia, social phobia, generalized anxiety disorder, obsessive compulsive disorder, major depressive disorder/dysthymia, bipolar spectrum disorder, alcohol abuse, alcohol dependence, drug abuse, drug dependence, intermittent explosive disorder, bulimia nervosa, and binge eating disorder.

Results

Associations of PTSD with Subsequent Onset/Diagnosis of Chronic Physical Conditions

PTSD had significant positive bivariate associations with subsequent onset/diagnosis of all 11 physical condition outcomes considered with ORs ranging from 1.4 (high blood pressure) to 2.6 (peptic ulcer) (see Table 6.5). Multivariate associations were more telling, as they show the ORs for PTSD controlling for comorbid mental disorders. Six of the 11 ORs of PTSD with the physical conditions remained significant in these models, albeit substantially reduced in magnitude from their respective bivariate association, again pointing to the role of comorbid mental disorders. The significant multivariate associations included the three pain outcomes (arthritis, chronic back/neck pain, and chronic headache) with ORs of 1.3–1.4. In addition, PTSD was significantly associated with asthma (OR = 1.5), peptic ulcer (OR = 1.7), and heart disease (OR = 1.5).

Discussion

Limitations similar to those noted above in the section on comorbidities involving mental disorders also apply to our analyses of comorbidities of PTSD with physical conditions. Retrospective recall of AOO of mental disorders is subject to bias and although the probing strategy employed in the WMH surveys has been shown to reduce bias (Knäuper et al., 1999), it is likely that some inaccuracy in onset timing remains. Recall of AOO of physical conditions may be more reliable (Pattaro et al., 2007), but it is nonetheless the case that the retrospective recall of trauma timing for both the predictor mental disorders and physical outcomes is a key limitation of these analyses. The cross-sectional design also raises the possibility

Table 6.5 Bivariate and multivariate associations of DSM-IV/CIDI PTSD with the subsequent onset/diagnosis of chronic physical conditions

	Bivariate[a]		Multivariate model[b]	
	OR	(95% CI)	OR	(95% CI)
Type of Chronic Physical Condition				
Arthritis	1.9*	(1.7–2.2)	1.4*	(1.2–1.6)
Asthma	2.1*	(1.6–2.7)	1.5*	(1.1–1.9)
Cancer	1.5*	(1.2–1.9)	1.3	(1.0–1.6)
Chronic back or neck pain	2.0*	(1.7–2.2)	1.3*	(1.1–1.4)
Chronic headache	2.0*	(1.7–2.3)	1.3*	(1.1–1.4)
Chronic lung disease	2.0*	(1.4–1.9)	1.1	(0.8–1.6)
Diabetes	1.5*	(1.1–2.0)	1.1	(0.8–1.6)
Heart disease	2.0*	(1.5–2.5)	1.5*	(1.1–2.0)
High blood pressure	1.4*	(1.2–1.6)	1.1	(0.9–1.2)
Peptic ulcer	2.6*	(2.1–3.1)	1.7*	(1.4–2.1)
Stroke	2.0*	(1.3–2.9)	1.4	(0.9–2.2)

*Significant at the 0.05 level, two-sided test.
[a]PTSD was estimated as a predictor of the physical condition in a discrete-time survival model, controlling for age cohorts, sex, person-year, and country, with a separate model estimated for each physical condition.
[b]The model was estimated with PTSD and all other assessed mental disorders entered simultaneously, including the controls specified above.

of spurious or inflated associations through mental disorders at the time of interview affecting self-report of physical conditions; however, sensitivity analyses excluding those with mental disorders at the time of interview found no meaningful alteration in associations (Scott et al., 2013a). Finally, retrospective assessment is known to lead to under-reporting of mental disorders, and, to a lesser extent, of physical conditions (Takayanagi et al., 2014). In addition, the assessment of physical conditions in the WMH surveys was less rigorous than the assessment of mental disorders, and self-report of physician-assigned diagnoses will miss conditions that are asymptomatic in early stages. These limitations will undoubtedly have resulted in some individuals with a true history of mental disorder and/or physical condition being misclassified as non-cases; although it is important to note that this kind of misclassification tends to bias associations towards the null, making the results conservative. Survival bias may also contribute to the conservative nature of these findings.

These findings are potentially quite important in documenting associations between PTSD and physical outcomes independent of a wide range of other mental disorders, although the design limitations mean that confirmation in prospective designs will be necessary. That said, it is noteworthy that those physical conditions that we found to be significantly associated with prior PTSD, independent of mental disorder comorbidity, are the same ones most reliably associated with PTSD in existing prospective research: heart disease and chronic pain conditions. We also found that PTSD was associated with adult onset asthma, consistent with one recent prospective study (de la Hoz et al., 2016), and we found it to be associated with ulcer, consistent with prior studies connecting PTSD with gastrointestinal distress (Pacella et al., 2013).

At this point, it is unclear why PTSD is associated with elevated risk of subsequent physical illness, but many potential mechanisms have been advanced. These include behavioral and lifestyle factors (e.g., smoking and alcohol use, poor diet, poor sleep, lack of physical activity) that are more common among those with PTSD and are also known to be on the causal pathway for many chronic physical conditions (Levine et al., 2014; Hall et al., 2015; Koenen et al., 2017). Many biological mechanisms have also been suggested, most of which relate to regulation of the physiological stress response pathways: the sympathetic-adrenal-medullary (SAM) axis and the hypothalamic-pituitary-adrenocortical (HPA) axis. Dysregulation of the HPA and SAM axes, associated with PTSD, has a range of adverse metabolic, cardiovascular, immune, and neurological effects (Miller et al., 2002; Yehuda, 2006; Chrousos & Kino, 2007; Levine et al., 2014). Effects of psychotropic medications such as antidepressants cannot be discounted as a contributing factor to the medical sequelae of PTSD, given the research linking the SSRIs with cardiovascular abnormalities (Licht et al., 2010; Shah et al., 2011; Brunoni et al., 2012). There may also be an important indirect contribution from health care inequalities that make it less likely for physical conditions to be both detected and treated in individuals with mental health problems (Lawrence & Kisely, 2010). Research has identified several reasons for these inequalities such as a lack of explicit allocation of responsibility for medical treatment of those with mental disorders, lack of service delivery integration, and pessimistic attitudes among treatment providers as to whether improved physical health is a priority – or even possible – among those with mental illness (Hyland et al., 2003). Finally, despite the many plausible causal mechanisms, it is also possible that the associations between PTSD and physical conditions instead reflect shared determinants stemming from a range of adverse social, biological, and psychological factors during fetal development or early childhood (Barker et al., 2002; Koenen et al., 2007; Scott, 2009).

Even if these associations between PTSD and physical conditions are not causal, they still highlight the need for improvements in service delivery to help ensure that risk factors for chronic disease are recognized and treated among those with PTSD. But it should also be understood that PTSD is not a special case in its links with subsequent chronic physical conditions; as noted earlier, there is a vast body of research on associations of depression with chronic physical condition outcomes. Moreover, WMH data indicate that virtually all mental disorders are associated with subsequent onset of at least some chronic physical conditions (Scott et al., 2016). Not only are the associations with physical outcomes common to all mental disorders but so are the hypothesized mediating mechanisms. These findings challenge traditional mind-body dichotomies and models of service delivery. Clinicians in all sectors and in all disciplines need greater awareness of the potential for mental disorders such as PTSD to affect physical health.

Acknowledgment

Portions of this chapter are based on Scott, K. M., Lim, C., Al-Hamzawi, A., et al. (2016). Association of mental disorders with subsequent chronic physical conditions: World Mental Health Surveys from 17 countries. *JAMA Psychiatry*, 73, 150–158, by permission of the American Medical Association.

References

Aguilar-Gaxiola, S., Loera, G., Geraghty, E. M., et al. (2016). Associations between DSM-IV mental disorders and subsequent onset of arthritis. *Journal of Psychosomatic Research*, 82, 11–16.

Alonso, J., Angermeyer, M. C., Bernert, S., et al. (2004). 12-month comorbidity patterns and associated factors in Europe: results from the European Study of the Epidemiology of Mental Disorders (ESEMeD) project. *Acta Psychiatrica Scandinavica. Supplementum*, 109, 28–37.

Alonso, J., de Jonge, P., Lim, C. C., et al. (2014). Association between mental disorders and subsequent adult onset asthma. *Journal of Psychiatric Research*, 59, 179–88.

Andrews, G., Goldberg, D. P., Krueger, R. F., et al. (2009). Exploring the feasibility of a meta-structure for DSM-IV and ICD-11: could it improve utility and validity? *Psychological Medicine*, 39, 1993–2000.

Angold, A., Costello, E. J., & Erkanli, A. (1999). Comorbidity. *Journal of Child Psychology and Psychiatry and Allied Disciplines*, 40, 57–87.

Barker, D. J. P., Eriksson, J. G., Forsen, T., & Osmond, C. (2002). Fetal origins of adult disease: strength of effects and biological basis. *International Journal of Epidemiology*, 31, 1235–9.

Beesdo-Baum, K., Höfler, M., Gloster, A., et al. (2009). The structure of common mental disorders: a replication study in a community sample of adolescents and young adults. *International Journal of Methods in Psychiatric Research*, 18, 204–20.

Bernhard, A., Martinelli, A., Ackermann, K., Saure, D., & Freitag, C. M. (2016). Association of trauma, posttraumatic stress disorder and conduct disorder: a systematic review and meta-analysis. *Neuroscience and Biobehavioral Reviews*, Dec 23 [Epub ahead of print].

Boscarino, J. A. (2008). A prospective study of PTSD and early-age heart disease mortality among Vietnam veterans: implications for surveillance and prevention. *Psychosomatic Medicine*, 70, 668–76.

Boyko, E. J., Seelig, A. D., Jacobson, I. G., et al. (2013). Sleep characteristics, mental health, and diabetes risk: a prospective study of US military service members in the Millennium Cohort Study. *Diabetes Care*, 36, 3154–61.

Brennstuhl, M. J., Tarquinio, C., & Montel, S. (2015). Chronic pain and PTSD: evolving views on their comorbidity. *Perspectives in Psychiatric Care*, 51, 295–304.

Bruffaerts, R., Demyttenaere, K., Kessler, R. C., et al. (2015). The associations between preexisting mental disorders and subsequent onset of chronic headaches: a worldwide epidemiologic perspective. *Journal of Pain*, 16, 42–52.

Brunoni, A. R., Lotufo, P. A., & Benseñor, I. M. (2012). Are antidepressants good for the soul but bad for the matter? Using noninvasive brain stimulation to detangle depression/antidepressants effects on heart rate variability and cardiovascular risk. *Biological Psychiatry*, 71, e27–8.

Burke, J. D., Loeber, R., Lahey, B. B., & Rathouz, P. J. (2005). Developmental transitions among affective and behavioral disorders in adolescent boys. *Journal of Child Psychology and Psychiatry and Allied Disciplines*, 46, 1200–10.

Campbell, R., Greeson, M. R., Bybee, D., & Raja, S. (2008). The co-occurrence of childhood sexual abuse, adult sexual assault, intimate partner violence, and sexual harassment: a mediational model of posttraumatic stress disorder and physical health outcomes. *Journal of Consulting and Clinical Psychology*, 76, 194–207.

Chamberlain, S. R., Blackwell, A. D., Fineberg, N. A., Robbins, T. W., & Sahakian, B. J. (2005). The neuropsychology of obsessive compulsive disorder: the importance of failures in cognitive and behavioural inhibition as candidate endophenotypic markers. *Neuroscience and Biobehavioral Reviews*, 29, 399–419.

Chrousos, G. P., & Kino, T. (2007). Glucocorticoid action networks and complex psychiatric and/or somatic disorders. *Stress*, 10, 213–19.

Copeland, W. E., Shanahan, L., Costello, E. J., & Angold, A. (2009). Childhood and adolescent psychiatric disorders as predictors of young adult disorders. *Archives of General Psychiatry*, 66, 764–72.

Costello, E. J., Mustillo, S., Erkanli, A., Keeler, G., & Angold, A. (2003). Prevalence and development of psychiatric disorders in childhood and adolescence. *Archives of General Psychiatry*, 60, 837–44.

Cox, B. J., & Swinson, R. P. (2002). Instrument to assess depersonalization-derealization in panic disorder. *Depression and Anxiety*, 15, 172–5.

Danovitch, I. (2016). Post-traumatic stress disorder and opioid use disorder: a narrative review of conceptual models. *Journal of Addictive Diseases*, 35, 169–79.

Davis, D. A., Luecjen, L. J., & Zautra, A. J. (2005). Are reports of childhood abuse related to the experience of chronic pain in adulthood? *Clinical Journal of Pain*, 21, 398–405.

de Jonge, P., Alonso, J., Stein, D. J., et al. (2014). Associations between DSM-IV mental disorders and diabetes mellitus: a role for impulse control disorders and depression. *Diabetologia*, 57, 699–709.

de la Hoz, R. E., Jeon, Y., Miller, G. E., Wisnivesky, J. P., & Celedón, J. C. (2016). Post-traumatic stress disorder, bronchodilator response, and incident asthma in World Trade Center rescue and recovery workers. *American Journal of Respiratory and Critical Care Medicine*, 194, 1383–91.

Demyttenaere, K., Bruffaerts, R., Posada-Villa, J., et al. (2004). Prevalence, severity, and unmet need for treatment of mental disorders in the World Health Organization World Mental Health Surveys. *JAMA*, 291, 2581–90.

Edmondson, D., & von Känel, R. (2017). Post-traumatic stress disorder and cardiovascular disease. *The Lancet Psychiatry*, 4, 320–9.

Efron, B. (1988). Logistic regression, survival analysis, and the Kaplan-Meier curve. *Journal of the American Statistical Association*, 83, 414–25.

Emdin, C. A., Odutayo, A., Wong, C. X., et al. (2016). Meta-analysis of anxiety as a risk factor for cardiovascular disease. *The American Journal of Cardiology*, 118, 511–19.

Fergusson, D. M., Horwood, L. J., & Ridder, E. M. (2007). Conduct and attentional problems in childhood and adolescence and later substance use, abuse and dependence: results of a 25-year longitudinal study. *Drug and Alcohol Dependence*, 88S, S14–26.

Flory, J. D., & Yehuda, R. (2015). Comorbidity between post-traumatic stress disorder and major depressive disorder: alternative explanations and treatment considerations. *Dialogues in Clinical Neuroscience*, 17, 141–50.

Geller, D. A., Biederman, J., Griffin, S., Jones, J., & Lefkowitz, T. R. (1996). Comorbidity of juvenile obsessive–compulsive disorder with disruptive behavior disorders. *Journal of the American Academy of Child and Adolescent Psychiatry*, 35, 1637–46.

Goldberg, D. P., Krueger, R. F., Andrews, G., & Hobbs, M. J. (2009). Emotional disorders: cluster 4 of the proposed meta-structure for DSM-IV and ICD-11. *Psychological Medicine*, 39, 2043–59.

Hall, K. S., Hoerster, K. D., & Yancy, W. S. (2015). Post-traumatic stress disorder, physical activity, and eating behaviors. *Epidemiologic Reviews*, 37, 103–15.

Harkness, J., Pennell, B. E., Villar, A., et al. (2008). Translation procedures and translation assessment in the World Mental Health Survey Initiative. In R. C. Kessler, & T. B. Üstün, eds., *The WHO World Mental Health Surveys: Global Perspectives on the Epidemiology of Mental Disorders*. New York, NY: Cambridge University Press, pp. 91–113.

Haro, J. M., Arbabzadeh-Bouchez, S., Brugha, T. S., et al. (2006). Concordance of the Composite International Diagnostic Interview Version 3.0 (CIDI 3.0) with standardized clinical assessments in the WHO World Mental Health Surveys. *International Journal of Methods in Psychiatric Research*, 15, 167–80.

Herpertz, S. C., Mueller, B., Qunaibi, M., et al. (2005). Response to emotional stimuli in boys with conduct disorder. *American Journal of Psychiatry*, 162, 1100–17.

Hoehn-Saric, R., & Barksdale, V. C. (1983). Impulsiveness in obsessive-compulsive patients. *British Journal of Psychiatry*, 143, 177–82.

Holley, A., Wilson, A., Noel, M., & Palermo, T. (2016). Post-traumatic stress symptoms in children and adolescents with chronic pain: a topical review of the literature and a proposed framework for future research. *European Journal of Pain*, 20, 1371–83.

Hyland, B., Judd, F., Davidson, S., Jolley, D., & Hocking, B. (2003). Case managers' attitudes to the physical health of their patients. *Australian and New Zealand Journal of Psychiatry*, 37, 710–14.

Jensen, P. S. (2003). Comorbidity and child psychopathology: recommendations for the next decade. *Journal of Abnormal Child Psychology*, 31, 293–300.

Jordan, H. T., Miller-Archie, S. A., Cone, J. E., Morabia, A., & Stellman, S. D. (2011). Heart disease among adults exposed to the September 11, 2001 World Trade Center disaster: results from the World Trade Center Health Registry. *Preventive Medicine*, 53, 370–6.

Kass, R. E., & Raftery, A. E. (1995). Bayes factors. *Journal of the American Statistical Association*, 90, 773–95.
Kessler, R. C., Amminger, G. P., Aguilar-Gaxiola, S., et al. (2007). Age of onset of mental disorders: a review of recent literature. *Current Opinion in Psychiatry*, 20, 359–64.
Kessler, R. C., Chiu, W. T., Demler, O., Merikangas, K. R., & Walters, E. E. (2005). Prevalence, severity, and comorbidity of 12-month DSM-IV disorders in the National Comorbidity Survey Replication. *Archives of General Psychiatry*, 62, 617–27.
Kessler, R. C., Ormel, J., Petukhova, M., et al. (2011a). Development of lifetime comorbidity in the World Health Organization World Mental Health Surveys. *Archives of General Psychiatry*, 68, 90–100.
Kessler, R. C., Petukhova, M., & Zaslavsky, A. M. (2011b). The role of latent internalizing and externalizing predispositions in accounting for the development of comorbidity among common mental disorders. *Current Opinion in Psychiatry*, 24, 307–12.
Knäuper, B., Cannell, C. F., Schwarz, N., Bruce, M. L., & Kessler, R. C. (1999). Improving accuracy of major depression age-of-onset reports in the US National Comorbidity Survey. *International Journal of Methods in Psychiatric Research*, 8, 39–48.
Koenen, K., Moffitt, T. E., Poulton, R., Martin, J., & Caspi, A. (2007). Early childhood factors associated with the development of post-traumatic stress disorder: results from a longitudinal birth cohort. *Psychological Medicine*, 37, 181–92.
Koenen, K., Sumner, J., Gilsanz, P., et al. (2017). Post-traumatic stress disorder and cardiometabolic disease: improving causal inference to inform practice. *Psychological Medicine*, 47, 209–25.
Kramer, M. D., Krueger, R. F., & Hicks, B. M. (2008). The role of internalizing and externalizing liability factors in accounting for gender differences in the prevalence of common psychopathological syndromes. *Psychological Medicine*, 38, 51–61.
Krueger, R. F. (1999). The structure of common mental disorders. *Archives of General Psychiatry*, 56, 921–6.
Krueger, R. F., Caspi, A., Moffitt, T. E., & Silva, P. A. (1998). The structure and stability of common mental disorders (DSM-III-R): a longitudinal-epidemiological study. *Journal of Abnormal Psychology*, 107, 216–27.
Krueger, R. F., Chentsova-Dutton, Y. E., Markon, K. E., Goldberg, D., & Ormel, J. (2003). A cross-cultural study of the structure of comorbidity among common psychopathological syndromes in the general health care setting. *Journal of Abnormal Psychology*, 112, 437–47.
Krueger, R. F., & Finger, M. S. (2001). Using item response theory to understand comorbidity among anxiety and unipolar mood disorders. *Psychological Assessment*, 13, 140–51.
Krueger, R. F., & Markon, K. E. (2006a). Reinterpreting comorbidity: a model-based approach to understanding and classifying psychopathology. *Annual Review of Clinical Psychology*, 2, 111–33.
(2006b). Understanding psychopathology: melding behavior genetics, personality, and quantitative psychology to develop an empirically based model. *Current Directions in Psychological Science*, 15, 113–17.
Kubzansky, L. D., Koenen, K. C., Jones, C., & Eaton, W. W. (2009). A prospective study of posttraumatic stress disorder symptoms and coronary heart disease in women. *Health Psychology*, 28, 125–30.
Kubzansky, L. D., Koenen, K. C., Spiro, A. I., Vokonas, P. S., & Sparrow, D. (2007). Prospective study of posttraumatic stress disorder symptoms and coronary heart disease in the normative aging study. *Archives of General Psychiatry*, 64, 109–16.
Lahey, B. B., Rathouz, P. J., Van Hulle, C., et al. (2008). Testing structural models of DSM-IV symptoms of common forms of child and adolescent psychopathology. *Journal of Abnormal Child Psychology*, 36, 187–206.
Lang, A. J., Laffaye, C., Satz, L. E., et al. (2006). Relationships among childhood maltreatment, PTSD, and health in female veterans in primary care. *Child Abuse and Neglect*, 30, 1281–92.
Lawrence, D., & Kisely, S. (2010). Review: inequalities in healthcare provision for people with severe mental illness. *Journal of Psychopharmacology*, 24, 61–8.
Lee, Y. C., Agnew-Blais, J., Malspeis, S., et al. (2016). Post-traumatic stress disorder and risk for incident rheumatoid arthritis. *Arthritis Care and Research*, 68, 292–8.
Levine, A. B., Levine, L. M., & Levine, T. B. (2014). Posttraumatic stress disorder and cardiometabolic disease. *Cardiology*, 127, 1–19.
Licht, C. M. M., de Geus, E. J. C., van Dyck, R., & Penninx, B. W. J. H. (2010). Longitudinal evidence for unfavorable effects of antidepressants on heart rate variability. *Biological Psychiatry*, 68, 861–8.
Markon, K. E. (2010). Modeling psychopathology structure: a symptom-level analysis of Axis I and II disorders. *Psychological Medicine*, 40, 273–88.
Marshall, R. D., & Garakani, A. (2002). Psychobiology of the acute stress response and its relationship to the psychobiology of post-traumatic stress disorder. *Psychiatric Clinics of North America*, 25, 385–95.
Matsunaga, H., Kiriike, N., Matsui, T., et al. (2005). Impulsive disorders in Japanese adult patients with obsessive-compulsive disorder. *Comprehensive Psychiatry*, 46, 43–9.
Miller, G. E., Cohen, S., & Ritchey, A. K. (2002). Chronic psychological stress and the regulation of pro-inflammatory cytokines: a glucocorticoid resistance model. *Health Psychology*, 21, 536–41.
Moffitt, T. E., Caspi, A., Taylor, A., et al. (2010). How common are common mental disorders? Evidence that lifetime prevalence rates are doubled by

prospective versus retrospective ascertainment. *Psychological Medicine*, 40, 899–909.
Newman, D. L., Moffitt, T. E., Caspi, A., et al. (1996). Psychiatric disorder in a birth cohort of young adults: prevalence, comorbidity, clinical significance, and new case incidence from ages 11 to 21. *Journal of Consulting and Clinical Psychology*, 64, 552–62.
O'Neill, S., Posada-Villa, J., Medina-Mora, M. E., et al. (2014). Associations between DSM-IV mental disorders and subsequent self-reported diagnosis of cancer. *Journal of Psychosomatic Research*, 76, 207–12.
Orr, S. P., & Roth, W. T. (2000). Psychophysiological assessment: clinical applications for PTSD. *Journal of Affective Disorders*, 61, 225–40.
Pacella, M. L., Hruska, B., & Delahanty, D. L. (2013). The physical health consequences of PTSD and PTSD symptoms: a meta-analytic review. *Journal of Anxiety Disorders*, 27, 33–46.
Paras, M. L., Murad, M. H., Chen, L. P., et al. (2009). Sexual abuse and lifetime diagnosis of somatic disorders: a systematic review and meta-analysis. *Journal of the American Medical Association*, 302, 550–61.
Pattaro, C., Locatelli, F., Sunyer, J., & de Marco, R. (2007). Using the age at onset may increase the reliability of longitudinal asthma assessment. *Journal of Clinical Epidemiology*, 60, 704–11.
Perneger, T. V. (1998). What's wrong with Bonferroni adjustments. *BMJ*, 316, 1236–8.
Petrakis, I. L., & Simpson, T. L. (2017). Posttraumatic stress disorder and alcohol use disorder: a critical review of pharmacologic treatments. *Alcoholism, Clinical and Experimental Research*, 41, 226–37.
Raphael, K. G., & Widom, C. S. (2011). Post-traumatic stress disorder moderates the relation between documented childhood victimization and pain 30 years later. *Pain*, 152, 163–9.
Rapsey, C. M., Lim, C. C., Al-Hamzawi, A., et al. (2015). Associations between DSM-IV mental disorders and subsequent COPD diagnosis. *Journal of Psychosomatic Research*, 79, 333–9.
SAS Institute Inc. (2002). *SAS/STAT® Software, Version 9.1 for Unix*. Cary, NC: SAS Institute Inc.
Schnurr, P. P., Spiro, A., & Paris, A. H. (2000). Physician-diagnosed medical disorders in relation to PTSD symptoms in older male military veterans. *Health Psychology*, 19, 91–7.
Scott, K. M. (2009). The development of mental-physical comorbidity. In M. Von Korff, K. M. Scott, & O. Gureje, eds., *Global Perspectives on Mental-Physical Comorbidity in the WHO World Mental Health Surveys*. New York, NY: Cambridge University Press, pp. 97–107.
(2014). Depression, anxiety and incident cardiometabolic diseases. *Current Opinion in Psychiatry*, 27, 289–93.
Scott, K. M., Alonso, J., de Jonge, P., et al. (2013a). Associations between DSM-IV mental disorders and onset of self-reported peptic ulcer in the World Mental Health Surveys. *Journal of Psychosomatic Research*, 75, 121–7.
Scott, K. M., de Jonge, P., Alonso, J., et al. (2013b). Associations between DSM-IV mental disorders and subsequent heart disease onset: beyond depression. *International Journal of Cardiology*, 168, 5293–9.
Scott, K. M., Lim, C., Al-Hamzawi, A., et al. (2016). Association of mental disorders with subsequent chronic physical conditions: World Mental Health Surveys from 17 countries. *JAMA Psychiatry*, 73, 150–8.
Seow, L. S., Ong, C., Mahesh, M. V., et al. (2016). A systematic review on comorbid post-traumatic stress disorder in schizophrenia. *Schizophrenia Research*, 176, 441–1.
Shaffer, J. P. (1995). Multiple hypothesis testing. *Annual Review of Psychology*, 46, 561–84.
Shah, A. J., Veledar, E., Shallenberger, L., et al. (2011). Association of antidepressant medications with carotid intima media thickness in middle aged veteran twins. *Journal of the American College of Cardiology*, 57, E1588.
Sharp, T. J., & Harvey, A. G. (2001). Chronic pain and posttraumatic stress disorder: mutual maintenance? *Clinical Psychology Review*, 21, 857–77.
Simon, G. E., & VonKorff, M. (1995). Recall of psychiatric history in cross-sectional surveys: implications for epidemiologic research. *Epidemiologic Reviews*, 17, 221–7.
Slade, T., & Watson, D. (2006). The structure of common DSM-IV and ICD-10 mental disorders in the Australian general population. *Psychological Medicine*, 36, 1593–600.
Spencer, A. E., Faraone, S. V., Bogucki, O. E., et al. (2016). Examining the association between posttraumatic stress disorder and attention-deficit/hyperactivity disorder: a systematic review and meta-analysis. *Journal of Clinical Psychiatry*, 77, 72–83.
Stein, D. J., Aguilar-Gaxiola, S., Alonso, J., et al. (2014). Associations between mental disorders and subsequent onset of hypertension. *General Hospital Psychiatry*, 36, 142–9.
Stein, M. B., Fuetsch, M., Muller, N., et al. (2001). Social anxiety disorder and the risk of depression: a prospective community study of adolescents and young adults. *Archives of General Psychiatry*, 58, 251–6.
Sterzer, P., Stadler, C., Krebs, A., Kleinschmidt, A., & Poustka, F. (2005). Abnormal neural responses to emotional visual stimuli in adolescents with conduct disorder. *Biological Psychiatry*, 57, 7–15.
Sumner, J., Kubzansky, L., Roberts, A., et al. (2016). Post-traumatic stress disorder symptoms and risk of hypertension over 22 years in a large cohort of younger and middle-aged women. *Psychological Medicine*, 46, 3105–16.

Sumner, J. A., Kubzansky, L. D., Elkind, M. S., et al. (2015). Trauma exposure and posttraumatic stress disorder symptoms predict onset of cardiovascular events in women. *Circulation*, 132, 251–9.

Swain, N. R., Lim, C. C., Levinson, D., et al. (2015). Associations between DSM-IV mental disorders and subsequent non-fatal, self-reported stroke. *Journal of Psychosomatic Research*, 79, 130–6.

Takayanagi, Y., Spira, A. P., Roth, K. B., *et al.* (2014). Accuracy of reports of lifetime mental and physical disorders: results from the Baltimore Epidemiological Catchment Area Study. *JAMA Psychiatry*, 71, 273–80.

Thomsen, P. H., & Jensen, J. (1991). Latent class analysis of organic aspects of obsessive-compulsive disorder in children and adolescents. *Acta Psychiatrica Scandinavica*, 84, 391–5.

Thurston, R. C., Rewak, M., & Kubzansky, L. D. (2013). An anxious heart: anxiety and the onset of cardiovascular diseases. *Progress in Cardiovascular Diseases*, 55, 524–37.

Vaccarino, V., Goldberg, J., Magruder, K. M., et al. (2014). Posttraumatic stress disorder and incidence of type-2 diabetes: a prospective twin study. *Journal of Psychiatric Research*, 56, 158–64.

Vaccarino, V., Goldberg, J., Rooks, C., et al. (2013). Posttraumatic stress disorder and incidence of coronary heart disease: a twin study. *Journal of the American College of Cardiology*, 62, 970–8.

Vollebergh, W. A., Iedema, J., Bijl, R. V., et al. (2001). The structure and stability of common mental disorders: the NEMESIS study. *Archives of General Psychiatry*, 58, 597–603.

Von Korff, M. R., Scott, K. M., & Gureje, O., eds. (2009). *Global Perspectives on Mental Physical Comorbidity in the WHO World Mental Health Surveys*. New York, NY: Cambridge University Press.

Wang, P. S., Angermeyer, M., Borges, G., et al. (2007). Delay and failure in treatment seeking after first onset of mental disorders in the World Health Organization's World Mental Health Survey Initiative. *World Psychiatry*, 6, 177–85.

Watson, D. (2005). Rethinking the mood and anxiety disorders: a quantitative hierarchical model for DSM-V. *Journal of Abnormal Psychology*, 114, 522–36.

Whooley, M. A., & Wong, J. M. (2013). Depression and cardiovascular disorders. *Annual Review of Clinical Psychology*, 9, 327–54.

Willett, J. B., & Singer, J. D. (1993). Investigating onset, cessation, relapse, and recovery: why you should, and how you can, use discrete-time survival analysis to examine event occurrence. *Journal of Consulting and Clinical Psychology*, 61, 952–65.

Wittchen, H. U. (1994). Reliability and validity studies of the WHO–Composite International Diagnostic Interview (CIDI): a critical review. *Journal of Psychiatric Research*, 28, 57–84.

Wittchen, H. U., Beesdo-Baum, K., Gloster, A., et al. (2009). The structure of mental disorders re-examined: is it developmentally stable and robust against additions? *International Journal of Methods in Psychiatric Research*, 18, 189–203.

Wolter, K. M. (1985). *Introduction to Variance Estimation*. New York, NY: Springer-Verlag.

Yehuda, R. (2006). Advances in understanding neuroendocrine alterations in PTSD and their therapeutic implications. *Annals of the New York Academy of Sciences*, 1071, 137–66.

Appendix

Table 6.A1 Unrotated eigenvalues of lifetime DSM-IV/CIDI disorders in exploratory factor analyses carried out in high-income and low- and middle-income WMH countries separately for internalizing and externalizing disorders[a]

Factor number	Eigenvalue			
	High-income countries		LMICs	
	Internal	External	Internal	External
1	4.8	4.9	4.3	4.2
2	1.0	1.2	1.2	1.4
3	0.9	0.7	0.9	0.8

[a]Results are based on principal axis factor analysis of tetrachoric correlation matrices estimated in person-year data sets.

Table 6.A2 Rotated (promax) factor pattern (standardized regression coefficients) of lifetime DSM-IV/CIDI disorders in high-income and low- and middle-income WMH countries for separate two-factor models of internalizing and externalizing disorders[a]

	Standardized regression coefficients							
	High-income countries				LMICs			
	Internalizing		Externalizing		Internalizing		Externalizing	
	I	II	I	II	I	II	I	II
I Internalizing Disorders								
MDD or dysthymic disorder	0.83	0.03			0.38	0.56		
BPD (broad definition)	0.49	0.16			0.15	0.66		
Panic disorder[b]	0.44	0.38			0.31	0.46		
Agoraphobia[c]	0.07	0.84			0.97	−0.22		
GAD	0.88	−0.11			0.56	0.30		
PTSD	0.69	0.07			−0.21	0.95		
Social phobia	0.19	0.69			0.68	0.15		
Specific phobia	−0.13	0.89			0.69	0.16		
Separation anxiety disorder	0.55	0.20			0.38	0.29		
OCD	0.25	0.43			0.35	0.43		
II Externalizing Disorders								
Attention-deficit disorder			−0.08	0.95			0.92	−0.15
Hyperactivity disorder			−0.08	0.95			0.96	−0.18
CD (overt)[d]			0.70	0.28			0.76	0.23
CD (covert)[e]			0.69	0.30			0.76	0.25
IED			0.36	0.47			0.61	0
ODD			0.42	0.58			0.66	0.15
Alcohol abuse or dependence			0.93	−0.10			−0.03	0.91
Drug abuse or dependence			0.95	−0.13			0.01	0.91
(n)[f]	(7,360)				(13,869)			

[a]Results are based on principal axis factor analysis of tetrachoric correlation matrices estimated in person-year data sets.
[b]With or without agoraphobia.
[c]With or without panic disorder.
[d]E.g., bullying, fighting, being physically cruel to people.
[e]E.g., lying, shoplifting.
[f]The n's are for the numbers of respondents. The numbers of person-years (every year of life of the respondents beginning at age four up to and including the age at interview) are 214,738 (high-income), 376,961 (low- and middle-income), and 591,699 (total).

Chapter 7

Functional Impairments Associated with Posttraumatic Stress Disorder

Ronald C. Kessler, Somnath Chatterji, Yanling He, Daphna Levinson, Elie G. Karam, and Jordi Alonso

Posttraumatic stress disorder (PTSD) exacts a high toll on populations not only because of its high prevalence and persistence, but also because it is associated with significant functional impairment (Atwoli et al., 2015). Although these secondary effects are seen most vividly in survivors of society-wide traumas, such as civilians or soldiers who have been exposed to war (Baker, 2014) and sectarian violence (Siriwardhana & Stewart, 2013), these effects also exist in PTSD cases resulting from other types of trauma such as sexual assault or intimate partner violence. The WMH surveys collected a good deal of data designed to document these social costs of mental disorders. In fact, an earlier volume in the WMH book series focused on these burdens (Alonso et al., 2013). In this chapter, we review the WMH results regarding the burdens of PTSD with a special focus on role impairments. Consistent with these earlier WMH analyses, we distinguish effects on life course role incumbency, timing, and transitions from effects on point-in-time role performance. Unlike most other chapters in this volume, we review data from several earlier WMH reports, each of which considered the joint predictive effects of a wide range of mental disorders on specific aspects of role impairment or quality of life. We highlight here the results in those earlier analyses involving PTSD.

Life Course Role Incumbency, Timing, and Transitions

Given that mental disorders typically have an early age-of-onset (AOO), they might be expected to have negative effects on critical developmental transitions, such as educational attainment and timing of marriage. A number of prior WMH reports examined these effects, with a focus on four domains: education, marital timing and stability, childbearing, and occupation.

Education

Several epidemiological studies prior to and coincident with the WMH surveys showed that early-onset mental disorders are associated with early termination of education (Kessler et al., 1995; Woodward & Fergusson, 2001; McLeod & Kaiser, 2004; Porche et al., 2011; Vaughn et al., 2011). Several WMH reports also examined this issue (Breslau et al., 2008, 2011b; Lee et al., 2009). While disruptive behavior disorders and bipolar disorder tended to have the strongest associations with low educational attainment in these studies, one cross-national WMH study found that anxiety disorders including PTSD (which was classified as an anxiety disorder in DSM-IV, the diagnostic system used in the WMH surveys) were associated with a significantly elevated risk of failure to complete secondary school in high income countries (Lee et al., 2009). However, these analyses did not have enough statistical power to detect effects of individual mental disorders beyond those in broad categories, making it impossible for us to determine whether PTSD is associated with effects on education different from those of other related internalizing disorders.

Marital Timing and Stability

A small number of epidemiological studies examined associations of premarital mental disorders with subsequent marriage (Forthofer et al., 1996; Whisman et al., 2007). A WMH analysis replicated and extended these studies (Breslau et al., 2011a). Early onset mental disorders were found to predict low probability of ever marrying, but to be positively associated (Forthofer et al., 1996) or unrelated (Breslau et al., 2011a) with early (before age 18) marriage, which often has a number of adverse outcomes, and to be negatively associated with on-time and late marriage, which often has a number of benefits (e.g., financial security, social support). These associations were largely the same for men and women and across countries. PTSD was one of the most important of these premarital mental disorders. A separate set of pre-WMH studies showed that premarital history of mental disorders predicts divorce (Kessler et al., 1998; Butterworth & Rodgers,

2008) and a subsequent WMH study of these associations showed that they are quite similar for men and women across all countries and that PTSD was among the most important disorders in this regard (Breslau et al., 2013).

Employment Status

Although common mental disorders are known to be associated with unemployment, most research on this association has emphasized the impact of job loss on mental illness rather than mental illness as a risk factor for job loss (Dooley et al., 1996; Rachiotis et al., 2015). However, an analysis of WMH data documented the latter association by showing that history of mental disorders as of the age of completing schooling predicted current (at the time of interview) unemployment and work disability (Kawakami et al., 2012). PTSD was important in this regard only in that it was associated with a 2.0 odds ratio of subsequent work disability. PTSD was not associated, in comparison, with employment status among those who were not disabled or with personal earnings among the employed, adjusting for level of education. Furthermore, the significant association of PTSD with disability was found only in high-income countries, raising the possibility that PTSD became more detrimental to work performance as the substantive complexity of work increased.

Role Performance

Comparative Global Role Impairments

A number of community surveys, most of them carried out in the United States, examined the comparative effects of diverse diseases on various aspects of role functioning (Verbrugge & Patrick, 1995; Kessler et al., 2001a; Stewart et al., 2003; Wang et al., 2003; Lerner et al., 2005; Merikangas et al., 2007; Barbaglia et al., 2017). Internalizing mental disorders were included in a number of these studies, and the results typically showed that these mental disorders were associated with among the highest levels of disability at the individual level all commonly occurring disorders assessed. The most compelling study of this sort outside the United States was based on the first 15 WMH surveys (Ormel et al., 2008). Disorder-specific disability scores were created based on the Sheehan Disability Scales (SDS; Leon et al., 1997). The SDS questions asked respondents to rate how much each of the mental disorders they reported having in the 12 months before interview interfered with their functioning in each of the four role domains (home management, ability to work, social life, and close personal relationships) using a 0–10 response scale of *None* (0), *Mild* (1–3), *Moderate* (4–6), *Severe* (7–9), and *Very Severe* (10) interference.

The SDS questions also asked about one chronic physical disorder from among those assessed with a chronic conditions checklist in the WMH surveys. As detailed in the original report of this analysis (Ormel et al., 2008), a weight was used to adjust for different probabilities of selection of physical conditions based on the extent of their comorbidities with each other. A global SDS score was created by assigning each respondent the highest SDS domain score across the four domains. PTSD and three other mental disorders (major depressive disorder, bipolar disorder, generalized anxiety disorder) were found to have the highest probabilities of being rated severely impairing (55% to 68% of respondents). This was true, even though the physical disorders included such severe conditions as cancer, diabetes, and heart disease.

Overall Days Out of Role

Considerable research has examined days out of role associated with various physical and mental disorders in an effort to produce data on comparative disease burden for health policy planning purposes (Alonso et al., 2004; Merikangas et al., 2007). These studies typically found that PTSD was associated with the highest mean number of days out of role of any physical or mental disorder (Wang et al., 2003; Collins et al., 2005; Munce et al., 2007). In the WMH surveys, for example, 62,971 respondents across 24 countries were assessed for a wide range of common physical and mental disorders as well as for days out of role (Alonso et al., 2011). PTSD was one of the three disorders associated with the highest mean numbers of days out of role in the 12 months before interview (42.7 days) along with panic disorder (42.9 days) and bipolar disorder (41.2 days).

Marital Functioning

It has long been known that marital dissatisfaction and discord are strongly related to symptoms of mental disorder (Whisman, 1999; Pankiewicz et al., 2012), although the symptoms considered in these analyses typically were those of nonspecific psychological distress, depression, or anxiety, making it impossible to know if PTSD was involved in a specific way. However, qualitative research

Table 7.1 Comparative impairments in close personal relationship role functioning associated with 12-month DSM-IV/CIDI PTSD vs. other 12-month chronic physical and mental disorders among married WMH respondents[a]

	Percent with severe impairment				Mean level of impairment				
	%	(SE)	OR	(95% CI)	Mean	(SE)	B	(SE)	(n)
I PTSD	30.5	(2.7)	1.0	–	4.5	(0.2)	0.0	–	(460)
II Mood Disorders									
MDD or dysthymic disorder	32.1	(1.3)	1.0	(0.7–1.3)	4.8	(0.1)	0.0	(0.1)	(2,283)
BPD (broad definition)	46.5	(2.7)	2.1*	(1.5–3.0)	5.6	(0.2)	1.1	(0.1)	(474)
III Anxiety Disorders									
Panic disorder	22.0	(2.2)	0.6*	(0.4–0.8)	3.5	(0.2)	−1.2	(0.1)	(579)
GAD	27.6	(1.5)	0.7*	(0.5–0.9)	4.3	(0.1)	−0.5	(0.1)	(1,130)
Social phobia	18.8	(1.3)	0.6*	(0.4–0.8)	3.7	(0.1)	−0.8	(0.1)	(1,328)
Specific phobia	7.8	(0.6)	0.2*	(0.1–0.2)	1.8	(0.1)	−2.7	(0.1)	(3,079)
IV Disruptive Behavioral Disorders									
ADHD	10.4	(2.4)	0.3*	(0.2–0.5)	2.8	(0.3)	−1.5	(0.1)	(178)
IED	16.0	(2.0)	0.5*	(0.3–0.7)	2.9	(0.2)	−1.6	(0.1)	(616)
ODD	32.0	(9.2)	0.8	(0.3–2.4)	5.5	(0.6)	0.8	(0.2)	(73)
V Chronic Physical Disorders									
Arthritis	6.9	(0.8)	0.1*	(0.1–0.2)	1.4	(0.1)	−3.3	(0.1)	(2,822)
Asthma	5.2	(1.2)	0.1*	(0.1–0.2)	1.0	(0.1)	−3.5	(0.1)	(994)
Back/neck pain	7.7	(0.6)	0.2*	(0.1–0.2)	1.6	(0.1)	−3.1	(0.1)	(3,864)
Cancer	6.6	(1.8)	0.1*	(0.1–0.3)	1.0	(0.2)	−3.5	(0.1)	(359)
Diabetes	10.2	(2.7)	0.2*	(0.1–0.4)	1.5	(0.2)	−3.3	(0.1)	(939)
Headaches	20.1	(1.2)	0.5*	(0.3–0.6)	3.1	(0.1)	−1.7	(0.1)	(2,968)
Heart disease	6.3	(1.4)	0.1*	(0.1–0.2)	1.5	(0.2)	−3.3	(0.1)	(856)
Hypertension	5.6	(1.0)	0.1*	(0.1–0.2)	1.1	(0.1)	−3.7	(0.1)	(2,569)
Other chronic pain conditions	11.3	(1.3)	0.2*	(0.2–0.3)	2.0	(0.1)	−2.7	(0.1)	(1,144)
Ulcer	7.0	(1.8)	0.1*	(0.1–0.3)	1.3	(0.2)	−3.5	(0.1)	(510)

*Significant difference from PTSD at the 0.05 level, two-sided test.
[a]Percent with severe impairment and mean level of impairment are reports of aggregate estimates across all surveys. The surveys included all those in Table 2.1 with the exception of Australia, which did not administer the SDS scales. Regression coefficients are based on pooled logistic (predicting severe impairment) and linear (predicting 0–10 impairment scores) regression models pooled across countries and stacking reports across disorders controlling for respondent age, sex, and survey.

carried out among veterans diagnosed with PTSD suggests that PTSD leads to substantial decrements in marital quality (Ray & Vanstone, 2009). Consistent with this observation, treatment for PTSD has been shown to improve marital satisfaction of spouses in studies of veterans with PTSD (Hojjat et al., 2016).

Disaggregated analyses of SDS scores for reports of married WMH respondents about impairments in close personal relationships are consistent with these earlier studies. We examined these data using data from all but one of the WMH surveys available at the time of preparing this volume (the exception being one Australian survey, which did not include the SDS). The proportion of married WMH respondents with 12-month PTSD who reported that their PTSD either severely or very severely impaired their close personal relationships was 30.5%. This compared to 5.2% to 20.1% severe impairment in this role domain associated with comparator chronic physical conditions and 7.8% to 46.5% with other mental disorders (see Table 7.1). The proportion of respondents reporting that their PTSD caused severe impairment in their close personal relationships was significantly higher than the percentages associated with all four other anxiety disorders included in the comparison, two of the three disruptive behavior disorders, and all 10 chronic physical disorders. Only bipolar disorder had a higher proportion of cases than PTSD reporting severe role impairment in this domain. Similar results were found for mean levels of impairment. The only disorders associated with significantly higher mean levels of impairment in close personal relationships were bipolar disorder and oppositional-defiant disorder.

Other research documents that physical violence in marital relationships is significantly associated with the mental illness of marital partners (Stith et al., 2004). While these studies generally focused on presumed mental health *consequences* of relationship violence

(Kim et al., 2008; Afifi et al., 2009; Renner, 2009), a growing body of research has suggested that marital violence is partly a consequence of pre-existing mental disorders (Riggs et al., 2000; Kessler et al., 2001b; Lorber & O'Leary, 2004; O'Leary et al., 2008). Indeed, longitudinal studies consistently find that premarital history of mental disorders, including PTSD, predict subsequent marital violence perpetration (Lorber & O'Leary, 2004) and victimization (Riggs et al., 2000; Stith et al., 2004; O'Leary et al., 2008). However, few of these studies adjusted for comorbidity. A WMH study on this issue (Miller et al., 2011) found that the association of premarital history of internalizing disorders with subsequent marital violence disappeared when controls were introduced for disruptive behavioral disorders and substance use disorders, suggesting that PTSD might be a risk marker that has no causal impact on marital violence rather than being a causal risk factor.

Work Role Functioning

Ten WMH surveys assessed work role functioning with the WHO Health and Work Performance Questionnaire (HPQ; Kessler et al., 2003, 2004), a validated self-report scale for employed individuals that assigned each respondent a score in the range of 0–100% for absenteeism and presenteeism (i.e., quality–quantity of work performance on days at work) over the 30 days before interview. The HPQ also included three yes–no questions about workplace successes ("*Did you experience any special work success or achievement at any time during the past 30 days?*"), failures ("*Did you have any special work failure at any time during the past 30 days?*"), and mistakes ("*Did you make any big mistake at work during the past 30 days that either caused an accident or that created a safety risk for yourself or for others?*"). The national surveys in which these questions were asked were those in Colombia, Mexico, Northern Ireland, Peru, Portugal, Romania, and the United States. The regional surveys were those in Colombia (Medellin), Japan, and Spain (Murcia). The total number of Part II employed respondents in these surveys was 13,362 (see Table 7.2).

In a previously unpublished analysis carried out specifically for this chapter, we examined the associations of PTSD with each of the above work functioning measures by estimating linear (for the absenteeism and presenteeism scales) or logistic (for the yes–no outcomes) regression models in which 12-month PTSD was used as a predictor, controlling for respondent age, sex, education, and survey. Workers with PTSD had significantly elevated rates of work absenteeism and presenteeism equal to 0.17–0.18 standard deviations on those outcome scales (see Table 7.3). Workers with PTSD had significantly elevated odds of work failure (2.1) and mistakes (3.0).

Table 7.2 Numbers of employed Part II respondents in the WMH surveys that used the WHO HPQ to assess the work performance of employed respondents

	Number of employed Part II respondents (*n*)
I High-Income Countries	
Japan	(1,059)
Northern Ireland	(1,161)
Portugal	(1,274)
Spain – Murcia	(724)
United States	(3,918)
II LMICs	
Colombia	(1,281)
Colombia – Medellin	(798)
Mexico	(1,233)
Peru	(1,119)
Romania	(795)
Total	(13,362)

Table 7.3 Associations of 12-month DSM-IV/CIDI PTSD with 30-day absenteeism, presenteeism, work successes, work failures, and work mistakes in the WMH surveys ($n = 13{,}362$)[a]

	Est	(95% CI)
Absenteeism[b]	0.2*	(0.0–0.3)
Presenteeism[b]	0.2*	(0.0–0.3)
Special work success	1.3	(1.0–1.8)
Special work failure	2.1*	(1.2–3.7)
Big mistake	3.0*	(1.0–9.1)

*Significant at the 0.05 level, two-sided test.
[a]Based on linear (for the 0–100 absenteeism and presenteeism scales) or logistic (for the dichotomous work success, failure, and mistake measures) regression models controlling respondent age, sex, education, and survey.
[b]Absenteeism and presenteeism were measured on 0–100 continuous scales in which higher scores represent higher rates of absenteeism (i.e., a higher proportion of days absent) and presenteeism (i.e., high levels of impaired performance while on the job).

Previously published disaggregated analyses of SDS scores for reports of employed WMH respondents about impairments in ability to work were consistent with the HPQ results. The proportion of employed WMH respondents with 12-month PTSD who reported that their PTSD either severely or very severely impaired their ability to work was 21.2%. This

Table 7.4 Comparative impairments in ability to work associated with 12-month DSM-IV/CIDI PTSD vs. other 12-month chronic physical and mental disorders among working (employed or self-employed) WMH respondents[a]

	Percent with severe impairment				Mean level of impairment				
	%	(SE)	OR	(95% CI)	Mean	(SE)	b	(SE)	(n)
I PTSD	21.2	(2.2)	1.0	–	3.8	(0.2)	0.0	–	(428)
II Mood Disorders									
MDD or dysthymic disorder	30.4	(1.2)	1.6*	(1.2–2.1)	4.6	(0.1)	0.6	(0.1)	(2,293)
BPD (broad definition)	34.7	(2.4)	2.1*	(1.6–3.0)	4.9	(0.2)	1.1	(0.1)	(609)
III Anxiety Disorders									
Panic disorder	20.2	(2.0)	0.9	(0.6–1.3)	3.6	(0.2)	−0.4	(0.1)	(560)
GAD	26.8	(1.8)	1.3	(1.0–1.8)	4.3	(0.1)	0.3	(0.1)	(1,058)
Social phobia	13.4	(1.2)	0.6*	(0.4–0.9)	3.0	(0.1)	−0.7	(0.1)	(1,547)
Specific phobia	8.4	(0.7)	0.3*	(0.3–0.5)	1.9	(0.1)	−1.9	(0.1)	(2,859)
IV Disruptive Behavioral Disorders									
ADHD	21.0	(4.7)	1.1	(0.6–2.1)	3.9	(0.3)	0.2	(0.2)	(220)
IED	11.4	(1.5)	0.5*	(0.3–0.8)	2.3	(0.1)	−1.5	(0.1)	(685)
ODD	21.2	(4.9)	0.7	(0.3–1.5)	3.5	(0.4)	−0.7	(0.3)	(92)
V Chronic Physical Disorders									
Arthritis	13.4	(1.2)	0.6*	(0.5–0.9)	2.4	(0.1)	−1.3	(0.1)	(1,921)
Asthma	5.9	(1.0)	0.2*	(0.2–0.4)	1.4	(0.2)	−2.5	(0.1)	(1,052)
Back/neck pain	23.0	(1.1)	1.2	(0.9–1.6)	3.6	(0.1)	−0.3	(0.1)	(3,372)
Cancer	15.5	(3.5)	0.7	(0.4–1.2)	1.8	(0.3)	−2.1	(0.1)	(265)
Diabetes	6.2	(1.6)	0.3*	(0.1–0.5)	1.5	(0.2)	−2.4	(0.1)	(619)
Headaches	28.9	(1.3)	1.5*	(1.1–2.0)	4.3	(0.1)	0.3	(0.1)	(2,757)
Heart disease	15.5	(3.1)	0.7	(0.4–1.2)	2.5	(0.3)	−1.5	(0.2)	(466)
Hypertension	8.3	(1.1)	0.3*	(0.2–0.5)	1.5	(0.1)	−2.4	(0.1)	(1,609)
Other chronic pain conditions	28.8	(2.2)	1.5*	(1.0–2.1)	4.1	(0.2)	0.1	(0.1)	(981)
Ulcer	13.8	(2.8)	0.7	(0.4–1.1)	2.4	(0.3)	−1.5	(0.1)	(409)

*Significant difference from PTSD at the 0.05 level, two-sided test.
[a]Percent with severe impairment and mean level of impairment are reports of aggregate estimates across all surveys. The surveys included all those in Table 2.1 with the exception of Australia, which did not administer the SDS scales. Regression coefficients are based on pooled logistic (predicting severe impairment) and linear (predicting 0–10 impairment scores) regression models pooled across countries and stacking reports across disorders controlling for respondent age, sex, and survey.

compares with 6.2% to 28.8% severe impairment in this role domain associated with comparator chronic physical conditions and 8.4% to 34.7% with other mental disorders (see Table 7.4). The proportion of respondents reporting that their PTSD caused severe impairment in their ability to work was significantly higher than the percentages associated with two of the four other anxiety disorders included in the comparison (specific and social phobia), one of the three disruptive behavior disorders (intermittent explosive disorder), and four of the ten chronic physical disorders (arthritis, asthma, diabetes, and hypertension). Only mood disorders, chronic headaches, and other chronic pain disorders had higher proportions of cases than PTSD reporting severe role impairment. Similar results were found for mean levels of impairment in ability to work. This impairment in this domain was significantly higher for PTSD than for three of the other four DSM-IV anxiety disorders (panic disorder, specific phobia, and social phobia), two of the three disruptive behavior disorders (intermittent explosive disorder and oppositional defiant disorder), and eight of the 10 chronic physical disorders (all other than headaches, which had higher mean impairment than PTSD, and other chronic pain conditions, which had mean impairment equivalent to that of PTSD). The mood disorders were the only mental disorders with higher mean impairments in ability to work than PTSD.

Suicidality

As discussed in Chapter 6, PTSD is significantly associated with the subsequent onset of many other mental disorders. As one would expect from this fact, PTSD is also associated with suicidality (Nock et al., 2009, 2012). An earlier WMH report examined this issue by studying the associations of temporally primary lifetime history of PTSD and other DSM-IV disorders with respondent reports about the subsequent onset of suicide ideation (*"Have you ever seriously thought*

Table 7.5 Multivariate associations of temporally primary DSM-IV/CIDI PTSD with subsequent first onset of suicidality in the Part II cross-national WMH sample ($n = 55,299$)[a]

	Multivariate model 1[b]		Multivariate model 2[b]		Multivariate model 3[b]	
	OR	(95% CI)	OR	(95% CI)	OR	(95% CI)
Ideation	1.8*	(1.6–2.2)	1.3*	(1.1–1.5)	2.2*	(1.8–2.6)
Plan	1.2	(0.9–1.4)	1.1	(0.9–1.3)	1.3	(1.0–1.7)
Attempt	2.0*	(1.7–2.2)	1.4*	(1.2–1.7)	3.0*	(2.4–3.7)
Planned attempt among ideators	1.2	(0.8–1.6)	1.2	(0.8–1.6)	1.5	(1.0–2.3)
Attempt among ideators without a plan	1.4	(0.9–2.0)	1.5*	(1.0–2.2)	1.7*	(1.1–2.8)

*Significant at the 0.05 level, two-sided test.
[a]Based on WMH surveys in 10 high-income countries (Belgium, France, Germany, Israel, Italy, Japan, Netherlands, New Zealand, Spain, United States) and 12 LMICs (Brazil – São Paulo, Bulgaria, Colombia, India, Lebanon, Mexico, Nigeria, PRC – Beijing/Shanghai/Shenzhen, Romania, South Africa).
[b]Analyses were based on discrete-time survival models with person-year, the unit of analysis. Multivariate model 1 controlled for CAs, time-varying lifetime history of other traumatic experiences, sex, time-varying socio-demographic characteristics (person-year, education, marital status), and survey. Multivariate model 2 additionally controlled for time-varying lifetime history of all other DSM-IV/CIDI disorders. Multivariate model 3 additionally controlled for number as well as type of the latter disorders.

about committing suicide?"), plans ("*Have you ever made a plan for committing suicide?*"), and attempts ("*Have you ever attempted suicide?*"). In addition to assessing AOO for each of these outcomes, the survey asked about recency, number of years with ideation and plans, and number of attempts. Discrete-time survival analysis with person-year as the unit of analysis and a logistic link function (Willett & Singer, 1993) was used to estimate time-lagged associations of PTSD with subsequent first onset of each of the suicidality outcomes. This analysis was carried out in pooled analyses of data from 22 WMH surveys.

A series of three models was estimated for each of the five outcomes: ideation, plans, attempts, planned attempts among ideators, and unplanned (presumably impulsive) attempts among ideators (Table 7.5). Model 1 controlled for childhood adversities, time-varying lifetime history of other traumas: sex, time-varying socio-demographic characteristics (person-year, education, marital status), and survey. Model 2 additionally controlled for time-varying lifetime history of all other DSM-IV/CIDI disorders. Model 3 additionally controlled for a number as well as type of the latter disorders. Temporally primary PTSD predicted subsequent suicide attempts in all three models, with ORs in the range of 1.4–3.0. Disaggregation through the intervening outcomes showed that the association of PTSD with attempts was due to a combination of a significant association with suicide ideation in the total sample (OR = 1.3–2.2) and a significant association with unplanned attempts among ideators (OR = 1.4–1.7). It is noteworthy that the ORs in Model 3 were larger than those in Model 2 because the controls for type-number of comorbid DSM-IV disorders documented significant interactions such that the incremental predictive effects of PTSD were strongest among respondents who had no other comorbid disorders. The ORs involving PTSD in Model 3 represent subgroup associations under the model among respondents with no other comorbid disorders.

This analysis was then extended to study predictors of the course of suicidality by using respondent reports about recency of ideation, plans, and attempts to estimate "time-to-next-event" models building on the work of demographers to study predictors of repeatable events (Yamaguchi, 2003; Scheike & Keiding, 2006; Keiding et al., 2011). As detailed elsewhere (Kessler et al., 2012), both backwards recurrence accelerated failure time models and discrete-time person-year survival models were estimated. No evidence was found in these models that temporally primary PTSD predicted the subsequent persistence of suicide ideation and plans among WMH respondents with lifetime ideation or plans. However, temporally primary PTSD was associated with statistically significant 1.7 OR of recurrent suicide attempts among respondents with a history of a first lifetime suicide attempt (Nock et al., 2012). As a point of comparison, PTSD was one of only four mental disorders that predicted recurrent suicide attempts, the others being additional anxiety disorders (panic disorder, social phobia, agoraphobia) with ORs comparable to the PTSD OR (1.6–2.0).

Discussion

The results reviewed in this chapter show clearly that PTSD is a seriously disabling disorder. This is true not only because current PTSD is associated with current role impairment, but also because a history of PTSD is associated with disadvantages in subsequent role situations and transitions. Coupled with the evidence of its high prevalence presented in Chapter 5 and independent evidence for the effectiveness of several PTSD treatments (Foa et al., 2008), these results argue strongly for the importance of both early detection and timely and effective treatment of PTSD. However, as shown in Chapter 8, PTSD treatment rates are disturbingly low. The data reported in the current chapter make this finding more alarming than it would be if PTSD were a less seriously disabling disorder.

References

Afifi, T. O., MacMillan, H., Cox, B. J., et al. (2009). Mental health correlates of intimate partner violence in marital relationships in a nationally representative sample of males and females. *Journal of Interpersonal Violence*, 24, 1398–17.

Alonso, J., Angermeyer, M. C., Bernert, S., et al. (2004). Disability and quality of life impact of mental disorders in Europe: results from the European Study of the Epidemiology of Mental Disorders (ESEMeD) project. *Acta Psychiatrica Scandinavica*, 109, 38–46.

Alonso, J., Chatterji, S., & He, Y., eds. (2013). *The Burdens of Mental Disorders: Global Perspectives from the WHO World Mental Health Surveys*. New York, NY: Cambridge University Press.

Alonso, J., Petukhova, M., Vilagut, G., et al. (2011). Days out of role due to common physical and mental conditions: results from the WHO World Mental Health surveys. *Molecular Psychiatry*, 16, 1234–46.

Atwoli, L., Stein, D. J., Koenen, K. C., & McLaughlin, K. A. (2015). Epidemiology of posttraumatic stress disorder: prevalence, correlates and consequences. *Current Opinion in Psychiatry*, 28, 307–11.

Baker, M. S. (2014). Casualties of the Global War on Terror and their future impact on health care and society: a looming public health crisis. *Military Medicine*, 179, 348–55.

Barbaglia, G., Adroher, N. C., Vilagut, G., et al. (2017). Health conditions and role limitation in three European Regions: a public-health perspective. *Gaceta Sanitaria*, 31, 2–10.

Breslau, J., Lane, M., Sampson, N., & Kessler, R. C. (2008). Mental disorders and subsequent educational attainment in a US national sample. *Journal of Psychiatric Research*, 42, 708–16.

Breslau, J., Miller, E., Jin, R., et al. (2013). Mental disorders, marriage, and divorce. In J. Alonso, S. Chatterji, & Y. He, eds., *The Burdens of Mental Disorders: Global Perspectives from the WHO World Mental Health Surveys*. New York, NY: Cambridge University Press, pp. 66–76.

Breslau, J., Miller, E., Jin, R., et al. (2011a). A multinational study of mental disorders, marriage, and divorce. *Acta Psychiatrica Scandinavica*, 124, 474–86.

Breslau, J., Miller, E., Joanie Chung, W. J., & Schweitzer, J. B. (2011b). Childhood and adolescent onset psychiatric disorders, substance use, and failure to graduate high school on time. *Journal of Psychiatric Research*, 45, 295–301.

Butterworth, P., & Rodgers, B. (2008). Mental health problems and marital disruption: is it the combination of husbands and wives' mental health problems that predicts later divorce? *Social Psychiatry and Psychiatric Epidemiology*, 43, 758–63.

Collins, J. J., Baase, C. M., Sharda, C. E., et al. (2005). The assessment of chronic health conditions on work performance, absence, and total economic impact for employers. *Journal of Occupational and Environmental Medicine*, 47, 547–57.

Dooley, D., Fielding, J., & Levi, L. (1996). Health and unemployment. *Annual Review of Public Health*, 17, 449–65.

Foa, E. B., Keane, T. M., Friedman, M. J., & Cohen, J. A. (2008). *Effective Treatments for PTSD: Practice Guidelines from the International Society for Traumatic Stress Studies*. New York, NY: Guilford Press.

Forthofer, M. S., Kessler, R. C., Story, A. L., & Gotlib, I. H. (1996). The effects of psychiatric disorders on the probability and timing of first marriage. *Journal of Health and Social Behavior*, 37, 121–32.

Hojjat, S. K., Hatami, S. E., Rezaei, M., Khalili, M. N., & Talebi, M. R. (2016). The efficacy of training of stress-coping strategies on marital satisfaction of spouses of veterans with post-traumatic stress disorder. *Electronic Physician*, 8, 2232–7.

Kawakami, N., Abdulghani, E. A., Alonso, J., et al. (2012). Early-life mental disorders and adult household income in the World Mental Health Surveys. *Biological Psychiatry*, 72, 228–37.

Keiding, N., Fine, J. P., Hansen, O. H., & Slama, R. (2011). Accelerated failure time regression for backward recurrence times and current durations. *Statistics & Probability Letters*, 81, 724–9.

Kessler, R. C., Ames, M., Hymel, P. A., et al. (2004). Using the World Health Organization Health and Work Performance Questionnaire (HPQ) to evaluate the indirect workplace costs of illness. *Journal of Occupational and Environmental Medicine*, 46, S23–S37.

Kessler, R. C., Barber, C., Beck, A., et al. (2003). The World Health Organization Health and Work Performance Questionnaire (HPQ). *Journal of Occupational and Environmental Medicine*, 45, 156–74.

Kessler, R. C., Foster, C. L., Saunders, W. B., & Stang, P. E. (1995). Social consequences of psychiatric disorders, I: educational attainment. *American Journal of Psychiatry*, 152, 1026–32.

Kessler, R. C., Greenberg, P. E., Mickelson, K. D., Meneades, L. M., & Wang, P. S. (2001a). The effects of chronic medical conditions on work loss and work cutback. *Journal of Occupational and Environmental Medicine*, 43, 218–25.

Kessler, R. C., Harkness, J., Heeringa, S. G., et al. (2012). Methods of the World Mental Health Surveys. In M. K. Nock, G. Borges, & Y. Ono, eds., *Suicide: Global Perspectives from the WHO World Mental Health Surveys*. New York, NY: Cambridge University Press, pp. 33–64.

Kessler, R. C., Molnar, B. E., Feurer, I. D., & Appelbaum, M. (2001b). Patterns and mental health predictors of domestic violence in the United States: results from the National Comorbidity Survey. *International Journal of Law and Psychiatry*, 24, 487–508.

Kessler, R. C., Walters, E. E., & Forthofer, M. S. (1998). The social consequences of psychiatric disorders, III: probability of marital stability. *American Journal of Psychiatry*, 155, 1092–6.

Kim, H. K., Laurent, H. K., Capaldi, D. M., & Feingold, A. (2008). Men's aggression toward women: a 10-year panel study. *Journal of Marriage and Family*, 70, 1169–87.

Lee, S., Tsang, A., Breslau, J., et al. (2009). Mental disorders and termination of education in high-income and low- and middle-income countries: epidemiological study. *British Journal of Psychiatry*, 194, 411–17.

Leon, A. C., Olfson, M., Portera, L., Farber, L., & Sheehan, D. V. (1997). Assessing psychiatric impairment in primary care with the Sheehan Disability Scale. *International Journal of Psychiatry in Medicine*, 27, 93–105.

Lerner, D., Allaire, S. H., & Reisine, S. T. (2005). Work disability resulting from chronic health conditions. *Journal of Occupational and Environmental Medicine*, 47, 253–64.

Lorber, M. F., & O'Leary, K. D. (2004). Predictors of the persistence of male aggression in early marriage. *Journal of Family Violence*, 19, 329–38.

McLeod, J. D., & Kaiser, K. (2004). Childhood emotional and behavioral problems and educational attainment. *American Sociological Review*, 69, 636–58.

Merikangas, K. R., Ames, M., Cui, L., et al. (2007). The impact of comorbidity of mental and physical conditions on role disability in the US adult household population. *Archives of General Psychiatry*, 64, 1180–8.

Miller, E., Breslau, J., Petukhova, M., et al. (2011). Premarital mental disorders and physical violence in marriage: cross-national study of married couples. *British Journal of Psychiatry*, 199, 330–7.

Munce, S. E., Stansfeld, S. A., Blackmore, E. R., & Stewart, D. E. (2007). The role of depression and chronic pain conditions in absenteeism: results from a national epidemiologic survey. *Journal of Occupational and Environmental Medicine*, 49, 1206–11.

Nock, M. K., Deming, C. A., Chiu, W. T., et al. (2012). Mental disorders, comorbidity, and suicidal behavior. In M. K. Nock, G. Borges, & Y. Ono, eds., *Suicide: Global Perspectives from the WHO World Mental Health Surveys*. New York, NY: Cambridge University Press, pp. 148–63.

Nock, M. K., Hwang, I., Sampson, N., et al. (2009). Cross-national analysis of the associations among mental disorders and suicidal behavior: findings from the WHO World Mental Health Surveys. *PLoS Medicine*, 6, e1000123.

O'Leary, K. D., Tintle, N., Bromet, E. J., & Gluzman, S. F. (2008). Descriptive epidemiology of intimate partner aggression in Ukraine. *Social Psychiatry and Psychiatric Epidemiology*, 43, 619–26.

Ormel, J., Petukhova, M., Chatterji, S., et al. (2008). Disability and treatment of specific mental and physical disorders across the world. *British Journal of Psychiatry*, 192, 368–75.

Pankiewicz, P., Majkowicz, M., & Krzykowski, G. (2012). Anxiety disorders in intimate partners and the quality of their relationship. *Journal of Affective Disorders*, 140, 176–80.

Porche, M. V., Fortuna, L. R., Lin, J., & Alegria, M. (2011). Childhood trauma and psychiatric disorders as correlates of school dropout in a national sample of young adults. *Child Development*, 82, 982–98.

Rachiotis, G., Stuckler, D., McKee, M., & Hadjichristodoulou, C. (2015). What has happened to suicides during the Greek economic crisis? Findings from an ecological study of suicides and their determinants (2003–2012). *BMJ Open*, 5, e007295.

Ray, S. L., & Vanstone, M. (2009). The impact of PTSD on veterans' family relationships: an interpretative phenomenological inquiry. *International Journal of Nursing Studies*, 46, 838–47.

Renner, L. M. (2009). Intimate partner violence victimization and parenting stress: assessing the mediating role of depressive symptoms. *Violence against Women*, 15, 1380–401.

Riggs, D. S., Caulfield, M. B., & Street, A. E. (2000). Risk for domestic violence: factors associated with perpetration and victimization. *Journal of Clinical Psychology*, 56, 1289–316.

Scheike, T. H., & Keiding, N. (2006). Design and analysis of time-to-pregnancy. *Statistical Methods in Medical Research*, 15, 127–40.

Siriwardhana, C., & Stewart, R. (2013). Forced migration and mental health: prolonged internal displacement, return migration and resilience. *International Health*, 5, 19–23.

Stewart, W. F., Ricci, J. A., Chee, E., & Morganstein, D. (2003). Lost productive work time costs from health conditions in the United States: results from the

American Productivity Audit. *Journal of Occupational and Environmental Medicine*, 45, 1234–46.

Stith, S. M., Smith, D. B., Penn, C. E., Ward, D. B., & Tritt, D. (2004). Intimate partner physical abuse perpetration and victimization risk factors: a meta-analytic review. *Aggression and Violent Behavior*, 10, 65–98.

Vaughn, M. G., Wexler, J., Beaver, K. M., et al. (2011). Psychiatric correlates of behavioral indicators of school disengagement in the United States. *Psychiatric Quarterly*, 82, 191–206.

Verbrugge, L. M., & Patrick, D. L. (1995). Seven chronic conditions: their impact on US adults' activity levels and use of medical services. *American Journal of Public Health*, 85, 173–82.

Wang, P. S., Beck, A., Berglund, P., et al. (2003). Chronic medical conditions and work performance in the Health and Work Performance Questionnaire calibration surveys. *Journal of Occupational and Environmental Medicine*, 45, 1303–11.

Whisman, M. A. (1999). Marital dissatisfaction and psychiatric disorders: results from the National Comorbidity Survey. *Journal of Abnormal Psychology*, 108, 701–6.

Whisman, M. A., Tolejko, N., & Chatav, Y. (2007). Social consequences of personality disorders: probability and timing of marriage and probability of marital disruption. *Journal of Personality Disorders*, 21, 690–5.

Willett, J. B., & Singer, J. D. (1993). Investigating onset, cessation, relapse, and recovery: why you should, and how you can, use discrete-time survival analysis to examine event occurrence. *Journal of Consulting and Clinical Psychology*, 61, 952–65.

Woodward, L. J., & Fergusson, D. M. (2001). Life course outcomes of young people with anxiety disorders in adolescence. *Journal of the American Academy of Child and Adolescent Psychiatry*, 40, 1086–93.

Yamaguchi, K. (2003). Accelerated failure-time mover-stayer regression models for the analysis of last-episode data. *Sociological Methodology*, 33, 81–110.

Chapter 8

Patterns of Treatment and Barriers to Care in Posttraumatic Stress Disorder

Graham Thornicroft, Sara Evans-Lacko, Karestan C. Koenen, Viviane Kovess-Masféty, David R. Williams, and Ronald C. Kessler

Most individuals with posttraumatic stress disorder (PTSD) never receive any treatment (Kantor et al., 2017), even though a few effective treatments exist (Cukor et al., 2010; Bisson et al., 2013). To date, much of the epidemiological research on treatment has been limited to studies on either of those exposed to particular types of trauma (e.g., natural disasters; Rodriguez & Kohn, 2008) or of special populations (e.g., members of the military; Hom et al., 2017). Most general population studies have focused on treatment for "worst" lifetime traumas (e.g., Roberts et al., 2011; Sheerin et al., 2016). In this chapter, we examine the World Mental Health (WMH) survey data related to patterns of treatment and barriers to obtaining treatment for PTSD.

Earlier WMH reports documented that many individuals throughout the world afflicted with mental disorders fail to benefit from proven treatments. Not only is the proportion of individuals with mental disorders who receive any treatment low, but the treatment provided also often fails to meet even minimal standards of adequacy (Wang et al., 2007a, 2007b; Thornicroft et al., 2017). It is unclear, though, whether these results also apply to PTSD, as individuals with PTSD tend to have greater access to treatment than those with other disorders. In particular, special treatment systems are often put in place to address the mental health needs of refugees (Mollica et al., 2004), combat veterans (Holdeman, 2009), and those exposed to natural or human-made disasters (Vernberg et al., 2008) and school shootings (Jordan, 2003). In addition, in contrast to those with other disorders, individuals with PTSD tend to face fewer psychological barriers to seeking treatment, since it is widely considered "normal" to have a difficulty coping with reactions to highly abnormal experiences (Mittal et al., 2013). As a result, we might expect that a higher proportion of individuals with PTSD would obtain treatment. We investigate this hypothesis in this chapter.

We also examine barriers to treatment. Most of the research on such barriers comes from high-income countries (Wells et al., 1994; Kessler et al., 1997) where attitudinal barriers to treatment, such as negative health beliefs (e.g., that treatments are not effective or that an individual cannot recover) (Prins et al., 2008), misinterpretations about the consequences of treatment, or stigma, are the most commonly reported barriers (Sareen et al., 2007; Jagdeo et al., 2009; Clement et al., 2015). Many individuals with severe mental disorders are unaware of available treatments that could be helpful (ten Have et al., 2010). Structural barriers, such as inconvenient location or inability to obtain an appointment, are less commonly reported (Alegria et al., 2000). However, Sareen et al. (2007) found that low-income respondents were significantly more likely to report a financial barrier to care in the United States than in either Canada or the Netherlands. While previous WMH studies have documented that low levels of perceived need and attitudinal barriers are the most commonly reported barriers by individuals with mental disorders who failed to obtain any treatment (Andrade et al., 2014), it is unclear whether these same patterns hold for PTSD.

Methods

We examined treatment after random traumas in the same 22 WMH surveys referred to in several other chapters that assessed lifetime PTSD after random traumas. Respondents who met DSM-IV/CIDI criteria for PTSD were asked whether they had ever *"talk(ed) to a medical doctor or other professional about"* the symptoms of PTSD reported in the survey. This question went on to define "other professionals" broadly to include *"psychologists, counselors, spiritual advisors, herbalists, acupuncturists, and other healing professionals."*

The respondents who reported receiving treatment were then asked two additional questions. The first asked if they had ever received treatment for their psychological reactions to the random trauma that *"you considered helpful or effective."* The second asked about the number of professionals seen. Respondents who reported helpful treatment were asked how many professionals they had seen *"up to and including"* the one who had helped them, whereas respondents who reported that the treatment was not helpful were asked how many professionals they had seen in total. Our intent in asking these questions was to learn both how often patients reported being helped by PTSD treatment, and how often obtaining helpful treatment required persistence in seeking out additional treatment providers, after one or more initial providers had proven unhelpful.

We used simple actuarial methods to calculate cumulative probabilities of obtaining helpful treatment by number of professionals seen. We then used logistic regression analysis to examine basic sociodemographic correlates of seeking treatment and among treatment-seekers, of being helped by the treatment. Although 1,575 respondents met criteria for PTSD associated with random traumas, only 1,106 were included in the analysis; that's because the cases in Brazil, Bulgaria, and South Africa were excluded due to a skip error that led to the random-trauma treatment questions being omitted in those countries. In addition, these questions were incorrectly skipped in a number of surveys when the random trauma was the same as the respondent's self-reported worst lifetime trauma, introducing a possible bias into the sample of excluding the most severe PTSD episodes.

We also carried out a separate analysis of more recent treatment by focusing on the subset of WMH respondents described in Chapter 5, who both met lifetime criteria for PTSD and reported that they continued to have PTSD in the 12 months before interview. These respondents were asked if they received any treatment for these symptoms in the past 12 months. As part of a broader assessment of 12-month service use in a separate section of the interview, we then asked the subset of these respondents who *did* receive 12-month treatment whether they were treated during that time period by any providers in four treatment categories: (1) *specialist mental health* treatment (psychiatrist, psychologist, other mental health professional in any setting, social worker or counselor in a mental health specialist treatment setting, used a mental health hotline); (2) *general medical* treatment (primary care doctor, other medical doctor, any other health-care professional seen in a general medical setting); (3) *human services* treatment (religious or spiritual advisor, social worker, or counselor in any setting other than specialist mental health); and (4) *complimentary and alternative medicine* (CAM) treatment (any other type of healer such as a chiropractor or participation in a self-help group).

We asked the respondents who received any treatment about the number of visits to providers in each of these four categories in the previous 12 months and about the content of treatment (psychotherapy, medication, or both). Responses to these questions enabled us to study treatment adequacy. Previous WMH analyses have shown that a substantial proportion of the individuals in community epidemiological surveys who report "receiving treatment" for mental health problems did not receive a type of treatment that met even the most minimal standards of adequacy (Wang et al., 2007a). Using evidence-based guidelines (Depression Guideline Panel, 1993; Lehman & Steinwachs, 1998; American Psychiatric Association, 2006), we defined minimally adequate treatment as receiving either pharmacotherapy ($\geq$1 month of a medication, plus $\geq$4 visits to any type of medical doctor) or psychotherapy ($\geq$8 visits with any professional). The decision to have four or more physician visits for pharmacotherapy was based on the fact that for medication assessment, initiation, and monitoring, four or more visits are generally recommended during the acute and continuation phases of treatment. We required at least eight sessions for psychotherapy, based on the fact that clinical trials showing efficacy have generally included eight or more visits. Any respondent in continuing treatment was regarded as having met this definition.

The subset of respondents with 12-month PTSD who did not receive treatment in the past 12 months were asked a different set of follow-up questions. This question series began by asking respondents whether there was ever a time in the past 12 months when they felt that they might have needed to see a professional for their problems with emotions, nerves, or mental health. Respondents who did not think they needed help, or who reported that their PTSD symptoms were not sufficiently distressing to warrant treatment, were coded as having "low perceived need." In contrast, respondents who reported having "perceived need" were asked additional questions about the structural barriers (e.g., financial) and attitudinal barriers (e.g., stigma) listed in Box 8.1.

Once we inspected the descriptive data for patterns of treatment, treatment adequacy, and barriers to treatment, we used logistic regression to examine the predictors of receiving treatment and of treatment in separate service sectors. We also carried out parallel analyses of the predictors of specific treatment barriers among those who did not receive treatment. Previous WMH analyses that studied 12-month treatment for any mental disorder found that both the proportion of cases in treatment (Wang et al., 2007a) and the barriers reported by those not in treatment (Andrade et al., 2014) varied significantly with disorder severity. As a result, we included a measure of 12-month disorder severity in the analysis of 12-month treatment for PTSD.

As in previous WMH studies, respondents with 12-month PTSD were classified as *severe* cases either if they made a suicide attempt in the 12 months before interview, or if they reported severe role impairment in the past 12 months in any domain of the expanded version of the Sheehan Disability Scales (SDS; Leon et al., 1997), or if they had a comorbid 12-month disorder that we considered prima facie evidence of severe disorder (either bipolar I disorder or substance dependence with a physiological dependence syndrome). Respondents not classified as severe were classified as *moderate* if they reported moderate impairment on any of the SDS dimensions, or if they met criteria for substance dependence without a physiological dependence syndrome. All other cases were classified as *mild*.

Box 8.1 The structural and attitudinal barriers to seeking treatment assessed in the WMH surveys

I **Structural Barriers**
- My health insurance would not cover this type of treatment.
- I was concerned about how much money it would cost.
- I was unsure about where to go or who to see.
- I thought it would take too much time or be inconvenient.
- I could not get an appointment.
- I had problems with things like transportation, child-care, or scheduling that would have made it hard to get to treatment.

II **Attitudinal Barriers**
- I thought the problem would get better by itself.
- I didn't think treatment would work.
- I was concerned about what others might think if they found out I was in treatment.
- I wanted to handle the problem on my own.
- I was scared about being put into a hospital against my will.
- I was not satisfied with available services.
- I received treatment before and it did not work.
- The problem didn't bother me very much.

Results

Treatment After Random Traumas

Broadly defined treatment of PTSD associated with random traumas was reported by 39.2% of respondents (see Table 8.1). This proportion was dramatically higher in high-income countries than in low- and middle-income countries (LMICs; 47.1% versus 14.3%; $\chi^2_1 = 58.5$, $p < 0.001$). Among the respondents who received treatment, 22.9% said that they were helped by

Table 8.1 Lifetime treatment and helpfulness among those with random lifetime DSM-IV/CIDI PTSD by country income

	Full sample			High-income countries			LMICs			
	%	(SE)	(*n*)	%	(SE)	(*n*)	%	(SE)	(*n*)	χ^2_1
I Obtained treatment	39.2	(1.9)	(1,209)	47.1	(2.1)	(891)	14.3	(2.5)	(318)	58.5*
II Treatment was helpful										
Helped by the first professional	22.9	(2.4)	(348)	21.0	(1.7)	(307)	45.2	(18.2)	(41)	2.3
Helped by the second professional[a]	22.3	(2.4)	(190)	21.5	(2.5)	(171)	36.5	(4.7)	(19)	8.6*
Helped by the third professional[a]	33.2	(5.4)	(107)	34.1	(5.8)	(97)	13.2	(6.0)	(10)	4.4*
Helped by a later professional[a]	13.2	(1.6)	(265)[b]	14.0	(1.7)	(211)[b]	3.5	(0.6)	(54)[b]	46.8*

*Significant at the 0.05 level, two-sided test.

[a]Among respondents who were not helped by the prior professional(s) and sought help from an additional professional. In the case of the last row, this percentage was averaged over all subsequent professionals visited beyond the first three.

[b]Some respondents sought treatment from up to six professionals. This number represents the number of professionals seen, not the number of individuals seeking treatment.

the first professional they saw. A comparable proportion of the remainder (22.3%) reported being helped by a second professional, conditional on not being helped by the first and seeing a second.

The conditional proportion being helped by a third professional was also comparable (33.2%), but decreased after the third visit (13.2%). The proportion of patients continuing to seek help from additional professionals after receiving unhelpful treatment declined after the third professional. It is unlikely that the patients who persisted in seeking help were comparable to those who gave up with regard to treatment response. But to the extent they were, these results suggest that close to 60% of patients would have been helped if they had persisted in seeing three professionals (see Figure 8.1).

Correlates of Treatment After Random Traumas

Consistent with the results in Table 8.1, the logistic regression analysis showed that respondents from high-income countries were significantly more likely to receive treatment after random traumas (OR = 6.2) (see Table 8.2) than those from LMICs. However, country income was unrelated to the odds of treatment being perceived as helpful. Women were somewhat more likely to receive treatment than men (OR = 1.4) and also somewhat more likely than men to believe that treatment helped (OR = 1.3). Respondent age at the time of trauma exposure was not associated either with odds of receiving treatment or odds of treatment being perceived as helpful. Respondent education at the time of trauma exposure was also not related significantly with odds of receiving treatment, but there was a significant nonlinear association of education with odds of treatment being perceived as helpful ($\chi^2_3 = 11.6$, $p = 0.010$) due to a significantly reduced OR for this perception among respondents with high-average levels of education (OR = 0.6).

Trauma category significantly predicted receiving treatment ($\chi^2_5 = 13.0$, $p = 0.020$) due to a significantly elevated OR of sexual violence victimization with receiving treatment (OR = 1.4), and a significantly reduced OR between physical violence victimization and treatment (OR = 0.7). Trauma category also predicted odds of treatment being perceived as helpful ($\chi^2_5 = 27.2$, $p = 0.020$), with significantly elevated ORs for physical and sexual violence victimization

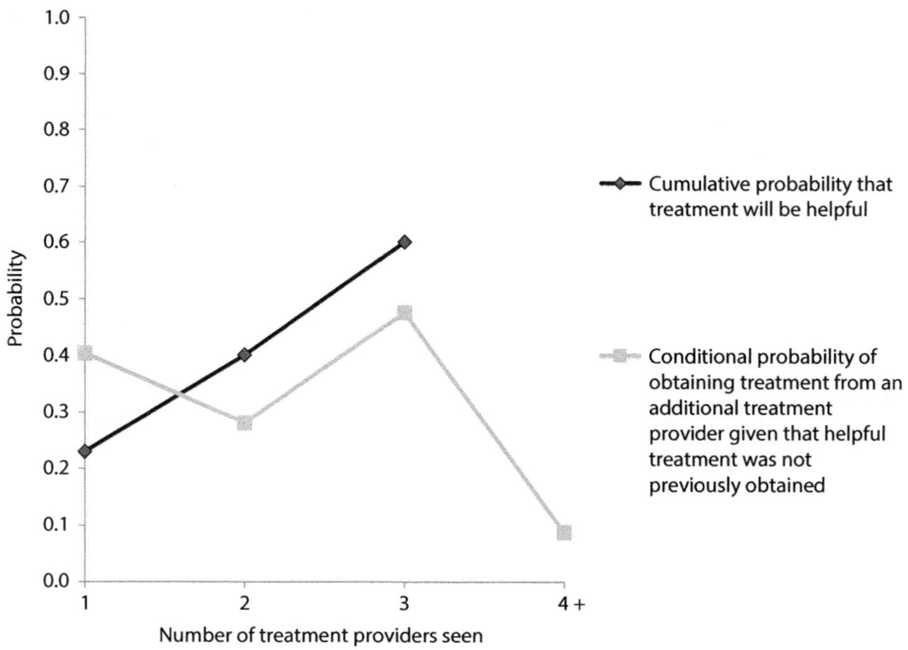

Figure 8.1 Cumulative probability of receiving helpful treatment as a function of number of treatment providers seen and conditional probabilities of continuing to seek treatment after prior unhelpful treatment

Table 8.2 Associations of lifetime treatment and helpful treatment among those with random lifetime DSM-IV/CIDI PTSD

	Received any treatment[a]		Treatment was helpful among those who received treatment[b]	
	OR	95% CI	OR	95% CI
I Country Income				
High income	6.2*	(4.1–9.3)	0.6	(0.2–1.9)
Low and middle income	1.0	–	1.0	–
II Age[c]	1.0	(0.8–1.3)	1.1	(0.9–1.2)
III Sex				
Female	1.4	(1.0–2.0)	1.3	(1.0–1.7)
Male	1.0	–	1.0	–
IV Education				
Low	1.0	–	1.0	–
Low average	1.2	(0.6–2.1)	1.2	(0.9–1.6)
High average	1.8*	(1.1–2.9)	0.7*	(0.5–1.0)
High	1.2	(0.5–2.5)	1.5	(0.7–3.1)
χ^2_3	5.8		11.6*	
V Random Trauma Category[d]				
Exposure to organized violence	1.0	(0.5–1.8)	0.6	(0.2–2.0)
Participation in organized violence	0.8	(0.5–1.4)	0.6*	(0.4–0.9)
Physical violence victimization	0.7*	(0.4–1.0)	1.5*	(1.1–2.1)
Sexual violence victimization	1.4*	(1.1–1.9)	1.7*	(1.2–2.2)
Accidents/injuries	1.1	(0.7–1.7)	0.9	(0.6–1.5)
Other	1.2	(0.8–1.9)	1.2	(0.8–1.8)
χ^2_5	13.0*		27.2*	
(*n*)	(1,209)		(492)	

*Significant at the 0.05 level, two-sided design-based test.
[a]Based on a logistic regression model to predict obtaining treatment controlling for survey.
[b]Based on a discrete patient-provider survival model for treatment helpfulness with controls for surveys and for number of prior treatment professionals seen. A total of 492 patients were included in the analysis and a total of 910 patient-provider observations.
[c]ORs are for a 10-year increase.
[d]ORs are relative to the average across all six trauma categories.

(OR = 1.5–1.7) and significantly reduced ORs for participation in organized violence (OR = 0.6).

Treatment Among 12-Month Cases

Slightly more than half (58.8%) of WMH respondents with 12-month PTSD in high-income countries and 25.4% in LMICs reported being in treatment for PTSD at some time in the 12 months before interview (see Table 8.3). Roughly two-thirds of these patients in high-income countries (40.3% of all respondents with 12-month PTSD) and 55% of those in LMICs (13.9% of all respondents with 12-month PTSD) were seen in the general medical (GM) sector; somewhat smaller proportions (53% of patients in high-income countries and 32% in LMICs) were seen in the specialty mental health (SMH) sector, and considerably smaller proportions in the human services (14% to 12% across country income groups) and CAM (15% to 11% across country income groups) sectors.

The proportion of cases receiving treatment was consistently much higher in high-income countries than in LMICs across treatment sectors. The sum of the proportions of cases in treatment in the separate treatment sectors was about 30.2% higher than the proportion receiving any treatment in high-income countries and 2.6% higher in LMICs, suggesting that a meaningful proportion of patients were seen in multiple treatment sectors. Nearly half (47.9%) of the patients in high-income countries and 24.6% of those in LMICs received minimally adequate treatment.

In high-income countries, a significant positive monotonic association was found between disorder severity and the proportion of cases receiving any treatment (between 73.0% for severe cases and 39.9% for mild cases; $\chi^2_2 = 50.8, p < 0.001$) as well as treatment

Table 8.3 Treatment of 12-month DSM-IV/CIDI PTSD by country income level and severity

	Any		SMH		GM		HS		CAM		Minimally Adequate		Minimally Adequate/Any		
	%	(SE)	%	(SE)	%	(SE)	%	(SE)	%	(SE)	%	(SE)	%	(SE)	(n)
I High-Income Countries[a]															
Severe	73.0	(2.8)	42.8	(3.1)	49.6	(3.4)	10.3	(1.9)	12.1	(1.9)	39.2	(3.5)	56.3	(4.7)	(405)
Moderate	56.1	(5.6)	31.2	(4.7)	36.8	(4.7)	6.8	(2.6)	9.0	(2.5)	26.3	(6.1)	42.6	(8.4)	(169)
Mild	39.9	(4.1)	14.0	(2.6)	29.2	(3.5)	7.0	(1.9)	4.8	(2.2)	13.6	(3.3)	32.0	(6.7)	(254)
Total	58.8	(2.6)	31.1	(2.0)	40.3	(2.2)	8.5	(1.2)	9.1	(1.3)	28.3	(2.3)	47.9	(3.6)	(828)
χ^2_2	50.8*		42.5*		16.3*		2.3		3.4		21.3*		11.6*		
II LMICs[b]															
Severe	32.6	(7.1)	13.7	(4.5)	13.8	(5.3)	5.9	(2.7)	2.0	(1.2)	15.2	(6.1)	39.0	(14.0)	(92)
Moderate	27.6	(8.8)	5.2	(3.9)	11.2	(4.2)	2.0	(1.4)	11.2	(7.9)	5.6	(5.4)	16.7	(15.4)	(54)
Mild	20.9	(6.1)	6.3	(3.4)	15.0	(5.5)	2.0	(1.1)	0.4	(0.4)	1.9	(1.5)	12.1	(4.6)	(115)
Total	25.4	(4.5)	8.1	(2.4)	13.9	(3.8)	3.1	(0.9)	2.9	(1.7)	6.4	(2.3)	24.6	(7.3)	(261)
χ^2_2	2.8		8.1*		1.9		2.3		6.9*		6.8*		0.7		

*Significant at the 0.05 level, two-sided test.

[a]High-income countries include: Belgium, France, Germany, Israel, Italy, Japan, Netherlands, New Zealand, Northern Ireland, Spain, Spain – Murcia, and the United States.

[b]LMICs include: Bulgaria, Colombia, Peru, Brazil – SãoPaulo, Ukraine, Lebanon, Colombia – Medellin, Mexico, Romania, and South Africa.

in the SMH (42.8.0–14.0%; χ^2_2 =42.5, $p < 0.001$) and GM (49.6–29.2; χ^2_2 =16.3, $p < 0.001$) sectors; receiving adequate treatment (39.2–13.6%; χ^2_2 = 21.3, $p < 0.001$); or receiving treatment classified as at least minimally adequate (56.3–32.0%; χ^2_2 = 11.6, $p = 0.003$). These patterns were less clear in LMICs, as severity was not significantly associated with the proportion of cases receiving any treatment (χ^2_2 =2.8, $p = 0.25$); GM treatment (χ^2_2 = 1.9, $p = 0.38$) HS (χ^2_2 = 2.3, $p = 0.32$); or minimally adequate treatment among those with any treatment (χ^2_2 = 0.7, $p = 0.70$). However, severity was significantly associated with treatment in the SMH sector (13.7–5.2%; χ^2_2 =8.1, $p = 0.017$) in the CAM sector (11.2–0.4%; χ^2_2 = 6.9, $p = 0.032$), and with receiving minimally adequate treatment (15.2–1.9; χ^2_2 =6.8, $p = 0.034$).

Correlates of 12-Month Treatment

Human services and CAM treatments were too rare in both high-income countries and LMICs and minimally adequate treatment was too low in LMICs to study their correlates with precision. Controlling for severity and comorbidity, age was not related significantly to any other treatment measures, either in high-income countries (χ^2_3 = 2.2–5.0, p = 0.53–0.17) or LMICs (χ^2_3 = 4.0, $p = 0.26$) other than for a statistically significant non-monotonic association with SMH treatment or in LMICs (see Table 8.4). Men were significantly less likely than women to receive any treatment, but only in high-income countries (OR = 0.6), and there was no sex difference in treatment within separate service sectors either in high-income countries or LMICs or in receipt of adequate treatment in high-income countries (χ^2_1 = 0.0–3.3, p = 0.87–0.7).

Education was unrelated to any of the treatment measures in high-income countries (χ^2_3 = 1.7–6.7, p = 0.65–0.08) and to all but one of the treatment measures in LMICs (χ^2_3 = 5.2–7.1, p = 0.16–0.07), the exception being a significantly positive association of education with SMH treatment (χ^2_3 = 10.5, $p = 0.015$). The other indicator of socio-economic status considered, family income, was unrelated to any of the treatment measures in either high-income countries (χ^2_3 = 2.2–4.1, p = 0.54–0.25) or LMICs (χ^2_3 = 1.0–7.1, p = 0.79–0.07). Finally, marital status was unrelated to any of the treatment measures in high-income countries (χ^2_2 = 0.1–3.7, p = 0.95–0.16) and to all but one in LMICs (χ^2_2 = 1.4–5.0, p = 0.50–0.08), the exception being a significant association with GM treatment (χ^2_2 = 7.9, $p = 0.019$) due to elevated ORs among the never married and previously married (OR = 3.1–3.6) relative to the married.

Barriers to 12-Month Treatment

The most commonly reported barriers to receiving 12-month treatment among respondents with severely impairing 12-month PTSD were attitudinal (53.4%), followed by low perceived need (43.6%) and structural barriers (31.1%) (see Table 8.5). In contrast, this rank ordering of barriers was quite different for respondents with moderate–mild 12-month PTSD, among whom low perceived need was by far the most commonly reported barrier to treatment (64.1%), followed by attitudinal barriers (34.0%) and structural barriers (9.1%). A significantly higher proportion of respondents with mild–moderate rather than severe PTSD reported low perceived need for treatment as a barrier to seeking treatment (χ^2_1 = 10.0, $p = 0.001$), whereas a significantly higher proportion of respondents with severe rather than mild–moderate PTSD reported structural and attitudinal barriers (χ^2_1 = 9.6–14.4, p = 0.001–< 0.001). The same basic patterns held when we looked separately at respondents in high-income countries and LMICs.

Given that low perceived need, unlike structural and attitudinal barriers, is a sufficient explanation for lack of treatment (unless treatment is involuntary, as it seldom is for PTSD), it is useful to examine the distribution of structural and attitudinal barriers among respondents who recognized a need for treatment but did not receive treatment (see Table 8.6). The vast majority of these individuals (94.6%) reported at least one attitudinal barrier. This was true regardless of level of disorder severity (94.5% to 94.8%).

By far the most common attitudinal barrier was the desire to handle the problem on their own (reported by 65.2% overall; 59.6–71.7% in subgroups defined by disorder severity). The next most common attitudinal barrier was related to perceived need: the belief that the problem would get better on its own (30.6% overall; 22.0–39.8% in subgroups), followed by perceived ineffectiveness (22.9%; 8.9–36.1%), stigma (17.8%; 5.7–37.1%), and the perception that the problem was not severe enough to need treatment (16.0%; 11.1–21.6%). The mean number of attitudinal barriers reported increased as severity decreased (from a low of 1.5 among severe cases to 1.9 among mild cases).

Table 8.4 Multivariable association of socio-demographic variables with 12-month treatment of DSM-IV/CIDI PTSD separately in high-income countries and LMICs[a]

	High-income countries								LMICs					
	Any		SMH		GM		Minimally Adequate		Any		SMH		GM	
	OR	(95% CI)	OR	(95% CI)	OR	(95% CI)	OR	(95% CI)	OR	(95% CI)	OR	(95% CI)	OR	(95% CI)
I Age														
18–34	0.8	(0.4–1.8)	0.9	(0.3–2.7)	0.7	(0.3–1.8)	1.1	(0.3–3.5)	0.7	(0.2–3.2)	0.1	(0.0–2.0)	0.7	(0.1–6.4)
35–49	1.3	(0.6–2.6)	1.4	(0.5–3.9)	1.2	(0.5–2.8)	1.6	(0.6–4.4)	1.1	(0.3–3.6)	0.8	(0.1–7.5)	0.8	(0.2–4.4)
50–64	1.3	(0.6–2.7)	1.2	(0.4–3.3)	1.2	(0.5–2.8)	1.1	(0.3–3.7)	1.9	(0.6–5.8)	1.9	(0.2–19.0)	1.9	(0.5–8.1)
65+	1.0	–	1.0	–	1.0	–	1.0	–	1.0	–	1.0	–	1.0	–
χ^2_3	4.5		3.0		5.0		2.2		4.0		9.2*		4.0	
II Sex														
Female	1.7*	(1.1–2.7)	1.3	(0.8–2.0)	1.6	(1.0–2.5)	1.2	(0.7–2.2)	0.9	(0.4–2.0)	0.9	(0.2–4.0)	0.5	(0.1–1.7)
Male	1.0	–	1.0	–	1.0	–	1.0	–	1.0	–	1.0	–	1.0	–
χ^2_1	5.1*		0.9		3.3		0.5		0.1		0.0		1.3	
III Education														
Low	0.6	(0.3-1.2)	0.8	(0.4–1.6)	1.1	(0.6–1.9)	0.8	(0.3–2.1)	1.0	(0.3–3.6)	0.0*	(0.0–0.4)	5.4	(0.8–38.4)
Low average	0.7	(0.4–1.1)	0.5*	(0.3–1.0)	0.9	(0.5–1.7)	0.4	(0.1–1.1)	0.8	(0.3–2.3)	0.2	(0.1–1.0)	3.7	(0.8–16.6)
High average	0.9	(0.5–1.6)	0.8	(0.4–1.5)	1.3	(0.7–2.1)	0.5	(0.2–1.2)	2.4	(0.9–6.6)	0.7	(0.2–3.6)	7.8*	(1.5–41.5)
High	1.0	–	1.0	–	1.0	–	1.0	–	1.0	–	1.0	–	1.0	–
χ^2_3	4.1		5.1		1.7		6.7		5.2		10.5*		7.1	
IV Marital Status														
Currently married	1.0	–	1.0	–	1.0	–	1.0	–	1.0	–	1.0	–	1.0	–
Previously married	1.4	(0.8–2.4)	1.3	(0.8–2.2)	1.1	(0.7–1.6)	1.9	(1.0–3.8)	2.2*	(1.0–4.9)	2.2	(0.6–8.8)	3.6*	(1.5–9.0)
Never married	1.0	(0.6–1.8)	1.0	(0.6–1.7)	1.1	(0.6–1.9)	1.5	(0.7–3.1)	2.2	(0.7–7.1)	1.1	(0.2–6.9)	3.1	(0.7–14.5)
χ^2_2	1.5		1.2		0.1		3.7		5.0		1.4		7.9*	
V Household Income														
Low	1.8	(0.9–3.7)	1.3	(0.6–2.7)	1.9	(1.0–3.8)	1.3	(0.4–4.0)	0.6	(0.2–1.7)	1.0	(0.2–4.5)	0.6	(0.2–2.0)
Low average	1.3	(0.6–2.6)	1.0	(0.4–2.1)	1.5	(0.8–2.9)	1.0	(0.3–2.8)	0.3	(0.1–1.1)	0.5	(0.1–3.3)	0.8	(0.2–2.9)
High average	1.3	(0.6–2.8)	0.8	(0.4–1.7)	1.6	(0.8–3.1)	1.7	(0.6–4.6)	0.9	(0.3–3.0)	0.2*	(0.0–0.9)	1.0	(0.3–3.7)
High	1.0	–	1.0	–	1.0	–	1.0	–	1.0	–	1.0	–	1.0	–
χ^2_3	3.6		3.0		4.1		2.2		7.1		5.7		1.0	
(*n*)	(795)									(261)				

*Significant at the 0.05 level, two-sided test.
[a]Based on logistic regression models among Part II respondents with one or more 12-month DSM-IV/CIDI disorders controlling for severity and survey.

Structural barriers were reported less often (36.8% overall; 23.1–55.3% in subgroups defined by disorder severity). The most common structural barriers were lack of availability (25.0%; 11.9–40.0%) and financial constraints (24.3%; 17.8–29.9%), followed by transportation (15.3%; 7.4–224%), and inconvenience (11.9%; 1.2–28.3%). As with attitudinal barriers, mean number of structural barriers reported increased as severity decreased (from a low of 0.5 among severe cases to 1.1 among mild cases).

Table 8.5 Barriers to treatment among all respondents with 12-month DSM-IV/CIDI PTSD who did not use services in that period, by the level of disorder severity

	Severe		Moderate/Mild		
	%	(SE)	%	(SE)	χ^2_1
I Total Sample					
Low perceived need	43.6	(5.1)	64.1	(3.8)	10.0*
Structural barriers	31.1	(5.0)	9.1	(1.9)	14.4*
Attitudinal barriers	53.4	(5.0)	34.0	(3.7)	9.7*
II High-Income Countries					
Low perceived need	42.5	(6.4)	63.0	(4.6)	6.7*
Structural barriers	27.6	(6.0)	6.8	(1.7)	9.9*
Attitudinal barriers	55.4	(6.4)	36.3	(4.6)	5.8*
III Upper-Middle-Income Countries					
Low perceived need	35.1	(10.4)	62.0	(7.6)	3.5
Structural barriers	50.9	(10.9)	14.6	(5.3)	6.1*
Attitudinal barriers	59.0	(9.0)	33.4	(7.7)	4.1*
IV Low- and Lower-Middle-Income Countries					
Low perceived need	57.5	(13.3)	76.3	(10.8)	1.2
Structural barriers	25.7	(14.0)	7.8	(3.9)	1.3
Attitudinal barriers	38.8	(12.8)	21.8	(10.7)	1.0
(*n*)	(89)		(138)		

*Significant at the 0.05 level, two-sided test.

Table 8.6 Barriers to seeking treatment among respondents with 12-month DSM-IV/CIDI PTSD who perceived a need for treatment but did not obtain treatment by disorder severity

	All cases		Severe		Moderate		Mild		
	%	(SE)	%	(SE)	%	(SE)	%	(SE)	χ^2_2
I Structural Barriers									
Financial	24.3	(3.4)	17.8	(4.2)	29.9	(9.5)	29.2	(5.4)	3.6
Availability	25.0	(3.7)	11.9	(3.7)	24.9	(9.3)	40.0	(6.6)	10.3*
Transportation	15.3	(3.0)	7.5	(2.8)	19.6	(9.0)	22.4	(5.4)	7.1*
Inconvenient	11.9	(3.2)	1.2	(0.9)	2.9	(2.4)	28.3	(7.4)	9.1*
Any structural barrier	36.8	(4.2)	23.2	(4.8)	30.8	(9.5)	55.1	(6.3)	11.5*
II Attitudinal Barriers									
Wanted to handle on own	65.2	(4.2)	71.7	(7.3)	59.6	(10.3)	60.2	(6.4)	1.7
Perceived ineffectiveness	23.0	(3.5)	8.9	(3.5)	29.4	(8.2)	36.2	(6.8)	12.0*
Stigma	17.8	(3.4)	5.7	(2.7)	5.7	(4.0)	37.1	(6.9)	12.9*
Thought would get better	30.7	(4.5)	22.0	(7.7)	32.5	(8.5)	39.8	(7.3)	2.5
Problem was not severe	16.0	(3.8)	21.6	(7.5)	11.1	(5.3)	11.9	(3.2)	1.4
Any attitudinal barrier	94.6	(1.7)	94.5	(2.6)	94.9	(3.0)	94.7	(3.0)	0.0
(*n*)	(227)		(89)		(38)		(100)		

*Significant at the 0.05 level, two-sided test.

Correlates of Barriers to 12-Month Treatment

Low perceived need for treatment was not significantly related to any of the socio-demographic variables we considered, including respondent age ($\chi^2_3 = 3.1$, $p=0.38$), sex ($\chi^2_1=0.3, p=0.56$), education ($\chi^2_6=12.5$, $p = 0.051$), income ($\chi^2_3 = 1.8$, $p = 0.60$), or marital status ($\chi^2_2 = 2.9$, $p = 0.23$) (see Table 8.7). Among respondents with a perceived need for treatment, marital status was the only significant socio-demographic predictor of structural barriers ($\chi^2_2 = 7.9$, $p = 0.019$) due to a significantly elevated OR among the married compared to the never married (5.4), although this barrier was more common among older respondents, among men, and among milder cases. Respondents with severe PTSD were more likely than respondents with mild PTSD to report a structural barrier (OR 1.6, 95% CI 1.2–2.2, $\chi^2_2 = 12.2, p = 0.002$).

Discussion

In addition to the limitations noted in other chapters, our analysis of treatment was limited by the fact that we had no corroborating data from administrative records. Earlier studies suggest that self-reported

Table 8.7 Multivariable analyses of the socio-demographic correlates of not seeking treatment because of low perceived need, any structural barriers or any attitudinal barriers among respondents with 12-month DSM-IV/CIDI PTSD (all countries)[a]

	Low perceived need		Any structural barrier given perceived need	
	OR	(95% CI)	OR	(95% CI)
I Age				
18–34	0.8	(0.3–2.0)	2.4	(0.3–16.4)
35–49	0.6	(0.2–1.4)	2.1	(0.3–12.6)
50–64	0.5	(0.2–1.2)	1.7	(0.2–12.7)
65+	1.0	–	1.0	–
χ^2_3	3.1		0.8	
II Sex				
Female	0.8	(0.5–1.5)	0.5	(0.2–1.4)
Male	1.0	–	1.0	–
III Education				
No education	0.2	(0.0–1.8)	0.0*	(0.0–0.6)
Some primary	2.6	(0.8–8.9)	0.4	(0.1–2.8)
Primary finished	2.1	(0.5–9.0)	0.6	(0.1–5.8)
Some secondary	0.6	(0.2–1.4)	0.5	(0.1–2.1)
Secondary finished	0.6	(0.3–1.5)	0.7	(0.2–2.8)
Some college	0.6	(0.3–1.5)	1.0	(0.4–3.0)
Completed college	1.0	–	1.0	–
χ^2_6	12.5		5.8	
IV Marital Status				
Married/cohabitating	1.2	(0.5–2.7)	5.4*	(1.3–23.1)
Separated/widowed/divorced	0.7	(0.3–1.7)	1.5	(0.3–7.7)
Never married	1.0	–	1.0	–
χ^2_2	2.9		7.9*	
V Household Income				
Low-income	1.2	(0.6–2.8)	0.5	(0.1–2.3)
Low-average-income	1.0	(0.4–2.4)	0.4	(0.1–1.3)
High-average-income	1.5	(0.6–3.6)	0.1*	(0.0–0.7)
High-income	1.0	–	1.0	–
χ^2_3	1.9		6.7	
(*n*)	(500)		(227)	

*Significant at the 0.05 level, two-sided test.
[a]Controlling for PTSD severity, number of comorbid 12-month mood, anxiety, substance and disruptive behavior disorders, and survey.

treatment overestimates actual treatment received as documented in administrative records (Rhodes & Fung, 2004). An additional limitation is that we did not ask about the types of professionals seen, the types of treatment received, or the patient ratings of adequacy of these treatments. Furthermore, since our analysis of barriers to treatment of 12-month PTSD relied on a list of barriers based on previous research in high-income countries, it might not have been sensitive to different national contexts. Finally, respondents were asked about barriers to treatment for any emotional problem, not just for PTSD; but even though responses were applied to respondents who failed to receive treatment for PTSD, this is a limitation because evidence exists that barriers to treatment are not uniform across diagnoses (Mojtabai et al., 2002).

Despite these limitations, the results reveal disturbingly high levels of unmet need for mental health treatment among individuals with PTSD after random traumas worldwide. Even in high-income countries, fewer than half of respondents with PTSD received treatment after random traumas, and only about one in five reported that the treatment provided by the first professional they saw was helpful (a total of only about 10% of cases that received helpful treatment from the first professional they saw). About 60% of those who persisted in seeking help from additional professionals were eventually helped. The situation was considerably worse in LMICs, where only 14.3% of individuals with PTSD sought treatment, of whom only a small minority received treatment that they considered helpful.

The finding that treatment rates for PTSD were much higher in high-income countries than in LMICs is consistent with prior WMH findings about patterns of treatment for any mental disorder (Wang et al., 2007b). And the finding that the treatment rate for PTSD after random traumas was slightly elevated among women is similar to WMH data on overall treatment of any mental disorder. However, the failure to find an age gradient in PTSD treatment is not consistent with the WMH results regarding overall treatment for any mental disorder, where we found a significant inverse association between age and odds of obtaining treatment. The finding that treatment rates were highest for PTSD associated with sexual assaults and lowest for PTSD associated with physical assaults might reflect differences in official recognition-reporting to law enforcement officials; in the case of sexual assault, the high treatment rates may be due to encouragement from law enforcement personnel. The finding of significantly higher rates of helpfulness reported by individuals receiving treatment after physical and sexual assaults could reflect either more intensive treatments, treatments that were specifically designed to address the special issues that emerge after these two types of trauma, or the greater effectiveness of PTSD treatments for these types of trauma. The WMH data provide no way of adjudicating among those and other possible explanations.

The findings for 12-month treatment of PTSD were somewhat different, as 58.8% of respondents were in treatment in high-income countries and 25% in LMICs. It is important to recognize that 12-month cases are different from lifetime cases in that 12-month cases over-represent people with chronic PTSD. In addition, 12-month treatment was defined as receiving treatment for any emotional problem rather than treatment specifically for PTSD. Importantly, the 12-month treatment rates we discovered were considerably higher than those found in other WMH analyses for mental disorders overall, consistent with our initial hypothesis that treatment for PTSD might be more common than for other mental disorders. For example, the 73.0% treatment rate for severely impairing 12-month PTSD in high-income countries was considerably higher than the 53% (48% to 58%) median (inter-quartile range) 12-month treatment rates found in earlier WMH analyses for all severely impairing 12-month mental disorders in those same countries (Wang et al., 2007a). The 32.6% treatment rate for severely impairing 12-month PTSD in LMICs was also higher than the 25% (20% to 26%) treatment rate for all severely impairing 12-month mental disorders found in earlier WMH analyses of those same countries.

As one might expect, we found a strong association between symptom severity and treatment in high-income countries. But this same association was not found in LMICs. This doubtlessly reflects differences in help-seeking behaviors, but could also be partly due to differences in the extent to which health-care providers place priorities on delivering care. An argument could be made that it could be cost-effective in terms of secondary prevention to motivate primary care physicians to recognize and treat mild and moderately severe PTSD and other mental disorders (McCrone & Knapp, 2007) or to implement models that make use of lay counselors to support primary care medical providers in treating these non-severe cases (Buttorff et al., 2012; Levin & Chisholm, 2015). The association of severity with treatment is related to the finding regarding barriers to treatment among the 12-month cases that did not receive treatment, which showed clearly that low perceived need for treatment was a critical barrier to seeking treatment of PTSD worldwide, even among individuals with severely impairing PTSD. This result is consistent with previous studies using WMH data (Andrade et al., 2014) as well as with other research (van Beljouw et al., 2010) showing that a substantial proportion of those with mental disorders do not define or recognize their distress as an "illness" that can be treated. Low perceived need was equally high in countries with various levels of economic development, although it is possible that a deeper analysis going beyond the WMH data might find that these perceptions differ in important ways across cultural settings.

It is plausible to imagine that the variation in mental health literacy – that is, in knowledge and beliefs about mental disorders – could be related to both perceived need for treatment and to service utilization. As mental disorders still are highly stigmatized, social and cultural factors might contribute to biased perceptions of need (Leventhal et al., 1984; Jorm, 2000; Gureje et al., 2006; Mojtabai, 2010; Lewer et al., 2015). Biased judgment due to the illnesses themselves might also have been involved, along with stigma and inaccurate beliefs (Mechanic, 2002; Prins et al., 2008; Schomerus & Angermeyer, 2008). Community campaigns aimed at increasing public awareness, raising mental health literacy, reducing the stigma and discrimination associated with mental illness, and bridging the gap between commonly held beliefs about treatment options and what mental health professionals actually have to offer, might be useful in reducing stigma and discrimination and improving awareness (Meadows & Burgess, 2009; Khandelwal et al., 2010; Thornicroft et al., 2016; Maulik et al., 2017).

Regarding those who did not seek treatment, it is noteworthy that attitudinal and structural barriers to treatment were more prevalent among those with severe than among those with mild–moderate PTSD. This difference presumably reflected the fact that individuals with severe PTSD were likely to recognize a need for help and would have a comparatively high probability of seeking treatment were it not for attitudinal and structural barriers. A desire to handle the problem by oneself was among the most common reasons reported by respondents who recognized a need. This result is consistent with other evidence that negative public attitudes, shame associated with mental illness (Mehta et al., 2009), and fear of being discriminated against in the workplace for revealing either a mental illness or psychiatric treatment (Thornicroft et al., 2009; Wheat et al., 2010; Lasalvia et al., 2013) often lead people to conceal mental health problems. Stigma has also been shown to be an important reason for not seeking treatment even among those with severe mental illness in both high-income countries and LMICs (Gureje et al., 2006; Saxena et al., 2007; Brohan et al., 2010; Clement et al., 2015).

We know from the dramatic increases in treatment rates of common mental disorders in high-income countries when direct-to-consumer advertisements for mental disorder treatments came into being that attitudinal barriers can be overcome with thoughtful public communication campaigns that help individuals with mental disorders recognize that their distress is a sign of illness, that the illness has a name, and that effective treatments exist to treat the illness (Ventola, 2011; Becker & Midoun, 2016). However, structural barriers have to be removed in order to enable individuals to act on these new realizations. Structural barriers such as financial constraints and lack of availability were commonly reported by WMH respondents with severe PTSD, even when they recognized a need for help. Even in high-income countries with well-funded health systems, individuals may lack insurance coverage for mental health treatment or the means to access services (Mechanic, 2002). In LMICs, the lack of trained mental health professionals and general scarcity of resources can reduce access to care much more (Andrade et al., 2008; Seedat et al., 2008). And in LMICs where mental health reform has been implemented, community-based services are often insufficient, the integration with primary care is weak, and inpatient beds are inadequate to meet population needs (e.g., Romero-Gonzalez et al., 2003; Andreoli et al., 2007; Caldas de Almeida & Horvitz-Lennon, 2010). In many LMICs, geographic distance from services in rural areas, population density, and lack of trained personnel also result in service deficiencies (Jacob et al., 2007). Health care policy planners need to address these structural barriers by improving service availability and accessibility in order to increase the proportion of individuals with PTSD and other mental disorders who receive treatment.

References

Alegria, M., Bijl, R. V., Lin, E., Walters, E. E., & Kessler, R. C. (2000). Income differences in persons seeking outpatient treatment for mental disorders: a comparison of the United States with Ontario and the Netherlands. *Archives of General Psychiatry*, 57, 383–91.

American Psychiatric Association (2006). *American Psychiatric Association Practice Guidelines for the Treatment of Psychiatric Disorders: Compendium 2006*. Arlington, VA: American Psychiatric Association.

Andrade, L. H., Viana, M. C., Tofoli, L. F., & Wang, Y. P. (2008). Influence of psychiatric morbidity and sociodemographic determinants on use of service in a catchment area in the city of São Paulo, Brazil. *Social Psychiatry and Psychiatric Epidemiology*, 43, 45–53.

Andrade, L. H., Alonso, J., Mneimneh, Z., et al. (2014). Barriers to mental health treatment: results from the WHO World Mental Health Surveys. *Psychological Medicine*, 44, 1303–17.

Andreoli, S. B., Almeida-Filho, N., Martin, D., Mateus, M. D., & Mari Jde, J. (2007). Is psychiatric reform a strategy for reducing the mental health budget? The case of Brazil. *Revista Brasileira de Psiquiatria*, 29, 43–6.

Bisson, J. I., Roberts, N. P., Andrew, M., Cooper, R., & Lewis, C. (2013). Psychological therapies for chronic post-traumatic stress disorder (PTSD) in adults. *Cochrane Database of Systematic Reviews*. 12. CD003388.

Becker, S. J., & Midoun, M. M. (2016). Effects of direct-to-consumer advertising on patient prescription requests and physician prescribing: a systematic review of psychiatry-relevant studies. *Journal of Clinical Psychiatry*, 77, e1293–e1300.

Brohan, E., Slade, M., Clement, S., & Thornicroft, G. (2010). Experiences of mental illness stigma, prejudice and discrimination: a review of measures. *BMC Health Services Research*, 10, 80.

Buttorff, C., Hock, R. S., Weiss, H. A., et al. (2012). Economic evaluation of a task-shifting intervention for common mental disorders in India. *Bulletin of the World Health Organization*, 90, 813–21.

Caldas de Almeida, J. M., & Horvitz-Lennon, M. (2010). Mental health care reforms in Latin America: an overview of mental health care reforms in Latin America and the Caribbean. *Psychiatric Services*, 61, 218–21.

Clement, S., Schauman, O., Graham, T., et al. (2015). What is the impact of mental health-related stigma on help-seeking? A systematic review of quantitative and qualitative studies. *Psychological Medicine*, 45, 11–27.

Cukor, J., Olden, M., Lee, F., & Difede, J. (2010). Evidence-based treatments for PTSD, new directions, and special challenges. *Annals of the New York Academy of Sciences*, 1208, 82–89.

Depression Guideline Panel. (1993). *Depression in primary care: detection, diagnosis and treatment. Clinical practice guideline, number 5*. Rockville, MD: U.S. Department of Health and Human Services, Public Health Service, Agency for Health Care Policy and Research. AHCPR publication no. 93-0552.

Gureje, O., Lasebikan, V. O., Kola, L., & Makanjuola, V. A. (2006). Lifetime and 12-month prevalence of mental disorders in the Nigerian Survey of Mental Health and Well-Being. *British Journal of Psychiatry*, 188, 465–71.

Holdeman, T. C. (2009). Invisible wounds of war: psychological and cognitive injuries, their consequences, and services to assist recovery. *Psychiatric Services*, 60, 272–273.

Hom, M. A., Stanley, I. H., Schneider, M. E., & Joiner, T. E., Jr. (2017). A systematic review of help-seeking and mental health service utilization among military service members. *Clinical Psychology Review*, 53, 59–78.

Jacob, K. S., Sharan, P., Mirza, I., et al. (2007). Mental health systems in countries: where are we now? *Lancet*, 370, 1061–77.

Jagdeo, A., Cox, B. J., Stein, M. B., & Sareen, J. (2009). Negative attitudes toward help seeking for mental illness in 2 population-based surveys from the United States and Canada. *The Canadian Journal of Psychiatry. La Revue Canadienne de Psychiatrie*, 54, 757–66.

Jordan, K. (2003). A trauma and recovery model for victims and their families after a catastrophic school shooting: focusing on behavioral, cognitive, and psychological effects and needs. *Brief Treatment and Crisis Intervention*, 3, 397–411.

Jorm, A. F. (2000). Mental health literacy. Public knowledge and beliefs about mental disorders. *British Journal of Psychiatry*, 177, 396–401.

Kantor, V., Knefel, M., & Lueger-Schuster, B. (2017). Perceived barriers and facilitators of mental health service utilization in adult trauma survivors: a systematic review. *Clinical Psychology Review*, 52, 52–68.

Kessler, R. C., Frank, R. G., Edlund, M., et al. (1997). Differences in the use of psychiatric outpatient services between the United States and Ontario. *New England Journal of Medicine*, 336, 551–7.

Khandelwal, S., Avode, G., Baingana, F., et al. (2010). Mental and neurological health research priorities setting in developing countries. *Social Psychiatry and Psychiatric Epidemiology*, 45, 487–95.

Lasalvia, A., Zoppei, S., Van Bortel, T., et al. (2013). Global pattern of experienced and anticipated discrimination reported by people with major depressive disorder: a cross-sectional survey. *Lancet*, 381, 55–62.

Lehman, A. F., & Steinwachs, D. M. (1998). Translating research into practice: the Schizophrenia Patient Outcomes Research Team (PORT) treatment recommendations. *Schizophrenia Bulletin*, 24, 1–10.

Leon, A. C., Olfson, M., Portera, L., Farber, L., & Sheehan, D. V. (1997). Assessing psychiatric impairment in primary care with the Sheehan Disability Scale. *International Journal of Psychiatry in Medicine*, 27, 93–105.

Leventhal, H., Nerenz, D. R., & Steele, D. F. (1984). Illness representations and coping with health threats. In A. Baum, S. E. Taylor, & J. E. Singer, eds., *A Handbook of Psychology and Health*. Hillsdale, NJ: Erlbaum, pp. 219–52.

Levin, C., & Chisholm, D. (2015). Cost-effectiveness and affordability of interventions, policies, and platforms for the prevention and treatment of mental, neurological, and substance use disorders. In V. Patel, D. Chisholm, T. Dua, R. Laxminarayan, & M. E. Medina-Mora, eds., *Mental, Neurological, and Substance Use Disorders: Disease Control Priorities, Third Edition (Volume 4)*. Washington, D.C.: The International Bank for Reconstruction and Development/the World Bank, pp. 219–36.

Lewer, D., O'Reilly, C., Mojtabai, R., & Evans-Lacko, S. (2015). Antidepressant use in 27 European countries: associations with sociodemographic, cultural and economic factors. *British Journal of Psychiatry*, 207, 221–6.

Maulik, P. K., Devarapalli, S., Kallakuri, S., et al. (2017). Evaluation of an anti-stigma campaign related to common mental disorders in rural India: a mixed methods approach. *Psychological Medicine*, 47, 565–75.

McCrone, P., & Knapp, M. (2007). Economic evaluation of early intervention services. *British Journal of Psychiatry*. Supplement 51, s19–s22.

Meadows, G. N., & Burgess, P. M. (2009). Perceived need for mental health care: findings from the 2007 Australian Survey of Mental Health and Wellbeing. *Australian and New Zealand Journal of Psychiatry*, 43, 624–34.

Mechanic, D. (2002). Removing barriers to care among persons with psychiatric symptoms. *Health Affairs*, 21, 137–47.

Mehta, N., Kassam, A., Leese, M., Butler, G., & Thornicroft, G. (2009). Public attitudes towards people with mental illness in England and Scotland, 1994–2003. *British Journal of Psychiatry*, 194, 278–84.

Mittal, D., Drummond, K. L., Blevins, D., et al. (2013). Stigma associated with PTSD: perceptions of treatment seeking combat veterans. *Psychiatric Rehabilitation Journal*, 36, 86–92.

Mojtabai, R., Olfson, M., & Mechanic, D. (2002). Perceived need and help-seeking in adults with mood, anxiety, or substance use disorders. *Archives of General Psychiatry*, 59, 77–84.

Mojtabai, R. (2010). Mental illness stigma and willingness to seek mental health care in the European Union. *Social Psychiatry and Psychiatric Epidemiology*, 45, 705–12.

Mollica, R. F., Cardozo, B. L., Osofsky, H. J., et al. (2004). Mental health in complex emergencies. *Lancet*, 364, 2058–67.

Prins, M. A., Verhaak, P. F., Bensing, J. M., & van der Meer, K. (2008). Health beliefs and perceived need for mental health care of anxiety and depression–the patients' perspective explored. *Clinical Psychology Review*, 28, 1038–58.

Rhodes, A. E., & Fung, K. (2004). Self-reported use of mental health services versus administrative records: care to recall? *International Journal of Methods in Psychiatric Research*, 13, 165–75.

Roberts, A. L., Gilman, S. E., Breslau, J., Breslau, N., & Koenen, K. C. (2011). Race/ethnic differences in exposure to traumatic events, development of post-traumatic stress disorder, and treatment-seeking for post-traumatic stress disorder in the United States. *Psychological Medicine*, 41, 71–83.

Rodriguez, J. J., & Kohn, R. (2008). Use of mental health services among disaster survivors. *Current Opinion in Psychiatry*, 21, 370–8.

Romero-Gonzalez, M., Gonzalez, G., & Rosenheck, R. A. (2003). Mental health service delivery following health system reform in Colombia. *The Journal of Mental Health Policy and Economics*, 6, 189–94.

Sareen, J., Jagdeo, A., Cox, B. J., et al. (2007). Perceived barriers to mental health service utilization in the United States, Ontario, and the Netherlands. *Psychiatric Services*, 58, 357–64.

Saxena, S., Thornicroft, G., Knapp, M., & Whiteford, H. (2007). Resources for mental health: scarcity, inequity, and inefficiency. *Lancet*, 370, 878–89.

Schomerus, G., & Angermeyer, M. C. (2008). Stigma and its impact on help-seeking for mental disorders: what do we know? *Epidemiologia e Psichiatria Sociale*, 17, 31–7.

Seedat, S., Stein, D. J., Herman, A., et al. (2008). Twelve-month treatment of psychiatric disorders in the South African Stress and Health Study (World Mental Health Survey Initiative). *Social Psychiatry and Psychiatric Epidemiology*, 43, 889–97.

Sheerin, C., Berenz, E. C., Knudsen, G. P., et al. (2016). A population-based study of help seeking and self-medication among trauma-exposed individuals. *Psychology of Addictive Behaviors*, 30, 771–7.

ten Have, M., de Graaf, R., Ormel, J., et al. (2010). Are attitudes towards mental health help-seeking associated with service use? Results from the European Study of Epidemiology of Mental Disorders. *Social Psychiatry and Psychiatric Epidemiology*, 45, 153–63.

Thornicroft, G., Brohan, E., Rose, D., Sartorius, N., & Leese, M. (2009). Global pattern of experienced and anticipated discrimination against people with schizophrenia: a cross-sectional survey. *Lancet*, 373, 408–15.

Thornicroft, G., Mehta, N., Clement, S., et al. (2016). Evidence for effective interventions to reduce mental-health-related stigma and discrimination. *Lancet*, 387, 1123–32.

Thornicroft, G., Chatterji, S., Evans-Lacko, S., et al. (2017). Undertreatment of people with major depressive disorder in 21 countries. *British Journal of Psychiatry*, 210, 119–24.

van Beljouw, I., Verhaak, P., Prins, M., et al. (2010). Reasons and determinants for not receiving treatment for common mental disorders. *Psychiatric Services*, 61, 250–7.

Ventola, C. L. (2011). Direct-to-consumer pharmaceutical advertising: therapeutic or toxic? *Pharmacy and Therapeutics*, 36, 669–84.

Vernberg, E. M., Steinberg, A. M., Jacobs, A. K., et al. (2008). Innovations in disaster mental health: psychological first aid. *Professional Psychology: Research and Practice*, 39, 381–8.

Wang, P. S., Aguilar-Gaxiola, S., Alonso, J., et al. (2007a). Use of mental health services for anxiety, mood, and substance disorders in 17 countries in the WHO world mental health surveys. *Lancet*, 370, 841–50.

Wang, P. S., Angermeyer, M., Borges, G., et al. (2007b). Delay and failure in treatment seeking after first onset of mental disorders in the World Health Organization's World Mental Health Survey Initiative. *World Psychiatry*, 6, 177–85.

Wells, J. E., Robins, L. N., Bushnell, J. A., Jarosz, D., & Oakley-Browne, M. A. (1994). Perceived barriers to care in St. Louis (USA) and Christchurch (NZ): reasons for not seeking professional help for psychological distress. *Social Psychiatry and Psychiatric Epidemiology*, 29, 155–64.

Wheat, K., Brohan, E., Henderson, C., & Thornicroft, G. (2010). Mental illness and the workplace: conceal or reveal? *Journal of the Royal Society of Medicine*, 103, 83–6.

Chapter 9

The Effects of Trauma Type, Timing, Accumulation, and Sequencing

Howard Liu, Laura Helena Andrade, Josep Maria Haro, Dan J. Stein, and Ronald C. Kessler

As we reported in Chapter 3, most individuals are exposed to trauma at some point in their life. Yet lifetime posttraumatic stress disorder (PTSD) prevalence is only 1.3% to 8.8% in community epidemiological surveys of the general population (Atwoli et al., 2015b). This discrepancy raises questions about the determinants of PTSD after trauma exposure. One line of research shows that PTSD prevalence is highest for traumas involving interpersonal violence (Breslau et al., 2008; Caramanica et al., 2015; Fossion et al., 2015). Another suggests that a history of prior trauma is a risk factor for subsequent PTSD, particularly any prior trauma involving interpersonal violence (Lowe et al., 2014; White et al., 2015; Smith et al., 2016). However, these studies did not examine prior traumas comprehensively, leaving numerous questions unanswered such as whether the special importance of prior traumas involving interpersonal violence is limited to personal victimization or includes witnessing violence (Atwoli et al., 2015a), and whether all types of prior traumas are equally important (Breslau et al., 2008; Breslau & Peterson, 2010) or only those involving interpersonal violence (Cougle et al., 2009). Likewise, it's also unclear whether re-exposure to similar traumas plays any role in the onset of subsequent PTSD (Green et al., 2000; Nishith et al., 2000), and whether some prior traumas may instead inoculate against future PTSD by building resilience (Shiri et al., 2008; Palgi et al., 2015). To address these assorted questions, we examined the associations of disaggregated trauma types and histories with PTSD in the large World Mental Health (WMH) sample.

Methods

The analyses focused on the 22 WMH surveys that assessed lifetime PTSD after *random* traumas, using the procedures described in Chapter 2. Logistic regression – with controls for surveys, respondent ages at both random trauma exposure and at interview, and for sex – was used to estimate associations of random trauma type and trauma history with PTSD. Logistic regression coefficients for random trauma types were scaled to have a sum of 0.0. As in other chapters, these coefficients and their design-based standard errors were exponentiated to create odds-ratios (ORs) and 95% confidence intervals (CIs). The scaling of the logistic regression coefficients led to the ORs for trauma types having a product of 1.0 and to ORs significantly different from 1.0 being significantly different from the average PTSD odds across all trauma types. This model was then elaborated to include information about prior trauma exposure. In an effort to evaluate the strength of overall model fit, a receiver operating characteristic (ROC) curve was calculated from each set of predicted probabilities (Zou et al., 2007) and area under the curve (AUC) computed to quantify overall prediction accuracy (Hanley & McNeil, 1983). The method of replicated tenfold cross-validation with 20 replicates (i.e., 200 separate estimates of model coefficients) was used to correct for over-estimation of prediction accuracy when both estimating and evaluating models in a single sample (Smith et al., 2014).

Results

Trauma Prevalence and Trauma-Specific PTSD Prevalence

Exposure to lifetime traumas was reported by a weighted 70.3% of Part II respondents in the WMH sample considered in this analysis ($n = 34{,}676$). Mean number of lifetime exposures among those with any exposure to trauma was 4.5. As in Chapter 3, the most common traumas were unexpected death of loved one (16.7% of all exposures) and direct exposure to death or serious injury (15.8%) (see Table 9.1). Accidents/injuries were the most common trauma group (25.0%) followed by traumas associated with participating in organized violence (20.4%).

PTSD occurred after a weighted 4.0% of random traumas. Being a relief worker is a war zone (0.3% of all

Table 9.1 Lifetime prevalence of exposure to specific trauma types, distribution of randomly selected trauma types among those with any lifetime trauma exposure, and associations of randomly selected trauma types with DSM-IV/CIDI PTSD across all WMH surveys ($n = 34{,}676$)

	Prevalence of lifetime trauma exposure		Percentage of trauma exposure/any		PTSD prevalence/ randomly selected traumas		Respondents with randomly selected traumas
	%	(SE)	%	(SE)	%	(SE)	(n)
I Exposure to Organized Violence							
Relief worker in war zone	0.9	(0.1)	0.3	(0.1)	0.0	–	(95)
Civilian in war zone	4.6	(0.2)	2.0	(0.2)	0.7	(0.4)	(886)
Civilian in region of terror	3.5	(0.1)	1.0	(0.1)	1.4	(0.6)	(449)
Refugee	2.2	(0.1)	0.6	(0.1)	5.0	(2.2)	(299)
Kidnapped	1.2	(0.1)	0.4	(0.1)	11.3	(3.2)	(127)
Any	9.5	(0.2)	4.3	(0.2)	2.4	(0.5)	(1,856)
II Participation in Organized Violence							
Witnessed death/dead body/ serious injury	23.3	(0.3)	15.8	(0.6)	1.6	(0.3)	(3,669)
Accidentally caused serious injury/ death	1.4	(0.1)	0.7	(0.1)	1.7	(0.8)	(168)
Combat experience	3.3	(0.1)	1.3	(0.1)	1.9	(0.7)	(355)
Purposely injured/tortured/killed someone	0.9	(0.1)	0.4	(0.1)	6.9	(5.1)	(60)
Witnessed atrocities	3.7	(0.1)	2.2	(0.3)	8.7	(5.7)	(297)
Any	26.1	(0.3)	20.4	(0.6)	2.5	(0.7)	(4,549)
III Physical Violence Victimization							
Beaten by caregiver	8.2	(0.2)	2.6	(0.1)	5.3	(1.2)	(1,467)
Beaten by someone else	5.9	(0.2)	3.3	(0.2)	2.8	(0.8)	(867)
Witnessed physical fight at home	7.9	(0.2)	2.4	(0.1)	4.0	(0.7)	(1,625)
Any	17.3	(0.3)	8.4	(0.3)	4.0	(0.5)	(3,959)
IV Sexual Violence Victimization							
Raped	3.2	(0.1)	1.8	(0.1)	17.4	(2.7)	(612)
Sexually assaulted	5.5	(0.1)	3.3	(0.2)	11.0	(1.7)	(1,084)
Stalked	5.3	(0.1)	2.9	(0.2)	8.4	(2.2)	(843)
Beaten by spouse/romantic partner	4.6	(0.1)	1.4	(0.1)	9.4	(1.6)	(1,019)
Trauma to loved one	5.5	(0.1)	2.5	(0.2)	7.2	(2.0)	(842)
Some other trauma	4.2	(0.1)	1.4	(0.1)	6.7	(1.2)	(694)
Private trauma[a]	5.1	(0.1)	1.5	(0.1)	8.0	(1.3)	(888)
Any	22.9	(0.3)	14.7	(0.4)	9.8	(0.8)	(5,982)
V Accidents/Injuries							
Natural disaster	7.1	(0.2)	4.0	(0.4)	0.2	(0.1)	(1,277)
Toxic chemical exposure	4.2	(0.1)	3.6	(0.3)	1.6	(0.8)	(517)
Automobile accident	14.1	(0.2)	6.2	(0.2)	2.1	(0.4)	(2,428)
Life-threatening illness	11.3	(0.2)	4.9	(0.2)	2.4	(0.6)	(2,194)
Child with serious illness	7.9	(0.2)	3.2	(0.2)	4.8	(0.7)	(1,468)
Other life-threatening accident	6.3	(0.2)	3.1	(0.3)	5.1	(2.5)	(870)
Any	35.8	(0.3)	25.0	(0.6)	2.5	(0.4)	(8,754)
VI Other							
Mugged/threatened with a weapon	15.5	(0.2)	8.5	(0.3)	2.0	(0.4)	(2,469)
Human-made disaster	3.9	(0.1)	1.9	(0.2)	2.7	(1.4)	(529)
UD of a loved one	31.5	(0.3)	16.7	(0.4)	4.8	(0.6)	(6,578)
Any	41.5	(0.4)	27.1	(0.5)	3.8	(0.4)	(9,576)
VII Total	**70.3**	**(0.3)**	**100.0**	**–**	**4.0**	**(0.2)**	**(34,676)**

[a]A *private* event is a trauma that some individuals reported in response to a question asked at the very end of the trauma section that asked if they ever had some other very upsetting experience they did not tell us about already (and this includes in response to a prior open-ended question about "any other" trauma) because they were too embarrassed or upset to talk about it. Respondents were told, before they answered, that if they reported such a trauma we would not ask them anything about what it was, only about their age when the trauma happened.

traumas) was the only trauma type not associated with any PTSD cases in the sample. Significant variation in PTSD prevalence was found across the remaining 28 trauma types ($\chi^2_{27} = 237.1, p < 0.001$), with highest weighted PTSD prevalence for rape (17.4%), kidnapped (11.3%), and other sexual assaults (11.0%) and lowest (other than for being a relief worker) for natural disasters (0.2%) and being a civilian in a war zone (0.7%) or region of terror (1.4%).

Differential Associations of Trauma Types with PTSD

The first model (Model 1, Table 9.2) estimated relative odds of PTSD across random trauma types when controlling for prior same-type exposures. Given the rarity of prior same-type exposures, the latter were coded at the level of the six trauma groups described in Chapter 3, with all respondents having prior same-type exposures in a single group collapsed into a group-level measure. Only five of the six such group-level measures were analyzed, though, because too few respondents previously experienced same-type traumas involving exposure to organized violence for analysis.

Odds of PTSD differed significantly across trauma types in Model 1 ($\chi^2_{27} = 224.1, p < 0.001$) due to a significant between-group difference in average odds ($\chi^2_5 = 73.9, p < 0.001$) and significant within-group differences in odds for traumas in each of the four groups: exposure to organized violence ($\chi^2_3 = 34.4, p < 0.001$); participation in organized violence ($\chi^2_4 = 14.0$, $p = 0.007$); accidents/injuries ($\chi^2_5 = 46.9, p < 0.001$); and the residual "other" trauma group ($\chi^2_2 = 6.9$, $p = 0.032$). In the two remaining groups, ORs were either not significant as a set (physical violence victimization; $\chi^2_3 = 4.5, p = 0.22$) or significant as a set, but not significantly different from each other (sexual violence victimization, with seven trauma types in the set; $\chi^2_7 = 65.1, p < 0.001$; $\chi^2_6 = 10.2, p = 0.12$).

Prior lifetime group-level same-type trauma exposure was a significant predictor of PTSD in Model 1 ($\chi^2_5 = 14.2$, $p = 0.014$) due to a significantly *higher* odds of PTSD after physical violence victimization in the presence vs. in the absence of a prior same-type trauma (OR = 3.2) and a significantly *lower* odds of PTSD after participation in organized violence in the presence vs. in the absence of a prior same-type trauma (OR = 0.2). The other three group-level ORs for prior same-type traumas were nonsignificant.

The predictors in Model 2 were based on Model 1 results to include each trauma type within the four groups having significant within-group OR differences in Model 1, a single measure for any sexual violence victimization, and measures of prior same-type participation in organized violence and physical violence victimization. Four random trauma types/groups had significantly elevated ORs and four others had significantly reduced ORs in Model 2. Three in each set of four were substantially elevated (OR = 2.7–4.7; kidnapped, witnessed atrocities, sexual violence) or reduced (OR = 0.1–0.3; civilian in a war zone or region of terror, natural disaster), while the other significant ORs were modest in magnitude, but associated with very common trauma types (unexpected death of loved one, 16.7% of all traumas; OR = 1.4; direct exposure to death/serious injury, 15.8% of all traumas; OR = 0.7). Based on these results, we estimated Model 3 with only the eight significant trauma measures in Model 2, plus dummy variables for prior same-type participation in organized violence and physical violence victimization. Model 3 (AIC = 2,943.3) was superior to Models 1 (AIC = 3,326.2) and 2 (AIC = 3,283.4). Results were similar to Model 2.

PTSD Risk Associated with Prior Lifetime Exposure to Other Traumas

Significant Model 3 predictors were used as controls in Model 4 (see Table 9.3), which evaluated associations of prior lifetime traumas other than the random trauma with random-trauma PTSD. Prior traumas were significant overall ($\chi^2_{28} = 165.6, p < 0.001$) and significantly different across types ($\chi^2_{27} = 56.7, p < 0.001$). ORs in the prior sexual violence group were significant overall ($\chi^2_7 = 37.1, p < 0.001$) and significantly different within the group ($\chi^2_6 = 17.4, p = 0.008$). ORs for two other trauma groups were significant overall, but not significantly different within the group: participation in organized violence ($\chi^2_5 = 15.5$, $p = 0.008$; $\chi^2_4 = 4.9, p = 0.30$); and physical violence victimization ($\chi^2_3 = 13.0, p = 0.005$; $\chi^2_2 = 0.6, p = 0.75$). Based on these results, Model 5 included a count of prior lifetime trauma types experienced in each of the two groups where the Model 4 trauma-specific ORs were significant overall, but not significantly different within the group. The model also included separate dummy variables for the two significant lifetime sexual violence victimization traumas in Model 4 (rape and other sexual assault). The fit of Model 5 was superior

Table 9.2 Associations of DSM-IV/CIDI PTSD associated with randomly selected trauma type and prior lifetime exposure of the same trauma type among people exposed to one or more lifetime traumas across all WMH surveys ($n = 34{,}581$)[a]

	Multivariate model 1[b]		Multivariate model 2		Multivariate model 3	
	OR	(95% CI)	OR	(95% CI)	OR	(95% CI)
I Exposure to Organized Violence						
Civilian in war zone	0.2*	(0.1–0.6)	0.3*	(0.1–0.7)	0.3*	(0.1–0.8)
Civilian in region of terror	0.3*	(0.1–0.6)	0.3*	(0.1–0.8)	0.3*	(0.1–0.8)
Refugee	1.5	(0.6–3.6)	1.9	(0.8–4.5)		
Kidnapped	3.8*	(2.0–7.1)	4.7*	(2.5–8.8)	4.9*	(2.6–9.3)
χ^2_4[c]	34.7*		37.5*		$\chi^2_3 = 37.0$*	
χ^2_5[d]	34.4*		35.1*		$\chi^2_2 = 34.9$*	
II Participation in Organized Violence						
Witnessed death/dead body/serious injury	0.5*	(0.4–0.8)	0.7*	(0.4–0.9)	0.7	(0.4–1.0)
Accidentally caused serious injury/death	0.6	(0.2–1.5)	0.7	(0.3–1.9)		
Combat experience	0.7	(0.3–1.7)	0.9	(0.4–2.1)		
Purposely injured/tortured/killed someone	2.2	(0.5–10.1)	2.8	(0.6–12.5)		
Witnessed atrocities	3.2	(0.8–12.8)	4.0*	(1.0–16.3)	4.2*	(1.0–17.8)
χ^2_5[c]	25.4*		17.0*		$\chi^2_2 = 9.0$*	
χ^2_2[d]	14.0*		14.4*		$\chi^2_1 = 6.3$*	
III Physical Violence Victimization			1.2	(0.8–1.7)		
Beaten by caregiver	1.5	(0.9–2.5)				
Beaten by someone else	0.7	(0.4–1.2)				
Witnessed physical fight at home	0.9	(0.6–1.4)				
χ^2_3[c]	4.5					
χ^2_2[d]	4.4					
IV Sexual Violence Victimization			2.7*	(2.0–3.6)	2.7*	(2.0–3.8)
Raped	3.8*	(2.5–5.8)				
Sexually assaulted	2.4*	(1.6–3.5)				
Stalked	2.0*	(1.1–3.7)				
Beaten by spouse/romantic partner	1.9*	(1.3–2.9)				
Trauma to loved one	1.7	(0.9–3.1)				
Some other trauma	1.6*	(1.1–2.4)				
Private trauma[e]	2.1*	(1.5–2.9)				
χ^2_7[c]	65.1*					
χ^2_6[d]	10.2					
V Accidents/Injuries						
Natural disaster	0.1*	(0.0–0.1)	0.1*	(0.0–0.2)	0.1*	(0.0–0.2)
Toxic chemical exposure	0.6	(0.2–1.6)	0.7	(0.3–2.0)		
Automobile accident	0.6*	(0.4–0.9)	0.7	(0.5–1.1)		
Life-threatening illness	0.6*	(0.3–0.9)	0.7	(0.4–1.1)		
Child with serious illness	1.1	(0.8–1.6)	1.4	(1.0–2.1)		
Other life-threatening accident	1.7	(0.6–4.6)	2.1	(0.8–5.9)		
χ^2_6[c]	62.2*		54.2*			
χ^2_5[d]	46.9*		49.1*			
VI Other						
Mugged/threatened with a weapon	0.6*	(0.4–0.9)	0.7	(0.5–1.2)		
Human-made disaster	0.6	(0.2–1.8)	0.8	(0.3–2.2)		
UD of a loved one	1.2	(0.8–1.6)	1.4*	(1.0–2.0)	1.5*	(1.0–2.0)
χ^2_3[c]	7.7*		7.1			
χ^2_2[d]	6.9*		6.7*			
VII Prior Lifetime Exposure to the Same Trauma Type						
Exposure to organized violence[f]						
Participation in organized violence	0.2*	(0.1–0.8)	0.2*	(0.1–0.9)	0.3*	(0.1–0.9)
Physical violence victimization	3.2*	(1.3–7.9)	2.5*	(1.0–6.4)	3.2*	(1.3–7.9)
Sexual violence victimization	0.8	(0.5–1.5)	0.9	(0.5–1.5)		
Accidents/injuries	0.4	(0.1–1.5)	0.5	(0.1–1.6)		

Table 9.2 *(cont.)*

	Multivariate model 1[b]		Multivariate model 2		Multivariate model 3	
	OR	(95% CI)	OR	(95% CI)	OR	(95% CI)
Other	0.7	(0.4–1.5)	0.8	(0.4–1.5)		
χ^2_5 [c]	14.2*		11.3*		$\chi^2_2 = 10.8^*$	
χ^2_4 [d]	13.4*		10.4*		$\chi^2_1 = 10.1^*$	
VIII Design-Adjusted AIC	**3,326.2**		**3,283.4**		**2,943.3**	

*Significant at the 0.05 level, two-sided test.
[a]Coefficients are based on multiple logistic regression equations with the 34,581 respondents who had a lifetime trauma (exclusive of the 95 whose randomly selected trauma was being a relief worker in a war zone) as the unit of analysis. All models control for respondent sex, age at interview, age at time of exposure to the trauma, and 21 dummy variables to distinguish among the 22 surveys.
[b]Given that all respondents experienced a trauma, a model containing a separate unrestricted OR for each of the 28 trauma types would be under-identified. The constraint we imposed to achieve identification was for the sum of the 28 logits to equal 0.0, which is equivalent to the product of the 28 ORs equaling 1.0. An OR significantly greater than 1.0 for a given trauma type in this model consequently can be interpreted as showing that the odds of PTSD associated with that trauma type are significantly greater than for the average trauma (noting that each trauma is given equal weight when defining the average).
[c]The joint significance of the set of ORs for traumas in the group.
[d]The significance of the differences among the ORs within the group.
[e]A *private* trauma is a trauma that some individuals reported in response to a question asked at the very end of the trauma section that asked if they ever had some other very upsetting experience they did not tell us about already (and this includes in response to a prior open-ended question about "any other" trauma) because they were too embarrassed or upset to talk about it. Respondents were told, before they answered, that if they reported such a trauma we would not ask them anything about what it was, only about their age when the trauma happened.
[f]There were no PTSD cases for those who had exposure to organized violence as their random event and experienced exposure to organized violence in the past.

to that of Model 4 (AIC = 2,933.2 vs. 3,528.4). All four ORs for prior trauma exposure in Model 5 were significantly elevated (OR = 1.3–1.4 for traumas involving participation in organized violence and physical violence victimization; OR = 2.5 for rape; OR = 1.6 for other sexual assault). We also evaluated the possibility that the four ORs associated with prior lifetime trauma exposure varied, depending on random trauma type, but that model (results not shown) performed less well than Model 5 (AIC = 3,076.9 vs. 2,933.2).

Sensitivity Analysis

Model 5 was estimated separately in subsamples defined by country income (high- vs. low- and middle-income [LMIC]), survey response rate (lower than vs. higher than 60%), and median length of recall (0–15 vs. 16+ years between age of random trauma occurrence and age at interview) (see Table 9.4). Three of the 14 coefficients in the model (eight random trauma types, two same-type prior traumas, and four other prior traumas) differed meaningfully across subgroups in at least one comparison. The significantly reduced OR for being a civilian in a region of terror was confined to respondents who subsequently immigrated to a high-income country (OR = 0.1; 95% CI, 0.0–0.4 vs. OR = 1.2; 95% CI, 0.4–3.7 in LMICs; $\chi^2_1 = 7.8$, $p = 0.005$). The significantly elevated OR for witnessing atrocities was confined to respondents in LMICs (OR = 18.6; 95% CI, 4.5–76.8 vs. OR = 0.5; 95% CI, 0.2–1.6 in high-income countries; $\chi^2_1 = 15.3$, $p < 0.001$). And the significantly elevated OR associated with prior history of participation in organized violence was confined to surveys with response rates higher than 60% (OR = 1.3; 95% CI, 1.1–1.6 vs. OR = 0.6; 95% CI, 0.4–1.0 in surveys with low response rates; $\chi^2_1 = 7.8$, $p = 0.005$).

Incremental Importance of Information about Prior Trauma Exposure

Incremental importance of information about prior trauma exposure in Model 5 was evaluated by estimating individual-level predicted probabilities of PTSD twice: once based on Model 5 and the second time on a model that excluded the Model 5 predictors for prior trauma exposure. An ROC curve for each set of predicted probabilities based on replicated tenfold cross-validation found AUC = 0.74 for Model 5 and AUC = 0.70 for the reduced model. Sensitivity among the 4% of respondents with highest predicted probabilities was 17.8% in Model 5 and 16.7% in the reduced model. (The 4% threshold was set because this is the prevalence of PTSD in the sample.)

Table 9.3 Associations of DSM-IV/CIDI PTSD associated with randomly selected trauma types as a function of prior lifetime trauma exposure across all WMH surveys ($n = 34{,}581$)[a]

	Multivariate model 4		Multivariate model 5	
	OR	(95% CI)	OR	(95% CI)
I Exposure to Organized Violence				
Civilian in war zone	0.8	(0.4–1.6)		
Civilian in region of terror	1.0	(0.5–1.8)		
Refugee	0.7	(0.3–1.9)		
Kidnapped	1.7	(0.9–3.2)		
$\chi^{2\,\mathrm{b}}_{4}$	3.9			
$\chi^{2\,\mathrm{c}}_{3}$	3.9			
II Participation in Organized Violence				
Witnessed death/dead body/serious injury	0.9	(0.6–1.4)		
Accidentally caused serious injury/death	1.2	(0.4–3.3)		
Combat experience	1.0	(0.5–2.3)		
Purposely injured/tortured/killed someone	1.5	(0.4–5.1)		
Witnessed atrocities	2.9*	(1.4–6.2)		
Number			1.3*	(1.0–1.6)
$\chi^{2\,\mathrm{b}}_{5}$	15.5*			
$\chi^{2\,\mathrm{c}}_{4}$	4.9			
III Physical Violence Victimization				
Beaten by caregiver	1.6*	(1.1–2.2)		
Beaten by someone else	1.3	(0.9–1.8)		
Witnessed physical fight at home	1.4	(1.0–2.0)		
Number			1.4*	(1.2–1.7)
$\chi^{2\,\mathrm{b}}_{3}$	13.0*			
$\chi^{2\,\mathrm{c}}_{2}$	0.6			
IV Sexual Violence Victimization				
Raped	2.3*	(1.5–3.5)	2.5*	(1.7–3.8)
Sexually assaulted	1.5	(1.0–2.2)	1.6*	(1.1–2.3)
Stalked	1.0	(0.5–1.8)		
Beaten by spouse/romantic partner	1.3	(0.8–2.0)		
Trauma to loved one	0.9	(0.5–1.4)		
Some other trauma	0.8	(0.3–1.7)		
Private trauma[d]	1.3	(0.8–2.1)		
$\chi^{2\,\mathrm{b}}_{7}$	37.1*		$\chi^2_2 = 23.8$*	
$\chi^{2\,\mathrm{c}}_{6}$	17.4*		$\chi^2_1 = 2.6$	
V Accidents/Injuries				
Natural disaster	1.0	(0.7–1.6)		
Toxic chemical exposure	0.8	(0.4–1.5)		
Automobile accident	1.0	(0.7–1.4)		
Life-threatening illness	1.1	(0.8–1.6)		
Child with serious illness	1.1	(0.7–1.9)		
Other life-threatening accident	0.8	(0.5–1.4)		
$\chi^{2\,\mathrm{b}}_{6}$	2.0			
$\chi^{2\,\mathrm{c}}_{5}$	1.8			
VI Other				
Mugged or threatened with a weapon	1.2	(0.9–1.6)		
Human-made disaster	0.9	(0.5–1.6)		
UD of a loved one	1.2	(0.8–1.8)		
$\chi^{2\,\mathrm{b}}_{3}$	3.5			
$\chi^{2\,\mathrm{c}}_{2}$	1.0			
VII Design-Adjusted AIC	**3,528.4**		**2,993.2**	

*Significant at the 0.05 level, two-sided test.

[a]Coefficients are based on multiple logistic regression equations with the 34,581 respondents who had a lifetime trauma (exclusive of the 95 whose randomly selected trauma was being a relief worker in a war zone) as the unit of analysis. Both models control for respondent sex, age at interview, age at time of exposure to the trauma, 21 dummy variables to distinguish among the 22 surveys, and the predictors in Table 9.2, Multivariate model 3.

[b]The joint significance of the set of ORs for traumas in the group.

[c]The significance of differences among the ORs within the group.

[d]A *private* trauma is a trauma that some individuals reported in response to a question asked at the very end of the trauma section that asked if they ever had some other very upsetting experience they did not tell us about already (and this includes in response to a prior open-ended question about "any other" trauma) because they were too embarrassed or upset to talk about it. Respondents were told, before they answered, that if they reported such a trauma we would not ask them anything about what it was, only about their age when the trauma happened.

Table 9.4 Associations of DSM-IV/CIDI PTSD among people exposed to randomly selected trauma in cross-national sample by country income, survey response rate, and length of recalls ($n = 34{,}581$)[a]

	Country income[b]				Survey response rate				Length of recalls			
	High-income[c]		Low- and middle-income[d]		Greater than or equal to 60%		Less than 60%		Greater than 15 years		Less than or equal to 15 years	
	OR	(95% CI)	OR	(95% CI)	OR	(95% CI)	OR	(95% CI)	OR	(95% CI)	OR	(95% CI)
I Randomly Selected Trauma												
Civilian in war zone	0.3	(0.1–1.2)	0.2*	(0.1–0.7)	0.3*	(0.1–1.0)	<0.001*	(<0.001–<0.001)	0.4	(0.1–1.2)	0.0	(<0.001–0.1)
Civilian in region of terror	0.1*	(0.0–0.4)	1.2	(0.4–3.7)	0.3*	(0.1–0.9)	0.5	(0.1–4.4)	0.2	(0.1–0.7)	0.8	(0.2–3.1)
Kidnapped	5.9*	(3.0–11.9)	3.7*	(1.3–10.5)	5.1*	(2.9–9.0)	<0.001*	(<0.001–0.0)	4.6*	(2.1–10.0)	4.6*	(1.8–11.5)
Witnessed death/dead body/ serious injury	0.6	(0.4–1.0)	0.9	(0.5–1.9)	0.8	(0.5–1.2)	0.3*	(0.1–1.0)	0.6	(0.4–1.1)	0.8	(0.4–1.6)
Witnessed atrocities	0.5	(0.2–1.6)	18.6*	(4.5–76.8)	4.4	(1.0–19.8)	0.3	(0.0–2.6)	6.1*	(1.4–26.3)	1.3	(0.2–7.5)
Sexual violence victimization	2.4*	(1.7–3.5)	2.8*	(1.5–4.9)	2.6*	(1.9–3.7)	2.0	(1.0–3.9)	2.2*	(1.5–3.3)	3.1*	(2.0–4.6)
Natural disaster	0.1*	(0.0–0.2)	0.0*	(0.0–0.3)	0.1*	(0.0–0.2)	<0.001*	(<0.001–<0.001)	0.1*	(0.0–0.2)	0.1*	(0.0–0.2)
UD of loved one	1.4	(0.9–2.2)	2.1*	(1.3–3.5)	1.7*	(1.2–2.4)	1.0	(0.4–2.2)	1.6*	(1.0–2.6)	1.6*	(1.1–2.4)
II Prior Lifetime Exposure to the Same Trauma Type												
Participation in organized violence	0.3	(0.1–1.2)	0.1	(0.0–1.0)	0.2*	(0.1–0.8)	0.2	(0.0–1.9)	0.1*	(0.0–0.9)	0.4	(0.1–1.5)
Physical violence victimization	0.9	(0.2–3.1)	4.3	(0.9–19.4)	1.5	(0.5–4.8)	4.6	(0.7–27.8)	0.5	(0.1–5.6)	3.5*	(1.2–10.2)
III Prior Lifetime Exposure to Other Traumas												
Participation in organized violence	1.4*	(1.1–1.7)	1.0	(0.7–1.5)	1.3*	(1.1–1.6)	0.6	(0.4–1.0)	1.2	(0.9–1.7)	1.3	(1.0–1.7)
Physical violence victimization	1.4*	(1.2–1.7)	1.5*	(1.0–2.1)	1.4*	(1.2–1.7)	1.4	(0.8–2.5)	1.4*	(1.1–1.8)	1.5*	(1.1–1.9)
Raped	2.5*	(1.6–4.1)	2.7*	(1.1–6.4)	2.6*	(1.7–4.1)	1.0	(0.4–2.5)	2.0*	(1.3–3.2)	3.0*	(1.6–5.6)
Sexually assaulted	1.3*	(0.9–2.0)	2.7*	(1.3–5.8)	1.6*	(1.0–2.4)	1.5	(0.6–3.4)	1.7*	(1.0–2.7)	1.4	(0.8–2.5)
IV Cross-Validated AUC	**0.76**		**0.70**		**0.73**		**0.73**		**0.68**		**0.73**	

*Significant at the 0.05 level, two-sided test.

[a]Coefficients are based on multiple logistic regression equations with the 34,581 respondents who had a lifetime trauma (exclusive of the 95 whose randomly selected trauma was being a relief worker in a war zone) as the unit of analysis. All models controls for respondent sex, age at interview, age at time of exposure to the trauma, and 21 dummy variables to distinguish among the 22 surveys.

[b]The World Bank (2012) Data. Accessed May 12, 2012 at: http://data.worldbank.org/country. Some of the WMH countries have moved into new income categories since the surveys were conducted. The income groupings above reflect the status of each country at the time of data collection. The current income category of each country is available at the preceding URL.

[c]High-income countries: Belgium, France, Germany, Israel, Italy, Japan, Netherlands, New Zealand, Northern Ireland, Spain, Spain–Murcia, United States.

[d]LMICs: Brazil–São Paulo, Bulgaria, Colombia, Colombia–Medellin, Mexico, Peru, Romania, South Africa, Ukraine.

Discussion

Our finding that PTSD was elevated after traumas involving extreme interpersonal violence is broadly consistent with previous research (Kessler et al., 1995; Bromet et al., 1998; Karam et al., 2014; Lowe et al., 2014; White et al., 2015; Smith et al., 2016). In contrast, our findings of lower-than-average ORs among civilians in a war zone/region of terror and victims of natural disaster are perplexing, given our finding regarding atrocities and numerous focused studies of high PTSD after disasters (Neria et al., 2008; North, 2014). However, further investigation provides plausible explanations. Many WMH respondents who were civilians in war zones/regions of terror were elderly residents reporting childhood experiences during World War II. Direct exposure to recent war-related traumas was rare among these respondents, and this factor may account for their low risk of PTSD. In contrast, studies of refugees from recent conflicts show that PTSD is often (Shaar, 2013; Bogic et al., 2015) but not always (Karam et al., 2008; Alhasnawi et al., 2009) common in populations exposed to war-related traumas. Our finding of low PTSD risk among such civilians consequently has to be interpreted narrowly. Likewise, the WMH finding of low PTSD prevalence after natural disasters is likely to differ from the results of disaster-focused studies because the latter studies over-represent highly traumatized survivors (Norris et al., 2006; Goldmann & Galea, 2014). Consistent with this possibility, rigorous studies of representative disaster survivor samples find PTSD prevalence comparable to the WMH estimate (Kessler et al., 2006; Bromet et al., 2017).

Our finding that prior participation in sectarian violence predicts low PTSD after random-trauma participation is indirectly consistent with research documenting low PTSD prevalence among policemen (Levy-Gigi et al., 2016) and other first responders (Levy-Gigi & Richter-Levin, 2014) and among Israeli settlers exposed to repeated bombings (Somer et al., 2009; Palgi et al., 2015). These results could be due either to selection bias and/or to prior exposures promoting resilience (Wilson et al., 2009). Both experimental animal studies (Liu, 2015) and observational human studies (Rutter, 2012) support the resilience possibility, although research showing that intervening psychopathology due to prior traumas mediates the association between trauma history and subsequent PTSD (Sayed et al., 2015) confirms that prior traumas are more likely to create vulnerability than resilience. Research on the "healthy warrior effect" supports the selection bias possibility (Larson et al., 2008; Wilson et al., 2009). These considerations suggest that both processes might be at work, although we have no way to assess their relative importance.

Our finding that prior physical violence victimization predicts elevated PTSD risk after re-victimization helps make sense of the fact that our initial models did not replicate previous findings that PTSD rates are especially high after physical violence victimization (Lowe et al., 2014; White et al., 2015; Smith et al., 2016). This failure presumably arose because the pattern applied only to *repeat* victimizations, which were controlled in our models. For sexual violence, in comparison, we found that prior victimization was not relevant. This might seem to contradict the results of studies showing that sexual assault *re-victimization* is associated with poor mental health (Classen et al., 2005; Miner et al., 2006; Das & Otis, 2016), but those studies typically focused on victims of childhood sexual assault who were – vs. those who were not – re-victimized as adults, whereas the WMH finding compared adult sexual assault victims who were – vs. those who were not – previously victimized.

We also found that prior exposure to some other traumas was associated with *generalized vulnerability* to subsequent PTSD. Although ongoing research is investigating pathways leading to such generalized vulnerability (Rutter, 2012; Daskalakis et al., 2013; Levy-Gigi et al., 2016), we know of no work on the differential effects of trauma types in leading to generalized vulnerability. However, suggestive related evidence exists on differences in associations of childhood adversities with adult mental disorders across different childhood adversity types (Pirkola et al., 2005; Kessler et al., 2010) and profiles (Putnam et al., 2013; McLafferty et al., 2015).

Our results are limited in several ways. First, the cross-sectional WMH design introduced the possibility of recall inaccuracy that could have biased estimates, as extensive research shows that individuals with PTSD differ significantly from others in their trauma memories (Moore & Zoellner, 2007; Brewin, 2014; Crespo & Fernández-Lansac, 2016). Second, PTSD was assessed with a fully structured diagnostic interview that had imperfect concordance with clinical diagnoses. Third, no attempt was made to assess individual differences in vulnerabilities that could have influenced trauma exposure or PTSD, possibly introducing bias into estimates of the relative importance of trauma types. Intervening mental disorders associated with prior traumas, which we will consider in Chapter 11, are special cases (Breslau et al., 2008; Cougle et al., 2009; Breslau & Peterson, 2010).

Within the context of these limitations, the analyses refined previous evidence that PTSD is especially common after traumas involving either experiencing or witnessing interpersonal violence, but that this is limited to *repeat* exposures. We also confirmed that prior exposure to some traumas is associated more with resilience than with vulnerability. Finally, we confirmed the finding of previous studies that a broad trauma history is associated with generalized vulnerability to PTSD, but that this is limited to prior traumas involving interpersonal violence. Although our results leave unanswered questions about causal pathways and mechanisms, they both document the complex ways specific trauma types and histories are associated with PTSD and provide an empirical foundation for more focused investigations of these associations in the future.

Acknowledgment

Portions of this chapter are based on Liu, H., Petukhova, M. V., Sampson, N. A., et al. (2017). Association of DSM-IV Posttraumatic Stress Disorder with Traumatic Experience Type and History in the World Health Organization World Mental Health Surveys. *JAMA Psychiatry*, 74, 270–81, by permission of the American Medical Association.

References

Alhasnawi, S., Sadik, S., Rasheed, M., et al. (2009). The prevalence and correlates of DSM-IV disorders in the Iraq Mental Health Survey (IMHS). *World Psychiatry*, 8, 97–109.

Atwoli, L., Platt, J., Williams, D. R., Stein, D. J., & Koenen, K. C. (2015a). Association between witnessing traumatic events and psychopathology in the South African Stress and Health Study. *Social Psychiatry and Psychiatric Epidemiology*, 50, 1235–42.

Atwoli, L., Stein, D. J., Koenen, K. C., & McLaughlin, K. A. (2015b). Epidemiology of posttraumatic stress disorder: prevalence, correlates and consequences. *Current Opinion in Psychiatry*, 28, 307–11.

Bogic, M., Njoku, A., & Priebe, S. (2015). Long-term mental health of war-refugees: a systematic literature review. *BMC International Health and Human Rights*, 15, 29.

Breslau, N., & Peterson, E. L. (2010). Assaultive violence and the risk of posttraumatic stress disorder following a subsequent trauma. *Behaviour Research and Therapy*, 48, 1063–6.

Breslau, N., Peterson, E. L., & Schultz, L. R. (2008). A second look at prior trauma and the posttraumatic stress disorder effects of subsequent trauma: a prospective epidemiological study. *Archives of General Psychiatry*, 65, 431–7.

Brewin, C. R. (2014). Episodic memory, perceptual memory, and their interaction: foundations for a theory of posttraumatic stress disorder. *Psychological Bulletin*, 140, 69–97.

Bromet, E. J., Atwoli, L., Kawakami, N., et al. (2017). Post-traumatic stress disorder associated with natural and human-made disasters in the World Mental Health Surveys. *Psychological Medicine*, 47, 227–41.

Bromet, E., Sonnega, A., & Kessler, R. C. (1998). Risk factors for DSM-III-R posttraumatic stress disorder: findings from the National Comorbidity Survey. *American Journal of Epidemiology*, 147, 353–61.

Caramanica, K., Brackbill, R. M., Stellman, S. D., & Farfel, M. R. (2015). Posttraumatic stress disorder after Hurricane Sandy among persons exposed to the 9/11 disaster. *International Journal of Emergency Mental Health and Human Resilience*, 17, 356–62.

Classen, C. C., Palesh, O. G., & Aggarwal, R. (2005). Sexual revictimization: a review of the empirical literature. *Trauma, Violence, &Abuse*, 6, 103–29.

Cougle, J. R., Resnick, H., & Kilpatrick, D. G. (2009). Does prior exposure to interpersonal violence increase risk of PTSD following subsequent exposure? *Behaviour Research and Therapy*, 47, 1012–7.

Crespo, M., & Fernández-Lansac, V. (2016). Memory and narrative of traumatic events: a literature review. *Psychological Trauma*, 8, 149–56.

Das, A., & Otis, N. (2016). Sexual contact in childhood, revictimization, and lifetime sexual and psychological outcomes. *Archives of Sexual Behavior*, 45, 1117–31.

Daskalakis, N. P., Bagot, R. C., Parker, K. J., Vinkers, C. H., & de Kloet, E. R. (2013). The three-hit concept of vulnerability and resilience: toward understanding adaptation to early-life adversity outcome. *Psychoneuroendocrinology*, 38, 1858–73.

Fossion, P., Leys, C., Kempenaers, C., et al. (2015). Beware of multiple traumas in PTSD assessment: the role of reactivation mechanism in intrusive and hyper-arousal symptoms. *Aging &Mental Health*, 19, 258–63.

Goldmann, E., & Galea, S. (2014). Mental health consequences of disasters. *Annual Review of Public Health*, 35, 169–83.

Green, B. L., Goodman, L. A., Krupnick, J. L., et al. (2000). Outcomes of single versus multiple trauma exposure in a screening sample. *Journal of Traumatic Stress*, 13, 271–86.

Hanley, J. A., & McNeil, B. J. (1983). A method of comparing the areas under receiver operating characteristic curves derived from the same cases. *Radiology*, 148, 839–43.

Karam, E. G., Friedman, M. J., Hill, E. D., et al. (2014). Cumulative traumas and risk thresholds: 12-month

PTSD in the World Mental Health (WMH) surveys. *Depression and Anxiety*, 31, 130–42.

Karam, E. G., Mneimneh, Z. N., Dimassi, H., et al. (2008). Lifetime prevalence of mental disorders in Lebanon: first onset, treatment, and exposure to war. *PLoS Medicine*, 5, e61.

Kessler, R. C., Galea, S., Jones, R. T., & Parker, H. A. (2006). Mental illness and suicidality after Hurricane Katrina. *Bulletin of the World Health Organization*, 84, 930–9.

Kessler, R. C., McLaughlin, K. A., Green, J. G., et al. (2010). Childhood adversities and adult psychopathology in the WHO World Mental Health Surveys. *British Journal of Psychiatry*, 197, 378–85.

Kessler, R. C., Sonnega, A., Bromet, E., Hughes, M., & Nelson, C. B. (1995). Posttraumatic stress disorder in the National Comorbidity Survey. *Archives of General Psychiatry*, 52, 1048–60.

Larson, G. E., Highfill-McRoy, R. M., & Booth-Kewley, S. (2008). Psychiatric diagnoses in historic and contemporary military cohorts: combat deployment and the healthy warrior effect. *American Journal of Epidemiology*, 167, 1269–76.

Levy-Gigi, E., & Richter-Levin, G. (2014). The hidden price of repeated traumatic exposure. *Stress*, 17, 343–51.

Levy-Gigi, E., Richter-Levin, G., Okon-Singer, H., Keri, S., & Bonanno, G. A. (2016). The hidden price and possible benefit of repeated traumatic exposure. *Stress*, 19, 1–7.

Liu, R. T. (2015). A developmentally informed perspective on the relation between stress and psychopathology: when the problem with stress is that there is not enough. *Journal of Abnormal Psychology*, 124, 80–92.

Lowe, S. R., Walsh, K., Uddin, M., Galea, S., & Koenen, K. C. (2014). Bidirectional relationships between trauma exposure and posttraumatic stress: a longitudinal study of Detroit residents. *Journal of Abnormal Psychology*, 123, 533–44.

McLafferty, M., Armour, C., McKenna, A., et al. (2015). Childhood adversity profiles and adult psychopathology in a representative Northern Ireland study. *Journal of Anxiety Disorders*, 35, 42–8.

Miner, M. H., Flitter, J. M., & Robinson, B. B. (2006). Association of sexual revictimization with sexuality and psychological function. *Journal of Interpersonal Violence*, 21, 503–24.

Moore, S. A., & Zoellner, L. A. (2007). Overgeneral autobiographical memory and traumatic events: an evaluative review. *Psychological Bulletin*, 133, 419–37.

Neria, Y., Nandi, A., & Galea, S. (2008). Post-traumatic stress disorder following disasters: a systematic review. *Psychological Medicine*, 38, 467–80.

Nishith, P., Mechanic, M. B., & Resick, P. A. (2000). Prior interpersonal trauma: the contribution to current PTSD symptoms in female rape victims. *Journal of Abnormal Psychology*, 109, 20–25.

Norris, F. H., Galea, S., Friedman, M. J., & Watson, P. J. (2006). *Methods for Disaster Mental Health Research*. New York, NY: Guilford Press.

North, C. S. (2014). Current research and recent breakthroughs on the mental health effects of disasters. *Current Psychiatry Reports*, 16, 481.

Palgi, Y., Gelkopf, M., & Berger, R. (2015). The inoculating role of previous exposure to potentially traumatic life events on coping with prolonged exposure to rocket attacks: a lifespan perspective. *Psychiatry Research*, 227, 296–301.

Pirkola, S., Isometsa, E., Aro, H., et al. (2005). Childhood adversities as risk factors for adult mental disorders: results from the Health 2000 study. *Social Psychiatry and Psychiatric Epidemiology*, 40, 769–77.

Putnam, K. T., Harris, W. W., & Putnam, F. W. (2013). Synergistic childhood adversities and complex adult psychopathology. *Journal of Traumatic Stress*, 26, 435–42.

Rutter, M. (2012). Resilience as a dynamic concept. *Development and Psychopathology*, 24, 335–44.

Sayed, S., Iacoviello, B. M., & Charney, D. S. (2015). Risk factors for the development of psychopathology following trauma. *Current Psychiatry Reports*, 17, 612.

Shaar, K. H. (2013). Post-traumatic stress disorder in adolescents in Lebanon as wars gained in ferocity: a systematic review. *Journal of Public Health Research*, 2, e17.

Shiri, S., Wexler, I. D., Alkalay, Y., Meiner, Z., & Kreitler, S. (2008). Positive and negative psychological impact after secondary exposure to politically motivated violence among body handlers and rehabilitation workers. *The Journal of Nervous and Mental Disease*, 196, 906–11.

Smith, G. C., Seaman, S. R., Wood, A. M., Royston, P., & White, I. R. (2014). Correcting for optimistic prediction in small data sets. *American Journal of Epidemiology*, 180, 318–24.

Smith, H. L., Summers, B. J., Dillon, K. H., & Cougle, J. R. (2016). Is worst-event trauma type related to PTSD symptom presentation and associated features? *Journal of Anxiety Disorders*, 38, 55–61.

Somer, E., Zrihan-Weitzman, A., Fuse, T., et al. (2009). Israeli civilians under heavy bombardment: prediction of the severity of post-traumatic symptoms. *Prehospital and Disaster Medicine*, 24, 389–94.

White, J., Pearce, J., Morrison, S., et al. (2015). Risk of post-traumatic stress disorder following traumatic events in a community sample. *Epidemiology and Psychiatric Sciences*, 24, 249–57.

Wilson, J., Jones, M., Fear, N. T., et al. (2009). Is previous psychological health associated with the likelihood of Iraq War deployment? An investigation of the "healthy warrior effect". *American Journal of Epidemiology*, 169, 1362–9.

Zou, K. H., O'Malley, A. J., & Mauri, L. (2007). Receiver-operating characteristic analysis for evaluating diagnostic tests and predictive models. *Circulation*, 115, 654–7.

Chapter 10

The Effects of Childhood Adversities

Katie A. McLaughlin, Oye Gureje, Norito Kawakami, Karestan C. Koenen, and Ronald C. Kessler

Child maltreatment has repeatedly been shown to predict posttraumatic stress disorder (PTSD) among adults exposed to traumas (Bremmer et al., 1993; Brewin et al., 2000; Schnurr et al., 2004; Koenen et al., 2007; Scott et al., 2010). However, there is less evidence about whether a broad set of childhood adversities (CAs) is similarly associated with increased vulnerability to PTSD following trauma exposure (McLaughlin et al., 2010), although studies show that the associations of stressful life events with anxiety, mood, and substance use disorders are elevated among individuals who have experienced a wide range of CAs (Hammen et al., 2000; Espejo et al., 2006; Harkness et al., 2006; McLaughlin et al., 2010; Roberts et al., 2010; Keyes et al., 2014; Myers et al., 2014). Prior analyses of the WMH data have documented that those CAs which are directly related to maladaptive family functioning (MFF) – such as child maltreatment, parent psychopathology, and family violence – are more strongly associated with the onset of mental disorders than other CAs and that the joint associations of MFF CAs with the onset of mental disorders are sub-additive (i.e., the incremental associations of additional CAs decrease as the number of CAs increases) (Kessler et al., 1997, 2010; Green et al., 2010; McLaughlin et al., 2012b). We also showed in Chapter 4 that MFF CAs are more powerful predictors of trauma exposure than are other CAs. Comparable analyses have not been carried out, though, with respect to the associations of CAs with the subsequent onset of PTSD in the wake of trauma exposure. It is also unclear whether CAs are associated with a generalized vulnerability to PTSD following any type of trauma exposure or whether these associations are more pronounced for specific types of trauma. As we saw in Chapter 9, PTSD risk varies markedly across trauma types, and prior exposure to certain trauma types is associated with elevated PTSD risk following exposure to subsequent traumas of the same type. In light of this evidence, it is plausible to think that the associations of CAs with PTSD might vary across trauma types. In addition, although earlier WMH analyses documented that CAs predict the onset of anxiety, mood, and substance use disorders at every stage of the life-span (Kessler et al., 1997, 2010; Green et al., 2010; McLaughlin et al., 2012b), these earlier studies did not determine whether vulnerability to PTSD among those with a history of CAs varies according to life-course stage. We consequently set out to examine the associations of CAs with PTSD as a function of type of CA, type of trauma, and life-course stage.

Methods

The analysis was carried out in the same subsample of the WMH surveys as used in Chapter 9, except that we excluded respondents from the surveys in Israel and New Zealand because those two surveys did not assess the CAs considered here. The analysis built on the final model in Chapter 9 by adding measures of 12 CAs to that model. These CAs, all of which were required to begin prior to age 18, included three types of interpersonal loss (parent death, parent divorce, and other loss of contact with parents or caregivers), four types of parent maladjustment (psychopathology, substance abuse, criminality, and family violence), three types of maltreatment (physical abuse, sexual abuse, and neglect), respondent serious physical illness, and economic adversity. Parent death and divorce were assessed only for biological parents, but other loss of contact with caregivers included any disruption of a caregiving relationship that lasted 6 months or longer. Respondents born to a single mother or adopted at birth were not coded as experiencing parent loss.

Physical abuse of the respondent by caregivers was assessed with a modified version of the Conflict Tactics Scale (CTS) (Straus, 1979) and with an item from the trauma section of the CIDI. Sexual abuse of the respondent by caregivers or other family members was assessed with questions from the CIDI regarding sexual assault, attempted rape, and rape, which asked whether these traumas were one-time experiences or repeat occurrences. Neglect was assessed with questions used in studies of child welfare that assessed the frequency of having inadequate food, clothing, medical care, or supervision, and being required to do age-inappropriate chores (Courtney et al., 2001).

Parent criminality was assessed with questions about whether a parent engaged in criminal activities or was ever arrested or sent to prison. Parent psychopathology (major depression, generalized anxiety disorder, panic disorder, or suicide attempt) and parent substance abuse were assessed with a revised version of the Family History Research Diagnostic Criteria Interview (Endicott et al., 1978; Kendler et al., 1991). Family violence was assessed with the modified CTS and a question in the trauma section of the CIDI about parent violence. Economic adversity was assessed with questions about whether the respondent's family received welfare or other government assistance or often did not have enough money to pay for basic necessities. Physical illness was assessed with a standard chronic conditions checklist.

Four of the above CAs are among the trauma types assessed in previous chapters: sexual abuse perpetrated by a family member; childhood physical abuse; witnessing family violence during childhood; and childhood physical illness. If the randomly selected trauma was one of these four CAs, it was not included among the CA measures. Several WMH countries omitted some CAs (neglect in South Africa; parent divorce and neglect in the six Western European countries). Rather than exclude these countries or exclude the missing CAs from analysis, we imputed individual-level missing values using multiple imputation (Klebanoff & Cole, 2008).

As noted above, our analysis built on the final model in Chapter 9. We began with a series of models (M1) examining each CA separately and controlling for all the predictors in the final Chapter 9 model. We then estimated a model that included the same controls and a separate predictor variable for each of the 12 CAs (M2), followed by a model that included predictor variables for number of CAs without variables for specific CA types (M3). The latter model included one variable for the number of MFF CAs (range: 0–4) and two dummy variables indicating exposure to exactly 1 or 2+ other CAs. Only MFF CAs that were significant in the bivariate models were included in the 0–4 count. We then estimated a model that included dummy variables for CA types in addition to variables for number of MFF and other CAs (M4). The next model deleted the four MFF CA type variables that were included in the MFF CA count variable, but retained the other type variables (M5). The next model (M6) included the same CA type variables as M5, but included dummy variables for exact numbers of MFF CAs rather than the count variable. A final model (M7) included only the MFF CA count variable and dropped all other CA variables.

Inspection of mean-squared error (MSE) and area under the receiver operating characteristic curve (AUC) based on tenfold cross-validation was used to select the best multivariate model among M2–M7 to predict PTSD in response to the randomly selected trauma. Additional models then examined whether associations of CAs with PTSD varied by trauma type and timing of trauma exposure, with interaction terms added to the best-fitting model. As in Chapter 9, the indeterminacy of the solution created by including an OR for each trauma type was resolved by scaling the product of all trauma-specific ORs to 1.0. Interactions were calculated between CAs and age of exposure to the randomly selected trauma classified age into five groups (0–12, 13–24, 25–44, 45–59, and 60+ years).

Results

CA Prevalence

Prevalence estimates of CAs associated with representative traumas are shown in Table 10.1. The proportions of traumas occurring to individuals with a history of CAs ranged from 3.8% (sexual abuse) to 20.9% (physical abuse). It is noteworthy that all prevalence estimates in the sample of traumas were higher than in the sample of respondents, indicating that CAs were positively associated with number of traumas experienced. For example, 10.7% of respondents reported exposure to physical abuse, but 20.9% of all random traumas occurred to individuals exposed to physical abuse. The most dramatically elevated CA prevalence estimates in the trauma sample relative to the sample of respondents involved the MFF CAs of family violence, physical abuse, and sexual abuse.

Associations of Childhood Adversities with PTSD

In bivariate models (M1), which considered one CA at a time, only MFF CAs were significant predictors of PTSD after the randomly selected trauma, with ORs in the range of 1.6–2.2 (see Table 10.2). MFF CAs

Table 10.1 Prevalence of CAs in the WMH surveys ($n = 27{,}017$)

	Percentage of random traumas occurring to respondents with a history of each CA[a]		Percentage of respondents with a history of each CA[b]	
	%	(SE)	%	(SE)
I MFF CAs				
Parent psychopathology	13.7	(0.6)	9.5	(0.3)
Parent substance misuse	7.8	(0.4)	6.0	(0.2)
Parent criminality	6.5	(0.4)	4.0	(0.2)
Family violence	16.3	(0.6)	9.7	(0.3)
Physical abuse	20.9	(0.7)	10.7	(0.3)
Sexual abuse	3.8	(0.2)	1.9	(0.1)
Neglect	8.2	(0.3)	5.7	(0.2)
II Other CAs				
Parent death	14.4	(0.5)	13.3	(0.3)
Parent divorce	9.7	(0.5)	8.0	(0.3)
Other parent loss	7.7	(0.4)	6.0	(0.2)
Serious physical illness	6.3	(0.4)	3.5	(0.2)
Economic adversity	6.1	(0.3)	4.7	(0.2)

[a]Given that randomly selected traumas were weighted by the inverse of their probabilities of selection and then multiplied by the Part II weight, the weighted sample of traumas represents the population of all traumas experienced in the population.
[b]Prevalence of CAs among the 27,017 respondents included in the analysis.

associated with PTSD included physical and sexual abuse, neglect, and parent psychopathology. The ORs for incremental associations of these four MFF CAs with PTSD were lower in the additive multivariate model (M2) that included all CA types. Three of the four MFF CAs remained significant in that model (parent psychopathology, sexual abuse, and neglect), with ORs in the range of 1.8–2.0. MFF CAs, as a set, were significantly associated with PTSD in M2 ($\chi^2_7 = 40.8$, $p < 0.001$), but other CAs were not ($\chi^2_5 = 5.8, p = 0.33$). In addition, the strength of the ORs varied significantly across the different types of MFF CAs ($\chi^2_6 = 18.5$, $p = 0.005$) but not other CAs ($\chi^2_4 = 5.8, p = 0.22$).

In multivariate model M3, which considered only number and not type of CAs, the number of MFF CAs was significantly associated with PTSD (OR = 1.7, $p < 0.001$), but the number of other CAs was not ($\chi^2_2 = 0.4$, $p = 0.84$). Subsequent models (M4–M6) included information about both type and number of CAs. We examined models including variables for number of MFF and other CAs as well as type variables for all CAs (M4), and type variables for CAs, excluding the four MFF CAs included in the count variable (M5). We also examined a model that included variables for exactly 1, 2, 3, and 4 MFF CAs rather than the 0–4 count (M6). However, the best-fitting model (M7) included only the count variable for the four individually significant MFF CAs (see Table 10.2). Consistent with M7 being the best model, neither the other MFF CAs not included in the count variable nor other CAs were associated with PTSD in M5 or M6, indicating an absence of meaningful associations of CAs other than physical and sexual abuse, neglect, and parent psychopathology with PTSD (see Table 10.2). In the best-fitting model (M7), number of MFF CAs was significantly associated with PTSD (OR = 1.8).

Differential Associations by Trauma Type and Timing of Trauma Exposure

To determine whether the association of number of MFF CAs with PTSD varied as a function of the type of trauma, we added interactions between this variable and nine indicators for trauma type to the best-fitting CA model (M7) (see Table 10.3). The association of number of MFF CAs with PTSD did not vary across trauma types ($\chi^2_8 = 13.9$, $p = 0.08$). The ORs for the interaction term were in the range of 0.8–1.6, except for natural disaster (OR = 0.3), witnessing atrocities (OR = 0.4), and being kidnapped (OR = 3.1).

Next, we examined interactions between number of MFF CAs and timing of trauma exposure. Here, the association of number of MFF CAs with PTSD varied, depending on age of trauma exposure ($\chi^2_4 = 16.4$, $p = 0.002$). Specifically, coefficients were positive and significant for traumas occurring during childhood

Table 10.2 Multivariate associations between CAs and DSM-IV/CIDI PTSD in response to a randomly selected trauma in the WMH surveys ($n = 27{,}017$)[a]

	M1[b]		M2[c]		M3[d]		M4[e]		M5[f]		M6[f]		M7[g]	
	OR	(95% CI)	OR	(95% CI)	OR	(95% CI)	OR	(95% CI)	OR	(95% CI)	OR	(95% CI)	OR	(95% CI)
I MFF CAs														
Parent psychopathology	2.2*	(1.6–3.0)	2.0*	(1.5–2.7)										
Parent substance misuse	1.2	(0.9–1.7)	0.9	(0.6–1.3)			0.9	(0.6–1.3)	0.9	(0.6–1.3)	0.9	(0.6–1.3)		
Parent criminality	1.4	(0.9–2.3)	1.1	(0.7–1.9)			1.1	(0.7–1.9)	1.1	(0.7–1.9)	1.1	(0.7–1.9)		
Family violence	1.1	(0.7–1.7)	1.0	(0.6–1.5)			1.0	(0.6–1.5)	1.1	(0.7–1.7)	1.1	(0.7–1.7)		
Physical abuse	1.6*	(1.1–2.3)	1.3	(0.9–2.0)			0.7	(0.4–1.1)						
Sexual abuse	2.0*	(1.2–3.4)	1.8*	(1.1–3.0)			0.9	(0.5–1.5)						
Neglect	2.2*	(1.4–3.2)	1.9*	(1.2–2.8)			0.9	(0.6–1.5)						
χ^2_7[h]			40.8*											
χ^2_6[i]			18.5*				3.4		$\chi^2_3 = 0.3$		$\chi^2_3 = 0.3$			
II Other CAs														
Parent death	1.4	(0.9–2.4)	1.4	(0.8–2.3)			1.4	(0.8–2.4)	1.4	(0.7–2.4)	1.4	(0.7–2.4)		
Parent divorce	0.9	(0.6–1.2)	0.9	(0.6–1.2)			0.9	(0.6–1.3)	0.8	(0.6–1.3)	0.9	(0.6–1.3)		
Other parent loss	0.9	(0.6–1.4)	0.8	(0.5–1.2)			0.7	(0.4–1.3)	0.7	(0.4–1.3)	0.7	(0.4–1.3)		
Serious physical illness	1.1	(0.8–1.7)	1.0	(0.7–1.5)			1.0	(0.7–1.6)	1.0	(0.6–1.6)	1.0	(0.7–1.6)		
Economic adversity	1.3	(0.8–2.0)	1.2	(0.7–1.8)			1.1	(0.6–1.9)	1.1	(0.6–2.0)	1.1	(0.6–2.0)		
χ^2_5[h]			5.8				6.1		6.7		6.8			
χ^2_4[i]			5.8				5.8		6.3		6.4			
χ^2_{12}[j]			63.8*				9.3		6.9		6.9			
III Number of MFF CAs														
0–4[k]					1.7*	(1.5–2.1)	2.0*	(1.5–2.7)	1.8*	(1.5–2.1)			1.8*	(1.5–2.1)
1											1.6*	(1.1–2.2)		
2											2.8*	(1.8–4.4)		
3											5.4*	(2.7–10.6)		
4											13.7*	(3.6–51.4)		
χ^2_4[l]											36.3*			
χ^2_3[m]											19.6*			

IV Number of Other CAs										
1		1.1	(0.7–1.6)							
2+		1.1	(0.8–1.7)	1.1	(0.6–2.1)	1.1	(0.6–2.2)	1.1	(0.6–2.2)	
X^2_2		0.4								
V Mean-Squared Error[n]	**0.039214**	**0.039162**		**0.039232**		**0.039206**		**0.039278**		**0.039146**
VI AUC[n]	**0.738**	**0.741**		**0.737**		**0.737**		**0.734**		**0.743**

*Significant at the 0.05 level, two-sided test.

[a]Models were estimated using logistic regression with PTSD in response to a randomly selected trauma as the outcome variable. Each model controlled for survey, age, sex, nine dummy variables for trauma type and six dummy variables for prior exposure to the same trauma type for trauma types shown in prior analysis to influence later risk of PTSD in response to a trauma of the same type (see Chapter 9 for details).

[b]Models were estimated with one CA at a time and the controls noted in footnote a.

[c]The model was estimated with all 12 CAs and the controls noted in footnote a.

[d]The model was estimated with dummy variables for the number of CAs without any information about CA type and the controls noted in footnote a.

[e]The model was estimated with dummy variables for both number and type of CAs plus the controls noted in footnote a.

[f]The model was estimated with dummy variables for both number and type of CAs, removing the variables for CA type for the four MFF CAs included in the 0–4 count variable (see footnote h), plus the controls noted in footnote a.

[g]The model was estimated with the 0–4 count variable (see footnote h), plus the controls noted in footnote a.

[h]The joint significance of the set of ORs for CAs in the group.

[i]The significance of the differences among the ORs within the group.

[j]The joint significance of all CAs in the model.

[k]The 0–4 variable is a count of the number of the following CAs experienced by the respondent: parent psychopathology, physical abuse, sexual abuse, and neglect.

[l]The joint significance of the set of ORs for the number of MFF CAs compared to none.

[m]The significance of the differences among the ORs for number of MFF CAs.

[n]These measures are based on replicated tenfold cross-validation with 10 replications.

Table 10.3 Variation in the associations of CAs and DSM-IV/CIDI PTSD in response to a randomly selected trauma and age of trauma exposure in the WHO WMH surveys ($n = 27{,}017$)[a]

	M8[b]		M9[c]	
	OR	(95% CI)	OR	(95% CI)
I Interaction of Number of MFF CAs with Trauma Types				
Civilian in war zone	0.8	(0.3–2.3)		
Civilian in region of terror	1.1	(0.6–2.0)		
Kidnapped	3.1*	(1.2–7.7)		
Witnessed death/dead body/serious injury	1.6*	(1.0–2.6)		
Witnessed atrocities	0.4	(0.1–1.6)		
Sexual violence victimization	1.2	(0.8–1.8)		
Natural disaster	0.3*	(0.1–0.9)		
UD of a loved one	1.4	(0.9–2.3)		
All other traumas	1.2	(0.8–1.7)		
χ^2_8	13.9			
II Interaction of Number of MFF CAs with Age of Trauma Exposure				
0–12 years			1.6*	(1.1–2.3)
13–24 years			1.8*	(1.3–2.6)
25–44 years			1.9*	(1.3–2.7)
45–59 years			1.5	(0.9–2.6)
60+			0.1*	(0.0–0.3)
χ^2_4			16.4*	

*Significant at the 0.05 level, two-sided test.
[a]See footnote a in Table 10.2 for a description of the overall modeling approach. CA and control variables are based on the best-fitting model of CAs in predicting PTSD in response to a randomly selected trauma (Table 10.2, Multivariate model 7).
[b]The model included nine dummy variables for the interaction of the 0–4 MFF CA count variable with trauma types in addition to CA and control variables from Table 10.2, Multivariate model 7. Trauma types are based on prior factor analysis in this sample (see Chapter 3 for details).
[c]The model included five dummy variables for the interaction of the 0–4 MFF CA count variable with age at trauma exposure in addition to CA and control variables from Table 10.2, Multivariate model 7.

(OR = 1.6), adolescence (OR = 1.8), and adulthood through age 44 (OR = 1.9), but not for traumas occurring in later-middle age, and the OR was significantly negative among respondents aged 60+ (OR = 0.1).

Discussion

We found that exposure to four types of CAs was associated with increased odds of developing PTSD. Of the wide range of CAs examined, physical and sexual abuse, neglect, and parent psychopathology were associated with elevated odds of developing PTSD following a trauma. The results thus document that both maltreatment and parent psychopathology – but not the other CA types considered here – are associated with increased risk of developing PTSD. These findings extend prior work documenting both a higher prevalence of past-year PTSD following a past-year trauma among individuals with high levels of exposure to CAs (McLaughlin et al., 2010) and a greater risk of developing PTSD among individuals who were maltreated as children (Bremmer et al., 1993; Brewin et al., 2000; Schnurr et al., 2004; Koenen et al., 2007; Scott et al., 2010).

Our finding of an association between parent psychopathology and PTSD is broadly consistent with evidence that parent psychopathology has robust, but largely nonspecific associations with offspring psychopathology (McLaughlin et al., 2012a; Caspi et al., 2014), which are likely mediated by both genetic and environmental factors (Goodman & Gotlib, 1999). Unlike prior research suggesting that the associations of CAs with mental disorders are sub-additive, such that the incremental effects of additional CAs get relatively smaller as the number of CAs increases (Green et al., 2010; Kessler et al., 2010; McLaughlin et al., 2012b), our results indicate that the associations of CAs involving maltreatment and parent psychopathology with PTSD are additive. That is, each additional exposure to specific CAs increases the odds of developing PTSD following a trauma – an association that is relatively consistent as the number of CAs increases.

The association of CAs involving child maltreatment and parent psychopathology with PTSD did not vary across a wide range of trauma types. This is surprising, given our results in Chapter 9 for significant variation in main effects of trauma type along with extensive other research showing that conditional risk of PTSD varies considerably across trauma types (Kessler et al., 1995; Breslau et al., 1998). Prior work on stress sensitization has produced conflicting findings about whether vulnerability to stressors among individuals with a history of CAs is general or specific to certain types of stressors. Some studies have shown that relatively mild stressors are more likely to trigger depression among those with a history of CA than those without (Hammen et al., 2000; Rudolph & Flynn, 2007), whereas other work indicates that CA exposure magnifies the association between relatively severe stressors and psychopathology (McLaughlin et al., 2010). Our failure to document variation in the associations of CAs with PTSD as a function of trauma type indirectly suggests that CAs produce a generalized vulnerability to PTSD following trauma exposure.

We found that the associations of CAs and PTSD vary by life-course stage, with the associations observable during childhood, adolescence, and early middle adulthood, but not during late-middle age or late adulthood. We are unaware of prior research examining this specification, although it is noteworthy that most prior studies documenting an interaction between CAs and later stressors in predicting mental disorders focused on adolescents or young adults (Hammen et al., 2000; Espejo et al., 2006; Harkness et al., 2006; Rudolph & Flynn, 2007; Breslau et al., 2014). There are two possible interpretations of this finding. Perhaps the association of CAs with PTSD wanes later in life due to increased temporal distance from the CA, variations in the features of traumas across the lifespan, or protective factors that increase in later life. Alternatively, recall biases in CA reports might be strongest among older adults, where the recall interval is longest. Under-reporting of CAs would attenuate CA-PTSD associations in the oldest group if PTSD symptoms are not under-reported. The fact that CAs were negatively associated with PTSD among older adults might be due to selective mortality favoring especially resilient individuals with CA histories in the later years of life.

Why might exposure to child maltreatment and parent psychopathology influence vulnerability to PTSD? And why were only these specific MFF CAs associated with PTSD? One potential mechanism involves heightened salience of threat cues and magnified emotional reactions to potential threats. Child maltreatment is associated with elevated emotional reactivity to negative stimuli, as measured using self-report (Hennessy et al., 1994; Heleniak et al., 2016), ecological momentary assessments (Wichers et al., 2009), and amygdala response (McCrory et al., 2011, 2013; Suzuki et al., 2014; McLaughlin et al., 2015). Similar patterns have been observed in children of parents with psychopathology (Davis et al., 2007; Feldman et al., 2009). Heightened amygdala reactivity to threat may be a key pathway through which maltreatment and parent psychopathology influence later risk for PTSD. Prospective studies in both adolescent and military samples have shown that elevated amygdala response to threat cues assessed prior to trauma exposure predicts the subsequent onset of PTSD symptoms following a trauma (Admon et al., 2009; McLaughlin et al., 2014a). Amygdala reactivity to threat cues decreases in old age (Mather et al., 2004), which may have contributed to the lack of CA-PTSD associations in older adults, although it is unclear if this would account for the negative CA-PTSD association among older respondents. The specificity of this pattern of neural response to CAs involving direct exposure to threat (McLaughlin et al., 2014b) or parent psychopathology (Davis et al., 2007; Feldman et al., 2009) may help explain why CAs involving interpersonal loss and economic adversity were not associated with PTSD vulnerability. Other mechanisms are also likely to play a role in the associations of these specific MFF CAs with PTSD, including habitual use of maladaptive emotional regulation strategies (e.g., rumination) and low social support, each of which is associated with child maltreatment and parent psychopathology as well as with risk for PTSD (Brewin et al., 2000; Kuyken et al., 2006; Heleniak et al., 2016; Jenness et al., 2016; Sheikh et al., 2016).

The above results are limited by the fact that the WMH data used retrospective reports of CAs, trauma exposures, and PTSD symptoms. Recall bias of CAs primarily involves under-reporting (Widom & Shepard, 1996; Widom & Morris, 1997; Hardt & Rutter, 2004), which might have either attenuated or increased associations of CAs with PTSD, depending on whether there is a significant positive association between recall bias involving CAs and recall bias involving PTSD. The absence of CA associations with PTSD in the oldest respondents could reflect under-reporting, which was most pronounced among respondents with the longest recall periods (Green et al., 2010). Additionally, assessment of PTSD with a fully structured diagnostic interview rather than a clinician-administered interview likely introduced imprecision. The CIDI diagnoses were relatively conservative, meaning that low-severity cases of PTSD may have been missed.

Despite these limitations, we replicated prior work indicating that child maltreatment is associated with heightened vulnerability to PTSD following traumas occurring later in development. We extended earlier findings by showing that a similar association existed with parent psychopathology, but not with other forms of CA, that the association of CAs involving child maltreatment and parent psychopathology with PTSD were additive and did not vary across trauma types, and that CA-PTSD associations were limited to childhood, adolescence, and early-middle adulthood. These results build on a growing body of evidence indicating that early experiences of adversity are associated with increased vulnerability to psychopathology following stressors later in development and suggest that CAs involving child maltreatment and parent psychopathology are associated with heightened risk for PTSD following a later trauma exposure.

Acknowledgments

Portions of this chapter are based on Mc Laughlin, K. A, Koenen, K. C., Bromet, E. J., et al. (2007) Childhood adversities and post-traumatic stress disorder: evidence for stress sensitization in the World Mental Health Surveys. *British Journal of Psychiatry*, 211, 280–8 by permission of the Royal College of Psychiatrists.

References

Admon, R., Lubin, G., Stern, O., et al. (2009). Human vulnerability to stress depends on amygdala's predisposition and hippocampal plasticity. *Proceedings of the National Academy of Sciences*, 106, 14120–5.

Bremmer, J. D., Southwick, S. M., Johnson, D. R., Yehuda, R., & Charney, D. S. (1993). Childhood physical abuse and combat-related posttraumatic stress disorder in Vietnam veterans. *American Journal of Psychiatry*, 150, 235–9.

Breslau, N., Kessler, R. C., Chilcoat, H. D., et al. (1998). Trauma and posttraumatic stress disorder in the community: the 1996 Detroit Area Survey of Trauma. *Archives of General Psychiatry*, 55, 626–32.

Breslau, N., Koenen, K. C., Luo, Z., et al. (2014). Childhood maltreatment, juvenile disorders and adult post-traumatic stress disorder: a prospective investigation. *Psychological Medicine*, 44, 1937–45.

Brewin, C. R., Andrews, B., & Valentine, J. D. (2000). Meta-analysis of risk factors for posttraumatic stress disorder in trauma-exposed adults. *Journal of Consulting and Clinical Psychology*, 68, 748–66.

Caspi, A., Houts, R. M., Belsky, D. W., et al. (2014). The p factor: one general psychopathology factor in the structure of psychiatric disorders? *Clinical Psychological Science*, 2, 119–37.

Courtney, M. E., Piliavin, I., Grogan-Kaylor, A., & Nesmith, A. (2001). Foster youth transitions to adulthood: a longitudinal view of youth leaving care. *Child Welfare*, 80, 685–717.

Davis, E. P., Glynn, L. M., Schetter, C. D., et al. (2007). Prenatal exposure to maternal depression and cortisol influences infant temperament. *Journal of the American Academy of Child & Adolescent Psychiatry*, 46, 737–46.

Endicott, J., Andreasen, N., & Spitzer, R. L. (1978). *Family History Research Diagnostic Criteria*. New York, NY: Biometrics Research, NY State Psychiatric Institute.

Espejo, E. P., Hammen, C., Connolly, N. P., et al. (2006). Stress sensitization and adolescent depressive severity as a function of childhood adversity: a link to anxiety disorders. *Journal of Abnormal Child Psychology*, 35, 287–99.

Feldman, R., Granat, A., Pariente, C., et al. (2009). Maternal depression and anxiety across the postpartum year and infant social engagement, fear regulation, and stress reactivity. *Journal of the American Academy of Child &Adolescent Psychiatry*, 48, 919–27.

Goodman, S. H., & Gotlib, I. H. (1999). Risk for psychopathology in the children of depressed mothers: a developmental model for understanding mechanisms of transmission. *Psychological Review*, 106, 458–90.

Green, J. G., McLaughlin, K. A., Berglund, P., et al. (2010). Childhood adversities and adult psychopathology in the National Comorbidity Survey Replication (NCS-R) I: associations with first onset of DSM-IV disorders. *Archives of General Psychiatry*, 62, 113–23.

Hammen, C., Henry, R., & Daley, S. E. (2000). Depression and sensitization to stressors among young women as a function of childhood adversity. *Journal of Consulting and Clinical Psychology*, 68, 782–7.

Hardt, J., & Rutter, M. (2004). Validity of adult retrospective reports of adverse childhood experiences: review of the evidence. *Journal of Child Psychology and Psychiatry*, 45, 260–73.

Harkness, K. L., Bruce, A. E., & Lumley, M. N. (2006). The role of childhood abuse and neglect in the sensitization to stressful life events in adolescent depression. *Journal of Abnormal Psychology*, 115, 730–41.

Heleniak, C., Jenness, J., Van der Stoep, A., McCauley, E., & McLaughlin, K. A. (2016). Childhood maltreatment exposure and disruptions in emotion regulation: a transdiagnostic pathway to adolescent internalizing

and externalizing psychopathology. *Cognitive Therapy and Research*, 40, 394–415.
Hennessy, K. D., Rabideau, G. J., Cicchetti, D., & Cummings, E. M. (1994). Responses of physically abused and nonabused children to different forms of interadult anger. *Child Development*, 65, 815–28.
Jenness, J., Jager-Hyman, S., Heleniak, C., et al. (2016). Catastrophizing, rumination, and reappraisal prospectively predict adolescent PTSD symptom onset following a terrorist attack. *Depression and Anxiety*, 33, 1039–47.
Kendler, K. S., Silberg, J. L., Neale, M. C., et al. (1991). The family history method: whose psychiatric history is measured? *American Journal of Psychiatry*, 148, 1501–4.
Kessler, R. C., Sonnega, A., Bromet, E., Hughes, M., & Nelson, C. B. (1995). Posttraumatic stress disorder in the National Comorbidity Survey. *Archives of General Psychiatry*, 52, 1048–60.
Kessler, R. C., Davis, C. G., & Kendler, K. S. (1997). Childhood adversity and adult psychiatric disorder in the US National Comorbidity Survey. *Psychological Medicine*, 27, 1101–19.
Kessler, R. C., McLaughlin, K. A., Green, J. G., et al. (2010). Childhood adversities and adult psychopathology in the WHO World Mental Health Surveys. *British Journal of Psychiatry*, 197, 378–85.
Keyes, K. M., Shmulewitz, D., Greenstein, E., et al. (2014). Exposure to the Lebanon War of 2006 and effects on alcohol use disorders: the moderating role of childhood maltreatment. *Drug and Alcohol Dependence*, 134, 296–303.
Klebanoff, M. A., & Cole, S. R. (2008). Use of multiple imputation in the epidemiologic literature. *American Journal of Epidemiology*, 168, 355–7.
Koenen, K. C., Moffit, T. E., Poulin, R., Martin, J., & Caspi, A. (2007). Early childhood factors associated with the development of post-traumatic stress disorder: results from a longitudinal birth cohort. *Psychological Medicine*, 37, 181–92.
Kuyken, W., Watkins, E., Holden, E., & Cook, W. (2006). Rumination in adolescents at risk for depression. *Journal of Affective Disorders*, 96, 39–47.
Mather, M., Canli, T., English, T., et al. (2004). Amygdala responses to emotionally valenced stimuli in older and younger adults. *Psychological Science*, 15, 259–63.
McCrory, E. J., De Brito, S. A., Sebastian, C. L., et al. (2011). Heightened neural reactivity to threat in child victims of family violence. *Current Biology*, 21, R947–8.
McCrory, E. J., De Brito, S. A., Kelly, P. A., et al. (2013). Amygdala activation in maltreated children during pre-attentive emotional processing. *British Journal of Psychiatry*, 202, 269–76.
McLaughlin, K. A., Conron, K. J., Koenen, K. C., & Gilman, S. E. (2010). Childhood adversity, adult stressful life events, and risk of past-year psychiatric disorder: a test of the stress sensitization hypothesis in a population-based sample of adults. *Psychological Medicine*, 40, 1647–58.
McLaughlin, K. A., Gadermann, A. M., Hwang, I., et al. (2012a). Parent psychopathology and offspring mental disorders: results from the WHO World Mental Health Surveys. *British Journal of Psychiatry*, 200, 290–9.
McLaughlin, K. A., Green, J. G., Gruber, M. J., et al. (2012b). Childhood adversities and first onset of psychiatric disorders in a national sample of adolescents. *Archives of General Psychiatry*, 69, 1151–60.
McLaughlin, K. A., Busso, D. S., Duys, A., et al. (2014a). Amygdala response to negative stimuli predicts PTSD symptom onset following a terrorist attack. *Depression and Anxiety*, 10, 834–42.
McLaughlin, K. A., Sheridan, M. A., & Lambert, H. K. (2014b). Childhood adversity and neural development: deprivation and threat as distinct dimensions of early experience. *Neuroscience and Biobehavioral Reviews*, 47, 578–91.
McLaughlin, K. A., Peverill, M., Gold, A. L., Alves, S., & Sheridan, M. A. (2015). Child maltreatment and neural systems underlying emotion regulation. *Journal of the American Academy of Child & Adolescent Psychiatry*, 54, 753–62.
Myers, B., McLaughlin, K. A., Wang, S., Blanco, C., & Stein, D. J. (2014). Associations between childhood adversity, adult stressful life events, and past-year drug use disorders in the National Epidemiological Study of Alcohol and Related Conditions (NESARC). *Psychology of Addictive Behaviors*, 28, 1117–26.
Roberts, A. L., McLaughlin, K. A., Conron, K. J., & Koenen, K. C. (2010). Adult stressors, history of childhood adversity, and risk of perpetration of intimate partner violence among men and women. *American Journal of Preventive Medicine*, 40, 128–38.
Rudolph, K. D., & Flynn, M. (2007). Childhood adversity and youth depression: influence of gender and pubertal status. *Development and Psychopathology*, 19, 497–521.
Schnurr, P. P., Lunney, C. A., & Sengupta, A. (2004). Risk factors for the development versus maintenance of posttraumatic stress disorder. *Journal of Traumatic Stress*, 17, 85–95.
Scott, K. M., Smith, D. R., & Ellis, P. M. (2010). Prospectively ascertained childhood maltreatment and its associations with DSM-IV mental disorders in young adults. *Archives of General Psychiatry*, 67, 712–19.
Sheikh, M. A., Abelsen, B., & Olsen, J. A. (2016). Clarifying associations between childhood adversity, social support, behavioral factors, and mental health, health, and well-being in adulthood: a population-based study. *Frontiers in Psychology*, 7, 727.
Straus, M. A. (1979). Measuring intrafamily conflict and violence: the Conflict Tactics (CT) Scales. *Journal of Marriage and the Family*, 41, 75–88.

Suzuki, H., Luby, J. L., Botteron, K. N., et al. (2014). Early life stress and trauma and enhanced limbic activation to emotionally valenced faces in depressed and healthy children. *Journal of the American Academy of Child & Adolescent Psychiatry*, 53, 800–13.

Wichers, M., Schrijvers, D., Geschwind, N., et al. (2009). Mechanisms of gene–environment interactions in depression: evidence that genes potentiate multiple sources of adversity. *Psychological Medicine*, 39, 1077–86.

Widom, C. S., & Shepard, R. L. (1996). Accuracy of adult recollections of childhood victimization: part 1. Childhood physical abuse. *Psychological Assessment*, 8, 412–21.

Widom, C. S., & Morris, S. (1997). Accuracy of adult recollections of childhood victimization: part 2. Childhood sexual abuse. *Psychological Assessment*, 9, 34–46.

Chapter 11

The Effects of Prior Psychopathology

Ronald C. Kessler, Evelyn J. Bromet, Beth-Ellen Pennell, and Elie G. Karam

Epidemiological research shows that prior psychopathology and prior trauma exposure are the two strongest pretrauma predictors of individual differences in post-traumatic stress disorder (PTSD) risk after subsequent trauma exposure (DiGangi et al., 2013). As noted in Chapter 4, prior trauma exposure is particularly interesting because, unlike prior psychopathology, earlier traumas are external to the individual and presumably predict future PTSD by creating biological or psychological vulnerabilities that could be the focus of study. Childhood family adversities (CAs) have been of special interest in this regard (Nemeroff, 2016) because CAs occur early in life and are associated with significantly increased risk of psychopathology throughout the life course (Kessler et al., 2010). We saw in Chapter 4 that comparable patterns are found in the World Mental Health (WMH) data. However, it is difficult to tease apart the environmental effects of CAs from the effects of preexisting risk and intervening psychopathology on vulnerability to subsequent PTSD. The reason is that CAs are strongly associated with parent psychopathology and, by extension, genetic risk (Green et al., 2010) and a high proportion of the most severe CAs are associated with both child- and adolescent-onset mental disorders and long-term neurobiological changes linked with a range of later disorders (McLaughlin et al., 2012), make it difficult to tease apart the environmental effects of CAs from the effects of preexisting risk and intervening psychopathology on vulnerability to subsequent PTSD.

The environmental effects of traumas not involving CAs would presumably be easier to study than those involving CAs due to the fact that other traumas (e.g., unexpected death of a loved one, accidents) are likely to be more independent than CAs of prior psychopathology and other individual-level risk factors for a range of subsequent mental disorders. A potential limitation in focusing on these traumas, though, is that some (Breslau et al., 2008; Breslau & Peterson, 2010), but not all (Cougle et al., 2009), epidemiological studies suggest that the associations of earlier traumas with PTSD after subsequent traumas are limited to individuals who developed PTSD due to the earlier traumas. If true, this specification would reintroduce the same complication as in research on the effects of CAs. Resolution of this uncertainty could have important implications for future research on the environmental determinants of individual differences in vulnerability to PTSD (Harkness et al., 2015).

Although the cross-sectional design of the WMH surveys does not lend itself to resolving this uncertainty definitively, we addressed it by investigating in more depth the associations reported in Chapter 9 between earlier traumas involving interpersonal violence (participation in organized violence, physical violence victimization, rape victimization, nonrape sexual assault victimization) and an increased odds of DSM-IV PTSD after subsequent traumas. We did not explore in Chapter 9 the possibility that these associations might vary depending on history of PTSD or other common DSM-IV disorders, but our subsequent analysis, which is reported in the current chapter, did precisely this.

Methods

The surveys considered in this analysis were the same as those in Chapter 9. We built on the final model in Chapter 9 by adding in information about lifetime occurrence of 14 DSM-IV disorders that had first onsets prior to the respondent's age at exposure to the random trauma. As described in more detail in Chapter 2, these disorders were assessed with the fully structured Composite International Diagnostic Interview (CIDI) (Kessler & Üstün, 2004). The disorders included two mood disorders (major depressive disorder/dysthymic disorder and broadly defined bipolar disorder [bipolar I and II and subthreshold bipolar disorder, defined using criteria described elsewhere]) (Kessler et al., 2006), six anxiety disorders (generalized anxiety disorder, panic disorder and/or agoraphobia, post-traumatic stress disorder, separation anxiety disorder, social phobia, and specific phobia), four disruptive behavior disorders (attention-deficit/hyperactivity disorder, conduct disorder, intermittent explosive disorder, and oppositional-defiant disorder), and two substance use disorders (alcohol and drug abuse with or without dependence). As noted in Chapter 2, PTSD was unique among these disorders in that it was assessed twice: once for the random trauma and a second time for the lifetime trauma nominated by the respondent as the worst trauma – that is, the trauma that caused the most distress impairment. Again as noted in Chapter 2, age of onset of each disorder was assessed using probing techniques shown experimentally to improve recall accuracy (Knäuper et al., 1999), enabling us to determine whether respondents had a history of each disorder prior to exposure to the random trauma. DSM-IV organic exclusion and diagnostic hierarchy rules were not used in making diagnoses.

We began with the final logistic regression model in Chapter 9 that estimated associations of earlier traumas and random traumas types with subsequent PTSD after random trauma exposure, controlling for sex and age at random trauma exposure, and survey. We expanded this model to evaluate associations of temporally prior (to the random trauma) lifetime DSM-IV/CIDI disorders with the outcome. The best-fitting model was then elaborated to consider interactions between earlier traumas and disorder history in predicting the outcome. As in other chapters, logistic regression coefficients and their design-based standard errors were exponentiated to create odds ratios (ORs) and 95% confidence intervals (CIs). Design-based Wald χ^2 tests were used to evaluate significance of predictor sets.

Results

Associations of DSM-IV/CIDI Disorder History with Subsequent PTSD after Random Traumas

All 14 prior lifetime DSM-IV/CIDI disorders were associated with increased odds of PTSD after random traumas in models that considered only one disorder at a time (see Table 11.1). The highest OR was associated with prior PTSD (OR = 5.7) and the lowest with prior conduct disorder (OR = 1.1). Also, 10 of the 14 ORs were statistically significant. In a multivariate model with all 14 prior disorders, only the anxiety disorders remained significant as a set ($\chi^2_6 = 112.1, p < 0.001$). The ORs for the individual anxiety disorders differed significantly among themselves ($\chi^2_5 = 26.8, p < 0.001$). Five of the six disorders had significant ORs (the exception was panic/agoraphobia) ranging between 4.3 for PTSD and 1.5 for social phobia (multivariate model 1 in Table 11.1).

A global interaction test for number of anxiety disorders was nonsignificant in an expanded model that included separate coefficients for history of each individually significant anxiety disorder and a count variable coded 0 for respondents with 0–1 such disorders and in the range 2–5 for respondents with multiple such disorders (OR = 0.9; 95% CI, 0.6–1.2). The interaction was also nonsignificant in a revised model that included separate dummy variables for respondents with histories of between two and all five significant anxiety disorders ($\chi^2_4 = 2.2, p = 0.70$). These results demonstrate clearly that the joint associations of prior anxiety disorders with PTSD after subsequent traumas are additive on a logistic scale.

Variation in Association of Trauma History with Later PTSD based on DSM-IV/CIDI Disorders

We next expanded the model to include interactions of the four significant earlier traumas with a three-category profile of the five significant anxiety disorders, where the categories were (1) prior PTSD regardless of presence/absence of one of the five anxiety disorders (2.8% of the sample, unweighted $n = 731$); (2) no prior PTSD, but one or more of the other significant anxiety disorders (16.1% of the sample, unweighted $n = 6{,}638$); and (3) no prior anxiety disorder (81.1% of the sample, unweighted $n = 27{,}307$). The ORs of the four earlier traumas with subsequent PTSD were examined in three models. Model 1 controlled for age at random trauma exposure, sex, survey, and random trauma type. Model 2 added history of anxiety disorders as a set of additional predictors. Model 3 added interactions of earlier traumas with the three-category disorder history profiles.

All four earlier traumas were found to have significant ORs in model 1 (between OR = 2.5 for rape victimization and OR = 1.3 for participation in organized violence; $\chi^2_4 = 63.7, p < 0.001$) (see Table 11.2). These ORs all became nonsignificant, though, in model 2

Table 11.1 The associations of DSM-IV/CIDI disorder history with PTSD due to subsequent random traumas ($n = 34{,}676$)[a]

	Prevalence		Bivariate		Multivariate model 1		Multivariate model 2		Multivariate model 3		Multivariate model 4	
	%	(SE)	OR	(95% CI)	OR	(95% CI)	OR	(95% CI)	OR	(95% CI)	OR	(95% CI)
I Mood Disorders												
MDD or dysthymic disorder	9.0	(0.3)	2.3*	(1.7-3.1)	1.3	(0.9–1.7)						
BPD (broad definition)	1.8	(0.2)	1.7	(0.9-3.3)	0.8	(0.5–1.4)						
Any	10.0	(0.4)	2.1*	(1.6-2.8)								
χ_2^{2b}					2.6							
χ_1^{2c}					1.8							
II Anxiety Disorders												
Panic disorder or agoraphobia	3.7	(0.3)	1.8*	(1.2–2.9)	1.0	(0.7–1.4)	1.0	–	1.0	–	1.0	–
GAD	3.5	(0.2)	4.1*	(2.3–7.2)	2.8*	(1.4–5.4)	3.4*	(1.5–7.5)	3.3*	(1.5–7.5)	3.0*	(1.6–5.5)
PTSD	2.8	(0.2)	5.7*	(3.8–8.6)	4.3*	(2.8–6.6)	4.9*	(2.8–8.4)	4.8*	(2.7–8.5)	4.3*	(2.8–6.6)
Social phobia	6.2	(0.3)	2.5*	(1.9–3.2)	1.5*	(1.1–2.0)	1.8*	(1.1–2.8)	1.8*	(1.1–2.8)	1.5*	(1.1–2.1)
Specific phobia	9.9	(0.4)	2.6*	(2.0–3.4)	1.9*	(1.4–2.5)	2.1*	(1.4–3.0)	2.1*	(1.4–3.0)	1.9*	(1.4–2.5)
Separation anxiety disorder	3.3	(0.2)	3.0*	(2.0–4.5)	2.1*	(1.5–3.1)	2.5*	(1.5–4.3)	2.6*	(1.5–4.4)	2.3*	(1.5–3.3)
χ_6^{2b}					112.1*		$\chi_5^2 = 35.8$*		$\chi_5^2 = 33.4$*		$\chi_5^2 = 130.7$*	
χ_5^{2c}					26.8*		$\chi_4^2 = 17.4$*		$\chi_4^2 = 16.0$*		$\chi_4^2 = 16.9$*	
Number(0–5)	20.3	(0.6)	2.3*	(1.9–2.6)			0.9	(0.6–1.2)				
1	13.8	(0.5)	2.5*	(1.6–3.7)								
2	3.6	(0.2)	4.8*	(3.2–7.3)					0.8	(0.4–1.6)		
3	1.2	(0.1)	9.7*	(5.5–17.1)					0.6	(0.2–1.9)		
4	0.2	(0.0)	50.8*	(19.8–130.5)					1.1	(0.2–5.7)		
5	0.0	(0.0)	48.5*	(3.0–774.2)					0.3	(0.0–10.0)		
χ_4^2			63.8*						2.2			

(cont.)

Table 11.1 *(cont.)*

	Prevalence		Bivariate		Multivariate model 1		Multivariate model 2		Multivariate model 3		Multivariate model 4	
	%	(SE)	OR	(95% CI)	OR	(95% CI)	OR	(95% CI)	OR	(95% CI)	OR	(95% CI)
III Disruptive Behavioral Disorders												
ADHD	2.2	(0.2)	2.4*	(1.5–3.8)	1.7*	(1.0–3.0)						
CD	2.1	(0.2)	1.1	(0.6–2.0)	0.6	(0.3–1.1)						
IED	2.8	(0.3)	1.4	(0.8–2.3)	0.8	(0.5–1.4)						
ODD	2.6	(0.2)	1.6	(0.9–3.1)	0.9	(0.5–1.7)						
Number	7.0	(0.4)	1.3*	(1.1–1.6)								
$\chi^{2\,b}_{4}$					5.3							
$\chi^{2\,c}_{3}$					5.3							
IV Substance Use Disorders												
Alcohol abuse or dependence	8.0	(0.4)	1.5*	(1.0–2.2)	1.0	(0.6–1.5)						
Drug abuse or dependence	3.2	(0.2)	1.9*	(1.1–3.3)	1.3	(0.7–2.3)						
Any	8.9	(0.5)	1.5*	(1.1–2.2)								
$\chi^{2\,b}_{2}$					1.0							
$\chi^{2\,c}_{1}$					0.5							
$\chi^{2\,d}_{14}$					136.8*							
$\chi^{2\,e}_{13}$					60.0*							

*Significant at the 0.05 level, two-sided test.
[a]Each model was estimated using logistic regression with controls for respondent age at random trauma exposure, sex, survey, and random trauma type.
[b]The joint significance for the set of ORs for mental disorders in the group.
[c]The significance of the differences among the ORs within the group.
[d]The joint significance of all mental disorders in the model.
[e]The significance of the differences among all mental disorders in the model.

Table 11.2 Variation in the associations of trauma history with DSM-IV/CIDI PTSD due to subsequent random traumas depending on history of DSM-IV/CIDI anxiety disorders ($n = 34{,}676$)[a]

	History of								
	Participation in organized violence		Physical violence victimization		Rape victimization		Other sexual assault victimization		
	OR	(95% CI)	OR	(95% CI)	OR	(95% CI)	OR	(95% CI)	χ^2_4
I Multivariate model 1 (no anxiety controls)	1.3*	(1.1–1.6)	1.4*	(1.2–1.7)	2.5*	(1.6–3.8)	1.6*	(1.1–2.3)	63.7*
II Multivariate model 2 (anxiety controls)[b]	1.1	(0.9–1.3)	1.2	(0.9–1.4)	1.6	(1.0–2.7)	1.2	(0.8–1.9)	7.1
III Multivariate model 3 (anxiety controls and interactions)[c]									
History of DSM-IV/CIDI PTSD	2.0*	(1.2–3.5)	0.7	(0.5–1.1)	1.1	(0.5–2.5)	1.3	(0.5–2.9)	7.3
History of other DSM-IV/CIDI anxiety disorders	0.9	(0.6–1.4)	1.1	(0.8–1.4)	1.0	(0.6–1.7)	1.3	(0.8–2.0)	1.5
No history of any DSM-IV/CIDI anxiety disorder	0.7	(0.5–1.0)	1.5*	(1.1–1.9)	3.4*	(1.6–7.0)	1.3	(0.6–2.4)	42.9*

*Significant at the 0.05 level, two-sided test.

[a]Each model was estimated using logistic regression with controls for respondent age at random trauma exposure, sex, survey, and random trauma type.

[b]All five prior (to the random trauma) lifetime anxiety disorders were significant, with ORs in the range between 4.3 for PTSD and 1.5 for social phobia, $\chi^2_5 = 130.5, p < 0.001$.

[c]The interaction between the three-category multivariate anxiety disorders history profile measure (history of DSM-IV/CIDI PTSD with or without other anxiety disorders, history of at least one other DSM-IV/CIDI anxiety disorder without PTSD, and no history of any DSM-IV/CIDI anxiety disorder) with the four prior (to the random trauma) lifetime traumas was significant ($\chi^2_8 = 29.7, p < 0.001$). The marginal effects of all five prior lifetime anxiety disorders were significant, with ORs in the range between 4.1 for PTSD and 1.7 for social phobia ($\chi^2_5 = 1204, p < 0.001$). The three subgroups have sample sizes of $n = 731$ (traumas that occurred to respondents with a history of DSM-IV/CIDI PTSD), $n = 6{,}638$ (traumas that occurred to respondents with a history of other DSM-IV/CIDI anxiety disorders but not PTSD), and $n = 27{,}307$ (traumas that occurred to other respondents).

($\chi^2_4 = 7.1, p = 0.13$). However, significant interactions between earlier traumas and history of anxiety disorders were found in model 3 ($\chi^2_8 = 29.7, p < 0.001$), resulting in earlier traumas having significant ORs among respondents with no history of anxiety disorders ($\chi^2_4 = 42.9, p < 0.001$), but not among respondents with a history of anxiety disorders ($\chi^2_4 = 7.3, p = 0.12$ among those with a history of PTSD; $\chi^2_4 = 1.5, p = 0.82$ among those with a history of other anxiety disorders, but not PTSD). Only two earlier traumas had significant ORs among respondents with no history of anxiety disorders: physical violence victimization (OR = 1.5) and rape victimization (OR = 3.4). The nonsignificance of the other two earlier traumas suggests that their significant ORs in model 1 were due to mediation through intervening anxiety disorders.

Population Distributions

It is instructive to project these results to the population by dividing the total WMH sample (i.e., including respondents with no history of trauma exposure) into the three subgroups of (1) individuals with a history of any anxiety disorder that predicts PTSD; (2) individuals without any such disorder, but with prior exposure to the earlier traumas found to predict PTSD after subsequent traumas (i.e., physical violence victimization and rape victimization); and (3) other respondents (see Table 11.3). These three subgroups made up 22.6%, 10.0%, and 67.4%, respectively, of the total sample. When we classified each WMH respondent using this scheme as of five years before interview and looked at trauma exposure over the next five years, we found a significantly higher rate of new trauma exposure among respondents in the first (71.1/100 respondents) and second (66.5/100) subgroups than in the third subgroup (23.5/100; $\chi^2_2 = 1796.6, p < 0.001$).

We also saw from the trauma-level sample that conditional PTSD prevalence after random traumas was much higher among respondents in the first (10.6%) than second (3.6%) or third (2.2%) subgroups ($\chi^2_2 = 185.3$, $p < 0.001$). Based on these distributions, we estimated that approximately 75.2% of PTSD cases occurred among individuals in the first subgroup, 10.3% in the second subgroup, and 14.5% in the third

Table 11.3 Estimated population distributions of traumas and DSM-IV/CIDI PTSD among WMH respondents (1) with prior PTSD or other anxiety disorders that predict PTSD, (2) with history of traumas that predict PTSD in the absence of anxiety disorders, and (3) other respondents ($n = 54{,}600$)[a]

	Prior PTSD or other anxiety disorders[b]		Earlier traumas but no prior anxiety disorders[c]		All others	
	%	(SE)	%	(SE)	%	(SE)
Percentage of respondents in the sample	22.6	(0.3)	10.0	(0.2)	67.4	(0.3)
Traumas/100 people over 5 years	74.1	(1.3)	66.5	(1.8)	23.5	(0.5)
PTSD prevalence associated with random traumas	10.6	(0.9)	3.6	(0.6)	2.2	(0.2)
Percentage of PTSD cases over 5 years	75.2	(2.1)	10.3	(1.5)	14.5	(1.3)
Number of PTSD cases/100 people over 5 years	7.8	(0.7)	2.4	(0.4)	0.5	(0.0)

[a]The results in the first two rows are based on the total weighted (to be representative of people in the population) Part II WMH sample of individuals ($n = 54{,}600$). The results in the third row are based on the weighted (to be representative of all traumas that occur in the population) random trauma sample ($n = 34{,}676$). The results in the last two rows are based on jackknife repeated replications simulations using the data in the first three rows.
[b]Limited to prior anxiety disorders found to predict PTSD. See the text for details.
[c]Limited to earlier traumas found to predict subsequent PTSD among respondents without any of the prior anxiety disorders that predict subsequent PTSD. See the text for details.

subgroup. We estimated that 7.8 new cases of PTSD would be found per 100 respondents by following respondents in the first subgroup over a period of 5 years compared to 2.4/100 in the second subgroup and 0.5/100 in the third subgroup. The roughly two-fold higher number of PTSD cases in the first than the second subgroup was due entirely to higher PTSD risk after trauma exposure. The nearly fourfold higher number of cases in the second than the third subgroup was due to a combination of substantially higher trauma exposure and significantly higher PTSD risk after trauma exposure.

Discussion

As in the other WMH analyses, the results reported in this chapter are limited by being based on retrospective self-reports and a lay-administered diagnostic interview. Within the context of these limitations, our finding that numerous mental disorders have significant gross associations with PTSD after subsequent traumas is broadly consistent with previous research (Ozer et al., 2003; DiGangi et al., 2013; Sayed et al., 2015). No previous study, though, examined the full range of disorders considered here, although studies of significant pretrauma biological and psychological vulnerabilities predicting subsequent PTSD are consistent with our finding that joint predictive effects are due largely to anxiety disorders (Bomyea et al., 2012; Sayed et al., 2015; Ogle et al., 2016). More direct evaluation of this issue is needed in future studies, though, possibly with a special focus on our unanticipated finding that history of prior anxiety disorders was associated with increased risk of subsequent trauma exposure.

Our finding that prior exposure to some (but not all) traumas is associated with generalized vulnerability to subsequent PTSD is broadly consistent with previous research showing that prior traumas involving interpersonal violence have the strongest associations with subsequent PTSD (Ozer et al., 2003). There are some exceptions to this general pattern, though, largely involving repeat exposures to the same trauma type (e.g., repeated natural disasters) (Caramanica et al., 2015) and also some evidence of variation in these associations depending on age of trauma exposure (Ogle et al., 2013).

The evidence is much thinner regarding whether only earlier traumas resulting in PTSD predict subsequent PTSD after later traumas. As noted in the introduction, Breslauet al. (2008) first documented this specification in a prospective epidemiological sample of young adults, showing that the significant association of a simple dichotomous measure of baseline trauma history with increased PTSD risk after subsequent trauma exposure between baseline and follow-up was limited to respondents with a baseline history of PTSD. No attempt was made to determine whether the association of baseline history of traumas without PTSD varied depending on baseline trauma type. Cougle et al. (2009) subsequently did this in a larger prospective adolescent survey about exposure to assaultive violence (physical or sexual). Among respondents with no baseline history of PTSD, those with a baseline history of assaultive violence victimization were significantly more likely than others to develop PTSD after subsequent trauma exposure during the follow-up interval. Breslau and Peterson (2010) subsequently reported a failure to replicate the Cougle et al. specification in a cross-sectional community epidemiological survey that, like the WMH surveys, assessed PTSD separately for a worst lifetime trauma and for a randomly selected lifetime trauma. However, trauma history was defined only in terms of worst lifetime trauma, which means that some respondents classified as having a history of only nonviolent trauma exposure had in fact been exposed to traumas involving assaultive violence.

Given the potential importance of this specification, it is somewhat surprising that we could not locate any subsequent published studies that carried out more definitive investigations. If the association between trauma history and PTSD after subsequent traumas is due entirely to the mediating effects of PTSD caused by earlier traumas, then trauma history cannot be considered an environmental risk factor for future PTSD. On the other hand, if history of at least some trauma types reliably predicts PTSD after subsequent traumas among individuals with no history of psychopathology, then these individuals could be targeted for intensive baseline evaluations and prospective study of premorbid modifiable biological and psychological vulnerabilities to PTSD after future traumas.

Our results provide the first evidence that at last two prior traumas – physical violence victimization and rape victimization – are associated with PTSD after subsequent trauma exposures even in the absence of a history of PTSD or other DSM-IV anxiety disorders. (PTSD, it should be noted, is no longer classified as an anxiety disorder in DSM-5.) We also showed that a meaningful proportion of the population falls into this subgroup, although only 10.3% of PTSD cases occur in this subgroup. The majority of PTSD cases occur among individuals with a history of prior PTSD or other DSM-IV anxiety disorders (75.2%). The investigation of environmental determinants of individual differences in vulnerability is complicated in the latter segment of the population due to the possibility that these individual differences are due to prior anxiety disorder severity comorbidity. Although this confounding can be addressed to some extent using prospective designs and multivariate analyses (e.g., Ogle et al., 2016), there could be considerable value in replicating results regarding predictive effects of biological and psychological vulnerabilities in prospective studies of individuals with a history of physical or sexual violence victimization, but no history of PTSD or other DSM-IV anxiety disorders.

Our finding that the gross association of trauma history with PTSD after subsequent traumas is due largely to mediating processes involving intervening anxiety disorders is important. We also found, though, that a meaningful part of the association is due to environmental influences on enduring biological and/or psychological vulnerabilities to PTSD after subsequent traumas among individuals with no history of either PTSD or the anxiety disorders that predict PTSD. This segment of the population, which our results suggest is made up largely of individuals with a history of exposure to physical or sexual violence, might be a useful distinct focus of future research on vulnerability to PTSD, given that the individuals in this segment of the population have some as-yet unspecified presumably environmentally caused vulnerabilities that are independent of anxiety disorders. In addition, given the interest in developing PTSD risk models to target preventive interventions (Galatzer-Levy et al., 2014; Kessler et al., 2014; Karstoft et al., 2015), both history of anxiety disorders and history of traumas involving interpersonal violence associated with PTSD among individuals without a history of anxiety disorders should be included as key predictors in such models.

Acknowledgment

Portions of this chapter are based on Kessler, R. C., Aguilar-Gaxiola, S., Alonso, J. et al. (In press). The Associations of Earlier Trauma Exposures and History of Mental Disorders with PTSD after Subsequent Traumas. *Molecular Psychiatry*, copyright Kessler, R. C., Aguilar-Gaxiola, S., Alonso, J. et al.

References

Bomyea, J., Risbrough, V., & Lang, A. J. (2012). A consideration of select pre-trauma factors as key vulnerabilities in PTSD. *Clinical Psychology Review*, 32, 630–41.

Breslau, N., & Peterson, E. L. (2010). Assaultive violence and the risk of posttraumatic stress disorder following a subsequent trauma. *Behaviour Research and Therapy*, 48, 1063–6.

Breslau, N., Peterson, E. L., & Schultz, L. R. (2008). A second look at prior trauma and the posttraumatic stress disorder effects of subsequent trauma: a prospective epidemiological study. *Archives of General Psychiatry*, 65, 431–7.

Caramanica, K., Brackbill, R. M., Stellman, S. D., & Farfel, M. R. (2015). Posttraumatic stress disorder after Hurricane Sandy among persons exposed to the 9/11 disaster. *International Journal of Emergency Mental Health and Human Resilience*, 17, 356–62.

Cougle, J. R., Resnick, H., & Kilpatrick, D. G. (2009). Does prior exposure to interpersonal violence increase risk of PTSD following subsequent exposure? *Behaviour Research and Therapy*, 47, 1012–17.

DiGangi, J. A., Gomez, D., Mendoza, L., et al. (2013). Pretrauma risk factors for posttraumatic stress disorder: a systematic review of the literature. *Clinical Psychology Review*, 33, 728–44.

Galatzer-Levy, I. R., Karstoft, K. I., Statnikov, A., & Shalev, A. Y. (2014). Quantitative forecasting of PTSD from early trauma responses: a Machine Learning application. *Journal of Psychiatric Research*, 59, 68–76.

Green, J. G., McLaughlin, K. A., Berglund, P. A., et al. (2010). Childhood adversities and adult psychiatric disorders in the National Comorbidity Survey Replication I: associations with first onset of DSM-IV disorders. *Archives of General Psychiatry*, 67, 113–23.

Harkness, K. L., Hayden, E. P., & Lopez-Duran, N. L. (2015). Stress sensitivity and stress sensitization in psychopathology: an introduction to the special section. *Journal of Abnormal Psychology*, 124, 1–3.

Karstoft, K. I., Galatzer-Levy, I. R., Statnikov, A., Li, Z., & Shalev, A. Y. (2015). Bridging a translational gap: using machine learning to improve the prediction of PTSD. *BMC Psychiatry*, 15, 30.

Kessler, R. C., Akiskal, H. S., Angst, J., et al. (2006). Validity of the assessment of bipolar spectrum disorders in the WHO CIDI 3.0. *Journal of Affective Disorders*, 96, 259–69.

Kessler, R. C., McLaughlin, K. A., Green, J. G., et al. (2010). Childhood adversities and adult psychopathology in the WHO World Mental Health Surveys. *British Journal of Psychiatry*, 197, 378–85.

Kessler, R. C., Rose, S., Koenen, K. C., et al. (2014). How well can post-traumatic stress disorder be predicted from pre-trauma risk factors? An exploratory study in the WHO World Mental Health Surveys. *World Psychiatry*, 13, 265–74.

Kessler, R. C., & Üstün, T. B. (2004). The World Mental Health (WMH) Survey Initiative version of the World Health Organization (WHO) Composite International Diagnostic Interview (CIDI). *International Journal of Methods in Psychiatric Research*, 13, 93–121.

Knäuper, B., Cannell, C. F., Schwarz, N., Bruce, M. L., & Kessler, R. C. (1999). Improving accuracy of major depression age-of-onset reports in the US National Comorbidity Survey. *International Journal of Methods in Psychiatric Research*, 8, 39–48.

McLaughlin, K. A., Greif Green, J., Gruber, M. J., et al. (2012). Childhood adversities and first onset of psychiatric disorders in a national sample of US adolescents. *Archives of General Psychiatry*, 69, 1151–60.

Nemeroff, C. B. (2016). Paradise lost: the neurobiological and clinical consequences of child abuse and neglect. *Neuron*, 89, 892–909.

Ogle, C. M., Rubin, D. C., Berntsen, D., & Siegler, I. C. (2013). The frequency and impact of exposure to potentially traumatic events over the life course. *Clinical Psychological Science*, 1, 426–34.

Ogle, C. M., Siegler, I. C., Beckham, J. C., & Rubin, D. C. (2016). Neuroticism increases PTSD symptom severity by amplifying the emotionality, rehearsal, and centrality of trauma memories. *Journal of Personality*, 85, 702–15.

Ozer, E. J., Best, S. R., Lipsey, T. L., & Weiss, D. S. (2003). Predictors of posttraumatic stress disorder and symptoms in adults: a meta-analysis. *Psychological Bulletin*, 129, 52–73.

Sayed, S., Iacoviello, B. M., & Charney, D. S. (2015). Risk factors for the development of psychopathology following trauma. *Current Psychiatry Reports*, 17, 612.

Chapter 12

Sexual Assault among Women

Kate Scott, Evelyn J. Bromet, Ronny Bruffaerts, Karestan C. Koenen, Yolanda Torres, and Ronald C. Kessler

Sexual assault, which includes child and adult sexual abuse, rape and intimate partner sexual violence, is a global public health concern (Dartnall & Jewkes, 2013; Abrahams et al., 2014; Benjet et al., 2016) as it is associated with a wide range of both mental and physical health consequences (Gilbert et al., 2009; Jina & Thomas, 2013), including the development of post-traumatic stress disorder (PTSD) (Kessler et al., 1995; Breslau et al., 1998; Maniglio, 2009; Chen et al., 2010). The fact that only a minority of sexual assault victims eventually develop PTSD has made identifying the predictors of PTSD among those exposed to sexual assault a research priority. Evidence of this sort could have both theoretical and practical applications such as the development of targeted interventions. Even though interventions can help prevent PTSD after sexual assault (Kearns et al., 2012; Rothbaum et al., 2012), these preventive interventions are resource-intensive, making it important to have accurate information about which individuals are most likely to benefit.

Prior research has identified a range of predictors of PTSD among sexual assault survivors, including socio-demographics (younger age, female, and less education), assault characteristics (perpetrator known to victim, high perceived threat, and violence), prior mental disorders, prior trauma history, and post-assault cognitions, including self-blame (Nishith et al., 2000; Ullman & Filipas, 2001; Ozer et al., 2003; Ullman et al., 2007; Maikovich et al., 2009; Najdowski & Ullman, 2009; Armour et al., 2012; Möller et al., 2014). However, methodological limitations may have biased assessments of these predictors as many studies were based on clinical or other self-selected samples (Ullman et al., 2007; Armour et al., 2012; Möller et al., 2014). Although community surveys lack this potential for bias, the majority of community surveys that assessed PTSD after traumas used the "worst trauma" method in which respondents were first asked whether they experienced a number of different traumas in their life and then asked to identify their worst trauma; this respondent-identified worst trauma then became the focal trauma. This approach overestimates the conditional risk of PTSD because worst traumas are atypical and presumably carry a higher risk of PTSD than other traumas (Breslau et al., 1998; Norris et al., 2003). As detailed in Chapter 2, the World Mental Health (WMH) surveys addressed this problem by assessing PTSD in relation to a computer-generated random trauma selected from all the lifetime traumas experienced by the respondent. One further limitation of prior population-based studies is that in contrast to the WMH surveys, the data came largely from high-income countries, limiting the generalizability of findings.

Methods

The analysis was carried out in the 12 WMH surveys in 11 countries that had a sufficient number of women with sexual assault identified as their random trauma. These included seven surveys in high-income countries (Belgium, Germany, the Netherlands, Northern Ireland, Spain [both the national survey and the regional survey in Murcia], and the United States) and five in low- and middle-income countries (LMICs; Medellin Colombia, Lebanon, Mexico, South Africa, and Ukraine). In addition to the standard question about age at exposure to the random trauma, these women were asked the identity of the perpetrator (spouse/partner, parent/guardian, step-relative, other relative, anyone else that the respondent knew, or a stranger), whether the assault was a repeated or one-time occurrence, and whether, as they looked back on it, *"realistically (emphasis in original) was there anything you could have done to prevent this from happening?"*

Data analysis used the same range of predictors as in Chapters 9–11: socio-demographics, prior lifetime exposure to other traumas and childhood adversities (CAs), and prior lifetime mental disorders. The analysis methods were also the same as in those other chapters: logistic regression in blocks of predictors with coefficients evaluated using design-based methods of significance testing. Once the final model was estimated, a predicted probability of PTSD was generated for each respondent from model coefficients and a receiver operating characteristic (ROC) curve was calculated from this summary predicted probability (Zou et al., 2007) to quantify overall prediction accuracy (Hanley & McNeil, 1983). As in other chapters, we used the method of replicated 10-fold cross-validation with 20 replicates (i.e., 200 separate estimates of model coefficients) to correct for the overestimation of prediction accuracy when both estimating and evaluating model fit in a single sample (Smith et al., 2014).

Results

Trauma Exposure

A total of 17,970 women in the 12 surveys were asked about lifetime trauma exposure. 12.1% of these women reported experiencing sexual assault at some time in their life, ranging from 1.8% in Spain to 26.1% in the United States, with a mean of 2.4 occurrences per respondent – 14.5% in high-income countries and 8.9% in LMICs (see Table 12.1). These women reported a mean of 2.4 lifetime occurrences (2.6 in high-income countries; 1.9 in LMICs), for a total of 28.8 occurrences per 100 women in the population and representing 10.2% of all lifetime traumas experienced by women in these surveys.

Prevalence of PTSD Associated with Sexual Assault

Prevalence of PTSD associated with sexual assaults averaged 20.2% across surveys (see Table 12.2) and was significantly higher in high-income countries than in LMICs (24.0% vs. 11.7%; $\chi^2_1 = 5.4, p = 0.020$).

Predictors of PTSD

Models 1 and 2

Respondent age, education, and marital status at time of assault were not significant predictors of PTSD (see Table 12.3). Two sexual assault characteristics were associated with elevated odds of PTSD: the identity of the perpetrator, with respondents refusing to disclose this identity (5.3% of respondents) having significantly elevated odds of PTSD (OR 4.8; 95% CI 1.0–23.7); and repeated occurrences (42.4% of respondents) associated with significantly elevated odds (OR 4.6; 95% CI 2.3–9.2). The distinction between rape and other sexual assault was not significant in model 2, although rape had higher odds of PTSD in the model that did not control for other assault characteristics. Perceived preventability was not a significant predictor of PTSD. We elaborated the model to control for the number of years between age at assault and age at interview (to adjust for biased recall related to length of the recall period) and found it was not significant (OR 0.9; 95% CI 0.7–1.2). (The distributions of all these and later predictors are reported in Appendix Table 12.A1.)

Model 3

Preliminary analyses of the joint associations of prior exposure to the 29 traumas and PTSD after the focal sexual assault found that the most stable specification had a single predictor for prior exposure to any trauma (71.6% of respondents). (Detailed results are reported in Appendix Table 12.A2.) Net of the predictors in model 2, this dichotomy had OR 2.1; 95% CI 1.0–4.4 predicting PTSD. Preliminary analyses of the joint associations of CAs with PTSD after the focal sexual assault found that a count of maladaptive family functioning CAs (27.5% of respondents had 1, and 29.7% 2+) was the most parsimonious measure, with OR 1.6; 95% CI 1.1–2.4. (Detailed results are reported in Appendix Table 12.A3.)

Model 4

Preliminary analyses of the joint associations of prior lifetime DSM-IV/CIDI disorders with PTSD after the focal sexual assault found that the number of mental disorders (57.4% of respondents had 0, 22.1% 1, and 20.4% 2+) was the most parsimonious measure, with OR 1.5; 95% CI 1.0–2.3. The introduction of this variable into model 4 led to the OR for prior traumas to become nonsignificant, suggesting that the association of prior traumas with PTSD was partly mediated by intervening mental disorders.

Model 5

We investigated interactions of trauma characteristics and perceived preventability with prior vulnerability factors. The only significant interaction was between prior mental disorders and perceived preventability of the assault ($\chi^2_1 = 6.0$, $p = 0.016$). Perceived preventability was associated with nonsignificantly reduced odds of PTSD among respondents with no history of prior mental disorders (OR 0.2; 95% CI 0.1–1.1) and nonsignificantly increased odds of PTSD among those

Table 12.1 Distribution of lifetime exposure to sexual assault among part II female respondents in the participating WMH surveys ($n = 17{,}970$)[a]

	Percentage of respondents exposed to any lifetime sexual assault		Mean number of sexual assaults among those exposed to any sexual assault		Sexual assaults as a percent of all lifetime traumas		Number of randomly selected sexual assaults
	%	(SE)	Mean	(SE)	%	(SE)	(*n*)
I High-Income Countries							
Belgium	6.5	(1.6)	2.2	(0.3)	7.0	(1.6)	(7)
Germany	13.5	(1.8)	2.1	(0.2)	11.7	(2.2)	(21)
The Netherlands	9.5	(1.2)	2.7	(0.2)	12.1	(1.7)	(22)
Northern Ireland	9.1	(0.8)	2.7	(0.4)	12.9	(1.9)	(18)
Spain	1.8	(0.5)	1.9	(0.1)	2.9	(0.7)	(7)
Spain – Murcia	4.0	(0.9)	3.3	(0.4)	8.9	(2.1)	(10)
United States	26.1	(1.3)	2.6	(0.1)	16.6	(0.6)	(201)
Total	14.5	(0.7)	2.6	(0.5)	13.9	(0.5)	(286)
II LMICs							
Colombia – Medellin	14.6	(1.5)	2.2	(0.2)	8.9	(1.3)	(57)
Lebanon	3.5	(0.7)	1.6	(0.1)	1.8	(0.4)	(6)
Mexico	12.7	(1.3)	2.1	(0.2)	10.8	(1.4)	(29)
South Africa	5.4	(0.6)	1.6	(0.1)	3.1	(0.4)	(11)
Ukraine	10.3	(1.2)	1.8	(0.2)	5.6	(0.8)	(22)
Total	8.9	(0.5)	1.9	(0.1)	5.9	(0.4)	(125)
III Total	12.1	(0.5)	2.4	(0.3)	10.2	(0.3)	(411)

[a] A total of 17,970 women were asked about lifetime trauma exposure in these 12 surveys. Eight additional surveys were excluded because there were no cases of PTSD associated with randomly selected sexual assaults in those surveys. The numbers of randomly selected sexual assaults were small in these surveys: Brazil – São Paulo ($n = 4$), Colombia ($n = 26$), Israel ($n = 13$), Japan ($n = 4$), Peru ($n = 17$), Romania ($n = 5$), France ($n = 8$), and Italy ($n = 7$). Male respondents were excluded because of the small number across surveys whose randomly selected trauma was a sexual assault victimization ($n = 32$).

with such a history (OR 1.2; 95% CI 0.4–4.0). However, the inverse association of perceived preventability with PTSD among respondents with no prior mental disorder was significant in the bivariate model (OR 0.2; 95% CI 0.1–0.7). Caution is needed in interpreting this result, though, as the set of six interactions was not significant overall ($F_{6,71} = 1.1$, $p = 0.36$) and the interaction between perceived preventability and prior mental disorder was only significant at the 0.14 level when we adjusted for multiple comparisons using the false discovery rate method (Benjamini & Hochberg, 1995). The distinction between rape and other sexual assault was also significant in this model.

Consistency and Strength of Overall Model Predictions

We compared overall model fit in subsamples by calculating individual-level predicted probabilities from model 5, estimating ROC curves from these predicted probabilities (see Figure 12.1) and calculating subsample AUCs. As noted in the discussion of analysis methods, we adjusted for overfitting by estimating AUC with 20 simulated replicates of 10-fold cross-validated predictions. AUC was 0.83 in the total observed sample, 0.64 in the total simulated sample, and 0.54–0.69 in simulated subsamples defined by respondent sex, age, and education. Although the latter AUCs are weak to intermediate, the steep slope of the simulated ROC curves when the false negative rate is low means that we would expect a high proportion of cases in other samples to be found among respondents with high predicted risk. Specifically, we estimate that 30.6% of all women with PTSD (sensitivity) would be found among the 10% of women with highest predicted risk if the model coefficients were applied to an independent sample (compared to an observed 40.3% in the WMH data; see Table 12.4). Among the 10% of women with highest predicted risk, we would expect 43.7% (49.6% in the WMH data) to develop PTSD in the absence of a targeted preventive intervention (positive predictive value).

Table 12.2 Prevalence of DSM-IV/CIDI PTSD associated with sexual assault among female respondents with random traumas of sexual assault by survey ($n = 411$)[a]

	PTSD prevalence		Number with PTSD[b]	Total sample size[b]
	%	(95% CI)	(*n*)	(*n*)
I High-Income Countries				
Belgium	96.9	(60.7–99.8)	(4)	(7)
Germany	5.3	(1.0–23.4)	(4)	(21)
The Netherlands	13.3	(3.6–38.9)	(5)	(22)
Northern Ireland	19.7	(6.0–48.4)	(4)	(18)
Spain	55.5	(23.9–83.2)	(4)	(7)
Spain – Murcia	17.2	(4.1–50.3)	(1)	(10)
United States	24.2	(15.2–33.1)	(68)	(201)
Total	24.0	(16.2–31.7)	(90)	(286)
II LMICs				
Colombia – Medellin	8.4	(3.1–20.8)	(6)	(57)
Lebanon	21.9	(4.8–60.9)	(1)	(6)
Mexico	11.1	(2.8–35.0)	(6)	(29)
South Africa	17.8	(5.0–47.3)	(3)	(11)
Ukraine	15.0	(3.6–45.4)	(2)	(22)
Total	11.7	(3.9–19.5)	(18)	(125)
III Total	20.2	(14.3–26.1)	(108)	(411)
χ^{2c}_1	5.4*			

*Significant at the 0.05 level, two-sided test.
[a]Each respondent who reported lifetime exposure to one or more traumas had one occurrence of one such experience selected at random for detailed assessment. Each of these randomly selected traumas was weighted by the inverse of its probability of selection at the respondent level to create a weighted sample of traumas that was representative of all traumas in the population. The random sexual assaults were the subset of these randomly selected traumas involving sexual assault. The sum of weights of the random sexual assaults was standardized within surveys to sum to the observed number of female respondents whose randomly selected trauma was a sexual assault. The *n* reported in the last column of this table represents that number of respondents. The results reported here are for the surveys where at least one female respondent with a randomly selected sexual assault met DSM-IV/CIDI criteria for PTSD related to that trauma. Eight surveys were excluded because there were no cases of PTSD associated with the randomly selected sexual assault: Brazil – São Paulo ($n = 4$), Colombia ($n = 26$), Israel ($n = 13$), Japan ($n = 4$), Peru ($n = 17$), Romania ($n = 5$), France ($n = 8$), and Italy ($n = 7$). Male respondents were excluded because of the small number of men across surveys whose randomly selected trauma was sexual assault ($n = 32$).
[b]The reported sample sizes are unweighted. The unweighted proportions of respondents with PTSD do not match the prevalence estimates in the first column because the latter were based on weighted data. Confidence intervals that include 0.0% as the lower bound were estimated using the Wilson-score method.
[c]The significance of the difference in PTSD prevalence between high-income countries and LMICs.

Sensitivity Analysis

Given that AUC was lower for respondents with adult than with child-adolescent ages of exposure and for those with low/low-average educations in LMICs, the final model, model 5 (see Table 12.3), includes interactions between each of these three potentially important specifiers and the significant predictors in that model. While global interactions were significant with both age-of-exposure and country income, only one interaction was significant in each set (prior trauma exposure with age of exposure of the focal trauma; could have prevented with country income) and both of those interactions were highly unstable (OR 42.7; 95% CI 3.5–525.5 for prior traumas × older age of exposure; OR 208.2; 95% CI 11.7–3721.0 for could have prevented × high country income) and replicated cross-validated model performance was not improved by using this more complex specification than model 5.

Discussion

These results should be considered in light of the same limitations noted in Chapters 9–11. But two of these limitations are especially important here. First, the sample of sexual assault survivors was not large enough to allow the development of a fine-grained prediction model; and second, the data were cross-sectional. Sexual assaults are known to be substantially underreported (Williams, 1994; Widom and Morris, 1997) with unknown effects on the estimates of associated mental health outcomes. The use of face-to-face interviews may have increased the likelihood of nondisclosure of sexual assaults. Retrospective reports of mental

Table 12.3 Associations of socio-demographic predictors, trauma characteristics, and prior stressors with DSM-IV/CIDI PTSD ($n = 411$)[a]

	Bivariate		Multivariate model 1		Multivariate model 2		Multivariate model 3		Multivariate model 4		Multivariate model 5	
	OR	(95% CI)	OR	(95% CI)	OR	(95% CI)	OR	(95% CI)	OR	(95% CI)	OR	(95% CI)
I Socio-Demographics												
Age in decades	0.8	(0.5–1.2)	0.8	(0.5–1.5)	0.9	(0.5–1.7)	0.8	(0.4–1.6)	0.7	(0.3–1.4)	0.7	(0.3–1.3)
Education[b]	0.8	(0.6–1.1)	0.8	(0.5–1.2)	0.9	(0.5–1.4)	1.0	(0.6–1.6)	0.9	(0.5–1.6)	1.0	(0.5–1.7)
Never (vs. ever) married	0.8	(0.3–2.0)	0.5	(0.2–1.4)	0.5	(0.2–1.5)	0.6	(0.2–1.8)	0.6	(0.2–1.8)	0.6	(0.2–1.9)
II Trauma Characteristics												
Rape (vs. sexual assault)	1.7*	(1.1–2.7)	1.7*	(1.1–2.7)	1.7	(0.9–3.4)	1.8	(0.9–3.7)	1.7	(0.8–3.5)	1.9*	(1.0–3.7)
Perpetrator refused (vs. other)	5.0	(1.0–26.1)			4.8*	(1.0–23.7)	4.9*	(1.0–24.0)	5.1*	(1.0–25.9)	5.4*	(1.1–26.7)
Repeated occurrence (vs. single)	4.7*	(2.5–8.6)			4.6*	(2.3–9.2)	4.8*	(2.3–9.8)	5.0*	(2.5–10.1)	4.5*	(2.1–9.4)
III Perceived Preventability												
Total	0.5			(0.2–1.3)	0.5	(0.2–1.4)	0.5	(0.2–1.5)	0.6	(0.2–1.6)		
Without prior mental disorders	0.2*	(0.1–0.7)									0.2	(0.0–1.1)
With at least one prior mental disorder	1.3	(0.5–3.6)									1.2	(0.4–4.4)
IV Prior Vulnerability Factors												
Prior exposure to any trauma	3.3*	(1.8–6.1)					2.1*	(1.0–4.4)	1.7	(0.8–3.7)	2.0	(0.9–4.1)
Number of MFF CAs	1.4*	(1.0–2.1)					1.6*	(1.1–2.4)	1.5	(1.0–2.3)	1.6*	(1.0–2.5)
Prior mental disorders	1.5*	(1.1–2.0)							1.5*	(1.0–2.3)	1.2	(0.8–2.0)
$F_{4,73}$			2.7*		$F_{7,70} = 3.8$*		$F_{9,68} = 5.0$*		$F_{10,67} = 4.6$*		$F_{11,66} = 6.5$*	
AUC			0.69		0.78		0.80		0.82		0.83	

*Significant at the 0.05 level, two-sided test.
[a]Models were based on weighted data. See the text for details. Each model included dummy variable controls for WMH survey.
[b]Values for education ranged from 1 to 4 (low, low-average, high-average, and high) using a country-specific coding scheme described elsewhere.

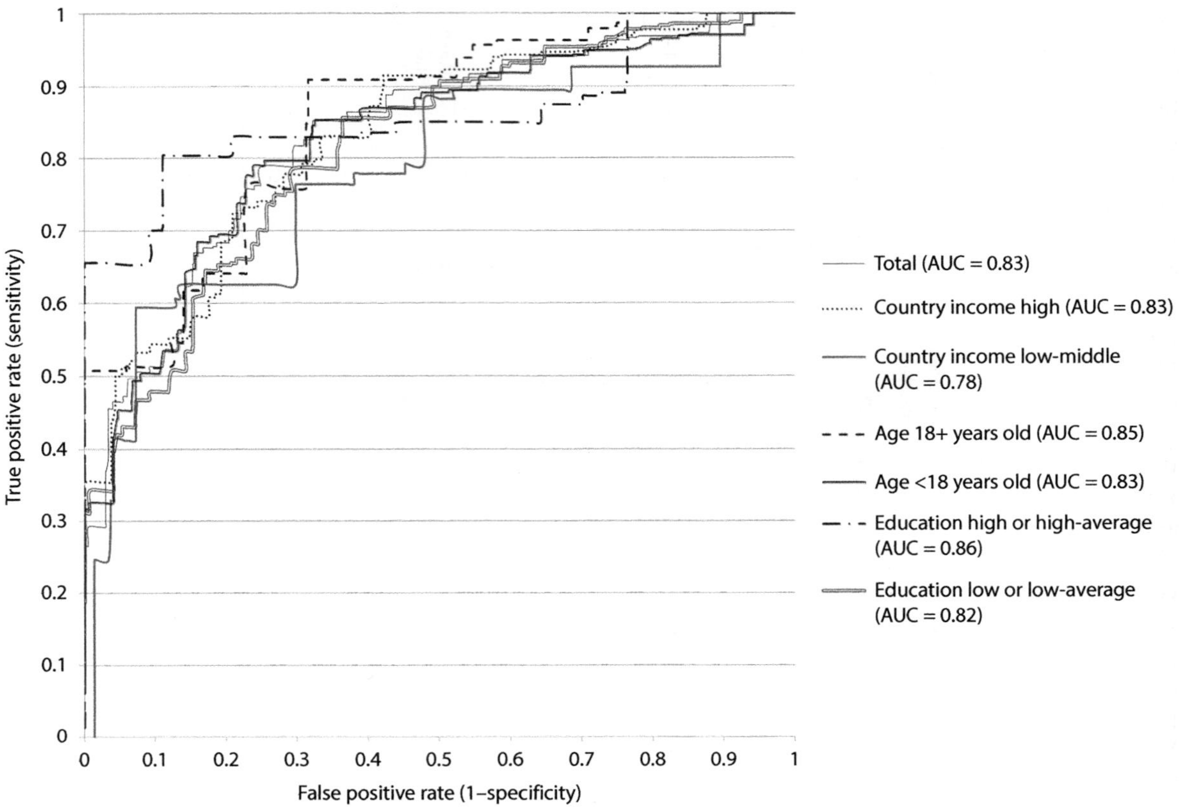

Figure 12.1 ROC curves for the prediction equation in the total sample and subsamples

Table 12.4 Observed sensitivity and positive predictive value of PTSD in the top 10th percentile of predicted PTSD in the total sample and projected values of these statistics in independent samples based on 20 replications of 10-fold cross-validation[a]

	Sensitivity[b]		Positive predictive value[c]	
	% PTSD	(SE)	% PTSD	(SE)
I Observed				
Total sample	40.3	(5.1)	49.6	(8.3)
II Simulated				
Total sample	30.6	(4.9)	43.7	(8.2)
Country income				
High-income	36.9	(5.0)	48.2	(8.7)
Low-and middle-income	1.3	(0.3)	3.2	(1.0)
Age (years)				
<18	36.8	(7.5)	47.9	(8.9)
≥18	8.5	(4.4)	18.4	(9.5)
Education				
Low/low-average	35.4	(6.1)	45.4	(8.5)
High/high-average	4.3	(1.5)	15.9	(8.5)

[a]As model fit would be weaker if the coefficients from this model were applied to an independent sample, 20 replicates of 10-fold cross-validation were used to simulate the expected values of sensitivity and positive predicted value in an independent sample if the coefficients estimated in the current sample were applied to that hypothetical sample.
[b]Sensitivity is the percentage of all PTSD found among the 10% of respondents with the highest predicted probabilities based on Table 12.3, multivariate model 5.
[c]Positive predictive value is the prevalence of PTSD among respondents in the row who are among the 10% in the total sample with the highest predicted probabilities based on Table 12.3, multivariate model 5.

disorders may also have resulted in underestimated prevalence (Takayanagi et al., 2014) and inaccuracies in onset timing (Simon & Von Korff, 1995). Recall of prior lifetime traumas and/or mental disorders may also have differed among those with PTSD versus those without PTSD (Zoellner et al., 2000; Brewin, 2011). In addition, and importantly for our finding about this variable, retrospective assessments of counterfactual preventability cognitions could vary with length of recall.

Despite these limitations, the results provide a rare portrait of PTSD associated with a *representative* sample of sexual assaults as the WMH surveys provide the largest such sample to date. We are aware of only one prior study of randomly selected traumas and PTSD: the Detroit Area Survey of Trauma (Breslau et al., 1998), which was based on 59 sexual assault survivors and found a PTSD prevalence of 49% among rape survivors and 24% among other sexual assault survivors, compared with 20.2% for rape and sexual assault survivors combined in this study. The somewhat higher prevalence of PTSD in the Detroit study may reflect its setting (urban Detroit) and the young age of the sample. The other important sample difference is that the WMH data are based on an international sample in which we found lower PTSD prevalence (in general, not just among sexual assault survivors) in LMICs than in high-income countries. It should be noted that this cross-national pattern is not confined to PTSD, but is also evident in the prevalence of many other mental disorders assessed in the WMH surveys, possibly reflecting a wide range of methodological and/or substantive factors (Scott et al., 2018).

We found that perpetrator identity was a significant predictor of PTSD, although only the undisclosed (refused) type. If we assume that refused disclosure is indicative of a perpetrator who is known to the victim, then this finding is consistent with prior research showing higher PTSD risk when perpetrators are intimates of victims (Ullman et al., 2006; Temple et al., 2007; Campbell et al., 2009). Although we did not find elevated PTSD risk associated with other known perpetrators (e.g., spouse, relatives), this may be due to the inclusion in models of an indicator of repeated occurrence of the assault as repeat assaults are usually perpetrated by intimates of victims.

It is notable that we did not find that a history of prior sexual assaults was associated with increased PTSD risk. While this is superficially inconsistent with prior studies (Nishith et al., 2000; Chen et al., 2010), it is noteworthy that we found that a wide range of prior traumas, including but not limited to prior sexual assaults, were significant predictors of PTSD after focal sexual assaults. It is also noteworthy that maladaptive family functioning CAs were independent predictors of PTSD; sexual assault by a family member was included in the composite scale of these CAs. But our detailed preliminary modeling of both the prior trauma data and the CA data suggests that the role of prior sexual assault history is difficult to disentangle from other related traumas and CAs. This finding is consistent with prior research (Mullen et al., 1993, 1996).

We found that the respondent perception that they could have prevented the assault was associated with a reduced risk of PTSD among women without prior mental disorder, but not among women with prior mental disorder. This is interesting in light of counterfactual theory (Roese, 1997), which suggests that after traumas that provoke negative emotions victims naturally reflect on how things might have been different. These reflections take the form of either "upward counterfactuals" that focus on how things could have turned out better ("if only ...") or "downwards counterfactuals" that focus on how things could have turned out worse ("at least ...") (Roese, 1997). Early research on counterfactual theory suggested that upward counterfactual thinking was distressing in the short term, but adaptive in the longer term because it led to the development of behavioral intentions that generated a sense of future control (Roese, 1997). However, subsequent research among sexual assault survivors has not supported this hypothesis, finding that upward counterfactual thinking, especially self-focused counterfactual preventability cognitions, is associated with increased self-blame and decreased well-being (Branscombe et al., 2003; Miller et al., 2010). Of particular relevance to the present study, however, is our finding that the extent to which upward counterfactuals are adaptive may depend on mental health status. In a study among students (not sexual assault survivors), those with severe depressive symptoms were more likely to engage in unhelpful counterfactuals that were more characterological and less reasonable (Markman & Miller, 2006) than those without depressive symptoms. This might explain why we found that positive endorsement of an item tapping counterfactual preventability thinking was associated with reduced risk of PTSD only among women without prior mental disorder. But this finding needs confirmation in a prospective study of sexual assault survivors that combines the more comprehensive assessment of counterfactual preventability cognitions undertaken in research focused on this topic (e.g., Miller et al., 2010) with the merits of the present study's relatively large general population sample with diagnostic assessment of mental disorders.

The final result of note is that we estimated that 30.6% of sexual assault victims with PTSD would be found among the 10% of victims with highest predicted risk if our model was applied to a different sample from the same composite population and that 43.7% in the simulation of those in the model-classified highest risk group would go on to develop PTSD. These findings are consistent with the more general WMH results reported in Chapter 5 that PTSD can be predicted in the peritraumatic period from information about pre-trauma risk factors, trauma characteristics, and early trauma responses. If this ability of multivariate modeling to predict those at risk of PTSD following sexual assault is borne out in prospective data, it could be of considerable practical value in the development of screening assessments to identify sexual assault survivors most in need of preventive interventions.

Acknowledgment

Portions of this chapter are based on Scott, K., Bromet, E., Bruffaerts, R. et al. (2018). Post-traumatic stress disorder associated with sexual assault among women in the World Mental Health surveys. *Psychological Medicine*, 48, 155–67, reproduced with permission.

References

Abrahams, N., Devries, K., Watts, C., et al. (2014). Worldwide prevalence of non-partner sexual violence: a systematic review. *The Lancet*, 383, 1648–54.

Armour, C., Shevlin, M., Elklit, A., & Mroczek, D. (2012). A latent growth mixture modeling approach to PTSD symptoms in rape victims. *Traumatology*, 18, 20–8.

Benjamini, Y., & Hochberg, Y. (1995). Controlling the false discovery rate: a practical and powerful approach to multiple testing. *Journal of the Royal Statistical Society. Series B (Methodological)*, 57, 289–300.

Benjet, C., Bromet, E., Karam, E., et al. (2016). The epidemiology of traumatic event exposure worldwide: results from the World Mental Health Survey Consortium. *Psychological Medicine*, 46, 327–43.

Branscombe, N. R., Wohl, M. J., Owen, S., Allison, J. A., & N'gbala, A. (2003). Counterfactual thinking, blame assignment, and well-being in rape victims. *Basic and Applied Social Psychology*, 25, 265–73.

Breslau, N., Kessler, R. C., Chilcoat, H. D. et al. (1998). Trauma and posttraumatic stress disorder in the community: the 1996 Detroit Area Survey of Trauma. *Archives of General Psychiatry*, 55, 626–32.

Brewin, C. R. (2011). The nature and significance of memory disturbance in posttraumatic stress disorder. *Annual Review of Clinical Psychology*, 7, 203–27.

Campbell, R., Dworkin, E., & Cabral, G. (2009). An ecological model of the impact of sexual assault on women's mental health. *Trauma, Violence, & Abuse*, 10, 225–46.

Chen, L. P., Murad, M. H., Paras, M. L., et al. (2010). Sexual abuse and lifetime diagnosis of psychiatric disorders: systematic review and meta-analysis. *Mayo Clinic Proceedings*, 85, 618–29.

Dartnall, E., & Jewkes, R. (2013). Sexual violence against women: the scope of the problem. *Best Practice & Research Clinical Obstetrics & Gynaecology*, 27, 3–13.

Gilbert, R., Widom, C. S., Browne, K., et al. (2009). Burden and consequences of child maltreatment in high-income countries. *The Lancet*, 373, 68–81.

Hanley, J. A., & McNeil, B. J. (1983). A method of comparing the areas under receiver operating characteristic curves derived from the same cases. *Radiology*, 148, 839–43.

Jina, R., & Thomas, L. S. (2013). Health consequences of sexual violence against women. *Best Practice & Research Clinical Obstetrics & Gynaecology*, 27, 15–26.

Kearns, M. C., Ressler, K. J., Zatzick, D., & Rothbaum, B. O. (2012). Early interventions for PTSD: a review. *Depression and Anxiety*, 29, 833–42.

Kessler, R. C., Sonnega, A., Bromet, E. J., Hughes, M., & Nelson, C. B. (1995). Posttraumatic stress disorder in the National Comorbidity Survey. *Archives of General Psychiatry*, 52, 1048–60.

Maikovich, A. K., Koenen, K. C., & Jaffee, S. R. (2009). Posttraumatic stress symptoms and trajectories in child sexual abuse victims: an analysis of sex differences using the National Survey of Child and Adolescent Well-Being. *Journal of Abnormal Child Psychology*, 37, 727–37.

Maniglio, R. (2009). The impact of child sexual abuse on health: a systematic review of reviews. *Clinical Psychology Review*, 29, 647–57.

Markman, K. D., & Miller, A. K. (2006). Depression, control, and counterfactual thinking: functional for whom? *Journal of Social and Clinical Psychology*, 25, 210–27.

Miller, A. K., Handley, I. M., Markman, K. D., & Miller, J. H. (2010). Deconstructing self-blame following sexual assault: the critical roles of cognitive content and process. *Violence Against Women*, 16, 1120–37.

Möller, A. T., Bäckström, T., Söndergaard, H. P., & Helström, L. (2014). Identifying risk factors for PTSD in women seeking medical help after rape. *PLoS One*, 9, e111136.

Mullen, P. E., Martin, J. L., Anderson, J. C., Romans, S. E., & Herbison, G. P. (1993). Childhood sexual abuse and mental health in adult life. *British Journal of Psychiatry*, 163, 721–32.

(1996). The long-term impact of the physical, emotional, and sexual abuse of children: a community study. *Child Abuse & Neglect*, 20, 7–21.
Najdowski, C. J., & Ullman, S. E. (2009). PTSD symptoms and self-rated recovery among adult sexual assault survivors: the effects of traumatic life events and psychosocial variables. *Psychology of Women Quarterly*, 33, 43–53.
Nishith, P., Mechanic, M. B., & Resick, P. A. (2000). Prior interpersonal trauma: the contribution to current PTSD symptoms in female rape victims. *Journal of Abnormal Psychology*, 109, 20.
Norris, F. H., Murphy, A. D., Baker, C. K., et al. (2003). Epidemiology of trauma and posttraumatic stress disorder in Mexico. *Journal of Abnormal Psychology*, 112, 646.
Ozer, E. J., Best, S. R., Lipsey, T. L., & Weiss, D. S. (2003). Predictors of posttraumatic stress disorder and symptoms in adults: a meta-analysis. *Psychological Bulletin*, 129, 52.
Roese, N. J. (1997). Counterfactual thinking. *Psychological Bulletin*, 121, 133–48.
Rothbaum, B. O., Kearns, M. C., Price, M., et al. (2012). Early intervention may prevent the development of posttraumatic stress disorder: a randomized pilot civilian study with modified prolonged exposure. *Biological Psychiatry*, 72, 957–63.
Scott, K. M., de Jonge, P., Stein, D. J., & Kessler, R. C., eds. (2018). *Mental Disorders Around the World: Facts and Figures from the World Mental Health Surveys*. Cambridge, England: Cambridge University Press.
Simon, G. E., & Von Korff, M. (1995). Recall of psychiatric history in cross-sectional surveys: implications for epidemiological research. *Epidemiological Reviews*, 17, 221–7.
Smith, G. C., Seaman, S. R., Wood, A. M., Royston, P., & White, I. R. (2014). Correcting for optimistic prediction in small data sets. *American Journal of Epidemiology*, 180, 318–24.
Takayanagi, Y., Spira, A. P., Roth, K. B., et al. (2014). Accuracy of reports of lifetime mental and physical disorders: results from the Baltimore Epidemiological Catchment Area Study. *JAMA Psychiatry*, 71, 273–80.
Temple, J. R., Weston, R., Rodriguez, B. F., & Marshall, L. L. (2007). Differing effects of partner and nonpartner sexual assault on women's mental health. *Violence Against Women*, 13, 285–97.
Ullman, S. E., & Filipas, H. H. (2001). Predictors of PTSD symptom severity and social reactions in sexual assault victims. *Journal of Traumatic Stress*, 14, 369–89.
Ullman, S. E., Filipas, H. H., Townsend, S. M., & Starzynski, L. L. (2006). The role of victim-offender relationship in women's sexual assault experiences. *Journal of Interpersonal Violence*, 21, 798–819.
(2007). Psychosocial correlates of PTSD symptom severity in sexual assault survivors. *Journal of Traumatic Stress*, 20, 821–31.
Williams, L. M. (1994). Recall of childhood trauma: a prospective study of women's memories of child sexual abuse. *Journal of Consulting and Clinical Psychology*, 62, 1167–76.
Widom, C. S., & Morris, S. (1997). Accuracy of adult recollections of childhood victimization, part 2: childhood sexual abuse. *Psychological Assessment*, 9, 34–46.
Zoellner, L. A., Foa, E. B., Brigidi, B. D., & Przeworski, A. (2000). Are trauma victims susceptible to "false memories"? *Journal of Abnormal Psychology*, 109, 517.
Zou, K. H., O'Malley, A. J., & Mauri, L. (2007). Receiver-operating characteristic analysis for evaluating diagnostic tests and predictive models. *Circulation*, 115, 654–7.

Appendix

Table 12.A1 Prevalence of DSM-IV/CIDI PTSD by selected respondent characteristics ($n = 411$)[a]

	Sample characteristics		PTSD prevalence		(n)[b]
	%	(SE)	%	(SE)	
I Age at Sexual Assault					
Children (≤9)	27.6	(3.8)	29.0	(6.2)	(117)
Adolescents (10–19)	51.8	(4.8)	17.8	(4.0)	(207)
Young adults and older (≥20)	20.5	(3.8)	14.7	(5.5)	(87)
χ^2_2			1.8		
II Age at Sexual Assault					
Children and adolescents (≤17)	74.1	(3.9)	21.3	(3.7)	(288)
Adults (≥18)	25.9	(3.9)	17.1	(5.0)	(123)
χ^2_1			0.3		

(cont.)

Table 12.A1 *(cont.)*

	Sample characteristics		PTSD prevalence		(n)[b]
	%	(SE)	%	(SE)	
III Education					
Low	53.6	(4.8)	26.5	(4.7)	(233)
Low-average	21.9	(3.8)	13.5	(4.5)	(82)
High-average	19.9	(4.2)	13.5	(5.9)	(71)
High	4.7	(2.3)	8.8	(7.6)	(25)
χ^2_3			1.1		
IV Marital History					
Ever married	8.9	(1.9)	22.5	(8.6)	(52)
Never married	91.1	(1.9)	20.0	(3.2)	(359)
χ^2_1			0.1		
V Subtype					
Sexual assault	62.3	(4.6)	18.2	(3.8)	(248)
Rape	37.7	(4.6)	23.5	(4.9)	(163)
χ^2_1			1.9		
VI Perpetrator					
Other	94.7	(2.3)	18.9	(2.9)	(397)
Refused	5.3	(2.3)	44.1	(21.4)	(14)
χ^2_1			4.2*		
VII Repeated vs. Single Occurrence					
Single	57.6	(4.8)	10.7	(2.3)	(282)
Repeated	42.4	(4.8)	33.2	(6.1)	(129)
χ^2_1			15.4*		
VIII Respondent could have Prevented					
No	72.5	(4.5)	22.5	(3.6)	(299)
Yes	27.5	(4.5)	14.4	(5.6)	(112)
χ^2_1			2.0		
IX Prior Sexual Assault					
No	92.8	(2.2)	18.3	(3.0)	(387)
Yes	7.2	(2.2)	44.7	(14.9)	(24)
χ^2_1			3.2		
X Prior Other Trauma					
No	35.6	(4.2)	17.6	(3.8)	(231)
Yes	64.4	(4.2)	21.7	(4.2)	(180)
χ^2_1			0.6		
XI MFF CAs					
0 or 1	70.3	(5.2)	18.1	(3.2)	(326)
2+	29.7	(5.2)	25.3	(7.1)	(85)
χ^2_1			1.6		
XII Number of Prior Mental Disorders					
0	57.4	(4.8)	14.1	(3.0)	(243)
1	22.1	(4.2)	27.6	(8.6)	(85)
2+	20.4	(4.0)	29.5	(7.8)	(83)
χ^2_2			3.1		
XIII Total			20.2	(3.0)	(411)

*Significant at the 0.05 level, two-sided design-based test.
[a]Estimates were weighted. Wald χ^2 statistics and *p*-values were estimated while controlling for country.
[b]Denominator *ns*.

Table 12.A2 Associations of individual prior traumas with DSM-IV/CIDI PTSD ($n = 411$)[a]

	Bivariate		Multivariate model 1[b]		Multivariate model 2	
	OR	(95% CI)	OR	(95% CI)	OR	(95% CI)
I Exposure to Organized Violence						
Relief worker in war zone						
Civilian in war zone	3.0	(0.3–30.4)	1.7	(0.1–34.7)		
Civilian in region of terror	1.4	(0.1–27.5)	1.7	(0.1–51.3)		
Refugee	0.0	(0.0–0.0)				
Kidnapped	39.3*	(1.2–1315.0)	34.1	(0.6–2026.0)		
Any	4.4*	(1.0–19.3)			4.8	(1.0–23.5)
II Participation in Organized Violence						
Witnessed death/dead body/serious injury	1.3	(0.5–3.7)	0.9	(0.2–4.7)		
Accidentally caused serious injury/death						
Combat experience						
Purposely injured/tortured/killed someone						
Witnessed atrocities	7.1	(0.6–84.9)	337.1*	(1.9–6114.0)		
Any	1.3	(0.5–3.4)			0.9	(0.3–2.5)
III Physical Violence Victimization						
Beaten by caregiver	1.4	(0.6–3.2)	1.6	(0.5–5.7)		
Beaten by someone else	1.9	(0.3–12.3)	1.5	(0.1–29.6)		
Witnessed physical fight at home	0.7	(0.3–1.6)	0.6	(0.2–2.0)		
Any	1.3	(0.6–2.8)			1.1	(0.5–2.4)
IV Sexual Violence Victimization						
Raped	0.8	(0.3–2.3)	1.0	(0.2–4.7)		
Sexually assaulted	3.8*	(1.1–13.1)	11.5*	(1.5–90.0)		
Stalked	15.9*	(2.5–101.6)	36.2*	(2.3–559.2)		
Beaten by spouse/partner	0.1*	(0.0–0.5)	0.0*	(0.0–0.7)		
Trauma to loved one	0.2*	(0.1–1.0)	0.5	(0.1–4.3)		
Some other trauma	43.5*	(1.1–1716.0)	3277.0*	(6.0–17804.0)		
Private trauma[c]	5.2	(0.4–71.5)	3.4	(0.1–86.2)		
Any	1.6	(0.8–3.4)			1.5	(0.7–3.4)
V Accident/Injuries						
Natural disaster	1.3	(0.5–3.9)	1.3	(0.3–5.7)		
Toxic chemical exposure	0.0	(0.0–0.0)				
Automobile accident	0.9	(0.3–3.1)	0.5	(0.1–3.2)		
Life-threatening illness	1.2	(0.4–3.9)	1.1	(0.2–5.5)		
Child with serious illness	8.3	(0.9–79.1)	1.8	(0.0–118.0)		
Other life-threatening accident	383.0	(0.0–9999.0)				
Any	1.4	(0.7–2.6)			1.3	(0.7–2.5)
VI Other Trauma						
Mugged/threatened with a weapon	3.3	(0.6–19.3)	0.8	(0.1–8.3)		
Human-made disaster	1.5	(0.4–5.6)	1.7	(0.3–10.8)		
UD of a loved one	1.0	(0.4–2.4)	0.5	(0.1–2.2)		
Any	1.4	(0.6–2.9)			1.1	(0.5–2.6)
VII Numbers of Prior Trauma Types						
Any	2.6*	(1.1–6.1)				
1	2.9*	(1.1–7.2)				
2	2.6	(0.8–7.9)				
3+	2.4	(0.9–6.2)				

*Significant at the 0.05 level, two-sided design-based test.

[a]Models controlled for age, education, marital history, trauma subtype, perpetrator, a dummy variable for single vs. repeated occurrence, a dummy variable for whether the respondent could have prevented the rape/sexual assault, and country.

[b]Only the prior traumas with at least one case of PTSD were carried forward into multivariate model 1. There were no respondents ($n = 0$) who reported being a "relief worker in war zone," having "combat experience," having "accidentally caused serious injury/death," or having "purposely injured/tortured/killed someone."

[c]A *private* event is a trauma that some individuals reported in response to a question asked at the very end of the trauma section that asked if they ever had some other very upsetting experience they did not tell us about already (and this includes in response to a prior open-ended question about "any other" trauma) because they were too embarrassed or upset to talk about it. Respondents were told, before they answered, that if they reported such a trauma we would not ask them anything about what it was, only about their age when the trauma happened.

Table 12.A3 Associations of individual CAs with DSM-IV/CIDI PTSD ($n = 411$)

	Bivariate		Multivariate model 1		Multivariate model 2	
	OR	(95% CI)	OR	(95% CI)	OR	(95% CI)
I MFF CAs						
Parent psychopathology	2.1*	(1.0–4.5)	2.0	(0.9–4.6)	2.1	(0.8–5.1)
Parent substance misuse	2.2	(0.9–5.5)	2.7	(0.9–8.2)	2.7	(0.9–8.5)
Parent criminality	1.2	(0.5–3.2)	0.5	(0.1–1.8)	0.5	(0.1–1.9)
Family violence	2.1*	(1.0–4.3)	1.5	(0.6–3.7)	1.5	(0.5–4.7)
Physical abuse	2.2*	(1.1–4.6)	1.8	(0.7–4.4)	1.8	(0.7–4.8)
Sexual abuse	1.8	(0.3–9.7)	1.1	(0.1–8.5)	1.1	(0.1–8.8)
Neglect	2.2	(0.9–5.4)	1.2	(0.4–3.8)	1.1	(0.3–3.9)
χ^{2a}_{7}			11.1		6.5	
χ^{2b}_{6}			4.5		4.3	
II Other CAs						
Parent death	1.4	(0.5–3.9)	1.9	(0.6–5.7)	1.7	(0.5–5.5)
Parent divorce	1.4	(0.6–3.1)	1.2	(0.5–3.0)	1.1	(0.4–3.0)
Other parent loss	1.4	(0.6–3.6)	1.0	(0.3–3.3)	0.8	(0.2–3.4)
Serious physical illness	2.1	(0.7–6.4)	1.5	(0.4–5.9)	1.4	(0.3–5.7)
Economic adversity	0.9	(0.4–2.0)	0.7	(0.2–1.7)	0.6	(0.2–1.7)
χ^{2a}_{5}			2.3		2.0	
χ^{2b}_{4}			2.1		2.0	
χ^{2c}_{12}			13.8		7.7	
χ^{2d}_{11}			7.4		6.9	
III Number of MFF CAs						
1	1.4	(0.6–3.2)				
2+	2.9*	(1.3–6.3)			1.0	(0.2–4.1)
χ^{2}_{2}	8.9*					
IV Number of Other CAs						
1	0.6	(0.3–1.3)				
2+	1.6	(0.6–4.1)			1.4	(0.3–5.8)
χ^{2}_{2}	0.6					

*Significant at the 0.05 level, two-sided test.
[a]The joint significance of the set of ORs for CAs in the group.
[b]The significance of the differences among the ORs within the group.
[c]The joint significance of all CAs in the model.
[d]The significance of the differences among all CAs in the model.

Table 12.A4 Associations of prior DSM-IV/CIDI mental disorders with DSM-IV/CIDI PTSD ($n = 411$)[a]

	Bivariate		Multivariate model 1a		Multivariate model 1b		Multivariate model 1c	
	OR	(95% CI)	OR	(95% CI)	OR	(95% CI)	OR	(95% CI)
I Mood Disorders								
MDD or dysthymic disorder	1.4	(0.6–3.3)	1.5	(0.5–4.5)	1.2	(0.4–3.8)		
BPD (broad definition)	0.1	(0.0–5.0)	0.1	(0.0–9.7)	0.1	(0.0–5.9)		
Any	1.2	(0.5–2.7)					1.0	(0.4–2.4)
II Anxiety Disorders								
Panic disorder or agoraphobia	2.1	(0.7–6.3)	1.0	(0.2–4.8)	0.8	(0.2–3.9)		
GAD	0.5	(0.1–3.3)	0.3	(0.0–2.1)	0.1	(0.0–1.4)		
PTSD	0.9	(0.3–3.1)	0.1*	(0.0–0.9)	0.1*	(0.0–0.7)		
Social phobia	3.7*	(1.5–9.2)	3.6*	(1.0–12.5)	2.5	(0.6–9.6)		
Specific phobia	2.8*	(1.4–5.8)	2.7*	(1.1–6.6)	1.9	(0.6–5.5)		
Separation anxiety disorder	2.1	(0.9–5.2)	1.6	(0.6–4.3)	1.4	(0.5–3.9)		
Any	1.5	(0.8–2.9)					1.5	(0.7–3.0)
III Disruptive Behavioral disorders								
ADHD	4.9*	(1.3–18.8)	4.2	(0.6–31.5)	4.6	(0.6–32.9)		
CD	3.0	(0.4–22.6)	0.6	(0.1–6.7)	0.4	(0.0–4.6)		

(cont.)

Table 12.A4 *(cont.)*

	Bivariate		Multivariate model 1a		Multivariate model 1b		Multivariate model 1c	
	OR	(95% CI)	OR	(95% CI)	OR	(95% CI)	OR	(95% CI)
IED	0.3	(0.0–1.5)	0.2	(0.0–1.3)	0.1*	(0.0–1.0)		
ODD	2.7	(0.6–11.9)	0.9	(0.1–6.6)	0.6	(0.1–4.7)		
Any	1.2	(0.4–3.1)					1.0	(0.3–2.7)
IV Substance Use disorders								
Alcohol abuse or dependence	4.7	(0.5–48.8)	0.4	(0.0–20.1)	0.3	(0.0–19.4)		
Drug abuse or dependence	32.4*	(1.4–727.7)	24.6	(0.3–1765)	27.3	(0.4–1945)		
Any	5.7	(0.7–44.0)					5.4	(0.7–41.7)
χ^{2b}_{14}			20.7		17.9		χ^2_4=4.3	
χ^{2c}_{13}			16.5		17.6		χ^2_3=2.4	
V Total								
Any disorder	1.8	(0.9–3.4)						
0–2+	1.7*	(1.2–2.6)						
1	1.8	(0.8–3.8)						
2+	3.0*	(1.4–6.8)			2.9	(0.5–15.0)		
χ^2_2	7.4*							

*Significant at the 0.05 level, two-sided test.
[a]Models controlled for age, education, marital history, trauma subtype, perpetrator, a dummy variable for single vs. repeated occurrence, a dummy variable for whether the respondent could have prevented the rape/sexual assault, and country.
[b]The joint significance of all mental disorders in the model.
[c]The significance of difference among all mental disorders in the model.

Table 12.A5 Associations of prior trauma or CA exposure with DSM-IV/CIDI PTSD ($n = 411$)[a]

	Multivariate model 3		Multivariate model 3a		Multivariate model 3b	
	OR	(95% CI)	OR	(95% CI)	OR	(95% CI)
I Socio-Demographics						
Age in decades	0.7	(0.3–1.9)	0.8	(0.3–2.0)	0.7	(0.3–1.7)
Education	0.8	(0.4–1.7)	0.8	(0.4–1.7)	0.8	(0.4–1.7)
Never (vs. ever) married	0.4	(0.1–1.7)	0.5	(0.1–1.8)	0.4	(0.1–1.3)
II Trauma Characteristics						
Rape (vs. sexual assault)	1.2	(0.5–2.9)	1.1	(0.5–2.6)	1.3	(0.6–3.0)
Perpetrator refused (vs. other)	4.8*	(1.2–18.9)	4.9*	(1.3–19.0)	5.1*	(1.3–20.5)
Repeated occurrence (vs. single)	4.9*	(2.1–11.6)	5.5*	(2.4–12.6)	3.9*	(1.7–9.1)
Respondent could have prevented rape or sexual assault	0.6	(0.2–1.7)	0.5	(0.2–1.6)	0.6	(0.2–1.7)
III Prior Trauma or CA Exposure						
Prior rape or sexual assault	7.7*	(1.5–40.8)	4.8	(0.9–24.7)	8.6*	(1.6–46.6)
Prior other trauma	1.8	(0.7–4.6)			2.2	(0.9–5.6)
Two or more MFF CAs	2.3	(1.0–5.5)	2.5*	(1.0–6.0)		

*Significant at the 0.05 level, two-sided test.
[a]Each model controlled for survey.

Chapter

13 Motor Vehicle Collisions

Dan J. Stein, Hristo Hinkov, Maria Elena Medina-Mora, and Ronald C. Kessler

Motor vehicle collisions (MVCs) are a substantial contributor to the global burden of disease, with recent estimates identifying them as the fifth leading contributor to disability-adjusted life-years (DALYs) worldwide (Murray et al., 2015). A growing literature based on evidence from MVC survivors recruited from emergency units and hospital wards suggests that MVCs are associated with high posttraumatic stress disorder (PTSD) prevalence (Kuch et al., 1996; Blanchard & Hickling, 2004; Beck & Coffey, 2007; Heron-Delaney et al., 2013; Craig et al., 2016). In contrast, community surveys, including the World Mental Health (WMH) surveys (see Chapter 9), find a low PTSD prevalence among MVC survivors (Kuch et al., 1996; Blanchard & Hickling, 2004; Beck & Coffey, 2007; Heron-Delaney et al., 2013). Nevertheless, as shown in Chapter 23, even a relatively low prevalence of MVC-related PTSD represents a significant global public health problem, given the enormous number of MVCs that occur across the world each year.

Many questions about MVC-related PTSD remain unaddressed. The most fundamental is that the vast majority of studies examining MVC-related PTSD come from a few high-income countries, leaving it unclear whether similar findings hold elsewhere. This is an especially important limitation, given that 90% of traffic deaths occur in low- and middle-income countries (LMICs) and fatality rates are more than twice as high in LMICs than in high-income countries (World Health Organization, 2015). We addressed this limitation in the WMH surveys by asking questions about MVC characteristics thought to predict PTSD (Norris, 1992; Kazantzis et al., 2012; Nickerson et al., 2013) to the subset of WMH respondents for whom an MVC was their random trauma. We also included in the models developed to predict PTSD among these respondents the predictors found to be significant in our other analyses of all traumas (see the other chapters in this section): socio-demographics, history of exposure to other traumas, and history of prior psychopathology.

Methods

The data included in the analysis came from the 13 WMH surveys with a sufficient number of respondents reporting life-threatening MVCs with at least one case of associated PTSD. These included five surveys in high-income countries (Germany, Israel, Spain, the United States, and the regional survey in Murcia Spain) and eight in LMICs (Bulgaria, Lebanon, Mexico, Peru, Romania, South Africa, Ukraine, and the regional survey in Medellin Colombia). Four questions were asked of respondents with random life-threatening MVCs about the circumstances of the trauma found in previous research to predict PTSD after MVCs: whether the respondent was the driver or passenger; the respondent's judgment about whether the MVC was caused by the respondent, someone else in the respondent's vehicle, someone not in the respondent's vehicle, and/or situational factors such as hazardous driving conditions or a mechanical error; whether anyone was killed and the relationship of that/those person(s) to the respondent; and whether anyone (including the respondent) was seriously injured and the relationship of that/those person(s) to the respondent. We also asked whether the respondent was a pedestrian, cyclist, or bystander, but these circumstances were seldom reported and were invariably not associated with PTSD in the small subsample of such individuals in our series. We consequently focused our analysis on cases where the respondent was either a driver or passenger in a motor vehicle.

We also included in the model information about a number of other predictor sets, each of which was more highly aggregated than in the earlier analyses of the total sample. This was because there were far fewer respondents whose random trauma was an MVC in the subset of surveys with a sufficient number of MVCs for analysis ($n = 649$). The first predictor set included socio-demographic characteristics, which consisted of age, education, and marital status – each defined at the time of the random trauma – and sex. Given the wide variation in education levels across countries, education was classified as high, high-average, low-average, or low, according to within-country norms. Details on this coding scheme are described in Chapter 5. The next predictor sets included the respondent's history of exposure to prior MVCs, other prior traumas, childhood adversities (CAs), and DSM-IV/CIDI mental disorders.

Logistic regression was used to examine predictors of PTSD pooled across surveys. Predictors were entered in blocks, beginning with socio-demographics (model 1), followed by MVC characteristics (model 2), prior traumas and CAs (model 3), and prior mental disorders (model 4). This sequence enabled us to examine the extent to which the significant coefficients in earlier models were explained statistically by predictors introduced in later models. As in the other chapters of this section, logistic regression coefficients and standard errors were exponentiated and are reported as odds ratios (ORs) with design-based 95% confidence intervals (CIs). Statistical significance was evaluated using 0.05-level two-sided tests. The design-based Taylor series method (Wolter, 1985) implemented in the SAS software system (SAS Institute Inc., 2008) was used to adjust for the weighting and clustering of observations. Because of the small sample size, design-based *F* tests were used to evaluate the significance of predictor sets; numerator degrees of freedom were equal to the number of variables in the set and denominator degrees of freedom were equal to the number of geographically clustered sampling error calculation units containing randomly selected MVCs across surveys ($n = 416$), minus the sum of primary sample units from which these sampling error calculation units were selected ($n = 284$) and one less than the number of variables in the predictor set (Korn & Graubard, 1990).

Once the final model was estimated, a predicted probability of PTSD was generated for each respondent from model coefficients. A receiver operating characteristic (ROC) curve was then calculated from this summary predicted probability (Zou et al., 2007). Area under the curve (AUC) was calculated to quantify overall prediction accuracy (Hanley & McNeil, 1983). We also evaluated sensitivity and positive predictive value of the model among the 5% of respondents with highest predicted probabilities to determine how well the model implies subsequent PTSD could be predicted if the model was applied as part of a screening effort in the immediate aftermath of the MVC. Sensitivity is the proportion of observed PTSD cases found among the 5% of respondents with highest predicted probabilities. Positive predictive value is the prevalence of PTSD among this 5% of respondents. We used the method of replicated 10-fold cross-validation with 20 replicates (i.e., 200 separate estimates of model coefficients) to correct for the overestimation of prediction accuracy when estimating and evaluating model fit in the same sample (Smith et al., 2014).

Results

Exposure to Life-Threatening MVCs

An average of 14.3% of respondents across the 13 surveys had a life-threatening MVC at some time in their life (see Table 13.1). Proportions were very similar in high-income countries (14.6%) compared to LMICs (14.1%). The typical respondent who had an MVC had more than 1, with means of 1.4 in high-income countries and 1.3 in LMICs. MVCs represented 6.0% of all the lifetime traumas reported in high-income countries and 6.6% in LMICs. A total of 649 respondents across the 13 surveys had an MVC selected as their random trauma, ranging from a low of 17 in Lebanon to a high of 168 in the United States. As an indication of the severity of these MVCs, a serious injury or death occurred in 41.8% of those MVCs in high-income countries and 38.1% in LMICs.

Prevalence of PTSD Associated with MVCs Perceived as Life-Threatening

Prevalence of MVC-related PTSD averaged 2.8% across the surveys that had at least one case of MVC-related PTSD, but was 2.5% when we also included surveys with no cases of MVC-related PTSD (see Table 13.2). A total of 36 respondents across surveys had PTSD associated with their randomly selected MVC. Prevalence did not vary significantly either over the full set of surveys with any cases ($\chi^2_{12} = 8.5$, $p = 0.75$), between surveys in high-income countries and those in LMICs ($\chi^2_1 = 0.1$, $p = 0.71$), within surveys in high-income countries ($\chi^2_4 = 3.7$, $p = 0.06$), or within surveys in LMICs ($\chi^2_7 = 4.7$, $p = 0.69$). It is noteworthy that the eight surveys that were excluded from further analysis because no cases of PTSD were observed (Belgium, Colombia, France, Italy, the Netherlands, and Northern Ireland; and regional surveys in Brazil and Japan) had numbers of respondents with randomly

Table 13.1 Distribution of lifetime exposure to any trauma and MVCs in the participating WMH survey ($n = 23{,}798$)

	Percentage of respondents exposed to any lifetime trauma		Percentage of respondents exposed to any lifetime MVC perceived as life-threatening		Mean number of reported MVCs among those with any		Reported MVCs as a proportion of all lifetime traumatic experiences		Number of respondents with randomly selected MVCs[a]
	%	(SE)	%	(SE)	Mean	(SE)	%	(SE)	(*n*)
I High-Income Countries									
Germany	67.3	(2.2)	9.1	(1.1)	1.1	(0.0)	3.8	(0.6)	(20)
Israel	74.8	(0.7)	11.6	(0.5)	1.3	(0.0)	4.7	(0.2)	(35)
Spain	54.0	(1.7)	14.1	(1.2)	1.3	(0.0)	12.3	(1.1)	(58)
Spain – Murcia	62.4	(1.9)	11.9	(0.7)	1.3	(0.1)	9.6	(1.1)	(39)
United States	82.7	(0.9)	19.2	(0.9)	1.5	(0.0)	6.0	(0.2)	(168)
Total	73.0	(0.6)	14.6	(0.4)	1.4	(0.0)	6.0	(0.1)	(320)
II LMICs									
Bulgaria	28.6	(1.3)	6.9	(0.9)	1.4	(0.1)	12.8	(1.4)	(31)
Lebanon	81.1	(2.7)	12.8	(1.4)	1.3	(0.1)	4.4	(0.5)	(17)
Colombia – Medellin	75.1	(2.6)	18.4	(1.7)	1.4	(0.1)	6.5	(0.6)	(52)
Mexico	68.8	(1.8)	15.3	(1.2)	1.3	(0.0)	6.8	(0.5)	(42)
Peru	83.1	(0.8)	20.1	(1.2)	1.4	(0.0)	7.4	(0.4)	(34)
Romania	41.5	(1.1)	9.3	(0.6)	1.4	(0.1)	10.2	(0.8)	(63)
South Africa	73.8	(1.2)	13.2	(0.6)	1.2	(0.0)	5.1	(0.2)	(52)
Ukraine	84.6	(1.7)	21.1	(1.3)	1.3	(0.0)	7.3	(0.6)	(38)
Total	65.6	(0.6)	14.1	(0.4)	1.3	(0.0)	6.6	(0.2)	(329)
III Total	69.1	(0.4)	14.3	(0.3)	1.4	(0.0)	6.3	(0.1)	(649)

[a]The surveys considered here are limited to the subset of WMH surveys that obtained information about trauma characteristics associated with one randomly selected lifetime traumatic experience for each respondent and in which a sufficient number of respondents with a randomly selected MVC was included for at least one such respondent to have met DSM-IV/CIDI criteria for PTSD associated with that MVC.

selected MVCs ($n = 9$–46) small enough that the 95% CI of PTSD prevalence after the MVC, based on the Wilson method – which allows the CI to be calculated for a sample prevalence of 0.0% (Reed, 2007) – in these surveys included the 2.8% prevalence observed in the five other surveys featured in the analysis.

Distributions of MVCs and PTSD by Socio-Demographic and Trauma Characteristics

The majority of random MVCs occurred to men (59.1%), a plurality (42.8%) during young adulthood (ages 18–29), and a majority during either childhood (11.7%; ages 1–12), adolescence (15.8%; ages 13–17), or middle age (24.7%; ages 30–44) (see Appendix Table 13.A1). Consistent with this age distribution, 66.9% of reported MVCs occurred to individuals who had never been married at the time of the MVC (25.1% currently married, 8.0% previously married). A higher proportion occurred to individuals with high-average (38.1%) than low (27.9%), low-average (20.5%), or high (13.5%) education. Sex, age, and education were not significantly related to PTSD risk, but PTSD prevalence was significantly lower among the never married (1.9%) than among either the currently married (5.0%) or previously married (4.3%).

More than half of the respondents with random MVCs were passengers (54.1%), and the remainder were drivers (45.9%). The majority said someone else was at fault (62.8%), and the others said that either they were at fault (20.6%) or there was no fault (16.6%). Someone was killed in 4.9% of the MVCs, the respondent was "seriously injured" (self-defined) in 31.4% of MVCs, and someone else was seriously injured in 20.5% of MVCs. The driver–passenger distinction and perceived fault were not significantly related to PTSD, but PTSD was significantly more prevalent when the MVC led to a death (11.6%), the respondent being seriously injured (5.6%), or someone else being seriously injured (5.2%) than otherwise.

Table 13.2 Prevalence of DSM-IV/CIDI PTSD after randomly selected MVCs perceived as life-threatening in the participating WMH surveys ($n = 649$)[a]

	PTSD prevalence		Number with PTSD	Total sample size
	%	(95% CI)[b]	(*n*)	(*n*)
I High-Income Countries				
Germany	1.0	(0.0–3.3)	(1)	(20)
Israel	5.5	(0.0–12.8)	(3)	(35)
Spain	1.2	(0.0–3.2)	(4)	(58)
Spain – Murcia	0.2	(0.0–0.6)	(1)	(39)
United States	4.2	(0.0–8.5)	(9)	(168)
Total	3.1	(0.7–5.6)	(18)	(320)
χ^{2c}_{4}	3.7			
II LMICs				
Bulgaria	6.7	(0.0–14.3)	(5)	(31)
Lebanon	2.0	(0.0–6.1)	(2)	(17)
Colombia – Medellin	1.8	(0.0–4.6)	(2)	(52)
Mexico	0.7	(0.0–1.9)	(2)	(42)
Peru	0.5	(0.0–1.6)	(1)	(34)
Romania	1.8	(0.0–5.3)	(1)	(63)
South Africa	5.6	(0.0–13.9)	(2)	(52)
Ukraine	1.5	(0.0–4.4)	(2)	(38)
Total	2.6	(0.8–4.3)	(17)	(329)
χ^{2c}_{7}	4.7			
III Total	2.8	(1.3–4.3)	(35)	(649)
χ^{2c}_{12}	8.5			
χ^{2d}_{1}	0.1			

*Significant at the 0.05 level, two-sided test.
[a]All results are based on weighted data that adjust for between-person differences in number of lifetime traumatic experiences within each survey. WMH surveys that had too few randomly selected MVCs (numbers of such cases are reported in parentheses) for any to meet criteria for PTSD were excluded. These surveys were those in Brazil – São Paulo (23), Colombia (25), Japan (25), Northern Ireland (25), Belgium (13), France (34), Italy (46), and the Netherlands (9).
[b]The Wilson interval method was used to calculate confidence intervals when the lower bound was less than 0.0.
[c]The significance of between-survey difference in PTSD prevalence among surveys in high-income countries, among surveys in LMICs, and across all 13 surveys.
[d]The significance of the difference in PTSD prevalence between high-income countries and LMICs.

Predictors of PTSD

Models 1 and 2

Respondent education was significantly and inversely related to odds of PTSD in the wake of a life-threatening MVC (model 1: OR 0.6; 95% CI 0.5–0.8), while the other socio-demographic characteristics considered (i.e., respondent age and marital status at the time of the MVC and sex) were not significant predictors (see Table 13.3). The OR of being married at the time of the MVC was high in substantive terms (5.7), but was not significant due to the low proportion of respondents who were married at the time of their MVC and the rarity of PTSD. (Prevalence of each predictor and the bivariate association of each predictor with PTSD are presented in Appendix Table 13.A1.) The design effects introduced by the weights also contributed to the wide CI of the OR for being married, although age, sex, and marital status remained insignificant when the model was estimated again, using unweighted data and a statistical control for the trauma-level weight.

Three MVC characteristics were positively and significantly associated with PTSD in model 2: someone dying in the collision (which occurred in 4.9% of MVCs; OR 7.7; 95% CI 4.4–13.4), the respondent being seriously injured (which occurred in 31.4% of MVCs; OR 3.5; 95% CI 1.4–8.8), and someone else being seriously injured (which occurred in 20.5% of MVCs; OR 3.1; 95% CI 1.5–6.3). The numbers of other people who died or were seriously injured were too small to distinguish effects depending on the relationship with the respondent. The other MVC characteristics – whether the respondent was the driver (45.9% of MVCs) or a passenger and perceived fault (20.6% respondent, 62.8% someone else, 16.6% circumstantial) – were not significant predictors.

Table 13.3 Predictors of DSM-IV/CIDI PTSD among WMH survey respondents after randomly selected MVCs perceived as life-threatening (n=649)[a]

	Multivariate model 1		Multivariate model 2		Multivariate model 3		Multivariate model 4	
	OR	(95% CI)	OR	(95% CI)	OR	(95% CI)	OR	(95% CI)
I Socio-demographics								
Age in decades	1.4	(0.9–2.4)	1.5	(0.8–2.6)	2.1*	(1.4–3.3)	2.2*	(1.4–3.5)
Sex								
Female	1.0	–	1.0	–	1.0	–	1.0	–
Male	0.6	(0.3–1.4)	0.6	(0.2–1.4)	0.7	(0.1–3.2)	1.2	(0.2–5.4)
Education[b]	0.6*	(0.5–0.8)	0.6*	(0.4–0.9)	0.7	(0.4–1.2)	0.7	(0.4–1.2)
Marital status								
Currently married	5.7	(0.5–60.0)	6.0	(0.6–61.1)	4.8	(0.6–37.0)	2.4	(0.5–13.2)
Previously married	1.4	(0.2–7.9)	2.1	(0.3–15.3)	1.8	(0.3–11.5)	1.6	(0.3–7.9)
Never married	1.0	–	1.0	–	1.0	–	1.0	–
χ^2_2	2.1		2.6		2.5		1.2	
II Trauma characteristics								
Respondent was the...[c]								
Driver			2.3	(0.5–10.7)	1.8	(0.3–9.1)	1.0	(0.2–6.1)
Passenger			1.0	–	1.0	–	1.0	–
Who was responsible for the MVC								
Fault of respondent			1.0	–	1.0	–	1.0	–
Fault of someone else			2.7	(0.5–14.7	2.3	(0.4–14.1)	2.2	(0.3–14.4)
No fault			3.7	(0.5–29.0)	3.9	(0.4–34.3)	2.3	(0.2–20.4)
χ^2_2			1.6		1.5		0.7	
Death/injury								
Someone died			7.7*	(1.3–45.6)	12.6*	(2.0–80.2)	9.9*	(2.1–45.7)
Respondent seriously injured			3.5*	(1.0–11.7)	3.1*	(1.0–9.2)	2.9*	(0.6–15.2)
Someone else seriously injured			3.1*	(1.1–8.9)	3.1*	(1.5–6.3)	3.9*	(1.9–8.0)
III Prior vulnerability factors								
Prior MVCs (0–2+)					3.2*	(1.2–8.5)	5.1*	(1.4–19.0)
Two or more CAs					10.2*	(1.8–55.9)	3.6	(0.4–31.3)
Number of prior anxiety disorders (0–3+)							4.7*	(2.0–11.2)

*Significant at the 0.05 level, two-sided test.
[a]Based on pooled logistic regression models with 12 dummy variable controls for the 13 surveys. Regression models were weighted and controls were included for survey.
[b]Values for education ranged from 1 to 4 (low, low-average, high-average, and high).
[c]The analysis was limited to respondents who were either drivers or passengers.

Model 3

Controlling for the predictors in model 2, a history of prior MVCs (19.3% of MVCs) was significantly associated with increased odds of PTSD (OR 3.2; 95% CI 1.4–7.7). In comparison, preliminary analysis found that prior exposure to other traumas (55.6% of all MVCs) was not associated consistently with PTSD either when we considered the 20 prior traumas (other than prior MVCs) found to be associated with at least one case of PTSD in a multivariate equation or when we created an aggregate measure of number of prior traumas (0, 1, 2, 3+). (Detailed results are presented in Appendix Table 13.A2.)

As noted in the section on measures, the WMH surveys assessed seven highly correlated CAs, which we labeled Maladaptive Family Functioning CAs (see also Chapter 10). Five other CAs were also assessed. Preliminary analyses showed that even though neither of these two sets of CAs predicted PTSD significantly when considered together, a summary measure of number of Maladaptive Family Functioning CAs had a significant and positive dose–response relationship with PTSD due to a very high OR for respondents who experienced 2+ such adversities (14.7% of all respondents). The OR for this measure of Maladaptive Family Functioning CAs in model 3 is 10.2 (95% CI 2.2–47.5). (Detailed results of preliminary analyses are presented in Appendix Table 13.A3.) One other noteworthy feature of model 3 is that the insignificant association between respondent age and PTSD in models 1 and 2 became significantly elevated in model 3 (OR 2.1; 95% CI 1.3–3.3). More detailed analysis showed that this occurred because age was inversely related to Maladaptive Family Functioning CAs, leading to a suppression of the significantly positive direct association of age with PTSD in model 3.

Model 4

Preliminary analyses found that half of the 14 prior mental disorders assessed in the surveys were associated with significantly elevated odds of PTSD after an MVC in models that added only one prior mental disorder at a time to the predictors in model 3. (Detailed results are presented in Appendix Table 13.A4.) Four of these seven were DSM-IV anxiety disorders – specific and social phobia, generalized anxiety disorder, and prior PTSD. (It should be noted that PTSD is no longer classified as an anxiety disorder in DSM-5.) Two were disruptive behavior disorders (attention-deficit hyperactivity disorder and oppositional-defiant disorder). And the other was major depression/dysthymia. These significant ORs were in the range 5.8–57.1, but had wide CIs due to the rarity of the individual disorders (which were present in 1.6–7.5% of respondents prior to their randomly selected MVC).

High comorbidity among these mental disorders resulted in the joint predictive associations of the 12 disorders other than conduct disorder and alcohol abuse being insignificant, despite many of the individual disorders being significant when considered one at a time. However, a reduced model that included four summary measures of major depression, number of anxiety disorders, number of disruptive behavior disorders other than conduct disorder, and drug abuse found significant joint associations due to a significant OR of number of anxiety disorders in conjunction with insignificant ORs of the other three summary disorder measures. (Detailed results are presented in Appendix Table 13.A4.) Based on this result, the only measure of prior mental disorders included in model 4 was number of anxiety disorders. Each additional anxiety disorder in the range 0–3 (the maximum number of prior anxiety disorders with sufficient numbers of respondents in the sample to estimate a stable OR) was associated with an incremental elevated OR of 4.7 (CI 2.5–8.9). It is noteworthy that the introduction of prior anxiety disorders into the model led to the coefficient for CAs becoming insignificant.

Consistency and Strength of Overall Model Predictions

Although the small sample sizes precluded estimating model coefficients separately in each survey, we were able to compare overall model fit in surveys carried out in high-income countries versus LMICs by generating individual-level predicted probabilities based on model 4 in the total sample and subsamples defined by country income level and respondent sex, age, and education. As noted in the section on analysis methods, the model was estimated 200 times, using 20 replicates of 10-fold cross-validation in order to adjust estimates of model fit for the optimistic bias that exists when estimating model coefficients and evaluating model fit in the same dataset (Smith et al., 2014). Estimated AUC based on this method was 0.75 in the total sample and 0.63–0.85 in the subsamples (see Figure 13.1), all of which represent intermediate levels of classification accuracy (Rice & Harris, 2005). The 5% of respondents with highest predicted probabilities of suicide included 32.0% of all cases of MVC-related PTSD (sensitivity) in the total sample, which is six times the concentration of risk expected by chance. Subgroup sensitivities range from a high of 49.8% in high-income countries to a low of 8.5% among men (see Table 13.4). Positive predictive value (the proportion of predicted positives who met criteria for PTSD) among the 5% of respondents with higher predicted probabilities was 15.7% in the total sample and ranged from a high of 26.4% among females to a low of 3.7% among males.

Discussion

Four limitations are noteworthy. First, traumas and mental disorders were assessed retrospectively. Although the WMH survey assessment procedure used a probing strategy shown experimentally to improve accuracy of timing estimates (Knäuper et al., 1999) and prospective evidence suggests that retrospective reports of traumas are valid (Dohrenwend et al., 2006), respondents with PTSD might nonetheless have been biased toward higher recall than other respondents of prior lifetime exposures and/or mental disorders (Roemer et al., 1998; Harvey & Bryant, 2000; Zoellner et al., 2000). Second, diagnoses were based on a fully structured lay-administered interview rather than on a semi-structured clinical interview. While

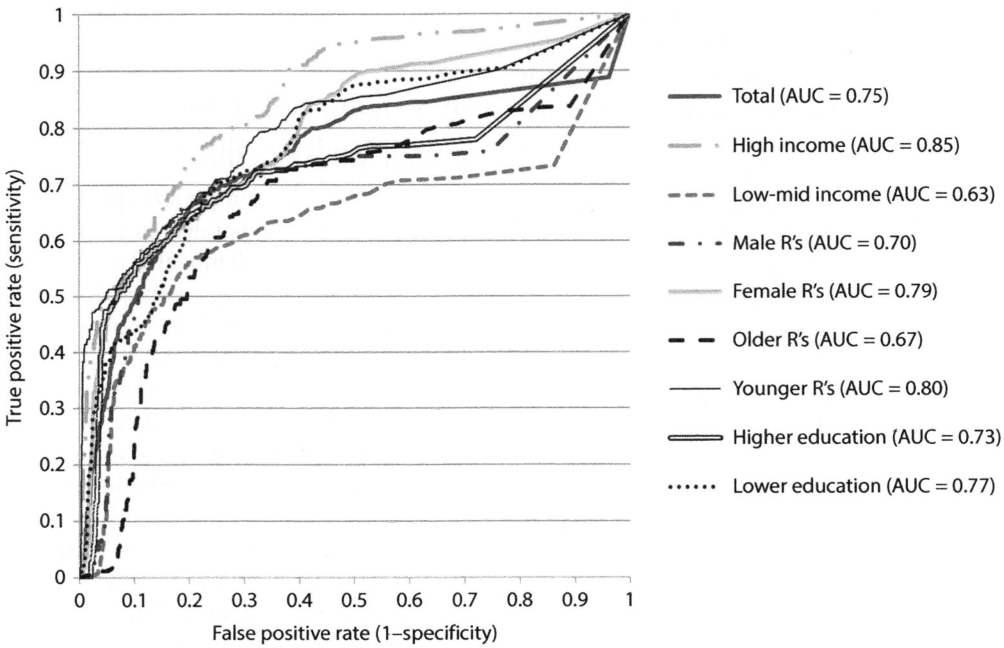

Figure 13.1 Area under the ROC curve for the final model (multivariate model 4 in Table 13.3) in the total sample and selected subsamples

the WMH survey clinical appraisal data are reassuring (Haro et al., 2006), such work was undertaken in only a minority of countries. Third, the definition of a "life-threatening" MVC was left up to the respondent. Although it has been suggested that even minor injuries after an MVC can have significant sequelae (Heron-Delaney et al., 2013; Kenardy et al., 2015), we were unable to investigate this threshold issue because of this imprecision. Nor were we able to examine other psychopathological consequences of MVCs due to the fact that PTSD was the only mental disorder assessed in relation to randomly selected MVCs.

The most serious limitation of the study involves the small number of respondents with PTSD ($n = 36$) in relation to the 14 predictors in the final model. The resulting 2.6 events-per-variable (EPV) ratio (where an "event" refers to the number of respondents with PTSD, not the number with an MVC) is well below the EPV of 10, which is typically recommended as the minimum to avoid biased OR estimates (Peduzzi et al., 1996). Even though more recent statistical evaluations show that this rule can often be relaxed (Vittinghoff & McCulloch, 2007) and that other considerations (e.g., number of predictors, correlations among predictors, clustering, magnitudes of regression coefficients, and selection rules used in building the model) are in many cases more important than EPV in determining model performance (Courvoisier et al., 2011; Steyerberg et al., 2011; Wynants et al., 2015), caution is nonetheless needed in interpreting model results because of the low EPV.

Despite these limitations, our results are valuable in providing the first large-scale cross-national data on prevalence and predictors of MVC-related PTSD. Three findings are particularly noteworthy. First, we found consistent evidence across surveys from different regions of the globe that PTSD is a relatively rare outcome of life-threatening MVCs. Pooled prevalence was 2.8% in the surveys with at least one case of PTSD and 2.5% when including surveys with no cases of PTSD. We are aware of only one previously published study that reported a prevalence estimate that could be compared to ours: the Detroit Area Survey of Trauma in the United States, which, like the WMH surveys, investigated PTSD associated with randomly selected traumas. Conditional risk of PSTD after an MVC in that study was 2.3% (Kenardy et al., 2015). This estimate is similar to the 2.5–2.8% in the current study. This focus on randomly selected traumas is important because more typical studies of PTSD after MVCs are based on samples recruited from patients in hospital emergency departments, among whom there is an

Table 13.4 Sensitivity and positive predictive value of a dichotomous classification distinguishing the 5% of respondents with highest predicted probabilities of DSM-IV/CIDI PTSD from other respondents based on replicated 10-fold cross-validation of the final model with 20 replications[a]

	Sensitivity[b]		Positive predictive value[c]	
	% PTSD	(SE)	% PTSD	(SE)
I Total	32.0	(3.2)	15.7	(2.0)
II Country Income				
High-income	49.8	(4.4)	24.2	(3.4)
Low- and middle-income	10.7	(2.4)	5.3	(1.3)
III Age at Collision (Years)				
<30	47.7	(4.9)	23.4	(3.8)
≥30	17.7	(2.6)	8.7	(1.4)
IV Sex				
Female	48.5	(4.1)	26.4	(3.3)
Male	8.5	(2.5)	3.7	(1.1)
V Education				
Low/low-average	41.7	(4.1)	19.1	(2.7)
High/high-average	14.2	(3.1)	8.1	(1.9)

[a]Ten-fold cross-validation involves dividing the sample into 10 separate random subsamples of equal size, estimating the model in each of the 10 separate 90% subsamples created by deleting 1 of the 10 subsamples, and applying predicted values based on each set of coefficients only to the remaining 10% of the sample. Replicated cross-validation involves repeating the cross-validation process some number of times (20 times in the current application), with a different random split of the sample into 10 equal-sized subsamples each time. Sensitivity and positive predictive value were calculated separately in each of these 200 subsamples and averaged to produce the results reported here.
[b]Sensitivity is the percentage of all PTSD found among the 5% of respondents with highest predicted probabilities based on the final model.
[c]Positive predictive value is the prevalence of PTSD among respondents in the row who are among the 5% in the total sample with the highest predicted probabilities based on the final model.

overrepresentation of MVC survivors with either serious injuries or high anxiety in the aftermath of their accidents (Kuch et al., 1996; Blaszczynski et al., 1998; Blanchard & Hickling, 2004; Beck & Coffey, 2007; Heron-Delaney et al., 2013). It is also noteworthy that PTSD prevalence estimates associated with a number of other traumas in the WMH surveys, most notably those involving interpersonal violence, were considerably higher than the prevalence estimate for PTSD after MVCs (e.g., 19.0% prevalence of PTSD associated with rape and 11.7% with intimate partner violence) (Kessler et al., 2014).

Second, the significant predictors found here were generally consistent with previous research. Exclusion from the analysis of surveys with no cases of MVC-related PTSD did not bias these results, as data from such surveys would not have contributed to estimates of pooled within-survey ORs. Our finding that low education was the only significant predictor of MVC-related PTSD is broadly consistent with a meta-analysis that found low education to be the most consistent socio-demographic predictor of all forms of PTSD (Brewin et al., 2000), although a more recent systematic review focusing specifically on PTSD after MVCs found no consistent socio-demographic predictors (Heron-Delaney et al., 2013). Our findings that death and serious injury predicted MVC-related PTSD are consistent with findings from both clinical (Heron-Delaney et al., 2013) and community epidemiological (Kazantzis et al., 2012) studies. Our findings that being the driver and perceived fault were not significant predictors are consistent with a systematic review of previous studies of MVC-related PTSD (Heron-Delaney et al., 2013), although other work on PTSD has found an association between trauma perpetration and PSTD (Stein et al., 2009), suggesting that more detailed study of the role of posttraumatic cognitions in MVC-related PTSD is needed (Nickerson et al., 2013).

Previous studies of MVC-related PTSD are not consistent with our findings that history of MVCs is a significant predictor of elevated PTSD risk, while history of other traumas is not a significant predictor (Beck & Coffey, 2007). The broader literature has generally found that history of traumas is associated with increased PTSD risk after subsequent re-traumatization (Brewin et al., 2000; Ozer et al., 2003; Kessler et al., 2014). Caution is consequently needed in interpreting our negative result in this regard. If true, our result regarding the lack of an association between history of exposure to traumas other than MVCs and MVC-related PTSD might mean that the trauma "sensitization" or "scarring" associated with MVCs is specific (Lissek & van Meurs, 2014). But another possibility is that the individuals involved in multiple MVCs have other vulnerability factors not captured in the measures of vulnerability included in our model (Stein et al., 1997; Benjet et al., 2015). In comparison, evidence from previous studies is consistent with our finding that CAs predict PTSD among individuals exposed to traumas (Brewin et al., 2000; Pratchett & Yehuda, 2011), although the specificity of this relationship may be low (Kessler et al., 2010). It is notable that in the current study, while CAs were associated with MVC-related PTSD, intervening anxiety disorders partially mediated this association.

Although we found that several prior mental disorders significantly predicted MVC-related PTSD, high comorbidities made it impossible to pinpoint specific disorders as being most important, resulting in the final best-fitting model including a count of DSM-IV anxiety disorders (including prior PTSD) as the measure of prior psychopathology. While meta-analyses of the broad PTSD literature have found that many prior mental disorders predict PTSD (Brewin et al., 2000; DiGangi et al., 2013), a recent systematic review of MVC-related PTSD showed that prior anxiety disorders were especially important predictors (Heron-Delaney et al., 2013). It has been suggested that anxious drivers engage in behaviors that increase risk of MVCs (Clapp et al., 2014). But we are unaware of previous research discussing the possibility that prior anxiety disorders are especially likely to predispose to PTSD after an MVC. One possibility is that the ubiquity of exposure to motor vehicles in the wake of an MVC makes avoidance especially difficult, with hyper-arousal in the face of re-exposure playing a more prominent role in posttraumatic reactions to MVCs than other traumas, possibly leading to prior anxiety disorders becoming especially important in leading to PTSD after MVCs.

Third, our finding that simulated sensitivity of post-MVC PTSD based on our model in an independent sample would be 32% (more than six times the expected value) among the 5% of respondents with highest predicted risk is broadly consistent with several recent more general studies showing that PTSD can be predicted significantly in the peritraumatic period from information about pretrauma risk factors, objective trauma characteristics, and early trauma responses (Galatzer-Levy et al., 2014; Kessler et al., 2014; Karstoft et al., 2015). We are also aware of one prior study that found good prediction accuracy of an index for subsequent PTSD among patients hospitalized after a severe injury (O'Donnell et al., 2008), although not all such injuries were sustained in an MVC. It is noteworthy that it was until recently thought that the effect sizes of individual predictors in epidemiological models predicting PTSD were too low and inconsistent to be clinically useful in targeting people for preventive interventions (Brewin, 2005a), making it necessary to use assessment tools in the aftermath of trauma that focused on current symptoms rather than on risk factors (Brewin, 2005b). The recent studies cited earlier demonstrate clearly, though, that predictions based on multivariate models can be quite robust, even when the coefficients for individual predictors are modest. Whether this prediction strength is high enough to be used in targeting preventive interventions is a more complex question that is beyond the scope of this chapter, as such a determination requires the consideration not only of sensitivity but also of positive predictive value, the costs of treatment, treatment effectiveness, and the valuation of reductions in DALYs associated with successful treatment.

It is important to note that the development of a practical model to predict MVC-related PTSD for targeting preventive intervention would require a much larger sample than the one examined in the current report. Such a sample should be prospective, should include data collected in the immediate aftermath of MVCs, and should follow participants over time to determine which ones developed PTSD. A richer set of predictors than those considered in the current report should be included in the baseline assessment. Machine learning methods should be used to develop the prediction model in order to maximize out-of-sample performance (Kessler et al., 2014). Given the growing literature on the effectiveness of pharmacological and cognitive-behavioral interventions for individuals in the immediate aftermath of trauma (Forneris et al., 2013; Kliem & Kroger, 2013; Amos et al., 2014; Bisson, 2014), including interventions that have specifically been undertaken in survivors of MVCs (Beck & Coffey, 2007; Wu et al., 2014; Guest et al., 2016), our preliminary results suggest that the development of such an optimal prediction model might be of considerable value.

Acknowledgment

Portions of this chapter are based on Stein, D. J., Karam, E. G., Shahly, V. et al. (2016). Post-traumatic stress disorder associated with life-threatening motor-vehicle collisions in the WHO World Mental Health Surveys. *BMC Psychiatry*, **16**, 257, by permission of Springer Nature.

References

Amos, T., Stein, D. J., & Ipser, J. C. (2014). Pharmacological interventions for preventing post-traumatic stress disorder (PTSD). *The Cochrane Database of Systematic Reviews*, Issue 7, CD006239.

Beck, J. G., & Coffey, S. F. (2007). Assessment and treatment of PTSD after a motor vehicle collision:

empirical findings and clinical observations. *Professional Psychology: Research and Practice*, 38, 629–39.

Benjet, C., Bromet, E., Karam, E. G., et al. (2016). The epidemiology of traumatic event exposure worldwide: results from the World Mental Health Survey Consortium. *Psychological Medicine*, 46, 1–17.

Bisson, J. I. (2014). Early responding to traumatic events. *British Journal of Psychiatry*, 204, 329–30.

Blanchard, E. B., & Hickling, E. J. (2004). *After the Crash: Psychological Assessment and Treatment of Survivors of Motor Vehicle Accidents*. Washington, DC: American Psychological Association.

Blaszczynski, A., Gordon, K., Silove, D., et al. (1998). Psychiatric morbidity following motor vehicle accidents: a review of methodological issues. *Comprehensive Psychiatry*, 39, 111–21.

Brewin, C. R. (2005a). Risk factor effect sizes in PTSD: what this means for intervention. *Journal of Trauma & Dissociation*, 6, 123–30.

(2005b). Systematic review of screening instruments for adults at risk of PTSD. *Journal of Traumatic Stress*, 18, 53–62.

Brewin, C. R., Andrews, B., & Valentine, J. D. (2000). Meta-analysis of risk factors for posttraumatic stress disorder in trauma-exposed adults. *Journal of Consulting and Clinical Psychology*, 68, 748–66.

Clapp, J. D., Baker, A. S., Litwack, S. D., Sloan, D. M., & Beck, J. G. (2014). Properties of the Driving Behavior Survey among individuals with motor vehicle accident-related posttraumatic stress disorder. *Journal of Anxiety Disorders*, 28, 1–7.

Courvoisier, D. S., Combescure, C., Agoritsas, T., Gayet-Ageron, A., & Perneger, T. V. (2011). Performance of logistic regression modeling: beyond the number of events per variable, the role of data structure. *Journal of Clinical Epidemiology*, 64, 993–1000.

Craig, A., Tran, Y., Guest, R., et al. (2016). Psychological impact of injuries sustained in motor vehicle crashes: systematic review and meta-analysis. *BMJ Open*, 6, e011993.

DiGangi, J. A., Gomez, D., Mendoza, L., et al. (2013). Pretrauma risk factors for posttraumatic stress disorder: a systematic review of the literature. *Clinical Psychology Review*, 33, 728–44.

Dohrenwend, B. P., Turner, J. B., Turse, N. A., et al. (2006). The psychological risks of Vietnam for U.S. veterans: a revisit with new data and methods. *Science*, 313, 979–82.

Forneris, C. A., Gartlehner, G., Brownley, K. A., et al. (2013). Interventions to prevent post-traumatic stress disorder: a systematic review. *American Journal of Preventive Medicine*, 44, 635–50.

Galatzer-Levy, I. R., Karstoft, K. I., Statnikov, A., & Shalev, A. Y. (2014). Quantitative forecasting of PTSD from early trauma responses: a Machine Learning application. *Journal of Psychiatric Research*, 59, 68–76.

Guest, R., Tran, Y., Gopinath, B., Cameron, I. D., & Craig, A. (2016). Psychological distress following a motor vehicle crash: a systematic review of preventative interventions. *Injury*, 47, 2415–23.

Hanley, J. A., & McNeil, B. J. (1983). A method of comparing the areas under receiver operating characteristic curves derived from the same cases. *Radiology*, 148, 839–43.

Haro, J. M., Arbabzadeh-Bouchez, S., Brugha, T. S., et al. (2006). Concordance of the Composite International Diagnostic Interview Version 3.0 (CIDI 3.0) with standardized clinical assessments in the WHO World Mental Health surveys. *International Journal of Methods in Psychiatric Research*, 15, 167–80.

Harvey, A. G., & Bryant, R. A. (2000). Memory for acute stress disorder symptoms: a two-year prospective study. *Journal of Nervous and Mental Disease*, 188, 602–7.

Heron-Delaney, M., Kenardy, J., Charlton, E., & Matsuoka, Y. (2013). A systematic review of predictors of posttraumatic stress disorder (PTSD) for adult road traffic crash survivors. *Injury*, 44, 1413–22.

Karstoft, K. I., Galatzer-Levy, I. R., Statnikov, A., et al. (2015). Bridging a translational gap: using machine learning to improve the prediction of PTSD. *BMC Psychiatry*, 15, 30.

Kazantzis, N., Kennedy-Moffat, J., Flett, R. A., et al. (2012). Predictors of chronic trauma-related symptoms in a community sample of New Zealand motor vehicle accident survivors. *Culture, Medicine and Psychiatry*, 36, 442–64.

Kenardy, J., Heron-Delaney, M., Warren, J., & Brown, E. (2015). The effect of mental health on long-term health-related quality of life following a road traffic crash: results from the UQ SuPPORT study. *Injury*, 46, 883–90.

Kessler, R. C., McLaughlin, K. A., Green, J. G., et al. (2010). Childhood adversities and adult psychopathology in the WHO World Mental Health Surveys. *British Journal of Psychiatry*, 197, 378–85.

Kessler, R. C., Rose, S., Koenen, K. C., et al. (2014). How well can post-traumatic stress disorder be predicted from pre-trauma risk factors? An exploratory study in the WHO World Mental Health Surveys. *World Psychiatry*, 13, 265–74.

Kliem, S., & Kroger, C. (2013). Prevention of chronic PTSD with early cognitive behavioral therapy. A meta-analysis using mixed-effects modeling. *Behaviour Research and Therapy*, 51, 753–61.

Knäuper, B., Cannell, C. F., Schwarz, N., Bruce, M. L., & Kessler, R. C. (1999). Improving accuracy of major depression age-of-onset reports in the US National Comorbidity Survey. *International Journal of Methods in Psychiatric Research*, 8, 39–48.

Korn, E., & Graubard, B. (1990). Simultaneous testing of regression coefficients with complex survey data:

use of the Bonferroni t statistics. *The American Statistician*, 44, 270–6.
Kuch, K., Cox, B. J., & Evans, R. J. (1996). Posttraumatic stress disorder and motor vehicle accidents: a multidisciplinary overview. *Canadian Journal of Psychiatry. Revue Canadienne de Psychiatrie*, 41, 429–34.
Lissek, S., & van Meurs, B. (2014). Learning models of PTSD: theoretical accounts and psychobiological evidence. *International Journal of Psychophysiology*, 98, 594–605.
Murray, C. J., Barber, R. M., Foreman, K. J., et al. (2015). Global, regional, and national disability-adjusted life years (DALYs) for 306 diseases and injuries and healthy life expectancy (HALE) for 188 countries, 1990–2013: quantifying the epidemiological transition. *Lancet*, 386, 2145–91.
Nickerson, A., Aderka, I. M., Bryant, R. A., & Hofmann, S. G. (2013). The role of attribution of trauma responsibility in posttraumatic stress disorder following motor vehicle accidents. *Depression and Anxiety*, 30, 483–8.
Norris, F. H. (1992). Epidemiology of trauma: frequency and impact of different potentially traumatic events on different demographic groups. *Journal of Consulting and Clinical Psychology*, 60, 409–18.
O'Donnell, M. L., Creamer, M. C., Parslow, R., et al. (2008). A predictive screening index for posttraumatic stress disorder and depression following traumatic injury. *Journal of Consulting and Clinical Psychology*, 76, 923–32.
Ozer, E. J., Best, S. R., Lipsey, T. L., & Weiss, D. S. (2003). Predictors of posttraumatic stress disorder and symptoms in adults: a meta-analysis. *Psychological Bulletin*, 129, 52–73.
Peduzzi, P., Concato, J., Kemper, E., Holford, T. R., & Feinstein, A. R. (1996). A simulation study of the number of events per variable in logistic regression analysis. *Journal of Clinical Epidemiology*, 49, 1373–79.
Pratchett, L. C., & Yehuda, R. (2011). Foundations of posttraumatic stress disorder: does early life trauma lead to adult posttraumatic stress disorder? *Development and Psychopathology*, 23, 477–91.
Reed, J. F. I. (2007). Better binomial confidence intervals. *Journal of Modern Applied Statistical Methods*, 6, 153–61.
Rice, M. E., & Harris, G. T. (2005). Comparing effect sizes in follow-up studies: ROC Area, Cohen's d, and r. *Law and Human Behavior*, 29, 615–20.
Roemer, L., Litz, B. T., Orsillo, S. M., Ehlich, P. J., & Friedman, M. J. (1998). Increases in retrospective accounts of war-zone exposure over time: the role of PTSD symptom severity. *Journal of Traumatic Stress*, 11, 597–605.
SAS Institute Inc. (2008). *SAS Software, Version 9.2*. Cary, NC: SAS Institute Inc.
Smith, G. C., Seaman, S. R., Wood, A. M., Royston, P., & White, I. R. (2014). Correcting for optimistic prediction in small data sets. *American Journal of Epidemiology*, 180, 318–24.
Stein, D. J., Boshoff, D., Traut, A., et al. (1997). Patients presenting with fresh trauma after interpersonal violence. Part II. Assault history. *South African Medical Journal*, 87, 999–1000.
Stein, D. J., Williams, S. L., Jackson, P. B., et al. (2009). Perpetration of gross human rights violations in South Africa: association with psychiatric disorders. *South African Medical Journal*, 99, 390–5.
Steyerberg, E. W., Schemper, M., & Harrell, F. E. (2011). Logistic regression modeling and the number of events per variable: selection bias dominates. *Journal of Clinical Epidemiology*, 64, 1464–65; author reply 1463–64.
Vittinghoff, E., & McCulloch, C. E. (2007). Relaxing the rule of ten events per variable in logistic and Cox regression. *American Journal of Epidemiology*, 165, 710–8.
Wolter, K. M. (1985). *Introduction to Variance Estimation*. New York, NY: Springer-Verlag.
World Health Organization (2015). *Global Status Report on Road Safety 2015*. Geneva, Switzerland: WHO.
Wu, K. K., Li, F. W., & Cho, V. W. (2014). A randomized controlled trial of the effectiveness of brief-CBT for patients with symptoms of posttraumatic stress following a motor vehicle crash. *Behavioural and Cognitive Psychotherapy*, 42, 31–47.
Wynants, L., Bouwmeester, W., Moons, K. G., et al. (2015). A simulation study of sample size demonstrated the importance of the number of events per variable to develop prediction models in clustered data. *Journal of Clinical Epidemiology*, 68, 1406–14.
Zoellner, L. A., Foa, E. B., Brigidi, B. D., & Przeworski, A. (2000). Are trauma victims susceptible to "false memories"? *Journal of Abnormal Psychology*, 109, 517–24.
Zou, K. H., O'Malley, A. J., & Mauri, L. (2007). Receiver-operating characteristic analysis for evaluating diagnostic tests and predictive models. *Circulation*, 115, 654–7.

Appendix

Table 13.A1 Sample distribution and prevalence of DSM-IV/CIDI PTSD by selected socio-demographic and collision-specific characteristics, weighted analysis ($n = 649$)[a]

	Distribution of PTSD			Sample characteristics	
	%	(SE)	(*n*)	%	(SE)
I Age at Collision					
Children (1–12)	0.0	–	(43)	11.7	(3.3)
Adolescents (13–17)	0.8	(0.6)	(99)	15.8	(3.2)
Young adult (18–29)	2.9	(1.3)	(271)	42.8	(4.1)
Middle age (30–44)	3.9	(1.8)	(156)	24.7	(4.2)
Older (45+)	10.5	(4.3)	(80)	5.0	(0.9)
χ^2_4	6.7				
II Sex					
Female	4.1	(1.5)	(331)	40.9	(4.2)
Male	2.0	(0.8)	(318)	59.1	(4.2)
χ^2_1	1.6				
III Education					
Low	2.7	(1.1)	(161)	27.9	(4.1)
Low average	5.3	(2.7)	(157)	20.5	(3.0)
High average	2.2	(1.1)	(224)	38.1	(4.2)
High	1.2	(0.8)	(107)	13.5	(2.5)
χ^2_3	4.6				
IV Marital Status					
Currently married	5.0	(2.4)	(183)	25.1	(4.1)
Previously married	4.3	(2.8)	(62)	8.0	(2.1)
Never married	1.9	(0.7)	(404)	66.9	(4.2)
χ^2_2	10.1*				
V Role of Respondent					
Passenger	2.3	(0.8)	(364)	54.1	(4.2)
Driver	3.5	(1.3)	(285)	45.9	(4.2)
χ^2_1	1.0				
VI Who was At Fault					
Respondent	1.3	(0.8)	(116)	20.6	(3.3)
Someone else	3.2	(1.1)	(404)	62.8	(4.0)
No fault/weather/missing	3.4	(1.6)	(129)	16.6	(2.9)
χ^2_2	1.5				
VII Anyone Killed?					
No	2.4	(0.6)	(609)	95.1	(1.7)
Yes	11.6	(7.4)	(40)	4.9	(1.7)
χ^2_1	6.8*				
VIII Respondent Injured?					
No	1.6	(0.5)	(415)	68.6	(3.9)
Yes	5.6	(2.2)	(234)	31.4	(3.9)
χ^2_1	8.3*				
IX Someone Else Injured?					
No	2.2	(0.8)	(522)	79.5	(3.7)
Yes	5.2	(2.2)	(127)	20.5	(3.7)
χ^2_1	4.3*				
X Prior Collisions					
0	2.3	(0.6)	(604)	80.7	(3.9)
1	1.4	(1.0)	(32)	13.0	(3.5)
2+	12.6	(8.9)	(13)	6.3	(2.3)
χ^2_2	7.9*				

(cont.)

Table 13.A1 *(cont.)*

	Distribution of PTSD			Sample characteristics	
	%	(SE)	(*n*)	%	(SE)
XI Prior Trauma Types					
0	2.3	(0.9)	(428)	44.4	(4.1)
1	1.7	(0.8)	(111)	32.3	(4.6)
2	5.5	(2.5)	(110)	23.2	(3.3)
χ^2_2	6.8*				
XII Number of CAs					
0	2.1	(0.7)	(502)	73.1	(3.6)
1	2.3	(1.6)	(87)	12.2	(2.3)
2	7.0	(3.8)	(60)	14.7	(3.2)
χ^2_2	7.9*				
XIII Number of Anxiety Disorders					
0	1.5	(0.6)	(525)	82.4	(3.0)
1	5.0	(2.2)	(91)	10.8	(2.1)
2	4.0	(3.4)	(18)	4.2	(2.1)
3+	33.8	(16.5)	(15)	2.6	(0.9)
χ^2_3	23.5*				
XIV Total	2.8	(0.8)	(649)		

*Significant at the 0.05 level, two-sided test.
[a]The analysis is limited to respondents who were either drivers or passengers in motor vehicles. All results are based on weighted data. See the text for a description of the weighting procedures. CIs for subgroups in which weighted prevalence estimates were less than two times the design-based SEs of these estimates were estimated using the Wilson score interval method.

Table 13.A2 Associations of individual prior traumas with DSM-IV/CIDI PTSD after randomly selected MVCs in the total sample (*n* = 649)[a]

	Bivariate		Multivariate model 1		Multivariate model 2	
	OR	(95% CI)	OR	(95% CI)	OR	(95% CI)
I Exposure to Organized Violence						
Relief worker in war zone						
Civilian in war zone	0.9	(0.3–3.0)	0.7	(0.1–3.5)		
Civilian in region of terror	0.9	(0.1–6.8)	1.2	(0.3–5.8)		
Refugee	1.4	(0.3–7.4)	0.3	(0.1–2.1)		
Kidnapped	0.0	(0.0–0.0)				
Any	1.0	(0.5–2.1)			0.8	(0.4–1.6)
II Participation in Organized Violence						
Witnessed death/dead body/serious injury	4.5*	(1.4–14.6)	0.7	(0.3–2.0)		
Accidentally cause injury/death	0.0	(0.0–0.0)				
Combat experience	0.0	(0.0–0.0)				
Purposefully injured/tortured/killed someone	0.0	(0.0–0.0)				
Witnessed atrocities	1.0	(0.1–12.3)	2.5	(0.4–17.8)		
Any	3.7	(1.1–12.5)			2.1	(0.7–5.9)
III Physical Violence Victimization						
Beaten by caregiver	5.3	(0.7–37.9)	0.6	(0.1–3.0)		
Beaten by someone else	0.0	(0.0–0.0)				
Witnessed physical fight at home	35.6*	(8.2–154.4)	54.1*	(9.5–309.0)		
Any	8.2*	(1.7–40.3)			5.4*	(1.4–21.6)
IV Sexual Violence Victimization						
Raped	10.4*	(2.0–55.3)	1.9	(0.4–8.4)		
Sexually assaulted	0.6	(0.1–5.4)	0.1	(0.0–0.2)		
Stalked	0.0	(0.0–0.0)				
Beaten by spouse/romantic partner	1.5	(0.0–44.4)	2.3	(0.2–27.6)		
Trauma to loved one	10.5*	(1.6–69.1)	1.4	(0.0–271.3)		
Some other trauma	0.0	(0.0–0.0)				
Private trauma[b]	2.8	(0.2–35.2)	57.0*	(2.0–1632)		
Any	2.2	(0.6–8.1)			1.3	(0.4–3.9)

(cont.)

Table 13.A2 *(cont.)*

	Bivariate		Multivariate model 1		Multivariate model 2	
	OR	(95% CI)	OR	(95% CI)	OR	(95% CI)
V Accident/Injuries						
Natural disaster	7.4*	(1.7–32.2)	3.7	(0.9–14.8)		
Toxic chemical exposure	0.5	(0.0–10.4)	0.1	(0.0–1.3)		
Automobile collision	3.9*	(1.6–9.6)	4.1*	(1.7–9.5)		
Life-threatening illness	9.3*	(2.6–33.7)	9.7*	(2.0–48.0)		
Child with serious illness	0.6	(0.0–12.7)	0.1	(0.0–21.1)		
Other life-threatening accident	0.3	(0.0–5.7)	0.2	(0.0–3.5)		
Any	1.4	(0.6–3.5)			1.0	(0.3–2.8)
VI Other						
Mugged/threatened with a weapon	2.9	(0.9–9.5)	1.4	(0.2–9.1)		
Human-made disaster	1.0	(0.1–9.6)	0.8	(0.0–36.7)		
UD of a loved one	1.2	(0.2–5.6)	2.4	(0.8–6.9)		
Any	1.5	(0.3–7.4)			1.5	(0.4–5.9)
$F_{21,112}$[c]			9.4*		$F_{6,127} = 2.0$	
$F_{20,113}$[d]			9.4*		$F_{5,128} = 1.5$	
VII Numbers of Prior Traumatic Experience Types						
Any	1.2	(0.6–2.4)				
1	0.7	(0.2–2.3)				
2	0.5	(0.1–1.9)				
3+	3.4	(1.4–6.0)				
$F_{3,130}$	3.8*					

*Significant at the 0.05 level, two-sided test.

[a]All models controlled for the predictors in multivariate model 2 in the main text. Multivariate models excluded prior traumatic experiences with no case of PTSD after the randomly selected MVC. Models were based on weighted data. See the text for a description of weighting procedures.

[b]A *private* event is a trauma that some individuals reported in response to a question asked at the very end of the trauma section that asked if they ever had some other very upsetting experience they did not tell us about already (and this includes in response to a prior open-ended question about "any other" trauma) because they were too embarrassed or upset to talk about it. Respondents were told, before they answered, that if they reported such a trauma we would not ask them anything about what it was, only about their age when the trauma happened.

[c]The joint significance of all the traumas in the model.

[d]The significance of differences among all traumas in the model.

Table 13.A3 Associations of CAs with DSM-IV/CIDI PTSD after randomly selected MVCs in the total sample ($n = 649$)[a]

	Bivariate		Multivariate model 1		Multivariate model 2	
	OR	(95% CI)	OR	(95% CI)	OR	(95% CI)
I MFF CA						
Parental psychopathology	1.7	(0.3–10.1)	0.5	(0.1–5.7)	0.5	(0.1–5.8)
Parental substance misuse	3.3	(0.6–18.0)	1.9	(0.2–15.8)	2.1	(0.2–29.1)
Parental criminality	10.6*	(1.9–60.3)	4.0*	(0.3–45.0)	2.6	(0.2–40.4)
Family violence	14.2*	(2.5–79.8)	5.4*	(0.6–48.5)	4.5	(0.3–62.7)
Physical abuse	6.4*	(1.2–33.1)	0.4	(0.0–4.8)	0.3*	(0.0–4.0)
Sexual abuse	12.8*	(2.0–83.5)	1.4	(0.1–22.8)	1.3	(0.1–21.8)
Neglect	20.9*	(3.4–128.9)	9.5*	(0.9–105.2)	7.7*	(0.6–95.0)
χ^{2b}_{7}			11.6		4.9	
χ^{2c}_{6}			4.7		4.3	
II Other CA						
Parent death	0.8	(0.1–4.3)	1.1	(0.1–8.7)	0.8	(0.1–8.0)
Parent divorce	6.0*	(1.1–32.1)	0.7	(0.1–10.1)	0.4	(0.0–9.4)
Other parent loss	0.0	(0.0–0.0)				
Serious physical illness	2.4	(0.4–12.8)	3.1	(0.3–28.0)	2.6	(0.3–26.2)

(cont.)

Table 13.A3 *(cont.)*

	Bivariate		Multivariate model 1		Multivariate model 2	
	OR	(95% CI)	OR	(95% CI)	OR	(95% CI)
Family economic adversity	0.6	(0.1–5.4)	0.6	(0.0–10.5)	0.3	(0.0–9.0)
χ^{2b}_{4}			1.2		1.5	
χ^{2c}_{3}			1.1		1.5	
χ^{2d}_{11}			15.6		7.4	
III Number of MFF CAs						
1	1.5	(0.2–13.7)				
2+	12.8*	(2.1–76.8)			1.8	(0.2–15.6)
χ^{2b}_{2}	8.1*				0.1	
IV Number of Other CAs						
1	0.4	(0.1–2.3)				
2+	4.3	(0.7–24.7)			4.5	(0.1–181.1)
χ^{2b}_{2}	5.4				0.6	

*Significant at the 0.05 level, two-sided test.
[a]All models controlled for the predictors in multivariate model 2 in the main text. Multivariate models excluded CAs associated with no case of PTSD after the randomly selected MVC. Models were based on weighted data. See the text for a description of weighting procedures.
[b]The joint significance of the set of ORs for CAs in the group.
[c]The significance of the differences among the ORs within the group.
[d]The joint significance of all CAs in the model.

Table 13.A4 Associations of prior DSM-IV/CIDI mental disorders with DSM-IV/CIDI PTSD after randomly selected MVCs in the total sample ($n = 649$)[a]

	Bivariate		Multivariate model 1		Multivariate model 2		Multivariate model 3		Multivariate model 4	
	OR	(95% CI)	OR	(95% CI)	OR	(95% CI)	OR	(95% CI)	OR	(95% CI)
I Mood Disorders										
MDD or dysthymia	5.8*	(1.6–21.0)	0.9	(0.1–9.0)	0.7	(0.1–7.1)				
BPD (broad definition)	0.9	(0.1–15.1)	7.8	(0.1–531.6)	5.9	(0.1–395.0)				
Any mood	4.1*	(1.1–15.0)					0.7	(0.1–4.7)	0.8	(0.1–5.2)
II Anxiety Disorders										
Panic disorder or agoraphobia	0.2	(0.0–5.3)	0.0*	(0.0–0.6)	0.0	(0.0–1.1)				
GAD	14.7*	(3.3–65.6)	2.8	(0.2–41.8)	1.7	(0.1–32.9)				
PTSD	14.1*	(2.6–75.3)	19.4*	(1.1–333.1)	14.0	(0.7–276.9)			1.0	(0.8–19.7)
Social phobia	57.1*	(6.7–488.0)	212.1*	(9.3–4830.0)	129.0*	(5.0–3346.0)				
Specific phobia	6.8*	(1.4–32.3)	2.1	(0.1–34.5)	2.6	(0.1–51.9)				
Separation anxiety disorder	3.9	(0.2–60.8)	0.2	(0.0–21.6)	0.3	(0.0–32.0)				
Number	4.5*	(2.1–9.5)					3.9*	(1.5–10.2)	3.9	(0.8–19.7)
III Disruptive Behavioral Disorders										
ADHD	18.9*	(3.0–118.1)	0.1	(0.0–84.7)	0.1	(0.0–131.6)				
CD	0.0	(0.0–0.0)								
IED	2.5	(0.3–23.7)	0.4	(0.0–17.8)	0.3	(0.0–11.0)				
ODD	30.6*	(4.9–191.9)	45.5	(0.4–5004.0)	41.5	(0.4–4698.0)				
Number	3.6*	(1.7–7.6)					1.9	(0.7–5.3)	2.3	(0.6–8.0)

(con

Table 13.A4 *(cont.)*

	Bivariate		Multivariate model 1		Multivariate model 2		Multivariate model 3		Multivariate model 4	
	OR	(95% CI)	OR	(95% CI)	OR	(95% CI)	OR	(95% CI)	OR	(95% CI)
IV Substance Use Disorders										
Alcohol abuse or dependence	0.0	(0.0–0.0)								
Drug abuse or dependence	3.1	(0.7–14.9)	0.0	(0.0–0.0)	0.0	(0.0–0.0)				
Any	2.7	(0.6–12.6)					1.0	(0.2–5.2)	1.1	(0.2–6.8)
$\chi^{2\,b}_{12}$			18.6		11.5		χ^2_4=15.8			
$\chi^{2\,c}_{11}$			13.3		11.1				χ^2_4=3.6	
V Total										
Any	8.9*	(2.4–30.4)								
1	4.9*	(0.9–17.7)								
2	27.3*	(3.7–187.8)			3.9	(0.2–78.9)			3.6	(0.2–52.1)
3+	35.0*	(7.3–443.7)			2.0	(0.0–265.2)			0.7	(0.0–93.3)
χ^{2d}_3	17.1*				0.8				2.4	

*Significant at the 0.05 level, two-sided test.
[a]All models controlled for the predictors in multivariate model 3 in the main text. Multivariate models excluded disorders associated with no case of PTSD after the randomly selected MVC. Models were based on weighted data. See the text for a description of weighting procedures.
[b]The joint significance of all mental disorders in the model.
[c]The significance of the differences among all mental disorders in the model.
[d]The joint significance of the three dummy variables for number of prior disorders.

Chapter 14

The Unexpected Death of a Loved One

Lukoye Atwoli, Dan J. Stein, Margreet ten Have, and Ronald C. Kessler

Unexpected death (UD) of a loved one is the most commonly reported trauma in the World Mental Health (WMH) surveys (see Chapter 3). It is also one of the traumas associated with the highest number of cases of posttraumatic stress disorder (PTSD) in the WMH surveys (see Chapter 9) as well as in several other epidemiological surveys (Breslau et al., 1998; Atwoli et al., 2013; Carmassi et al., 2014; Olaya et al., 2015). UD is also associated with a significantly elevated risk of first onset of other mental disorders (Keyes et al., 2014). But given that the research documenting PTSD in the wake of UD is relatively recent (Zisook et al., 1998), few epidemiological studies have yet addressed questions about the prevalence and correlates of PTSD associated with this type of trauma. The WMH surveys provide a unique opportunity to do so.

In this chapter, we report on the prevalence and predictors of UD-related DSM-IV PTSD. The predictors considered are those found to be significant in previous studies of PTSD (DiGangi et al., 2013; Ferry et al., 2014) as well as in previous studies of bereavement and complicated grief (Lobb et al., 2010; Kristensen et al., 2012), including socio-demographics, characteristics of the death, childhood adversities (CAs), history of prior traumas, and history of prior psychopathology. As in the other chapters, in this chapter, we focus on the subset of WMH respondents for whom the trauma under consideration was their random trauma.

Methods

The data in this chapter come from the 19 WMH surveys that used an expanded PTSD assessment to determine PTSD prevalence associated with random traumas, where 2,813 respondents were selected to have UD as their random trauma. The respondent's age at the time of the UD was recorded, along with responses to five questions about the circumstances surrounding the death: the respondent's relationship to the deceased (spouse, parent, child, sibling, other relative, or nonrelative); the cause of death (homicide, suicide, accident/medical error, or illness); length of illness if the death was due to illness; the age of the deceased at the time of death; and the respondent's perception of whether he/she could have prevented the death assessed as a yes–no answer to the question: *"Looking back on it now, is there any way you could have prevented the death from happening?"*

As in all the chapters in this section, we examined five classes of predictors in addition to the characteristics of the focal trauma. The first two pertained to socio-demographics including age, education, and marital status at the time of the death as well as sex. Age was coded in quartiles, as was education, which was classified as low, low-average, high-average, or high (coded as a continuous 1–4 score) according to within-country norms described in Chapter 5. The next three classes of predictors assessed the respondent's history of trauma prior to the UD, including previous UD, exposure to each of the other 28 lifetime trauma types assessed in the surveys, and exposure to each of 12 CAs. We distinguished between CAs in a highly correlated set of seven that we labeled Maladaptive Family Functioning CAs (parent mental disorder, parent substance abuse, parent criminality, family violence, physical abuse, sexual abuse, and neglect) and other CAs (parent divorce, parent death, other parent loss, serious physical illness, and family economic adversity) (see Chapter 10). The final set of predictors consisted of the respondent's history of the same 14 DSM-IV/CIDI mood disorders, anxiety disorders, disruptive behavior disorders, and substance disorders.

As in other chapters in this section of the volume, logistic regression was used to examine predictors of PTSD pooled across surveys. Predictors were entered in blocks, beginning with socio-demographics, followed sequentially by characteristics of the death, prior trauma and CA exposure, and prior mental disorders. All models included dummy control variables for surveys, meaning that the reported coefficients represent pooled within-survey coefficients. Logistic regression coefficients and standard errors were exponentiated and are reported as odds ratios (ORs) with design-based 95% confidence intervals (CIs), with statistical significance evaluated using 0.05-level two-sided tests. Design-based *F* tests were used to evaluate the significance of each block of predictor, with numerator degrees of freedom equal to number of predictors and denominator degrees of freedom equal to number of geographically clustered sampling error calculation units containing random UDs across surveys ($n = 1{,}062$) minus the sum of primary sample units from which these sampling error calculation units were selected ($n = 569$) and one less than the number of variables in the predictor set (Reed III, 2007). This resulted in 493 denominator degrees of freedom in evaluating bivariate associations and fewer in evaluating multivariate associations.

Once the final model was estimated, a predicted probability of PTSD was generated for each respondent from model coefficients. A receiver operating characteristic (ROC) curve was then calculated from this summary predicted probability (Zou et al., 2007). Area under the ROC curve (AUC) was calculated to quantify overall prediction accuracy of the model (Hanley & McNeil, 1983). We also evaluated *concentration of risk* of PTSD among the 5% of respondents with highest predicted risk of PTSD based on the final model, which we defined as the proportion of all observed cases of PTSD found among this 5% of respondents. This was done to determine how well subsequent PTSD could have been predicted in the immediate aftermath of the UD using our model. We also calculated *positive predictive value,* the proportion of the 5% of respondents with highest predicted risk that actually developed PTSD. Given that a number of different predictors were examined, the possibility of false positives and overfitting was taken into consideration in two ways. First, we evaluated the simultaneous significance of predictor blocks and interpreted individually significant coefficients only when the overall block was significant. Second, we used the method of replicated 10-fold cross-validation with 20 replicates (i.e., 200 separate estimates of model coefficients) to correct for the overestimation of overall model prediction accuracy when estimating AUC, concentration of risk, and positive predictive value (Smith et al., 2014).

Results

Prevalence of UD and Association with PTSD

Prevalence of UD was 30.2% (2,813 respondents) across surveys (interquartile range [IQR] across surveys was 24.4–33.0%), with an average 1.6 lifetime occurrences per respondent with any and representing 16.4% of all traumas in the population (IQR 15.3–17.5% across surveys) (see Table 14.1). PTSD prevalence associated with random UDs averaged 5.2% across surveys and was comparable in high-income countries versus low- and middle-income countries (LMICs) (4.8% vs. 5.9%; $\chi^2_1 = 0.6, p = 0.45$) (see Table 14.2). However, prevalence varied significantly across all surveys ($\chi^2_{18} = 35.4, p = 0.010$) and among surveys in high-income countries ($\chi^2_9 = 19.0,$ $p = 0.030$), but not among surveys in LMICs ($\chi^2_8 =$ $15.3, p = 0.06$).

Predictors of PTSD Associated with UD

Respondents who were in the oldest age quartile (35+; 28.1% of respondents with random UD) at the time they experienced the UD had significantly elevated bivariate PTSD odds compared to those in the youngest quartile (ages 1–17; 25.4% of respondents) (OR 2.5; 95% CI 1.1–5.9) (see Table 14.3). PTSD was also significantly more common among women (58.2% of respondents) than men (OR 3.0; 95% CI 1.5–6.0) and among the currently (at the time of the UD) married (31.1% of respondents; OR 2.1; 95% CI 1.3–3.6) and previously married (6.5% of respondents; OR 3.2; 95% CI 1.3–7.7) than among the never married in bivariate models, but was not significantly associated with respondent education. (See Appendix Table 14.A1 for distributions of all predictors.)

Model 1

However, sex was the only socio-demographic variable that remained significant in a multivariate model that included all the socio-demographic characteristics (see Table 14.3, model 1). We subsequently elaborated on that model to include a methodological control for the number of years between respondent age at the time of UD and age at interview to investigate the possibility of time-related recall bias, but that association was nonsignificant (OR 1.1; 95% CI 0.9–1.3).

Model 2

The respondent's relationship to the deceased was a significant predictor of PTSD ($F_{4,490} = 12.6, p < 0.001$) in the model that added characteristics of the UD to the socio-demographic predictors (see Table 14.3, model 2), with highest odds of PTSD associated with UD of the respondent's spouse (4.8% of respondents; OR 9.6; 95% CI 4.1–22.3) or son or daughter (5.4% of respondents; OR 8.7; 95% CI 4.2–18.0) followed by UD

Table 14.1 Distribution of lifetime exposure to UD of a loved one in the participating WMH surveys ($n = 40,067$)[a]

	Percentage of respondents exposed to any lifetime UD of a loved one		Mean number of UDs of a loved one among those exposed to any		UD of a loved one as a proportion of all lifetime traumas		Number of randomly selected UDs of a loved one
	%	(SE)	Mean	(SE)	%	(SE)	(*n*)
I High-Income Countries							
Belgium	24.4	(2.2)	1.5	(0.1)	28.1	(2.6)	(74)
France	28.2	(1.9)	1.5	(0.1)	26.5	(2.1)	(107)
Germany	27.2	(2.0)	1.6	(0.1)	29.0	(2.1)	(73)
Italy	20.4	(1.2)	1.5	(0.0)	23.8	(1.4)	(104)
Japan	23.7	(1.4)	1.6	(0.1)	31.5	(2.0)	(114)
The Netherlands	25.4	(2.1)	1.6	(0.1)	31.3	(2.2)	(82)
Northern Ireland	26.7	(1.2)	1.6	(0.1)	30.5	(1.3)	(139)
Spain	20.6	(1.4)	1.4	(0.1)	32.2	(1.9)	(172)
Spain – Murcia	29.6	(2.3)	1.3	(0.1)	40.2	(1.5)	(202)
United States	41.9	(1.1)	2.0	(0.1)	31.9	(0.7)	(516)
Total	29.8	(0.6)	1.7	(0.0)	30.8	(0.5)	(1,583)
II LMICs							
Brazil – São Paulo	31.0	(1.1)	1.5	(0.0)	25.2	(0.9)	(85)
Bulgaria	11.0	(1.0)	1.4	(0.1)	35.0	(3.9)	(72)
Colombia	39.7	(1.5)	1.8	(0.1)	27.6	(1.2)	(121)
Colombia – Medellin	33.0	(2.3)	2.0	(0.1)	29.6	(1.5)	(162)
Lebanon	36.6	(2.5)	1.6	(0.1)	27.0	(1.4)	(68)
Peru	31.6	(1.0)	1.4	(0.1)	22.2	(1.2)	(92)
Romania	10.5	(0.7)	1.4	(0.0)	21.0	(1.3)	(92)
South Africa	39.2	(1.2)	1.6	(0.0)	33.2	(0.8)	(374)
Ukraine	41.0	(2.1)	1.4	(0.1)	27.5	(1.3)	(164)
Total	30.5	(0.5)	1.6	(0.0)	28.0	(0.4)	(1,230)
III Total	30.2	(0.4)	1.6	(0.0)	29.3	(0.3)	(2,813)

[a]Two surveys were excluded for the following reasons: Mexico for low frequency of outcome ($n = 94$) and Israel for having no respondents experiencing UD of a loved one as a trauma ($n = 0$).

Table 14.2 Prevalence of DSM-IV/CIDI PTSD associated with UD of a loved one among respondents for whom UD of a loved one was their randomly selected trauma by survey ($n = 2,813$)[a]

	PTSD prevalence		Number with PTSD[b]	Total sample size[b]
	%	(95% CI)[c]	(*n*)	(*n*)
I High-Income Countries				
Belgium	6.8	(2.2–19.3)	(6)	(74)
France	2.7	(0.8–4.6)	(14)	(107)
Germany	8.1	(2.5–23.4)	(7)	(73)
Italy	5.3	(3.0–7.6)	(12)	(104)
Japan	1.4	(0.1–2.6)	(8)	(114)
The Netherlands	3.8	(1.3–6.2)	(8)	(82)
Northern Ireland	12.6	(3.7–21.5)	(27)	(139)
Spain	4.1	(1.2–7.0)	(18)	(172)
Spain – Murcia	1.7	(0.5–5.4)	(8)	(202)
United States	4.5	(1.3–7.7)	(50)	(516)
Total	4.8	(3.3–6.2)	(158)	(1,583)
χ^2_9	19.0*			
II LMICs				
Brazil – São Paulo	7.1	(2.3–11.9)	(10)	(85)
Bulgaria	13.8	(4.0–38.0)	(15)	(72)
Colombia	0.7	(0.1–4.4)	(4)	(121)
Colombia – Medellin	11.7	(4.0–29.5)	(21)	(162)
Lebanon	4.0	(1.3–11.6)	(6)	(68)
Peru	1.4	(0.3–3.1)	(4)	(92)
Romania	3.3	(0.9–7.8)	(6)	(92)

(*cont.*)

Table 14.2 *(cont.)*

	PTSD prevalence		Number with PTSD[b]	Total sample size[b]
	%	(95% CI)[c]	(*n*)	(*n*)
South Africa	3.3	(0.2–6.4)	(8)	(374)
Ukraine	10.4	(3.1–17.7)	(20)	(164)
Total	5.9	(3.3–8.4)	(94)	(1,230)
χ^2_8	15.3			
III Total	5.2	(3.9–6.6)	(252)	(2,813)
χ^2_{18} [d]	35.4*			
χ^2_1 [e]	0.6			

*Significant at the 0.05 level, two-sided test.
[a]Each respondent who reported lifetime exposure to one or more traumas had one occurrence of one such experience selected at random for detailed assessment. Each of these randomly selected traumas was weighted by the inverse of its probability of selection at the respondent level to create a weighted sample of traumas that was representative of all traumas in the population. The randomly selected UDs of a loved one were the subset of these randomly selected traumas involving UD of a loved one. The sum of weights of the randomly selected UDs of a loved one was standardized within surveys to sum to the observed number of respondents whose randomly selected trauma was UD of a loved one. The *n* reported in the last column of this table represents that number of respondents. The results reported here are for the surveys where at least one respondent with a randomly selected UD of a loved one met DSM-IV/CIDI criteria for PTSD related to that trauma. Two surveys were excluded: Mexico for low frequency of outcome ($n = 94$) and Israel for having no respondents experiencing UD of a loved one as a trauma ($n = 0$).
[b]The reported sample sizes are unweighted. The unweighted percentages of respondents with PTSD do not match the prevalence estimates in the first column because the latter were based on weighted data.
[c]Confidence intervals that include 0.0% as the lower bound were estimated using the Wilson score method. This method was used for the following countries: Belgium, Germany, Spain – Murcia, Bulgaria, Colombia – Medellin, Lebanon, Peru, and Romania.
[d]The significance of between-survey difference in PTSD prevalence among surveys in high-income countries, among LMICs, and across all 19 surveys.
[e]The significance of the difference in PTSD prevalence between high-income countries and LMICs.

of any other child (4.1% of respondents; OR 4.2; 95% CI 1.7–10.2) and of the respondent's parent (19.9% of respondents; OR 2.2; 95% CI 1.1–4.4) compared to others. Cause of death was not a significant predictor ($F_{3,491} = 0.8$, $p = 0.49$). The respondent's perception that he/she could have done something to prevent the death was also a significant predictor (7.1% of respondents; OR 2.8; 95% CI 1.2–6.6).

Model 3

Preliminary analysis found that prior lifetime exposure to traumas predicted PTSD significantly, but that this association was mainly due to traumas involving interpersonal violence or human-made disasters, which were found to be significantly intercorrelated in an exploratory factor analysis reported elsewhere (Benjet et al., 2016). (Detailed results are reported in Appendix Table 14.A2.) Multivariate analysis showed that those reporting these traumas had significantly increased odds of PTSD after the UD (OR 2.6; 95% CI 1.2–5.9 per trauma in the range 0–3) (see Table 14.3, Model 3). Preliminary analysis also showed that Maladaptive Family Functioning CAs predicted PTSD related to UD, while further analysis showed that these gross associations were due to three particular CAs – parent mental illness, parent alcohol abuse, and sexual abuse (OR 2.8; 95% CI 1.7–4.8 per trauma in the range 0–2). (Detailed results are reported in Appendix Table 14.A3.) The respondent's perception that he/she could have done something to prevent the death was nonsignificant in model 3.

Model 4

Preliminary analysis showed that each of the 14 temporally primary lifetime DSM-IV/CIDI disorders assessed in the surveys had an elevated OR (10 of them significant at the 0.05 level) when considered one at a time, but that few remained significant in a multivariate model due to high comorbidity among the disorders. (Detailed results are reported in Appendix Table 14.A4.) Further analysis (see Table 14.3, Model 4) then showed that the most parsimonious characterization of these joint associations was provided by a composite variable that summed up the number of anxiety disorders (0–3+), ADHD, and the number of substance abuse disorders (0–2) (OR 1.8; 95% CI 1.5–2.3 per disorder in the range 0–8).

Strength and Consistency of Overall Model Predictions

Estimated AUC based on 20 replicates of 10-fold cross-validated predictions (as described in the "Methods"

Table 14.3 Associations of socio-demographic variables, trauma characteristics, and prior stressors with DSM-IV/CIDI PTSD after randomly selected UD of a loved one ($n = 2{,}813$)[a]

	Bivariate		Multivariate model 1		Multivariate model 2		Multivariate model 3		Multivariate model 4	
	OR	(95% CI)	OR	(95% CI)	OR	(95% CI)	OR	(95% CI)	OR	(95% CI)
I Socio-demographics at Time of Trauma										
Respondent age at trauma exposure										
Child/adolescent (1–17)	1.0	–	1.0	–	1.0	–	1.0	–	1.0	–
Young adult (18–24)	0.7	(0.3–1.9)	0.7	(0.2–2.1)	0.8	(0.3–2.1)	0.9	(0.3–2.5)	0.6	(0.2–1.5)
Lower middle age (25–34)	1.4	(0.5–3.8)	1.1	(0.3–3.9)	1.1	(0.4–3.3)	1.2	(0.4–3.7)	0.7	(0.2–2.3)
Upper middle-older age (35+)	2.5*	(1.1–5.9)	1.7	(0.5–6.2)	1.2	(0.4–3.9)	1.6	(0.5–5.3)	0.9	(0.2–3.1)
$F_{3,491}$	5.1*		1.5		0.4		0.5		0.6	
Sex										
Female	3.0*	(1.5–6.0)	2.7*	(1.3–5.6)	2.1*	(1.0–4.3)	1.9*	(1.1–3.5)	2.2*	(1.2–3.9)
Male	1.0	–	1.0	–	1.0	–	1.0	–	1.0	–
Education	1.0	(0.7–1.3)	1.0	(0.7–1.5)	1.0	(0.7–1.4)	1.0	(0.7–1.3)	1.0	(0.8–1.4)
Marital status										
Currently married	2.1*	(1.3–3.6)	1.4	(0.6–3.1)	1.1	(0.5–2.4)	1.1	(0.5–2.5)	1.5	(0.6–3.9)
Previously married	3.2*	(1.3–7.7)	1.7	(0.5–5.4)	2.2	(0.6–7.5)	1.7	(0.5–5.2)	0.8	(0.5–6.2)
Never married	1.0	–	1.0	–	1.0	–	1.0	–	1.0	–
$F_{2,492}$	5.3*		0.4		0.9		0.5		0.5	
II Trauma Characteristics										
Who died										
Spouse	12.3*	(5.6–27.0)			9.6*	(4.1–22.3)	10.3*	(4.5–23.6)	13.0*	(5.3–31.9)
Son or daughter	12.1*	(5.8–25.3)			8.7*	(4.2–18.0)	11.7*	(1.4–6.7)	15.1*	(7.2–31.5)
Some other child (0–12 years old)	5.9*	(1.5–22.2)			4.2*	(1.7–10.2)	3.1*	(1.4–6.7)	2.0*	(1.1–3.9)
Parent	2.3*	(1.2–4.3)			2.2*	(1.1–4.4)	2.5*	(1.3–4.9)	3.3*	(1.7–6.6)
Other relative or nonfamily member	1.0	–			1.0	–	1.0	–	1.0	–
$F_{4,490}$	15.7*				12.6*		17.1*		15.4*	

Cause of death									
Homicide	0.7	(0.2–2.6)		1.3	(0.5–3.5)	1.7	(0.6–4.5)	2.1	(0.8–5.4)
Suicide	0.4	(0.1–1.3)		0.5	(0.2–1.4)	0.5	(0.2–1.4)	0.4	(0.1–1.5)
Accident, natural disaster, or medical mishap	0.7	(0.4–1.3)		1.0	(0.6–1.8)	1.1	(0.6–2.0)	1.4	(0.7–2.5)
Illness or other	1.0	–		1.0	–	1.0	–	1.0	–
$F_{3,491}$	0.9			0.8		1.0		1.9	
III Perceived Preventability									
Respondent could have prevented death	3.4*	(1.2–10.2)		2.8*	(1.2–6.6)	1.9	(0.7–4.9)	1.5	(0.5–4.0)
IV Prior Vulnerability Factors									
Prior stresses									
Prior exposure to any trauma (0–3)[b]	2.5*	(1.4–4.5)				2.6*	(1.2–5.9)	1.7	(1.0–3.1)
Number of MFF CAs (0–2)[c]	3.5*	(2.2–5.6)				2.8*	(1.7–4.8)	2.2*	(1.3–3.8)
Prior mental disorders (0–8)[d]	1.8*	(1.5–2.2)						1.8*	(1.5–2.3)
$F_{7,487}$[e]			5.6*	$F_{15,479} = 7.6$*		$F_{17,477} = 11.4$*		$F_{18,476} = 11.1$*	

*Significant at the 0.05 level, two-sided test.
[a]Models were based on weighted data. See the text for details. Each model included dummy variable controls for WMH survey.
[b]Number of prior traumas (values = 0–3+) was calculated as the sum of four individual prior traumas (beaten by caregiver, beaten by someone else, witnessed physical fight at home, and human-made disaster) from Appendix Table 14.A2.
[c]Number of MFF CAs (values = 0–2+) was calculated as the sum of three significant individual MFF CAs (parent psychopathology, parent substance abuse, and sexual abuse) from Appendix Table 14.A3.
[d]Number of mental disorders was calculated as the weighted sum of ADHD, drug abuse or dependence, and alcohol abuse or dependence from Appendix Table 14.A4.
[e]Design-based *F* tests were used to evaluate significance of predictor sets, with numerator degrees of freedom equal to number of predictors and denominator degrees of freedom equal to number of geographically clustered sampling error calculation units containing randomly selected UDs of a loved one across surveys ($n = 1{,}062$) minus the sum of primary sample units from which these sampling error calculation units were selected ($n = 569$) and one less than the number of variables in the predictor set, resulting in 493 denominator degrees of freedom in evaluating bivariate associations and fewer in evaluating multivariate associations.

section) was 0.80 in the total sample and 0.74–0.86 in subsamples defined by respondent sex, age, and education (see Figure 14.1). The 5% of respondents with highest predicted risk included 30.6% of all cases of UD-related PTSD. This is six times the proportion expected by chance (see Table 14.4). Subgroup values of this concentration of risk ranged from 36.8% among those with high/high-average education to 14.7% among men. Positive predictive value among the 5% of respondents with highest predicted risk was 25.3% in the total sample and ranged from 36.6% among respondents from LMICs to 18.2% among respondents from high-income countries.

Discussion

These results are limited in a number of ways. First, although prospective evidence suggests that retrospective trauma reports are valid (Dohrenwend et al., 2006), respondents with PTSD may have been biased toward higher recall of prior lifetime traumas and/or mental disorders (Roemer et al., 1998; Zoellner et al., 2000). Second, PTSD might have led respondents to perceive that they could have done something to prevent the death, resulting in the significant positive association between that "predictor" and PTSD. Third, diagnoses were based on a fully structured lay-administered interview rather than on a semi-structured clinical interview. While the WMH clinical appraisal data are reassuring (Haro et al., 2006), only a small number of countries carried out clinical reappraisal studies, potentially limiting generalizability. Fourth, although the combined sample size of the WMH surveys is large, the number of respondents selected for in-depth UD assessment was relatively small, reducing statistical power to carry out subtle analyses. In particular, with only 252 respondents meeting criteria for PTSD and 20 predictors, the resulting 12.6 events-per-variable (EPV) ratio, is well above the 10.0 EPV recommended to avoid biased OR estimates in an additive model (Peduzzi et al., 1996), where "events" refer to the number of people with PTSD, not the number of people with UD. As a result of this sample size problem, we were unable to consider interactions of trauma characteristics with preexisting vulnerabilities or other interactions. Fifth, the WMH interview schedule was developed before the DSM-5 criteria for persistent complex bereavement disorder (PCBD) were codified (American Psychiatric Association, 2013). As a result, no information was obtained in the surveys on PCBD

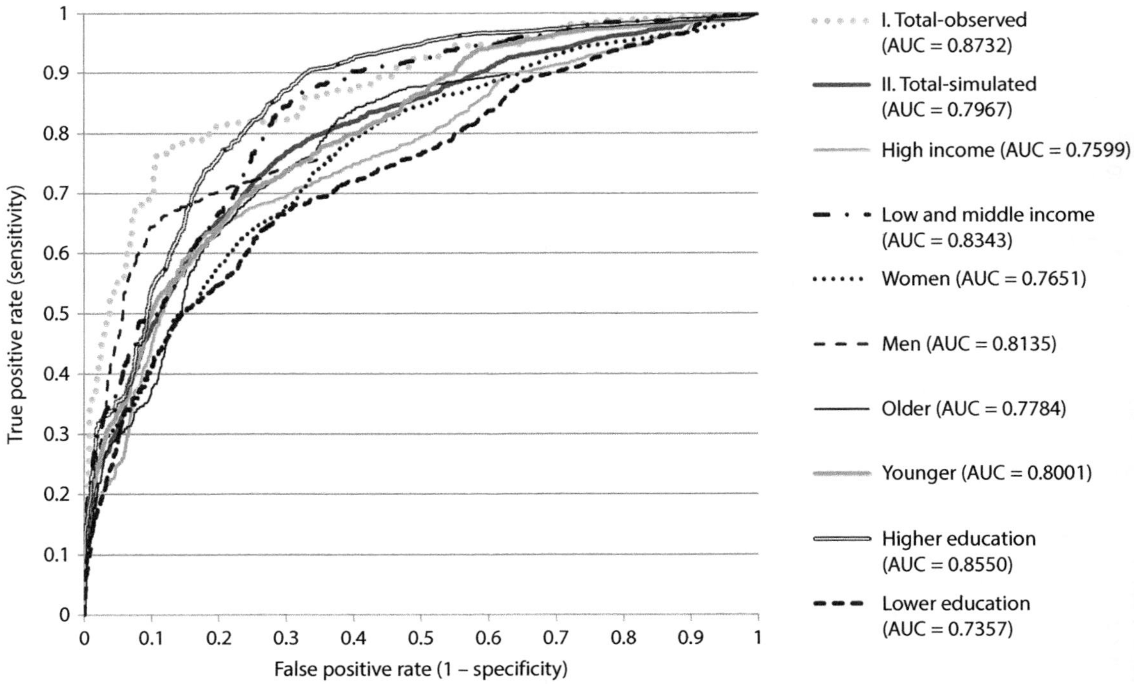

Figure 14.1 AUC of PTSD model, total sample, and by selected subgroups, "unexpected death of a loved one," weight analysis

Table 14.4 Concentration of risk and positive predictive value of observed DSM-IV/CIDI PTSD among the 5% of respondents assessed for PTSD after randomly selected UD of a loved one with highest predicted risk of PTSD in the total sample and stratified by subgroups

	Simulated sample[a] ($n = 56,260$)				Observed sample[b] ($n = 2,813$)			
	Concentration of risk		Positive predictive value[c]		Concentration of risk		Positive predictive value[c]	
	% PTSD	(SE)	% PTSD	(SE)	% PTSD	(SE)	% PTSD	(SE)
I Total	30.6	(6.2)	25.3	(5.3)	53.7	(6.5)	37.2	(5.9)
II Country Income								
High-income	26.7	(4.3)	18.2	(3.2)	50.5	(7.8)	37.7	(7.6)
Low- and middle-income	34.6	(11.4)	36.6	(11.1)	57.0	(10.3)	36.8	(8.9)
III Age (Years)								
<30	25.0	(12.0)	32.8	(14.8)	45.6	(10.6)	40.0	(10.7)
≥30	35.7	(6.5)	22.0	(3.2)	61.1	(8.2)	35.5	(6.1)
IV Sex								
Female	35.2	(7.6)	25.6	(5.8)	55.3	(7.2)	36.1	(6.1)
Male	14.7	(4.0)	22.6	(9.7)	48.2	(15.0)	42.5	(15.2)
V Education								
Low/low-average	24.6	(5.4)	22.9	(5.6)	45.0	(9.2)	27.5	(7.1)
High/high-average	36.8	(10.7)	27.2	(8.3)	62.7	(8.3)	50.5	(8.6)

[a]Estimates calculated from 20 replicates of 10-fold cross-validation of the final model.
[b]Estimates calculated from the final model.
[c]Positive predictive value is the prevalence of PTSD among respondents in the row who are among the 5% in the total sample with the highest predicted probabilities based on the final model.

or other complicated grief syndromes (Cozza et al., 2016), making it impossible for us to evaluate the extent to which our results would have been different if they had been adjusted for comorbidity or the confounding of our PTSD diagnoses with these syndromes (Maercker & Znoj, 2010).

Despite these limitations, our findings make several significant contributions to knowledge on the sequelae of UD. First, no previous cross-national study has reported on the prevalence of PTSD after UD, which we found to average 5.2%. This figure is somewhat higher than the 4.0% mean prevalence for any randomly selected trauma across the WMH surveys (Kessler et al., 2014), although the prevalence of UD-related PTSD varied widely across surveys. It is unclear why this variation exists, but the higher mean prevalence of UD-related PTSD than for PTSD related to other types of traumas points to the public health importance of UD-related PTSD (Breslau et al., 1998; Atwoli et al., 2013; Carmassi et al., 2014; Ferry et al., 2014; Kawakami et al., 2014; Keyes et al., 2014; Olaya et al., 2015).

Second, we found a number of significant predictors of UD-related PTSD. While the literature on these predictors is sparse, our results are consistent with evidence about the predictors of PTSD after other types of traumas (Brewin et al., 2000; Ozer et al., 2003; DiGangi et al., 2013; Ferry et al., 2014) and our findings about the relationship with the deceased, earlier lifetime traumas, and history of mental disorders are consistent with prior studies of complicated grief, including those on bereavement symptoms after the loss of a spouse or child (Lobb et al., 2010; Kristensen et al., 2012). Overlap of predictors of UD-related PTSD with the predictors found in studies of complicated grief highlights important commonalities and supports inclusion in the same chapter of the psychiatric nosology (Maercker & Znoj, 2010), but again raises concerns about how our results might have changed if data had been available in the WMH surveys to distinguish UD-related PTSD from PCBD.

Third, the lack of an association between cause of death and PTSD is relevant to a key debate about the DSM-5 diagnostic criteria for PTSD. While DSM-IV (American Psychiatric Association, 2000) identified UD as a qualifying trauma for PTSD, DSM-5 (American Psychiatric Association, 2013) developed a more stringent threshold for criterion A1, requiring that in cases of actual or threatened death of a family member or friend, the trauma(s) must have been directly witnessed, violent, or accidental. The WMH interview did not ask whether the respondent witnessed the death, making it impossible for us to know if the UD qualified as a DSM-5 trauma. However, PTSD symptoms can occur after a nonviolent/nonwitnessed death (Zisook et al., 1998) and this narrowing of the definition of qualifying death in DSM-5 has been questioned (Friedman, 2013; Keyes et al., 2014; Larsen & Pacella, 2016). It is relevant that our analysis found that the specific manner of death of a loved one has little impact on the risk of subsequent DSM-IV PTSD. This is true, furthermore, even though some deaths reported by respondents were not completely unexpected – that is, they were due to long-standing physical illnesses, and it was only the exact time of death that came as a surprise (e.g., a relative, who the respondent knew had only a short time to live, but was seemingly in stable condition, suddenly died at a holiday dinner).

One of the most striking results in our study was that 30.6% of people who experienced UD-related PTSD were among the 5% of respondents with the highest predicted risk scores in our cross-validated model. This result is broadly consistent with the more general WMH finding in Chapter 22 showing that PTSD can be predicted with good accuracy, using predictor data collected in the immediate aftermath of trauma. It is noteworthy that the high concentration of risk of PTSD we found was based on a replicated cross-validated simulation designed to adjust for overfitting. This finding provides robust evidence that useful models could be developed in future prospective studies to target prevention and treatment of UD-related PTSD (Maercker & Znoj, 2010; Simon, 2013; Endo et al., 2015).

Acknowledgment

Portions of this chapter are based on Atwoli, L., Stein, D. J., King, A. et al. (2017). Posttraumatic stress disorder associated with unexpected death of a loved one: cross-national findings from the world mental health surveys. *Depression and Anxiety*, **34**, 315–26, by permission of Wiley-Blackwell.

References

American Psychiatric Association. (2000). *Diagnostic and Statistical Manual of Mental Disorders, Fourth Edition, Text Revision. DSM-IV-TR*. Washington, DC: American Psychiatric Association.

American Psychiatric Association. (2013). *Diagnostic and Statistical Manual of Mental Disorders, Fifth Edition. DSM-5*. Arlington, VA: American Psychiatric Association.

Atwoli, L., Stein, D. J., Williams, D. R., et al. (2013). Trauma and posttraumatic stress disorder in South Africa: analysis from the South African Stress and Health Study. *BMC Psychiatry*, 13, 182.

Benjet, C., Bromet, E., Karam, E. G., et al. (2016). The epidemiology of traumatic event exposure worldwide: results from the World Mental Health Survey Consortium. *Psychological Medicine*, 46, 327–43.

Breslau, N., Kessler, R. C., Chilcoat, H. D., et al. (1998). Trauma and posttraumatic stress disorder in the community: the 1996 Detroit Area Survey of Trauma. *Archives of General Psychiatry*, 55, 626–32.

Brewin, C. R., Andrews, B., & Valentine, J. D. (2000). Meta-analysis of risk factors for posttraumatic stress disorder in trauma-exposed adults. *Journal of Consulting and Clinical Psychology*, 68, 748–66.

Carmassi, C., Dell'Osso, L., Manni, C., et al. (2014). Frequency of trauma exposure and Post-Traumatic Stress Disorder in Italy: analysis from the World Mental Health Survey Initiative. *Journal of Psychiatric Research*, 59, 77–84.

Cozza, S. J., Fisher, J. E., Mauro, C., et al. (2016). Performance of DSM-5 persistent complex bereavement disorder criteria in a community sample of bereaved military family members. *The American Journal of Psychiatry*, 173, 919–29.

DiGangi, J. A., Gomez, D., Mendoza, L., et al. (2013). Pretrauma risk factors for posttraumatic stress disorder: a systematic review of the literature. *Clinical Psychology Review*, 33, 728–44.

Dohrenwend, B. P., Turner, J. B., Turse, N. A., et al. (2006). The psychological risks of Vietnam for U.S. veterans: a revisit with new data and methods. *Science*, 313, 979–82.

Endo, K., Yonemoto, N., & Yamada, M. (2015). Interventions for bereaved parents following a child's death: a systematic review. *Palliative Medicine*, 29, 590–604.

Ferry, F., Bunting, B., Murphy, S., et al. (2014). Traumatic events and their relative PTSD burden in Northern Ireland: a consideration of the impact of the 'Troubles'. *Social Psychiatry and Psychiatric Epidemiology*, 49, 435–46.

Friedman, M. J. (2013). Finalizing PTSD in DSM-5: getting here from there and where to go next. *Journal of Traumatic Stress*, 26, 548–56.

Hanley, J. A., & McNeil, B. J. (1983). A method of comparing the areas under receiver operating characteristic curves derived from the same cases. *Radiology*, 148, 839–43.

Haro, J. M., Arbabzadeh-Bouchez, S., Brugha, T. S., et al. (2006). Concordance of the Composite International Diagnostic Interview Version 3.0 (CIDI 3.0) with standardized clinical assessments in the WHO World Mental Health surveys. *International Journal of Methods in Psychiatric Research*, 15, 167–80.

Kawakami, N., Tsuchiya, M., Umeda, M., Koenen, K. C., & Kessler, R. C. (2014). Trauma and posttraumatic stress

disorder in Japan: results from the World Mental Health Japan Survey. *Journal of Psychiatric Research*, 53, 157–65.
Kessler, R. C., Rose, S., Koenen, K. C., et al. (2014). How well can post-traumatic stress disorder be predicted from pre-trauma risk factors? An exploratory study in the WHO World Mental Health Surveys. *World Psychiatry*, 13, 265–74.
Keyes, K. M., Pratt, C., Galea, S., et al. (2014). The burden of loss: unexpected death of a loved one and psychiatric disorders across the life course in a national study. *The American Journal of Psychiatry*, 171, 864–71.
Kristensen, P., Weisaeth, L., & Heir, T. (2012). Bereavement and mental health after sudden and violent losses: a review. *Psychiatry*, 75, 76–97.
Larsen, S. E., & Pacella, M. L. (2016). Comparing the effect of DSM-congruent traumas vs. DSM-incongruent stressors on PTSD symptoms: a meta-analytic review. *Journal of Anxiety Disorders*, 38, 37–46.
Lobb, E. A., Kristjanson, L. J., Aoun, S. M., et al. (2010). Predictors of complicated grief: a systematic review of empirical studies. *Death Studies*, 34, 673–98.
Maercker, A., & Znoj, H. (2010). The younger sibling of PTSD: similarities and differences between complicated grief and posttraumatic stress disorder. *European Journal of Psychotraumatology*, 1, 5558.
Olaya, B., Alonso, J., Atwoli, L., et al. (2015). Association between traumatic events and post-traumatic stress disorder: results from the ESEMeD-Spain study. *Epidemiology and Psychiatric Sciences*, 24, 172–83.
Ozer, E. J., Best, S. R., Lipsey, T. L., & Weiss, D. S. (2003). Predictors of posttraumatic stress disorder and symptoms in adults: a meta-analysis. *Psychological Bulletin*, 129, 52–73.
Peduzzi, P., Concato, J., Kemper, E., Holford, T. R., & Feinstein, A. R. (1996). A simulation study of the number of events per variable in logistic regression analysis. *Journal of Clinical Epidemiology*, 49, 1373–79.
Reed III, J. F. (2007). Better binomial confidence intervals. *Journal of Modern Applied Statistical Methods*, 6, 15.
Roemer, L., Litz, B. T., Orsillo, S. M., Ehlich, P. J., & Friedman, M. J. (1998). Increases in retrospective accounts of war-zone exposure over time: the role of PTSD symptom severity. *Journal of Traumatic Stress*, 11, 597–605.
Simon, N. M. (2013). Treating complicated grief. *JAMA*, 310, 416–23.
Smith, G. C., Seaman, S. R., Wood, A. M., Royston, P., & White, I. R. (2014). Correcting for optimistic prediction in small data sets. *American Journal of Epidemiology*, 180, 318–24.
Zisook, S., Chentsova-Dutton, Y., & Shuchter, S. R. (1998). PTSD following bereavement. *Annals of Clinical Psychiatry*, 10, 157–63.
Zoellner, L. A., Foa, E. B., Brigidi, B. D., & Przeworski, A. (2000). Are trauma victims susceptible to "false memories"? *Journal of Abnormal Psychology*, 109, 517–24.
Zou, K. H., O'Malley, A. J., & Mauri, L. (2007). Receiver-operating characteristic analysis for evaluating diagnostic tests and predictive models. *Circulation*, 115, 654–7.

Appendix

Table 14.A1 Sample distribution and prevalence of DSM-IV/CIDI PTSD associated with randomly selected UD of a loved one by selected respondent characteristics ($n = 2{,}813$)[a]

	Sample distribution		PTSD prevalence		(n)[b]
	%	(SE)	%	(95% CI)	
I Socio-demographics at Time of Trauma					
Age					
Children and adolescents (1–17)	25.4	(2.1)	4.4	(1.1–7.7)	(584)
Young adult (18–24)	23.9	(1.8)	2.8	(1.4–4.2)	(621)
Lower middle age (25–34)	22.6	(1.7)	4.9	(2.8–7.0)	(605)
Older (35+)	28.1	(1.7)	8.3	(5.3–11.4)	(1,003)
χ^2_4			15.3*		
Sex					
Female	58.2	(2.3)	7.0	(4.9–9.0)	(1,980)
Male	41.8	(2.3)	2.8	(1.3–4.3)	(833)
χ^2_1			9.9*		
Education					
Low	24.9	(1.5)	5.7	(3.0–8.5)	(711)
Low-average	31.9	(2.0)	3.9	(2.1–5.7)	(840)
High-average	32.2	(1.8)	6.3	(3.3–9.2)	(947)
High	11.1	(1.3)	4.9	(1.9–8.0)	(315)
χ^2_3			4.5		

(cont.)

Table 14.A1 *(cont.)*

	Sample distribution		PTSD prevalence		(*n*)[b]
	%	(SE)	%	(95% CI)	
Marital status					
Currently married	31.1	(1.8)	7.0	(4.5–9.5)	(1,028)
Previously married	6.5	(0.9)	9.9	(2.7–17.1)	(198)
Never married	62.4	(1.8)	3.9	(2.3–5.5)	(1,587)
χ^2_2			10.6*		
II Trauma Characteristics					
Who died					
Spouse	4.8	(0.7)	24.0	(12.6–35.3)	(254)
Son or daughter	5.4	(0.7)	17.5	(8.9–26.2)	(232)
Some other child (ages 0–12)	4.1	(0.7)	11.9	(0.0–28.3)	(115)
Parent	19.9	(1.4)	5.2	(3.2–7.2)	(583)
Other relative or nonfamily member	65.7	(1.8)	2.5	(1.4–3.5)	(1,629)
χ^2_4			62.5*		
Cause of death					
Homicide	10.9	(1.2)	6.1	(2.8–9.5)	(295)
Suicide	9.9	(1.1)	2.5	(0.0–4.9)	(257)
Accident, natural disaster, or medical mishap	35.2	(2.1)	4.8	(2.6–6.9)	(952)
Illness or other	44.8	(2.1)	6.0	(3.8–8.3)	(1,309)
χ^2_3			2.6		
III Perceived Preventability					
Respondent could have prevented death					
Yes	7.1	(1.1)	11.4	(0.9–21.9)	(202)
No	92.9	(1.1)	4.8	(3.5–6.0)	(2,611)
χ^2_1			5.0*		
IV Prior Vulnerability Factors					
Number of prior exposure to any traumas[c]					
0	77.5	(1.9)	4.5	(3.3–5.7)	(2,514)
1	17.1	(1.7)	5.2	(2.4–8.1)	(236)
2	4.8	(1.0)	12.2	(0.0–27.0)	(59)
3+	0.6	(0.3)	46.3	(0.0–100.0)	(4)
χ^2_3			13.7*		
Number of MFF CAs[d]					
0	84.1	(1.5)	4.0	(2.8–5.1)	(2,464)
1	13.8	(1.4)	8.4	(4.6–12.3)	(302)
2+	2.1	(0.5)	35.4	(9.8–61.0)	(47)
χ^2_2			29.4*		
Number of prior mental disorders[e]					
0	73.3	(1.6)	4.0	(2.7–5.3)	(2,080)
1	13.6	(1.3)	4.1	(2.2–6.0)	(410)
2	6.1	(0.8)	5.6	(1.4–9.7)	(177)
3	3.1	(0.6)	16.9	(6.4–27.4)	(87)
4	0.9	(0.2)	10.8	(1.7–19.8)	(31)
5	2.2	(0.1)	4.3	(0.0–8.9)	(10)
6	0.5	(0.4)	74.5	(30.8–100.0)	(9)
7	0.4	(0.2)	73.8	(38.4–100.0)	(8)
8	0.0	(0.0)	100.0	(100.0–100.0)	(1)
χ^2_8			35.8*		
V Total			5.2	(3.9–6.6)	(2,813)

*Significance based on 0.05 level, two-sided test.
[a]Prevalence estimates are based on weighted data. See the text for a description of the weighting procedures. Significance tests are design-based tests of bivariate associations of each characteristic with PTSD based on logistic regression models with dummy controls for survey. Estimates were calculated from weighted data. Wald χ^2 statistics and *p*-values were estimated while controlling for country.
[b]Reported sample sizes are unweighted.
[c]Traumas include those involving interpersonal violence and human-made disasters (beaten by caregiver, beaten by someone else, witnessed physical fight at home, and human-made disaster), identified as significant from Appendix Table 14.A2.
[d]MFF CAs include parent mental illness, parent substance disorder, and sexual abuse, identified as significant from Appendix Table 14.A3.
[e]Mental disorders include anxiety disorders, ADHD, alcohol abuse or dependence, and drug abuse or dependence.

Table 14.A2 Associations of prior lifetime traumas with DSM-IV/CIDI PTSD associated with UD of a loved one ($n = 2,813$)[a]

	Bivariate		Multivariate model 1[b]		Multivariate model 2		Multivariate model 3		Multivariate model 4		Multivariate model 5	
	OR	(95% CI)	OR	(95% CI)	OR	(95% CI)	OR	(95% CI)	OR	(95% CI)	OR	(95% CI)
I Exposure to Organized Violence												
Relief worker in war zone	0.0	(0.0–0.0)										
Civilian in war zone	0.4	(0.1–2.2)	0.3	(0.0–2.3)								
Civilian in region of terror	1.1	(0.4–2.7)	0.8	(0.2–2.9)								
Refugee	2.4	(0.8–7.1)	2.0	(0.5–8.4)								
Kidnapped	1.9	(0.2–16.1)	0.3	(0.0–2.3)								
Number (0–2)	0.9	(0.5–1.7)			0.6	(0.3–1.2)						
$F_{4,490}$[c]			0.9									
$F_{3,491}$[d]			1.1									
II Participation in Organized Violence												
Witnessed death/dead body/serious injury	2.0	(0.9–4.2)	1.5	(0.7–3.2)								
Accidentally caused serious injury/death	17.0*	(2.2–131.2)	5.4*	(1.3–22.0)								
Combat experience	1.0	(0.1–8.9)	1.1	(0.1–22.1)								
Purposely injured/tortured/killed someone	65.2*	(4.7–912.7)	12.9*	(1.6–104.3)								
Witnessed atrocities	0.8	(0.1–6.9)	0.7	(0.0–15.3)								
Number (0–2)	1.9	(1.0–3.8)			1.6	(0.9–3.0)						
$F_{5,489}$[c]			3.1*									
$F_{4,490}$[d]			1.7									
III Physical Violence Victimization												
Beaten by caregiver	4.1*	(1.4–12.6)	2.3*	(1.0–5.1)								
Beaten by someone else	3.3	(0.4–25.3)	0.8	(0.2–2.9)								
Witnessed physical fight at home	3.2*	(1.4–7.2)	2.6	(0.9–7.9)								
Number (0–2)[e]	3.2*	(1.4–7.1)			2.4*	(1.3–4.6)	2.8*	(1.5–5.2)			0.9	(0.2–4.3)
$F_{3,491}$[c]			2.9*									
$F_{2,492}$[d]			1.5									
IV Sexual Violence Victimization												
Raped	3.4*	(1.3–8.8)	2.3	(0.7–7.2)								
Sexually assaulted	2.9*	(1.3–6.6)	2.1	(0.9–5.1)								
Stalked	0.9	(0.2–4.6)	0.7	(0.1–5.0)								
Beaten by spouse/partner	2.5*	(1.0–5.8)	2.7*	(1.2–6.4)								
Trauma to loved one	2.0	(0.6–6.1)	1.9	(0.5–7.0)								
Some other event	2.7	(0.8–8.5)	1.8	(0.5–7.0)								
Private trauma[f]	0.3	(0.1–1.1)	0.2*	(0.0–0.7)								
Number (0–5)	1.6*			(1.1–2.2)	1.4	(1.0–2.1)						
$F_{7,487}$[c]			2.1*									
$F_{6,488}$[d]			1.6									
V Accident/Injuries												
Natural disaster	0.5	(0.1–1.5)	0.3	(0.1–1.2)								
Toxic chemical exposure	6.7*	(1.0–44.5)	1.2	(0.4–4.3)								

(*cont.*)

Table 14.A2 *(cont.)*

	Bivariate		Multivariate model 1[b]		Multivariate model 2		Multivariate model 3		Multivariate model 4		Multivariate model 5	
	OR	(95% CI)	OR	(95% CI)	OR	(95% CI)	OR	(95% CI)	OR	(95% CI)	OR	(95% CI)
Automobile accident	2.3	(0.9–5.5)	2.1	(0.9–4.8)								
Life-threatening illness	2.7	(0.9–8.3)	1.2	(0.5–3.1)								
Child with serious illness	1.1	(0.4–3.5)	1.0	(0.3–3.2)								
Other life-threatening accident	1.8	(0.2–12.7)	0.3	(0.1–1.1)								
Number (0–3)	1.6	(0.9–2.7)			1.1	(0.7–1.6)						
$F_{6,488}$[c]			1.4									
$F_{5,489}$[d]			1.7									
VI Other Trauma												
Mugged/threatened with a weapon	1.8	(0.6–5.6)	0.8	(0.3–2.2)								
Human-made disaster	7.0*	(1.7–28.8)	4.2*	(1.3–13.3)	4.9*	(1.6–15.3)	5.2*	(1.8–15.0)			1.8	(0.6–5.5)
UD of a loved one	1.4	(0.8–2.5)	1.0	(0.6–1.8)								
Number (0–3)	1.7	(0.9–3.3)										
$F_{3,491}$[c]			2.9*									
$F_{2,492}$[d]			3.9*									
VII Total Traumas												
$F_{28,466}$[g]			2.9*		$F_{5,489} = 4.0$*							
$F_{27,467}$[h]			2.3*		$F_{4,490} = 2.6$*						$F_{2,492} = 0.6$	
VIII Composite of Physical Violence Victimization and Human-Made Disaster												
Number (0–3)	3.3*	(1.7–6.2)							3.3*	(1.7–6.2)	2.9*	(1.1–7.2)
IX Any Trauma												
0–3+	1.4*	(1.2–1.6)										
1	1.4	(0.8–2.5)										
2	1.2	(0.6–2.4)										
3+	2.4*	(1.2–4.6)										
$F_{3,491}$	3.1*											

*Significant at the 0.05 level, two-sided design-based test.

[a]All results are based on weighted data. See the text for a description of the weighting procedures. Coefficients come from logistic regression models controlling for the socio-demographic variables and characteristics of UD of a loved one in Table 14.3, multivariate model 2 and dummy variables for survey predicting PTSD.

[b]Only the traumas associated with at least one case of PTSD were carried forward into the multivariate models.

[c]The joint significance of the set of ORs for traumas in the group.

[d]The significance of the differences among the ORs within the group.

[e]The OR of 0.9 (0.2–4.3) in multivariate model 5 comes from a dummy variable for exactly two of the count of the three physical violence traumas and human-made disaster.

[f]A *private* event is a trauma that some individuals reported in response to a question asked at the very end of the trauma section that asked if they ever had some other very upsetting experience they did not tell us about already (and this includes in response to a prior open-ended question about "any other" trauma) because they were too embarrassed or upset to talk about it. Respondents were told, before they answered, that if they reported such a trauma we would not ask them anything about what it was, only about their age when the trauma happened.

[g]The joint significance of all traumas in the model.

[h]The significance of the differences among all traumas in the model.

Table 14.A3 Associations of CAs with DSM-IV/CIDI PTSD associated with UD of a loved one ($n = 2{,}813$)[a]

	Bivariate		Multivariate model 1		Multivariate model 2		Multivariate model 3		Multivariate model 4		Multivariate model 5	
	OR	(95% CI)	OR	(95% CI)	OR	(95% CI)	OR	(95% CI)	OR	(95% CI)	OR	(95% CI)
I MFF CAs												
Parent psychopathology	4.0*	(2.2–7.2)	3.2*	(1.5–6.7)	3.0*	(1.4–6.4)	3.6*	(1.9–6.7)			0.8	(0.3–2.1)
Parent substance misuse	3.4*	(1.4–8.1)	2.7*	(1.0–7.2)	2.8*	(1.1–7.2)	2.5*	(1.1–5.7)			0.6	(0.2–1.7)
Parent criminality	1.2	(0.5–2.9)	0.5	(0.2–1.3)	0.5	(0.2–1.3)						
Family violence	2.4*	(1.1–5.1)	1.1	(0.3–3.6)	1.0	(0.3–3.4)						
Physical abuse	3.3*	(1.3–8.3)	2.2	(0.7–6.4)	2.3	(0.7–7.7)						
Sexual abuse	6.1*	(2.4–15.3)	5.0*	(2.1–11.9)	4.7*	(1.9–11.4)	4.6*	(1.9–11.2)				
Neglect	3.1*	(1.4–7.1)	1.0	(0.3–3.2)	1.2	(0.5–3.1)						
$F_{7,487}$[b]			6.5*		7.2*		$F_{3,491} = 11.9$*				$F_{2,492} = 0.6$	
$F_{6,488}$[c]			3.0*		3.0*							
Number of selected MFF CAs (0–2)	3.6*	(2.4–5.3)							3.6*	(2.4–5.3)	4.9*	(2.0–12.1)
II Other CAs												
Parent death	0.9	(0.5–1.7)	0.8	(0.4–1.5)								
Parent divorce	1.6	(0.6–4.5)	1.1	(0.5–2.7)								
Other parent loss	2.7	(0.7–11.1)	2.4	(0.5–10.4)								
Serious physical illness	0.4	(0.1–1.6)	0.2	(0.0–1.1)								
Economic adversity	1.3	(0.3–5.3)	0.8	(0.2–2.8)								
$F_{5,489}$[b]			1.1									
$F_{4,490}$[c]			1.3									
III Total CAs (MFF and Other)												
$F_{12,482}$[d]			4.1*									
$F_{11,483}$[e]			2.2*									
IV Number of MFF CAs												
1	4.1*	(1.9–8.8)										
2+	4.3*	(2.3–8.3)										
$F_{2,492}$	12.0											
V Number of Other CAs												
1	1.2	(0.7–2.0)										
2+	1.3	(0.2–9.6)										
$F_{2,492}$	0.3											

*Significant at the 0.05 level, two-sided test.
[a]All results are based on weighted data. See the text for a description of the weighting procedures. Coefficients come from logistic regression models controlling for the socio-demographic variables and characteristics of UD of a loved one in Table 14.3, multivariate model 2 and dummy variables for survey predicting PTSD.
[b]The joint significance of the differences among the ORs within the group.
[c]The significance of the differences among the ORs within the group.
[d]The joint significance of all CAs in the model.
[e]The significance of the differences among all CAs in the model.

Table 14.A4 Associations of prior lifetime DSM-IV/CIDI mental disorders with DSM-IV/CIDI PTSD associated with UD of a loved one ($n = 2{,}813$)[a]

	Bivariate		Multivariate model 1		Multivariate model 2		Multivariate model 3		Multivariate model 4	
	OR	(95% CI)	OR	(95% CI)	OR	(95% CI)	OR	(95% CI)	OR	(95% CI)
I Mood Disorders										
MDD or dysthymic disorder	2.1*	(1.1–3.8)	1.1	(0.6–2.2)						
BPD (broad definition)	10.1*	(1.7–58.5)	2.3	(0.5–10.4)						
Number	2.4*	(1.3–4.1)			1.4	(0.8–2.4)				
$F_{2,492}$[b]			0.6							
$F_{1,493}$[c]			0.7							
II Anxiety Disorders										
Panic disorder or agoraphobia	1.3	(0.5–3.6)	0.6	(0.2–1.7)						
GAD	3.6*	(1.5–8.5)	2.6*	(1.1–6.0)						
PTSD	3.2*	(1.1–9.2)	1.8	(0.5–6.5)						
Social phobia	3.3*	(1.5–7.2)	2.9*	(1.3–6.7)						
Specific phobia	1.4	(0.8–2.7)	0.9	(0.5–1.7)						
Separation anxiety disorder	3.7*	(1.3–10.5)	1.5	(0.6–3.8)						
Number (0–3)	1.8*	(1.4–2.4)			1.5*	(1.1–2.1)	5.1	(0.5–51.9)		
$F_{6,488}$[b]			2.5*							
$F_{5,489}$[c]			1.7							
III Disruptive Behavioral Disorders										
ADHD	6.1*	(2.5–14.4)	6.7*	(2.3–19.7)	6.6*	(2.5–17.1)	21.4*	(1.6–294.9)	1.5	(0.4–5.4)
CD	1.4	(0.2–8.4)	0.3	(0.0–2.2)						
IED	1.1	(0.1–9.4)	0.9	(0.1–12.3)						
ODD	4.3*	(1.5–12.5)	3.2	(0.8–12.9)						
Number (0–3)	2.1*	(1.2–3.8)								
$F_{4,490}$[b]			4.6*							
$F_{3,491}$[c]			3.2*							

IV Substance Use Disorders										
Alcohol abuse or dependence	5.7*	(2.3–14.6)	2.4	(0.7–8.4)						
Drug abuse or dependence	18.1*	(4.3–75.1)	7.9*	(1.3–47.2)						
Number	4.7*	(2.2–9.9)			3.9*	(1.8–8.3)	10.3*	(1.3–84.5)	1.5	(0.6–4.0)
$F_{2,492}$[b]			5.6*						0.4	
$F_{1,493}$[c]			0.8							
$F_{14,480}$[d]			3.1*							
$F_{13,481}$[e]			1.9*							
VI Composite of Anxiety, ADHD, and Substance Use Disorders										
Score (0–8)	1.8*	(1.5–2.3)							1.6*	(1.2–2.2)
VII Total										
Any disorder	2.3*	(1.4–3.8)								
1	0.9	(0.5–1.6)								
2	2.3	(0.9–5.7)								
3	5.2*	(1.9–13.9)								
4+	7.4*	(2.8–19.1)								
$F_{4,490}$	7.1*									

*Significant at the 0.05 level, two-sided design-based test.
[a]All results are based on weighted data. See the text for a description of the weighting procedures. Coefficients come from logistic regression models controlling for the socio-demographic variables, characteristics of the UD, and prior stressors in Table 14.3, multivariate model 3 and dummy variables for survey predicting PTSD.
[b]The joint significance of the set of ORs for mental disorders in the group.
[c]The significance of the differences among the ORs within the group.
[d]The joint significance of all mental disorders in the model.
[e]The significance of the differences among all mental disorders in the model.

Chapter

15 Natural and Human-Made Disasters

Evelyn J. Bromet, Silvia Florescu, Giovanni de Girolamo, Fernando Navarro-Mateu, and Elie G. Karam

Natural and human-made disasters are common occurrences around the globe (Lopes et al., 2014; Warsini et al., 2014). Systematic research on the development of posttraumatic stress disorder (PTSD) following disasters has been undertaken for more than three decades, but most studies report only short-term consequences. Recent reviews suggest that between 20% (North, 2014) and 40% (Neria et al., 2008) of disaster survivors develop PTSD, but the range across studies is extremely broad (5–60% following natural disasters; 25–75% following human-made disasters) (Galea et al., 2005) due to both differences in the characteristics and locations of disasters and to methodological differences in studies (Norris et al., 2006; Goldmann & Galea, 2014).

A handful of general population epidemiological surveys before the World Mental Health (WMH) surveys retrospectively assessed lifetime exposure to disasters and prevalence of postdisaster PTSD. The first such study, the National Comorbidity Survey (Kessler et al., 1995), reported that a much lower proportion of disaster survivors developed PTSD (3.7% of men, 5.4% of women) than did the above-mentioned disaster-focused studies. This finding is broadly consistent with the WMH results reported in Chapter 9. Other recent community epidemiological surveys in Europe (Ferry et al., 2014; Olaya et al., 2015) and the United States (Breslau et al., 1998, 2013) reported similar results. Importantly, PTSD prevalence estimates in these surveys were considerably higher for some other lifetime traumas (Molnar et al., 2001; Darves-Bornoz et al., 2008; Olaya et al., 2015), suggesting that the low postdisaster PTSD prevalence estimates were not due to recall bias. The discrepancy between these low prevalence estimates in representative community samples and the much higher estimates in postdisaster surveys raises the question of whether demand characteristics and unrepresentative samples led to upwardly biased estimates in postdisaster surveys (Bonanno et al., 2010).

We attempted to address this question by carrying out a focused analysis of the WMH data on disaster-related PTSD. Measures capturing the severity of disaster-related stressors that are among the strongest risk factors for PTSD in postdisaster surveys (Fergusson et al., 2014; Goldmann & Galea, 2014; Bromet et al., 2016) were assessed among WMH respondents whose random trauma was a disaster. Other predictors of postdisaster PTSD in the literature are predisaster history of mental disorder, female sex, young age at the time of the disaster, and childhood adversities (CAs) (Sayed et al., 2015). As in all the other chapters in this section, all these variables are included in models to predict PTSD after disasters in the WMH data.

Methods

Data were analyzed from the 18 WMH surveys that had a sufficient number of respondents with random disasters for analysis. Respondents whose random trauma was a disaster were asked whether they were seriously injured in the disaster, whether they were displaced (i.e., forced to leave their home) by the disaster, whether anyone close to them was seriously injured or died in the disaster, and whether they witnessed anyone die during the disaster. As in the other chapters in this section, we examined five classes of predictors in addition to disaster characteristics. The first were socio-demographics: age, education, and marital status – each defined as of the time of the disaster – as well as sex. As in earlier chapters, education was classified as low, low-average, high-average, or high (coded as a continuous 1–4 score) according to within-country norms. (See Chapter 5 for details on this coding scheme.) Missing values, which were rare, were imputed using regression-based imputation. The next three classes of predictors assessed whether the respondent had been in one or more previous disasters, exposed to other prior lifetime traumas, and exposed to CAs. As in earlier chapters, we distinguished between CAs in a highly correlated set of seven that we labeled Maladaptive Family Functioning (MFF) CAs (parent mental disorder, parent substance abuse, parent criminality, family violence, physical abuse, sexual abuse, and neglect) and other CAs (parent divorce, parent death, other parent loss, serious physical illness, and family economic adversity). (See Chapter 10 for details on CA measurement.) CAs that were in broader classes of traumas (e.g., sexual assaults perpetrated by a family member versus other sexual assaults) were included both in the trauma inventory and the CA inventory in order to evaluate the incremental importance of exposure in the family context. Missing CA reports, which were rare, were coded conservatively as the CAs being absent. The final set of predictors consisted of the same DSM-IV/CIDI disorders examined in previous chapters.

As in previous chapters, logistic regression was also used to examine predictors of postdisaster PTSD pooled across surveys, with predictors entered in blocks beginning with socio-demographics, followed by disaster characteristics, prior trauma and CA exposure, and prior mental disorders. All models included dummy control variables for surveys. Logistic regression coefficients and their design-based standard errors were exponentiated and are reported as odds ratios (ORs) with 95% confidence intervals (CIs). Design-based *F* tests were used to evaluate significance of predictor sets, with numerator degrees of freedom equal to number of predictors and denominator degrees of freedom equal to number of geographically clustered sampling error calculation units containing randomly selected disasters across surveys ($n = 138$), minus the sum of primary sample units from which these sampling error calculation units were selected ($n = 100$) and one less than the number of variables in the predictor set (Reed, 2007). This resulted in 38 denominator degrees of freedom in evaluating bivariate predictions and fewer in evaluating multivariate predictions.

Once the final model was estimated, a predicted probability of PTSD was generated for each respondent from model coefficients. A receiver operating characteristic (ROC) curve was calculated from these predicted probabilities (Zou et al., 2007), and area under the ROC curve (AUC) was calculated to quantify overall prediction accuracy (Hanley & McNeil, 1983). We then evaluated sensitivity and positive predictive value among the 5% of respondents with highest predicted probabilities to determine how well the model implies that subsequent PTSD could be predicted if the model was applied in the immediate aftermath of a future disaster. Sensitivity was the proportion of observed PTSD cases found among the 5% of respondents with highest predicted probabilities. Positive predictive value was the prevalence of PTSD among this 5% of respondents. We used the method of replicated 10-fold cross-validation with 20 replicates (i.e., 200 separate estimates of model coefficients) to correct for the overestimation of prediction accuracy when both estimating and evaluating model fit in a single small sample (Smith et al., 2014).

Results

Prevalence of Disaster-Related PTSD

Disaster exposure was the randomly selected trauma for 661 respondents across the 18 surveys. In 10 surveys, none of the respondents met DSM-IV/CIDI criteria for PTSD, while in the remaining 8 surveys, mean-weighted PTSD prevalence was 2.5% (18 observed PTSD cases across surveys; see Table 15.1). Six of the latter eight surveys (accounting for 86.3% of respondents across all eight) were done in high-income countries and the other two in low- and middle-income countries (LMICs). PTSD prevalence estimates were, on average, higher in high-income countries than in LMICs (2.8% vs. 0.4%; $t = 1.9, p = 0.051$).

Predictors of Disaster-Related PTSD

The number of respondents with disaster-related PTSD in the two LMICs was too small ($n = 2$ of $n = 60$ respondents) to estimate logistic regression equations separately. We consequently excluded LMICs from further analysis. Median (interquartile range) number of years between the index disaster and the WMH interview in the remaining six surveys was 14 (3–35) years.

Model 1

Although respondent age and education at time of disaster both had significant positive bivariate associations with disaster-related PTSD (age: OR 1.2; 95% CI 1.0–1,4; education: OR 2.1; 95% CI 1.1–3.9), neither association remained significant in the multivariate model (model 1) (see Table 15.2). A methodological control for number of years between respondent age at disaster and age at interview to investigate the possibility of time-related recall bias added to the model was nonsignificant (OR 1.4; 95% CI 0.8–2.2).

Model 2

Human-made disasters (reported by 26.6% of respondents) were associated with significantly higher odds of

Table 15.1 Prevalence of DSM-IV/CIDI disaster-related PTSD among respondents with randomly selected disasters by survey ($n = 438$)[a]

	PTSD prevalence		Number with PTSD[b]	Total sample size[b]
	%	(95% CI)	(*n*)	(*n*)
I High-Income Countries				
Belgium	0.5	(0.0–1.7)	(1)	(7)
Italy	3.8	(0.0–11.2)	(1)	(35)
Northern Ireland	0.5	(0.0–1.5)	(1)	(23)
Spain	0.1	(0.0–0.2)	(1)	(14)
Spain – Murcia	2.6	(0.0–5.4)	(9)	(141)
United States	3.4	(0.0–8.0)	(3)	(158)
Total	2.8	(0.5–5.1)	(16)	(378)
χ_5^{2c}	3.9			
II LMICs				
Colombia	0.5	(0.0–1.5)	(1)	(21)
Mexico	0.3	(0.0–0.9)	(1)	(39)
Total	0.4	(0.0–0.9)	(2)	(60)
χ_1^{2c}	0.1			
III Total	**2.5**	**(0.5–4.4)**	**(18)**	**(438)**
χ_7^{2c}	5.0			
χ_1^{2d}	3.5			

*Significant at the 0.05 level, two-sided test.
[a]Each respondent who reported lifetime exposure to one or more traumas had one occurrence of one such trauma selected at random for detailed assessment. Each of these randomly selected traumas was weighted by the inverse of its probability of selection at the respondent level to create a weighted sample of traumas that was representative of all traumas in the population. The randomly selected disasters were the subset of these randomly selected traumas involving either natural or human-made disasters. The sum of weights of the randomly selected disasters was standardized within surveys to sum to the observed number of respondents whose randomly selected trauma was a disaster. The *n* reported in the last column of this table represents that number of respondents. The results reported here are for the surveys where at least one respondent with a randomly-selected disaster met DSM-IV/CIDI criteria for PTSD related to that trauma. None of the respondents with randomly selected disasters in the other WMH surveys met criteria for disaster-related PTSD. These included 21 respondents in France, 13 in Germany, 21 in Japan, 19 in Lebanon, 26 in Colombia – Medellin, 11 in the Netherlands, 39 in Peru, 29 in Romania, 29 in South Africa, and 15 in Ukraine.
[b]The reported sample sizes are unweighted. The unweighted proportions of respondents with PTSD do not match the prevalence estimates in the first column because the latter were based on weighted data.
[c]The significance of between-survey difference in PTSD prevalence among surveys in high-income countries, among LMICs, and across all eight countries.
[d]The significance of the difference in PTSD prevalence between high-income countries and LMICs.

PTSD than natural disasters (OR 3.3; 95% CI 1.1–9.7) in the multivariate model of disaster characteristics (model 2). Serious injury or death of someone close (reported by 4.3% of respondents) was also a significant predictor (OR 21.5; 95% CI 2.1–222.8), although the wide CI and much higher OR than in the bivariate model signaled model instability. This instability was due to high intercorrelations among disaster characteristics (see Table 15.3). Being displaced by the disaster (reported by 27.8% of respondents) was also a significant predictor in the multivariate model (OR 6.6; 95% CI 1.9–22.3), even though it was not significant in the bivariate model. Serious injury to the respondent (reported by 1.1% of respondents), while a significant bivariate predictor, was not significant in the multivariate model. Finally, witnessing death (reported by 7.8% of respondents) was not a significant bivariate or multivariate predictor. (Distributions of all predictors are reported in Appendix Table 15.A1.)

Model 3

Preliminary analysis of associations of prior traumas with disaster-related PTSD showed prior traumas involving exposure to sectarian, interpersonal, or sexual violence were the only ones consistently associated with increased risk of disaster-related PTSD, when controlling for model 3 predictors. (Detailed results are reported in Appendix Table 15.A2.) The most parsimonious characterization of those associations used a single dichotomous variable for whether the respondent was previously exposed to any such trauma (reported by 25.1% of respondents; OR 16.4; 95% CI 2.6–101.6). Preliminary analysis of the associations of CAs with disaster-related PTSD showed numerous significant

Table 15.2 Associations of socio-demographics, disaster characteristics, and prior vulnerabilities with DSM-IV/CIDI disaster-related PTSD ($n = 378$)[a]

	Bivariate[b]		Multivariate model 1		Multivariate model 2		Multivariate model 3		Multivariate model 4	
	OR	(95% CI)	OR	(95% CI)	OR	(95% CI)	OR	(95% CI)	OR	(95% CI)
I Socio-demographics										
Age at disaster (in decades)	1.2*	(1.0–1.4)	1.4	(0.9–2.1)	1.8	(1.0–3.2)	1.4	(0.7–2.6)	0.9	(0.3–3.0)
Sex (female)	1.0	(0.3–4.1)	1.4	(0.3–5.6)	0.9	(0.2–3.8)	1.4	(0.5–3.5)	0.9	(0.3–2.8)
Education[c]	2.1*	(1.1–3.9)	2.7	(0.9–8.0)	2.7	(0.7–10.8)	3.2	(0.8–12.4)	2.5*	(1.5–4.2)
Ever (vs. never) married	0.8	(0.2–2.8)	0.2	(0.0–3.9)	0.1	(0.0–1.3)	0.2*	(0.0–0.6)	0.2	(0.0–1.2)
II Disaster Characteristics										
Human-made (vs. natural) disaster	5.3*	(1.4–19.3)			3.3*	(1.1–9.7)	2.9*	(1.3–6.7)	3.1	(0.9–10.0)
Serious injury to respondent	8.6*	(2.2–33.9)			0.6	(0.1–3.0)	0.6	(0.1–6.6)	0.3	(0.0–2.4)
Respondent witnessed death	6.4	(0.4–108.2)			1.3	(0.0–57.0)	1.2	(0.2–6.6)	0.3	(0.1–1.5)
Serious injury/UD of a loved one	15.3*	(1.6–143.1)			21.5*	(2.1–222.8)	88.2*	(13.0–596.7)	165.9*	(26.7–1,031.0)
Respondent displaced from home	4.3	(0.8–22.9)			6.6*	(1.9–22.3)	9.3*	(5.1–16.9)	6.2*	(3.2–12.2)
III Prior Vulnerability Factors										
Any prior violent traumas[d]	7.7*	(3.3–18.0)					16.4*	(2.6–101.6)	5.0*	(1.2–21.5)
Number of CAs[e]	2.2*	(1.2–4.0)					2.9*	(1.4–6.2)	3.6*	(2.0–6.7)
Prior mental disorders										
1	1.7	(0.5–6.5)							9.8	(0.5–192.4)
2+	38.4*	(15.5–95.0)							60.0*	(21.1–170.5)
$F_{2,37}$	214.1*								52.5*	
$F_{4,35}$[f]			1.9		$F_{9,30} = 72.3$*		$F_{11,28} = 69.9$*		$F_{13,26} = 133.1$*	

*Significant at the 0.05 level, two-sided test.
[a]All models were estimated in weighted data pooled across the six surveys in high-income countries. See footnote a of Table 15.1 for a description of the weighting. All models included dummy variable controls for surveys. This means that the reported ORs should be interpreted as pooled within-survey coefficients.
[b]The bivariate associations are based on a separate model for each row, with the variable in the row and the dummy controls for survey the only predictors in the model.
[c]Education was treated as a continuous variable coded 1–4 (low, low-average, high-average, high).
[d]Any prior violent trauma includes exposure to any of four types of organized violence (e.g., civilian in war zone, relief worker in war zone, refugee); three types of interpersonal violence (e.g., witnessed physical fight at home, beaten by caregiver, beaten by someone else); and seven types of sexual violence (e.g., raped, sexually assaulted, beaten by romantic partner).
[e]A count in the range 0–3+ of MFF CAs experienced by the respondent in childhood from a total of seven assessed in the surveys that included parent psychopathology, parent substance abuse, parent criminality, family violence, physical abuse, sexual abuse, and physical neglect.
[f]The joint significance of all the predictors of the model.

Table 15.3 Tetrachoric correlations among disaster characteristics ($n = 378$)[a]

	Human-made vs. natural disaster	Serious injury to respondent	Respondent witnessed death	Serious injury/UD of a loved one	Respondent displaced from home
Human-made vs. natural disaster	1.0	0.25	0.58	0.32	0.05
Serious injury to respondent	0.25	1.0	−1.0	0.81	0.35
Respondent witnessed death	0.58	−1.0[b]	1.0	0.55	−0.22
Serious injury/UD of a loved one	0.32	0.81	0.55	1.0	0.03
Respondent displaced from home	0.05	0.35	−0.22	0.03	1.0

[a]Based on weighted data pooled across the six surveys in high-income countries. See footnote a of Table 15.1 for a description of the weighting.
[b]None of the respondents who witnessed death were themselves injured.

positive bivariate associations that could best be summarized with a 0–3+ count for number of MFF CAs (15.4% for 1, 6.5% for 2, 13.3% for 3+; OR 2.9; 95% CI 1.4–6.2). (Detailed results are reported in Appendix Table 15.A3.) The multivariate ORs of both traumas and CAs were larger than the bivariate ORs and had wide CIs. In addition, the OR of serious injury/death of someone close became dramatically higher in model 3 than in model 2.

Model 4

Preliminary analysis showed that 13 of the 14 temporally primary lifetime DSM-IV/CIDI disorders had elevated bivariate ORs predicting disaster-related PTSD (11 of them significant at the 0.05 level), but that only a handful were significant in a multivariate model due to high comorbidity. (Detailed results are reported in Appendix Table 15.A4.) The most parsimonious characterization of these associations used dummy variables for exactly 1 (17.6%; OR 9.8; 95% CI 0.5–192.4) and 2+ (14.1%; OR 60.0; 95% CI 21.1–170.5) prior lifetime DSM-IV/CIDI disorders as predictors. The significant OR of prior lifetime traumas in model 3 decreased substantially, while the significant OR of serious injury or death of someone close to the respondent increased substantially in model 4, as compared to model 3, when controlling for mental disorders.

Strength and Consistency of Overall Model Predictions

Although the small sample size precluded estimating model coefficients separately in each survey, we could compare overall model fit in subsamples by calculating individual-level predicted probabilities from model 4 with 20 replicates of 10-fold cross-validation, estimating subsample ROC curves from these predicted probabilities, and calculating AUC based on these curves. Estimated AUC based on 20 replicates of 10-fold cross-validated predictions was 0.63 in the total sample and 0.48–0.75 in subsamples defined by respondent sex, age, and education (see Figure 15.1). These are weak to intermediate levels of overall classification accuracy (Roemer et al., 1998). However, the 5% of respondents with highest predicted probabilities of PTSD included a substantial proportion (44.5%) of all disaster-related PTSD (sensitivity) in the total sample. This is nine times the concentration of risk expected by chance alone (see Table 15.4). Subgroup sensitivities among this 5% of respondents with highest predicted risk ranged from 56.4% among men to 22.4% among respondents with low-average/low education. Positive predictive value (the proportion of predicted positives who met criteria for PTSD) among the 5% of respondents with higher predicted risk was 20.4% in the total sample and between 39.5% among respondents with high-average/high education to 3.9% among respondents with low-average/low education.

Discussion

Several limitations of the results are noteworthy. First, traumas and mental disorders were assessed retrospectively, although special recall probes used in WMH surveys have been shown experimentally to improve retrospective recall accuracy (Knauper et al., 1999). Second, diagnoses were based on a fully structured lay-administered interview rather than on semi-structured clinical interviews, although WMH clinical appraisal data are reassuring (Haro et al., 2006). Third, given that

Table 15.4 Concentration of risk of observed DSM-IV/CIDI PTSD in the top 5th percentile of predicted PTSD, total sample and stratified by subgroups ($n = 378$)[a]

	Sensitivity[b]		Positive predictive value[c]	
	% PTSD	(SE)	% PTSD	(SE)
I Total	44.5	(18.0)	20.4	(9.5)
II Age (Years)				
<25	52.9	(26.3)	32.4	(20.7)
≥25	34.0	(13.6)	11.8	(1.3)
III Sex				
Female	27.9	(23.8)	10.9	(8.8)
Male	56.4	(24.3)	29.4	(19.6)
IV Education				
Low/low-average	22.4	(14.9)	3.9	(0.5)
High/high-average	50.3	(20.3)	39.5	(16.4)

[a]Based on weighted data pooled across the six surveys in high-income countries. See footnote a of Table 15.1 for a description of the weighting. Ten-fold cross-validation involves dividing the sample into 10 separate random subsamples of equal size, estimating the model in each of the 10 separate 90% subsamples created by deleting 1 of the 10 subsamples, and applying predicted values based on each set of coefficients only to the remaining 10% of the sample. Replicated cross-validation involves repeating the cross-validation process some number of times (20 times in the current application), with a different random split of the sample into 10 equal-sized subsamples each time. Sensitivity and positive predictive value were calculated separately in each of these 200 subsamples and averaged to produce the results reported here.

[b]Sensitivity is the percentage of all PTSD found among the 5% of respondents with highest predicted probabilities based on the final model.

[c]Positive predictive value is the prevalence of PTSD among respondents in the row who are among the 5% in the total sample with the highest predicted probabilities based on the final model.

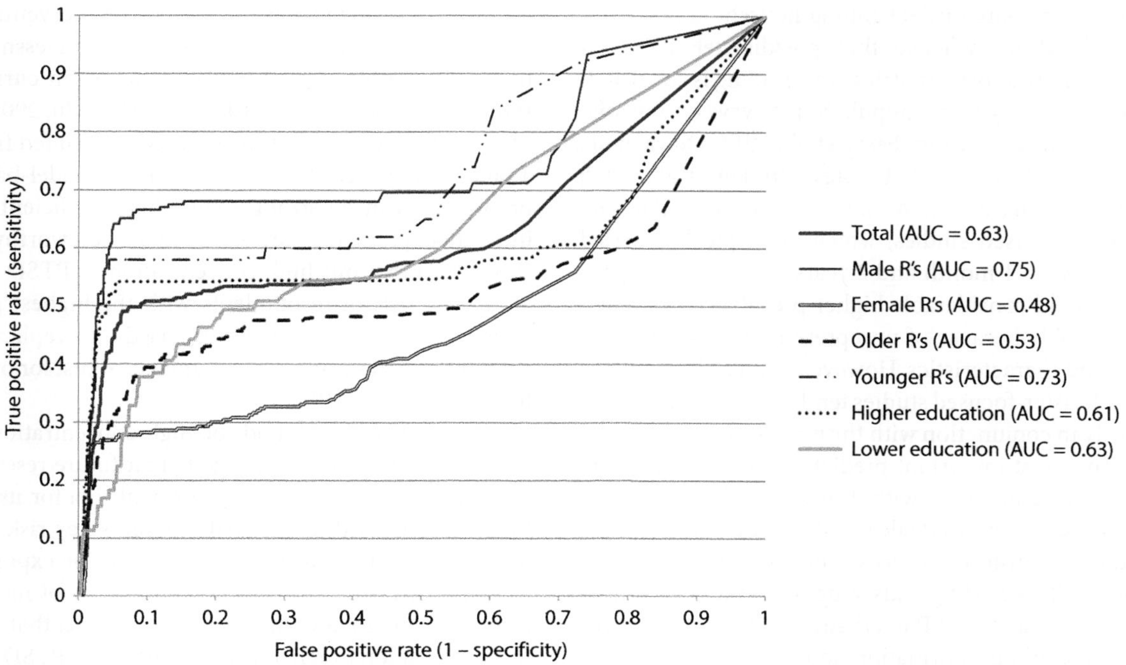

Figure 15.1 AUC of predicted probabilities based on multivariate model 4 overall and in selected subgroups

disasters were only one of many traumas assessed in the WMH surveys, information on potentially important predictors of postdisaster PTSD was much more limited than in disaster-focused surveys.

The sampling restrictions are of special importance. The vast majority of disasters occur in LMICs (Roy et al., 2011), but our analyses were carried out exclusively in high-income countries. In addition, the samples were restricted to household residents, which means we excluded people living in displacement camps and other group quarters. This limitation is particularly serious, given that displacement was a significant predictor of disaster-related PTSD. While the 378 respondents assessed for randomly selected disasters constituted a large enough sample for us to estimate prevalence of postdisaster PTSD with good precision, the fact that PTSD was an uncommon outcome (n = 16) meant that we lacked statistical power to estimate multivariate predictor coefficients with precision. Indeed, with 13 model coefficients, the 1.2 events-per-variable (EPV) ratio was well below the value recommended to avoid biased OR estimates (Peduzzi et al., 1996). Caution is consequently needed in interpreting our results because of low EPV and the clear evidence of model instability noted in Table 15.2.

Despite these limitations, the WMH results, which constitute the first cross-national data on prevalence of disaster-related PTSD among household residents, provide clear evidence that postdisaster PTSD is uncommon across countries. This finding is consistent with previous general population surveys on postdisaster PTSD in Europe (Ferry et al., 2014; Olaya et al., 2015) and in the United States (Breslau et al., 1998; Breslau et al., 2013). As noted in the introduction, disaster-focused studies, which are typically carried out between 1 month and 2 years after disasters, generally yield considerably higher prevalence estimates, presumably because of unrepresentative samples and demand characteristics. However, it must also be noted that disaster-focused studies tend to be carried out primarily in conjunction with the most severe disasters.

The most important predictors in our study were generally consistent with those found in previous postdisaster studies (Galea et al., 2005): prior psychopathology, disaster severity, and history of previous trauma. This finding adds support to the recommendation of North and Pfefferbaum (2013), which advocates including information about these three classes of risk factors in needs assessment surveys of disaster survivors. It is noteworthy that the WMH surveys also found that human-made disasters have more pernicious psychological effects than natural disasters. This result is consistent with several previous epidemiological studies (Galea et al., 2005). However, we observed that this association became much less pronounced when we controlled for disaster-related characteristics, suggesting that at least part of the reason why human-made disasters were associated with higher rates of PTSD than natural disasters is that the former were objectively more severe. Caution is needed in interpreting this result, though, as the exploratory factor analysis of trauma associations in Chapter 3 found that the human-made disasters reported in the WMH surveys included a mix of accidents caused by human error and acts of terrorism (Benjet et al., 2016). We had no way of distinguishing between these two types of human-made disasters to determine if they have similar associations with PTSD.

Perhaps our most striking result was that nearly half of disaster-related PTSD occurred among the 5% of respondents with the highest predicted risk scores in our model. This result is broadly consistent with the more general results in Chapter 22. These findings contradict the previously held view that the individual predictors in epidemiological models of PTSD have ORs that are too weak and inconsistent to be clinically useful in targeting people for preventive interventions (Brewin, 2005a), making it necessary to use assessment tools in the aftermath of trauma focused on current symptoms rather than on risk factors (Brewin, 2005b). The error in this earlier way of thinking resulted from a failure to appreciate that multivariate model-based predictions can be strong even when coefficients of individual predictors are weak. It is noteworthy in this regard that our high concentration of PTSD risk among the 5% of respondents with the highest predicted risk from our model was based on a replicated cross-validated simulation designed to adjust for overfitting due to low EPV.

The evidence we found for high concentration of risk based on our model suggests that future research is needed both to create an assessment tool for use in the aftermath of disasters that measures key risk factors (i.e., disaster-related experiences, prior exposure to highly stressful experiences, and history of mental disorders) and to develop a prediction model that uses this information to generate individual-level PTSD risk scores so as to target high-risk survivors for preventive interventions. While the WMH results provide strong suggestive evidence that a useful model of this sort could be developed from self-report data, the WMH model itself is inadequate because it was based on coarse measures assessed retrospectively in a small sample.

At the same time, the WMH results were sufficiently consistent with prior evidence that one could imagine developing a triage screening system based loosely on these consistent risk factors. This is the approach taken in the PsySTART system adopted by the American Red Cross to target rapid delivery of psychological first aid and referral for mental health services to disaster survivors judged to be at high risk of postdisaster mental disorders in the immediate aftermath of a disaster (Schreiber et al., 2014). PsySTART is different from previous postdisaster risk evaluation schemes in that it does not focus on current psychological distress (other than acute suicidality), which is an unreliable predictor of postdisaster mental disorders (Norris et al., 2002), but on evidence-based predictors of those disorders (disaster-related experiences, prior disaster exposure, prior trauma exposure, and history of prior mental disorders) evaluated by trained Red Cross disaster mental health workers.

The approach proposed here could be seen as a next step in the PsySTART program designed to refine the selection of risk factors and to optimize the weighting scheme used to combine information about these risk factors into a composite risk score. These refinements would require data to be collected from a much larger sample than the one used in the WMH analysis. The sample should include a baseline assessment of a broad range of risk factors obtained in the immediate aftermath of disaster. Participants should be followed over time to determine who develops PTSD or other postdisaster mental disorders. Much more sophisticated data analysis methods should be used to analyze these data than in the WMH analysis. In particular, machine learning methods of the sort used in Chapter 22 should be used to maximize out-of-sample prediction accuracy in the final model (Kessler et al., 2014), leading to optimal selection of the risk factors to include in subsequent assessments and to optimal weighting of these measures to assess risk of postdisaster psychopathology. We were unable to use these methods in the current study because of our small sample size. Given the growing literature documenting the value of interventions in the immediate aftermath of trauma (Forneris et al., 2013; Kliem & Kroger, 2013; Amos et al., 2014; Bisson, 2014), the development of such an optimal prediction model could be of considerable practical value.

Acknowledgment

Portions of this chapter are based on Bromet, E. J., Atwoli, L., Navarro-Mateu, F., et al. (2017). Posttraumatic stress disorder associated with natural and human-made disasters in the World Mental Health Surveys. *Psychological Medicine*, **47**, 227–41, by permission of Cambridge University Press.

References

Amos, T., Stein, D. J., & Ipser, J. C. (2014). Pharmacological interventions for preventing post-traumatic stress disorder (PTSD). *The Cochrane Database of Systematic Reviews*, Issue 7, CD006239.

Bisson, J. I. (2014). Early responding to traumatic events. *The British Journal of Psychiatry*, 204, 329–30.

Benjet, C., Bromet, E., Karam, E. G., et al. (2016). The epidemiology of traumatic event exposure worldwide: results from the World Mental Health Survey Consortium. *Psychological Medicine*, 46, 327–43.

Bonanno, G. A., Brewin, C. R., Kaniasty, K., & La Greca, A. M. (2010). Weighing the costs of disaster: consequences, risks, and resilience in individuals, families, and communities. *Psychological Science in the Public Interest*, 11, 1–49.

Breslau, N., Kessler, R. C., Chilcoat, H. D., et al. (1998). Trauma and posttraumatic stress disorder in the community: the 1996 Detroit Area Survey of Trauma. *Archives of General Psychiatry*, 55, 626–32.

Breslau, N., Troost, J. P., Bohnert, K., & Luo, Z. (2013). Influence of predispositions on post-traumatic stress disorder: does it vary by trauma severity? *Psychological Medicine*, 43, 381–90.

Brewin, C. R. (2005a). Risk factor effect sizes in PTSD: what this means for intervention. *Journal of Trauma & Dissociation*, 6, 123–30.

(2005b). Systematic review of screening instruments for adults at risk of PTSD. *Journal of Traumatic Stress*, 18, 53–62.

Bromet, E. J., Hobbs, M. J., Clouston, S. A., et al. (2016). DSM-IV post-traumatic stress disorder among World Trade Center responders 11–13 years after the disaster of 11 September 2001 (9/11). *Psychological Medicine*, 46, 771–83.

Darves-Bornoz, J. M., Alonso, J., de Girolamo, G., et al. (2008). Main traumatic events in Europe: PTSD in the European study of the epidemiology of mental disorders survey. *Journal of Traumatic Stress*, 21, 455–62.

Fergusson, D. M., Horwood, L. J., Boden, J. M., & Mulder, R. T. (2014). Impact of a major disaster on the mental health of a well-studied cohort. *JAMA Psychiatry*, 71, 1025–31.

Ferry, F., Bunting, B., Murphy, S., et al. (2014). Traumatic events and their relative PTSD burden in Northern Ireland: a consideration of the impact of the 'Troubles'. *Social Psychiatry and Psychiatric Epidemiology*, 49, 435–46.

Forneris, C. A., Gartlehner, G., Brownley, K. A., et al. (2013). Interventions to prevent post-traumatic stress disorder: a systematic review. *American Journal of Preventive Medicine*, 44, 635–50.

Galea, S., Nandi, A., & Vlahov, D. (2005). The epidemiology of post-traumatic stress disorder after disasters. *Epidemiologic Reviews*, 27, 78–91.

Goldmann, E., & Galea, S. (2014). Mental health consequences of disasters. *Annual Review of Public Health*, 35, 169–83.

Hanley, J. A., & McNeil, B. J. (1983). A method of comparing the areas under receiver operating characteristic curves derived from the same cases. *Radiology*, 148, 839–43.

Haro, J. M., Arbabzadeh-Bouchez, S., Brugha, T. S., et al. (2006). Concordance of the Composite International Diagnostic Interview Version 3.0 (CIDI 3.0) with standardized clinical assessments in the WHO World Mental Health surveys. *International Journal of Methods in Psychiatric Research*, 15, 167–80.

Kessler, R. C., Rose, S., Koenen, K. C., et al. (2014). How well can post-traumatic stress disorder be predicted from pre-trauma risk factors? An exploratory study in the WHO World Mental Health Surveys. *World Psychiatry*, 13, 265–74.

Kessler, R. C., Sonnega, A., Bromet, E., Hughes, M., & Nelson, C. B. (1995). Posttraumatic stress disorder in the National Comorbidity Survey. *Archives of General Psychiatry*, 52, 1048–60.

Kliem, S., & Kroger, C. (2013). Prevention of chronic PTSD with early cognitive behavioral therapy. A meta-analysis using mixed-effects modeling. *Behaviour Research and Therapy*, 51, 753–61.

Knauper, B., Cannell, C. F., Schwarz, N., Bruce, M. L., & Kessler, R. C. (1999). Improving accuracy of major depression age-of-onset reports in the US National Comorbidity Survey. *International Journal of Methods in Psychiatric Research*, 8, 39–48.

Lopes, A. P., Macedo, T. F., Coutinho, E. S., Figueira, I., & Ventura, P. R. (2014). Systematic review of the efficacy of cognitive-behavior therapy related treatments for victims of natural disasters: a worldwide problem. *PLoS One*, 9, e109013.

Molnar, B. E., Buka, S. L., & Kessler, R. C. (2001). Child sexual abuse and subsequent psychopathology: results from the National Comorbidity Survey. *American Journal of Public Health*, 91, 753–60.

Neria, Y., Nandi, A., & Galea, S. (2008). Post-traumatic stress disorder following disasters: a systematic review. *Psychological Medicine*, 38, 467–80.

Norris, F. H., Friedman, M. J., Watson, P. J., et al. (2002). 60,000 disaster victims speak: part I. An empirical review of the empirical literature, 1981–2001. *Psychiatry*, 65, 207–39.

Norris, F. H., Galea, S., Friedman, M. J., & Watson, P. J. (2006). *Methods for Disaster Mental Health Research*. New York, NY: Guilford Press.

North, C. S. (2014). Current research and recent breakthroughs on the mental health effects of disasters. *Current Psychiatry Reports*, 16, 481.

North, C. S., & Pfefferbaum, B. (2013). Mental health response to community disasters: a systematic review. *JAMA*, 310, 507–18.

Olaya, B., Alonso, J., Atwoli, L., et al. (2015). Association between traumatic events and post-traumatic stress disorder: results from the ESEMeD-Spain study. *Epidemiology and Psychiatric Sciences*, 24, 172–83.

Peduzzi, P., Concato, J., Kemper, E., Holford, T. R., & Feinstein, A. R. (1996). A simulation study of the number of events per variable in logistic regression analysis. *Journal of Clinical Epidemiology*, 49, 1373–9.

Reed, J. F., III. (2007). Better binomial confidence intervals. *Journal of Modern Applied Statistical Methods*, 6, 153–161.

Roemer, L., Litz, B. T., Orsillo, S. M., Ehlich, P. J., & Friedman, M. J. (1998). Increases in retrospective accounts of war-zone exposure over time: the role of PTSD symptom severity. *Journal of Traumatic Stress*, 11, 597–605.

Roy, N., Thakkar, P., & Shah, H. (2011). Developing-world disaster research: present evidence and future priorities. *Disaster Medicine and Public Health Preparedness*, 5, 112–6.

Sayed, S., Iacoviello, B. M., & Charney, D. S. (2015). Risk factors for the development of psychopathology following trauma. *Current Psychiatry Reports*, 17, 70.

Schreiber, M. D., Yin, R., Omaish, M., & Broderick, J. E. (2014). Snapshot From Superstorm Sandy: American Red Cross mental health risk surveillance in lower New York State. *Annals of Emergency Medicine*, 64, 59–65.

Smith, G. C., Seaman, S. R., Wood, A. M., Royston, P., & White, I. R. (2014). Correcting for optimistic prediction in small data sets. *American Journal of Epidemiology*, 180, 318–24.

Warsini, S., West, C., Ed Tt, G. D., et al. (2014). The psychosocial impact of natural disasters among adult survivors: an integrative review. *Issues in Mental Health Nursing*, 35, 420–36.

Zou, K. H., O'Malley, A. J., & Mauri, L. (2007). Receiver-operating characteristic analysis for evaluating diagnostic tests and predictive models. *Circulation*, 115, 654–7.

Appendix

Table 15.A1 The distribution and bivariate associations of each predictor considered in the analysis with DSM-IV/CIDI PTSD ($n = 378$)[a]

	Prevalence of DSM-IV/CIDI PTSD		Distribution of the predictor in the total sample	
	% PTSD	(95% CI)	%	(SE)
I Age at Time of Disaster				
Children (0–9)	0.8	(0.0–2.4)	14.1	(5.7)
Adolescents (10–19)	2.4	(0.0–7.1)	22.5	(6.0)
Young adults (20–29)	3.2	(0.0–8.8)	33.2	(10.6)
Older (30+)	3.5	(0.6–6.5)	30.2	(5.9)
χ^2_3	2.1			
II Sex				
Female	2.9	(0.7–5.2)	40.1	(7.4)
Male	2.7	(0.0–6.2)	59.9	(7.4)
χ^2_1	0.0			
III Education at Time of Disaster				
Low	0.8	(0.0–1.7)	42.0	(8.2)
Low-average	1.7	(0.0–4.3)	14.1	(3.1)
High-average	6.3	(0.0–14.4)	33.0	(10.7)
High	1.4	(0.0–4.0)	10.8	(3.1)
χ^2_3	6.6			
IV Marital Status at Time of Disaster				
Never married	2.9	(0.0–6.1)	66.1	(6.6)
Ever married	2.6	(0.0–5.1)	33.9	(6.6)
χ^2_1	0.1			
V Subtype				
Human-made disaster	5.5	(0.0–12.5)	26.6	(5.7)
Natural disaster	1.8	(0.3–3.4)	73.4	(5.7)
χ^2_1	5.2*			
VI Serious Injury to Respondent				
No	2.7	(0.4–4.9)	98.9	(0.5)
Yes	15.8	(0.0–36.7)	1.1	(0.5)
χ^2_1	5.1*			
VII Respondent Witnessed Death				
No	2.5	(0.3–4.6)	92.2	(3.3)
Yes	6.6	(0.0–19.9)	7.8	(3.3)
χ^2_1	2.1			
VIII Serious Injury/UD of a Loved One				
No	1.8	(0.0–3.7)	95.7	(1.6)
Yes	23.9	(0.0–50.2)	4.3	(1.6)
χ^2_1	8.6*			
IX Respondent Displaced from Home				
No	1.6	(0.0–3.4)	72.2	(5.6)
Yes	6.1	(0.1–12.0)	27.8	(5.6)
χ^2_1	2.8			
X Number of Prior Traumas				
0	1.3	(0.0–2.6)	74.9	(6.1)
1+	7.3	(0.0–15.2)	25.1	(6.1)
χ^2_2	10.9*			
XI Number of MFF CAs				
0	1.8	(0.1–3.4)	64.9	(7.7)
1	1.4	(0.0–3.6)	15.4	(5.1)
2	8.1	(0.0–24.0)	6.5	(2.7)
3+	6.8	(0.0–19.5)	13.3	(5.7)
χ^2_3	11.5*			

(cont.)

Table 15.A1 *(cont.)*

	Prevalence of DSM-IV/CIDI PTSD		Distribution of the predictor in the total sample	
	% PTSD	(95% CI)	%	(SE)
XII Number of Prior DSM-IV/CIDI Mental Disorders				
0	1.0	(0.0–2.2)	68.3	(7.0)
1	0.8	(0.0–2.1)	17.6	(5.9)
2+	14.0	(1.0–26.9)	14.1	(3.4)
χ^2_3	30.1*			
XIII Total	2.8	(0.5–5.1)		

*Significant at the 0.05 level, two-sided test.
[a]Results are based on weighted data pooled across the six surveys in high-income countries. See footnote a of Table 15.1 for a description of the weighting. χ^2 estimates were based on multivariate models that controlled for survey dummy variables and exactly one of the predictors in the table in predicting PTSD.

Table 15.A2 Detailed associations of prior traumas with DSM-IV/CIDI PTSD controlling for the predictors in Table 15.2, multivariate model 2 ($n = 378$)[a]

	Bivariate[b]		Multivariate model 1[c]		Multivariate model 2	
	OR	(95% CI)	OR	(95% CI)	OR	(95% CI)
I Exposure to Organized Violence						
Relief worker in war zone	0.0	(0.0–0.0)				
Civilian in war zone	118.4*	(11.5–1,217.0)	0.4	(0.0–128.6)		
Civilian in region of terror	0.0	(0.0–0.0)				
Refugee						
Kidnapped	0.0	(0.0–0.0)				
Any	58.6*	(8.8–390.6)			13.3*	(3.5–50.5)
II Participation in Organized Violence						
Witnessed death/dead body/serious injury	2.6	(0.5–13.4)	0.0*	(0.0–0.1)		
Accidentally caused serious injury/death	0.0	(0.0–0.0)				
Combat experience	7.8*	(1.1–57.2)	2.4	(0.9–6.5)		
Purposely injured/tortured/killed someone	0.0	(0.0–0.0)				
Witnessed atrocities	10.2	(0.8–132.3)	521.1	(0.4–6,697.0)		
Any	2.4	(0.5–12.4)			0.4	(0.1–1.1)
III Physical Violence Victimization						
Beaten by caregiver	40.7*	(5.2–317.2)	0.1	(0.0–183.2)		
Beaten by someone else	58.8*	(11.6–299.0)	2.3	(0.3–19.3)		
Witnessed physical fight at home	37.6*	(3.5–407.0)	51.5	(0.1–4,563.5)		
Any	19.3*	(5.1–73.0)			9.5*	(3.1–28.8)
IV Sexual Violence Victimization						
Raped	1.3	(0.1–13.9)	0.0*	(0.0–0.4)		
Sexually assaulted	2.5	(0.1–48.4)	60.2	(0.1–24,723.0)		
Stalked	2.2	(0.0–119.9)	1.6	(0.0–5,131.0)		
Beaten by spouse/romantic partner	2.8	(0.3–28.4)	0.3	(0.0–16.0)		
Trauma to loved one	152.6*	(15.7–1,486.0)	1.0	(0.0–368.1)		
Some other trauma	0.0	(0.0–0.0)				
Private trauma[d]	8.0	(1.8–36.3)	8.8*	(1.2–65.0)		
Any	59.7*	(4.5–783.8)			26.2*	(2.1–327.1)
V Accidents/Injuries						
Natural disaster	6.3	(0.8–48.4)	0.3	(0.0–44.0)		
Toxic chemical exposure	53.7*	(5.9–490.7)	1,050.0	(0.2–4,824.0)		
Automobile accident	1.2	(0.2–5.5)	1.2	(0.0–40.7)		
Life-threatening illness	0.0	(0.0–0.0)				
Child with serious illness	0.0	(0.0–0.0)				
Other life-threatening accident	0.0	(0.0–0.0)				
Any	2.1	(0.7–6.5)			1.5	(0.4–6.6)

Table 15.A2 *(cont.)*

	Bivariate[b]		Multivariate model 1[c]		Multivariate model 2	
	OR	(95% CI)	OR	(95% CI)	OR	(95% CI)
VI Other Trauma						
Mugged/threatened with a weapon	6.7	(0.5–94.4)	4.4	(0.0–1,452.0)		
Human-made disaster	0.0	(0.0–0.0)				
UD of a loved one	4.4	(0.9–21.8)	2.7	(0.1–76.0)		
Any other trauma	2.9	(0.2–37.8)			1.5	(0.1–30.7)
$F_{18,21}$[e]			528.1*		$F_{6,33} = 7.9$*	
$F_{17,22}$[f]			303.4*		$F_{5,34} = 9.7$*	
VII Any Trauma	2.1	(0.2–18.3)				
1	1.1	(0.1–10.3)				
2	0.5	(0.0–55.8)				
3+	10.8*	(1.5–76.8)				
$F_{3,36}$	6.4*					

*Significant at the 0.05 level, two-sided test.
[a]All models were estimated in weighted data pooled across the six surveys in high-income countries. See footnote a of Table 15.1 for a description of the weighting.
[b]The bivariate associations are based on a separate model for each row, with the variable in the row and the predictions in multivariate model 2 from Table 15.2 the predictors in the model.
[c]Only traumas associated with at least one case of PTSD were carried forward into the multivariate models.
[d]A *private* event is a trauma that some individuals reported in response to a question asked at the very end of the trauma section that asked if they ever had some other very upsetting experience they did not tell us about already (and this includes in response to a prior open-ended question about "any other" trauma) because they were too embarrassed or upset to talk about it. Respondents were told, before they answered, that if they reported such a trauma we would not ask them anything about what it was, only about their age when the trauma happened.
[e]The joint significance of all traumas in the model.
[f]The significance of differences among all traumas in the model.

Table 15.A3 Detailed associations of CAs with DSM-IV/CIDI PTSD controlling for the predictors in Table 15.2, multivariate model 3 ($n = 378$)[a]

	Bivariate[b]		Multivariate model 1		Multivariate model 2	
	OR	(95% CI)	OR	(95% CI)	OR	(95% CI)
I MFF CAs						
Parent psychopathology	123.3*	(6.7–2,271.0)	189.4*	(15.6–2,306.0)		
Parent substance misuse	20.9*	(2.9–149.3)	0.8	(0.3–2.1)		
Parent criminality	40.9*	(1.7–973.6)	2.1	(0.3–14.1)		
Family violence	38.5*	(2.9–510.5)	14.7*	(2.6–83.2)		
Physical abuse	23.8*	(3.1–182.9)	0.1	(0.0–0.8)		
Sexual abuse	1.0	(0.1–11.5)	2.9	(0.3–31.5)		
Neglect	69.1*	(2.9–1,627.0)	19.8*	(6.2–63.5)		
$F_{7,32}$[c]			22.4*			
II Other CAs						
Parent death	5.2	(1.9–13.8)	10.2*	(5.1–20.4)		
Parent divorce	56.2*	(3.5–903.6)	5.0*	(1.7–14.2)		
Other parent loss	0.6	(0.0–7.7)	0.6	(0.1–2.5)		
Serious physical illness	0.0	(0.0–0.0)	–[d]	–		
Economic adversity	77.5*	(6.0–1,010.0)	22.5*	(5.9–86.3)		
$F_{4,35}$[c]			13.7*			
$F_{11,28}$[e]			14.0*			
III Number of MFF CAs						
0–3+	6.0*	(1.9–18.8)			4.2*	(2.1–8.3)
1	12.1	(0.8–173.9)				
2	36.9*	(3.1–442.0)				
3+	233.4*	(16.7–3,272.0)				
$F_{3,36}$	11.8*					

(cont.)

Table 15.A3 *(cont.)*

	Bivariate[b]		Multivariate model 1		Multivariate model 2	
	OR	(95% CI)	OR	(95% CI)	OR	(95% CI)
IV Number of Other CAs						
0–2+					3.5	(0.9–13.6)
1	6.3*	(1.5–26.3)				
2+	29.0*	(5.9–142.4)				
$F_{2,37}$	9.9*					

*Significant at the 0.05 level, two-sided test.
[a]All models were estimated in weighted data pooled across the six surveys in high-income countries. See footnote a of Table 15.1 for a description of the weighting.
[b]The bivariate associations are based on a separate model for each row, with the variable in the row and the predictions in Table 15.2, multivariate model 2 the predictors in the model.
[c]The joint significance of the set of ORs for CAs in the group.
[d]Only CAs associated with at least one case of PTSD were carried forward into the multivariate model.
[e]The joint significance of all CAs in the model.

Table 15.A4 Detailed associations of prior DSM-IV/CIDI mental disorders with DSM-IV/CIDI PTSD controlling for the predictors in Table 15.2, multivariate model 4 ($n = 378$)[a]

	Bivariate[b]		Multivariate model 1		Multivariate model 2		Multivariate model 3	
	OR	(95% CI)	OR	(95% CI)	OR	(95% CI)	OR	(95% CI)
I Mood Disorders								
MDD or dysthymic disorder	23.0*	(7.0–75.8)	6.5*	(1.3–34.0)	47.7*	(6.2–365.3)		
BPD (broad definition)	0.2	(0.0–11.8)	0.0	(0.0–2,883.0)	0.0*	(0.0–0.1)		
Any	10.4*	(3.4–32.1)					3.2*	(1.3–7.9)
II Anxiety Disorders								
Panic disorder or agoraphobia	3.3	(0.4–27.6)	3.0	(0.2–49.7)	20.8*	(4.7–91.3)		
GAD	10.8*	(1.3–91.3)	1.8	(0.6–5.6)	13.1*	(5.0–34.6)		
PTSD	8.5*	(3.1–24.0)	1.4	(0.3–7.2)	15.4*	(1.7–138.1)		
Social phobia	10.0	(0.8–124.3)	2.4	(0.8–7.4)	5.0*	(1.1–22.4)		
Specific phobia	31.5*	(13.8–71.7)	2.6	(0.7–10.2)	11.2*	(1.0–124.6)		
Separation anxiety disorder	43.1*	(4.0–463.1)	6.2	(0.7–57.2)	51.1*	(11.1–234.9)		
Any	51.5*	(19.6–135.4)					10.8*	(1.7–68.1)
III Disruptive Behavioral Disorders								
ADHD	20.0*	(2.6–154.7)	1.3	(0.0–3,154.0)	0.6	(0.0–181.7)		
CD	44.6*	(3.8–522.8)	0.9	(0.1–8.3)	8.1	(0.6–110.9)		
IED	204.2*	(23.4–1,779.0)	83.2*	(4.6–1,511.0)	20.4*	(1.5–270.7)		
ODD	78.8*	(11.9–519.9)	75.7*	(1.3–4,289.0)	227.8*	(2.0–26,146.0)		
Any	289.2*	(12.5–6,665.0)					43.1*	(12.5–148.4)
IV Substance Use Disorders								
Alcohol abuse or dependence	54.3*	(4.1–719.7)	40.5*	(15.9–102.7)	349.2*	(2.9–41,683.0)		
Drug abuse or dependence	19.7*	(2.4–159.2)	0.0	(0.0–5.2)	0.0*	(0.0–0.0)		
Any	54.0*	(3.9–738.7)					16.5*	(1.8–153.2)
$F_{14,25}$[c]			76.5*		$F_{4,35} = 79.7$*		$F_{4,35} = 53.7$*	
$F_{13,26}$[d]			85.5*		$F_{3,36} = 59.1$*		$F_{3,36} = 7.5$*	

Table 15.A4 *(cont.)*

	Bivariate[b]		Multivariate model 1		Multivariate model 2		Multivariate model 3	
	OR	(95% CI)	OR	(95% CI)	OR	(95% CI)	OR	(95% CI)
V Total								
Any disorder	26.9*	(8.7–83.6)						
1	9.8	(0.5–192.4)						
2+	60.0*	(21.1–170.5)			0.0	(0.0–14.8)		
$F_{2,37}$	52.5*							

*Significant at the 0.05 level, two-sided test.
[a]All models were estimated in weighted data pooled across the six surveys in high-income countries. See footnote a of Table 15.1 for a description of the weighting.
[b]The bivariate associations are based on a separate model for each row, with the variable in the row and the predictions in multivariate model 2 of Table 15.2 predictors in the model.
[c]The joint significance of all mental disorders in the model.
[d]The significance of differences among all mental disorders in the model.

Chapter 16

Patterns and Predictors of the Course of Posttraumatic Stress Disorder

Anthony J. Rosellini, John Fayyad, Karestan C. Koenen, and Ronald C. Kessler

Little research has been conducted on the predictors of the long-term course of posttraumatic stress disorder (PTSD) (Steinert et al., 2015). The literature suggests that even though a substantial proportion of cases recover within a few months, at least one-third of cases persist for many years (Kessler et al., 1995; Breslau et al., 1998; Pietrzak et al., 2011; Chapman et al., 2012), and that chronic PTSD can lead to both secondary disorders (Perkonigg et al., 2005) and suicidality (Tarrier & Gregg, 2004). To date, retrospective studies have focused on three predictors of PTSD recovery: trauma type characteristics, PTSD symptom severity, and history of comorbid mental disorders (Breslau et al., 1998; Pietrzak et al., 2011; Chapman et al., 2012), while prospective naturalistic studies have identified socio-demographic factors and childhood adversities (CAs) as important predictors (Steinert et al., 2015).

Previous studies of PTSD recovery were based on relatively small samples, making it impossible to investigate fine-grained associations. We address this limitation by presenting data on patterns and predictors of PTSD recovery in a sample of 1,575 respondents with a history of PTSD in the World Mental Health (WMH) surveys (Kessler & Üstün, 2008).

Methods

Analyses are based on the same 22 WMH surveys that assessed PTSD due to randomly selected traumas and are described in other chapters. The predictors considered were: respondent age at trauma exposure, sex, trauma type and history (see Chapter 9), childhood adversities (CAs; see Chapter 10), and prior psychopathology (see Chapter 12). Number of months with PTSD was defined as the minimum of the number of months (or years) the respondent reported having re-experiencing (DSM-IV criterion B), avoidance/numbing (criterion C), and hyperarousal (criterion D) symptoms. If symptoms within all three clusters persisted at the time of interview, the respondent was classified as not having experienced recovery. PTSD recovery was assessed using a discrete-time survival model framework (Willett & Singer, 1993), with person-month the unit of analysis and a logistic link function in SAS version 9.3 (SAS Institute Inc., 2010). The outcome was coded 0 for each person-month until the retrospectively reported month of recovery. Respondents were censored after the month of recovery. The actuarial method (Halli & Rao, 1992) was used to generate descriptive information about the distribution of speed of recovery.

All models included dummy variables for person-month and survey location so that coefficients for other predictors could be interpreted as pooled within-survey coefficients. This approach implicitly assumed that within-survey slopes were constant across surveys. We made this decision because we wanted to focus on central tendencies in the data rather than on analysis of between-survey differences. These associations would have been difficult to interpret because of the small number of countries represented in the series.

Model 1 examined associations of recovery with sex, age at trauma exposure, and number of years between age at exposure and age at interview. These variables were also controlled for in all subsequent models. Model 2 then added dummy variables for the random trauma type. Model 3 added information about history of prior (to the random trauma) trauma exposure. Model 4 added information about history of CAs, and Model 5 added information about prior DSM-IV/CIDI mental disorders. Significant predictors were carried forward across models. Logistic regression coefficients and standard errors were exponentiated and are reported as odds ratios (ORs) with 95% confidence intervals (CIs). In model 2, the logistic regression coefficients were scaled to have a sum of 0 across the 28 trauma types, resulting in the ORs for these trauma types having a product of 1.0. Therefore, the ORs that are significantly different from 1.0 can be interpreted as meaning that PTSD due to the associated trauma types has either a significantly more rapid (ORs >1.0) or more slow (ORs <1.0) odds of recovery than PTSD due to the average trauma. (Our definition of "average" was derived by giving each trauma type equal weight and ignoring the relative prevalence of the different trauma types.) Statistical significance was consistently evaluated using 0.05-level two-sided tests. The design-based Taylor series linearization method (Wolter, 1985) implemented in the SAS software system (SAS Institute Inc., 2008) was used to adjust for the weighting and clustering of observations. Design-based Wald χ^2 tests were used to evaluate statistical significance of predictor sets.

In order to examine overall final model performance, we generated individual-level predicted probabilities of recovery and examined observed recovery curves separately within the first two quartiles and the latter half of the distribution of predicted probability of recovery. The method of replicated 10-fold cross-validation with 20 replicates (i.e., 200 separate estimates of model coefficients) was used to correct for the overestimation of prediction accuracy when, as in this analysis, model coefficients are both estimated and evaluated in the same sample (Smith et al., 2014).

Results

Observed Speed-of-Recovery Distributions by Age-of-Onset

A total of 1,404 respondents out of 1,575 eventually recovered. The slope of the recovery curve was steepest in the first 6 months, with 20% of cases recovering within 3 months and 27% within 6 months (see Figure 16.1). Fifty percent of cases recovered within 24 months and 77% within 10 years (120 months; the longest follow-up period for which a sufficient number of cases were observed for stable estimation of conditional probability of remission). The lowest projected recovery rate was among cases with onsets at ages 60+ (48%), and the highest among cases with onsets at ages 25–44 (89%).

Predictors of Recovery

Socio-demographics and Length of Recall

Sex was not associated with recovery overall ($\chi^2_1 = 1.0$, $p = 0.31$), and age at trauma exposure was significant along the lines seen in Figure 16.1 ($\chi^2_4 = 34.3$,

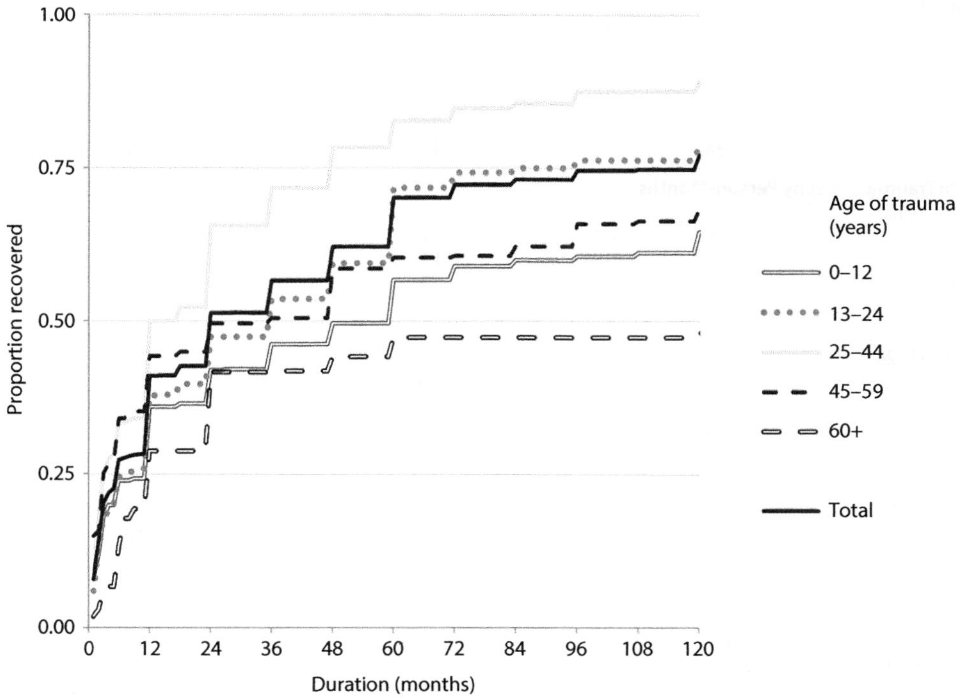

Figure 16.1 Speed of recovery from random trauma PTSD, in the total sample and age of trauma exposure subgroups

$p < 0.001$) (see Table 16.1, model 1). Length of recall between respondent age at trauma exposure and age at interview was also significant; this association is most plausibly interpreted as evidence of time-related recall bias. Length of recall was divided into quartiles (low = 0–7, low-average = 8–16, high-average = 17–30, and high = 31+ years) and its association with recovery was found to differ by time to recovery, where the latter was collapsed to capture meaningful interactions. Length of recall did not predict recovery in the first 12 months after onset ($\chi^2_3 = 4.3, p = 0.23$), by which time, as seen in Figure 16.1, roughly one-fourth of cases had recovered. Length of recall was significant in months 13–24 ($\chi^2_3 = 10.8, p = 0.013$), by which time roughly half of cases had recovered due to a single significantly reduced OR associated with low-average length of recall (OR = 0.5), but odds of recovery were equivalent for cases with both lower and higher length of recall. It was only in months 25+ that a consistently strong monotonic inverse association emerged between length of recall and odds of recovery (ORs in the range 0.5–0.2 for low-average to high length of recall; $\chi^2_3 = 95.5, p < 0.001$).

Based on these results, all subsequent analyses were carried out separately for months 1–24 and 25+, with a recognition that results in the latter subsample might be biased due to recall error. Women had a significantly elevated odds of early recovery (OR = 1.4) and a significantly decreased odds of later recovery (OR = 0.8) compared to men (see Table 16.1, models 1a and 1b). Both models found a significantly elevated odds of recovery among respondents whose traumas occurred

Table 16.1 Associations of sex, age at trauma exposure, and length of recall with recovery from DSM-IV/CIDI PTSD in the WMH surveys ($n = 1{,}575$)[a]

	Multivariate model 1		Multivariate model 1a		Multivariate model 1b	
	OR	(95% CI)	OR	(95% CI)	OR	(95% CI)
I Sex						
Female	1.1	(0.9–1.3)	1.4*	(1.0–2.0)	0.8*	(0.7–1.0)
Male	1.0	–	1.0	–	1.0	–
II Age of Trauma						
0–12	0.8	(0.7–1.1)	0.8	(0.6–1.2)	0.9	(0.7–1.1)
13–24	1.0	–	1.0	–	1.0	–
25–44	1.4*	(1.1–1.6)	1.4*	(1.1–1.8)	1.4*	(1.1–1.9)
45–59	0.9	(0.7–1.2)	1.1	(0.7–1.5)	0.8	(0.6–1.1)
60+	0.7	(0.5–1.0)	0.6*	(0.4–1.0)	1.0	(0.6–1.6)
χ^2_4	34.3*		24.1*		33.4*	
III Years from Trauma Onset by Person-Months						
Person-months 1–12						
High	0.6	(0.4–1.0)	0.7	(0.4–1.1)		
High-average	1.1	(0.8–1.5)	1.1	(0.8–1.6)		
Low-average	1.1	(0.8–1.5)	1.1	(0.8–1.5)		
Low	1.0	–	1.0	–		
χ^2_3	4.3		5.6			
Person-months 13–24						
High	0.8	(0.4–1.5)	0.9	(0.5–1.5)		
High-average	0.9	(0.5–1.5)	0.9	(0.5–1.5)		
Low-average	0.5*	(0.3–0.7)	0.5*	(0.3–0.8)		
Low	1.0	–	1.0	–		
χ^2_3	10.8*		9.0*			
Person-months 25+						
High	0.2*	(0.1–0.4)			0.2*	(0.1–0.4)
High-average	0.3*	(0.2–0.3)			0.3*	(0.2–0.5)
Low-average	0.5*	(0.4–0.7)			0.6*	(0.5–0.7)
Low	1.0	–			1.0	–
χ^2_3	95.5*				42.9*	

*Significant at the 0.05 level, two-sided test.
[a]Coefficients in the first pair of columns are based on a multivariate discrete-time person-month survival model controlling for number of follow-up person-months and survey location among the 1,575 respondents with PTSD associated with random traumas (a total of $n = 111{,}355$ person-months). The coefficients in the next columns are based on separate subgroups in multivariate discrete-time person-month survival models for early recovery (months 1–24) and later recovery (months 25–120) among the same 1,575 respondents.

in middle age (OR = 1.4), whereas odds of early recovery were significantly decreased among respondents whose traumas occurred at ages 60+ (OR = 0.6).

Trauma Type

Distribution of random trauma types ranged from a high of 19.8% for unexpected death of a loved one to 0.2% for natural disasters. This wide variation was a joint function of differences in population prevalence (Benjet et al., 2016) and PTSD risk (Liu et al., 2017). Controlling for the predictors in models 1a and 1b, random trauma type significantly predicted both early ($\chi^2_{26} = 87.8, p < 0.001$) and later ($\chi^2_{26} = 201.3, p < 0.001$) recovery (see Table 16.2, models 2a and 2b). As none of the respondents whose random trauma was purposefully injuring/torturing/killing someone recovered within 24 months of onset, we removed those respondents from the early-recovery sample. Other traumas in five of the six trauma groups were significant in both the early-recovery and later-recovery models, sexual violence victimization being the exception in both cases. Two of five within-group OR differences were nonsignificant in the early-recovery model, leading us to collapse traumas in these groups in that model. We retained individually significant traumas otherwise. Neither collapsed group (exposure to organized violence, and accidents/injuries) had early-recovery odds significantly different from the omitted category (OR = 1.0–1.5). Being beaten up by someone other than a caregiver or romantic partner was the only trauma that had significantly elevated odds of recovery in the early-recovery (OR = 2.3) model, and two other traumas had significantly reduced odds (witnessed atrocities and mugged/threatened with a weapon; OR = 0.2–0.5). The reduced later-recovery model, in comparison, had four traumas with elevated odds of recovery (accidentally caused serious injury/death, witnessed physical fights at home in childhood, other life-threatening accident, and human-made disaster; OR = 1.7–5.0) and two additional traumas with significantly reduced odds (kidnapped and automobile accident; OR = 0.3–0.6).

Prior Traumas

Controlling for the predictors in models 2c and 2d, prior (to age at random trauma exposure) lifetime trauma exposure significantly predicted both early ($\chi^2_{28} = 114.1$, $p < 0.001$) and later ($\chi^2_{28} = 348.2$, $p < 0.001$) recovery (see Table 16.3, models 3a and 3b). Three of the six prior trauma sets were significant in the early-recovery model, in each case with ORs differing significantly within the group, whereas five trauma sets were significant in the later-recovery model (the exception being exposure to organized violence). In one of the latter groups (sexual assault victimization), within-group ORs did not differ significantly from each other, and we consequently entered a count variable of all prior lifetime traumas in that group in the reduced model.

In the reduced early-recovery model, three traumas had significantly elevated odds (witnessed death/dead body/serious injury, combat experience, and the residual "other" trauma category; OR = 1.4–2.9) and four others had significantly reduced odds (refugee, witnessed atrocities, raped, and trauma to loved one; OR = 0.3–0.7). In the reduced later-recovery model (model 3d), five traumas had significantly elevated odds (witnessed death/dead body/serious injury, beaten up by someone other than a caregiver or romantic partner, automobile accident, life-threatening illness, and unexpected death of loved one; OR = 1.4–1.9) and two other significantly reduced odds (accidentally caused serious injury/death and number of sexual violence victimizations; OR = 0.3–0.9).

Childhood Adversities

Controlling for the predictors in models 3c and 3d, CAs significantly predicted both early ($\chi^2_{12} = 44.9$, $p < 0.001$) and later ($\chi^2_{12} = 50.8$, $p < 0.001$) recovery (see Table 16.4, models 4a and 4b) In both cases, this was due to maladaptive family functioning (MFF) CAs ($\chi^2_7 = 36.9–39.3$, $p < 0.001$) rather than other CAs ($\chi^2_5 = 5.2–5.6$, $p = 0.35–0.40$). One MFF CA, witnessing family violence, was associated with significantly elevated odds of recovery in both early-recovery and later-recovery models (OR = 1.4–1.9) and three others with significantly reduced odds in either the early-recovery (neglect; OR = 0.6) or later-recovery (physical and sexual abuse; OR = 0.6) models.

Mental Disorders

Controlling for earlier predictors, prior (to age at random trauma exposure) lifetime DSM-IV/CIDI disorders significantly predicted both early ($\chi^2_{14} = 66.3$, $p < 0.001$) and later ($\chi^2_{14} = 78.4$, $p < 0.001$) recovery. Mood and anxiety disorders were significant as sets in both models, although ORs did not vary within either group in the early-recovery model, but did in the later-recovery model (see Table 16.5, models 5a and 5b). Disruptive behavior disorders were also significant as a set (with significant within-group differences in ORs)

Table 16.2 Associations between randomly selected trauma type with recovery from DSM-IV/CIDI PTSD in the WMH surveys ($n = 1,575$)[a]

	Model 2a Months 1–24		Model 2b Months 25+		Model 2c Months 1–24		Model 2d Months 25+	
	OR	(95% CI)	OR	(95% CI)	OR	(95% CI)	OR	(95% CI)
I Exposure to Organized Violence					1.5	(0.9–2.3)		
Civilian in war zone	2.9	(0.7–11.3)	1.6	(0.8–3.0)				
Civilian in region of terror	2.2*	(1.1–4.6)	1.4	(0.9–2.2)				
Refugee	2.2*	(1.1–4.4)	0.5	(0.2–1.0)				
Kidnapped	0.9	(0.5–1.9)	0.3*	(0.2–0.4)			0.3*	(0.2–0.5)
χ^{2b}_{4}	12.5*		58.3*					
χ^{2c}_{3}	4.0		27.5*					
II Participation in Organized Violence								
Witnessed death/dead body/injury	1.2	(0.8–1.9)	0.7	(0.5–1.0)				
Accidentally caused injury/death	1.4	(0.6–2.8)	2.7*	(1.3–5.7)			3.4*	(1.9–6.3)
Combat experience	0.2*	(0.1–1.0)	1.6	(0.9–2.7)	0.2	(0.1–1.0)		
Purposely injured/tortured/killed someone			0.6*	(0.4–0.9)			0.6	(0.3–1.0)
Witnessed atrocities	0.2*	(0.0–0.8)	1.2	(0.6–2.3)	0.2*	(0.0–0.9)		
χ^{2b}_{5}	10.9*		12.5*		$\chi^2_2 = 8.2$*		$\chi^2_2 = 21.5$*	
χ^{2c}_{4}	10.9*		12.3*		$\chi^2_1 = 0.1$		$\chi^2_1 = 19.4$*	
III Physical Violence Victimization								
Beaten by caregiver	0.8	(0.3–2.1)	0.9	(0.7–1.3)				
Beaten by someone else	2.4*	(1.6–3.6)	1.8*	(1.0–3.3)	2.3*	(1.6–3.5)	1.9	(1.0–3.8)
Witnessed physical fight at home	0.6	(0.4–1.0)	1.7*	(1.2–2.4)			1.7*	(1.2–2.4)
χ^{2b}_{3}	22.2*		14.0*				$\chi^2_2 = 10.8$*	
χ^{2c}_{2}	18.0*		11.8*				$\chi^2_1 = 0.1$	
IV Sexual Violence Victimization								
Raped	1.0	(0.6–1.6)	1.1	(0.8–1.6)				
Sexually assaulted	1.0	(0.5–1.9)	0.9	(0.6–1.3)				
Stalked	1.0	(0.5–1.7)	1.4	(0.8–2.2)				
Beaten by spouse/romantic partner	0.7	(0.5–1.0)	0.7	(0.5–1.0)				
Trauma to loved one	0.8	(0.4–1.5)	0.8	(0.6–1.1)				
Some other trauma	1.3	(0.9–1.9)	0.6*	(0.3–1.0)				
Private trauma[d]	1.1	(0.7–1.6)	1.0	(0.6–1.6)				
χ^{2b}_{7}	7.5		13.3					
χ^{2c}_{6}	7.3		12.0					

V Accidents/Injuries					1.0	(0.7–1.3)		
Natural disaster	2.6*	(1.3–5.3)						
Toxic chemical exposure	0.7	(0.2–2.3)	0.6*	(0.5–0.9)			0.6	(0.4–1.0)
Automobile accident	1.6*	(1.0–2.6)	0.5*	(0.4–0.7)			0.6*	(0.4–0.9)
Life-threatening illness	0.9	(0.5–1.6)	0.7	(0.4–1.1)				
Child with serious illness	1.4	(1.0–2.0)	0.7*	(0.5–1.0)			0.8	(0.5–1.2)
Other life-threatening accident	0.6	(0.2–1.9)	1.8*	(1.4–2.3)			1.9*	(1.3–2.7)
χ^{2b}_{6}	14.5*		76.1*				$\chi^2_1 = 60.0$*	
χ^{2c}_{5}	9.4		76.1*				$\chi^2_3 = 59.9$*	
VI Other								
Mugged/threatened with a weapon	0.5*	(0.3–0.9)	0.7*	(0.6–1.0)	0.5*	(0.3–0.9)	0.8	(0.6–1.1)
Human-made disaster	0.9	(0.2–3.0)	5.1*	(3.1–8.4)			5.0*	(3.1–8.1)
UD of a loved one	1.3	(1.0–1.7)						
χ^{2b}_{3}	9.6*		49.5*				51.7*	
χ^{2c}_{2}	9.5*		48.8*				48.7*	
χ^{2e}_{27}	87.8*		201.3*		$\chi^2_5 = 37.3$*		$\chi^2_{11} = 265.0$*	

*Significant at the 0.05 level, two-sided test.
[a]Coefficients are based on multivariate discrete-time person-month survival models for early recovery (months 1–24) and later recovery (months 25–120) among the 1,575 respondents with PTSD associated with random traumas (a total of $n = 111{,}355$ person-months) controlling for number of follow-up person-months, survey location, and all significant variables in Table 18.1 multivariate models 1a and 1b.
[b]The joint significance of the set of ORs for traumas in the group.
[c]The significance of differences among the ORs within the group.
[d]A *private* trauma is a trauma that some individuals reported in response to a question at the very end of the trauma section that asked if they ever had some other very upsetting experience they did not tell us about already because they were too embarrassed or upset to talk about it. Respondents were told, before they answered, that if they reported such a trauma we would not ask them anything about what it was, only about their age when the trauma happened.
[e]The joint significance of all traumas in the model.

Table 16.3 Associations of history of prior trauma with recovery from DSM-IV/CIDI PTSD in the WMH surveys ($n = 1,575$)[a]

	Multivariate model 3a Months 1–24		Multivariate model 3b Months 25+		Multivariate model 3c Months 1–24		Multivariate model 3d Months 25+	
	OR	(95% CI)	OR	(95% CI)	OR	(95% CI)	OR	(95% CI)
I Exposure to Organized Violence								
Civilian in war zone	0.6	(0.4–1.1)	1.0	(0.7–1.6)				
Civilian in region of terror	0.8	(0.5–1.4)	1.4	(0.9–2.0)				
Refugee	0.3*	(0.1–1.0)	1.7*	(1.1–2.8)	0.3*	(0.1–0.9)		
Kidnapped	2.3*	(1.1–4.6)	1.0	(0.6–1.9)	1.6	(0.8–3.3)		
χ_4^{2b}	13.9*		9.3		$\chi_2^2 = 7.4$*			
χ_3^{2c}	10.9*		3.0		$\chi_1^2 = 7.2$*			
II Participation in Organized Violence								
Witnessed death/dead body/serious injury	1.5*	(1.2–2.0)	1.5*	(1.1–2.0)	1.4*	(1.0–2.0)	1.6*	(1.2–2.1)
Accidentally caused serious injury/death	0.6	(0.2–2.3)	0.4*	(0.2–1.0)			0.3	(0.1–0.8)
Combat experience	2.8*	(1.4–5.7)	0.3	(0.1–1.1)	2.9*	(1.5–5.7)		
Purposely injured/tortured/killed someone	0.8	(0.2–3.6)	0.7	(0.1–4.9)				
Witnessed atrocities	0.4*	(0.2–0.8)	1.2	(0.8–1.8)	0.3*	(0.2–0.6)		
χ_5^{2b}	22.2*		14.1*		$\chi_3^2 = 21.1$*		$\chi_2^2 = 12.8$*	
χ_4^{2c}	14.8*		10.8*		$\chi_2^2 = 19.3$*		$\chi_1^2 = 10.0$*	
III Physical Violence Victimization								
Beaten by caregiver	0.9	(0.7–1.2)	0.8	(0.6–1.1)				
Beaten by someone else	1.4	(1.0–2.1)	1.4*	(1.1–1.9)			1.4*	(1.0–1.9)
Witnessed physical fight at home	1.2	(0.9–1.6)	1.2	(0.9–1.7)				
χ_3^{2b}	6.5		13.0*					
χ_2^{2c}	4.4		11.0*					
IV Sexual Violence Victimization								
Raped	0.7*	(0.5–1.0)	0.8	(0.6–1.1)	0.7*	(0.5–0.9)		
Sexually assaulted	0.8	(0.6–1.2)	1.0	(0.8–1.3)				
Stalked	1.1	(0.7–1.7)	1.2	(0.8–1.8)				
Beaten by spouse/romantic partner	0.8	(0.5–1.2)	0.8	(0.6–1.1)				
Trauma to loved one	0.6*	(0.3–1.0)	0.7	(0.4–1.1)	0.5*	(0.3–0.8)		
Some other trauma	2.8*	(1.3–6.2)	1.2	(0.9–1.6)	2.2*	(1.1–4.2)		
Private trauma[d]	1.1	(0.7–1.8)	1.1	(0.9–1.5)				
Number							0.9*	(0.8–1.0)
χ_7^{2b}	26.4*		14.7*		$\chi_3^2 = 22.8$*			
χ_6^{2c}	15.2*		10.2		$\chi_2^2 = 10.8$*			
V Accidents/Injuries								
Natural disaster	1.1	(0.6–1.8)	1.3	(0.8–2.0)				
Toxic chemical exposure	0.4	(0.1–1.1)	1.0	(0.7–1.5)				
Automobile accident	1.3	(0.9–1.9)	2.0*	(1.4–3.0)			1.9*	(1.3–2.7)
Life-threatening illness	1.2	(0.7–2.1)	1.5*	(1.1–2.1)			1.6*	(1.2–2.0)

Table 16.3 *(cont.)*

	Multivariate model 3a Months 1–24		Multivariate model 3b Months 25+		Multivariate model 3c Months 1–24		Multivariate model 3d Months 25+	
	OR	(95% CI)	OR	(95% CI)	OR	(95% CI)	OR	(95% CI)
Child with serious illness	0.7	(0.4–1.2)	1.3	(0.7–2.6)				
Other life-threatening accident	1.1	(0.6–2.0)	0.9	(0.5–1.5)				
χ^{2b}_{6}	9.9		66.2*				$\chi^2_2 = 46.4$*	
χ^{2c}_{5}	9.9		12.4*				$\chi^2_1 = 0.4$	
IV Other								
Mugged/threatened with a weapon	0.9	(0.6–1.4)	0.8	(0.6–1.0)				
Human-made disaster	0.6	(0.3–1.0)	1.0	(0.7–1.4)				
UD of a loved one	1.1	(0.8–1.5)	1.7*	(1.3–2.2)			1.6*	(1.2–2.0)
χ^{2b}_{3}	4.2		25.1*					
χ^{2c}_{2}	3.8		22.2*					
χ^{2e}_{28}	114.1*		348.2*					

*Significant at the 0.05 level, two-sided test.

[a]Coefficients are based on multivariate discrete-time person-month survival models for early recovery (months 1–24) and later recovery (months 25–120) among the 1,575 respondents with PTSD associated with random traumas (a total of $n = 111{,}355$ person-months) controlling for number of follow-up person-months, survey location, and all significant variables in Table 16.2, multivariate models 2c and 2d.

[b]The joint significance of the set of ORs for traumas in the group.

[c]The significance of the differences among the ORs within the group.

[d]A *private* trauma is a trauma that some individuals reported in response to a question asked at the very end of the trauma section that asked if they ever had some other very upsetting experience they did not tell us about already (and this includes in response to a prior open-ended question about "any other" trauma) because they were too embarrassed or upset to talk about it. Respondents were told, before they answered, that if they reported such a trauma we would not ask them anything about what it was, only about their age when the trauma happened.

[e]The joint significance of all traumas in the model.

Table 16.4 Associations between CAs and recovery from DSM-IV/CIDI PTSD in the WMH surveys ($n = 1{,}575$)[a]

	Multivariate model 4a Months 1–24		Multivariate model 4b Months 25+		Multivariate model 4c Months 1–24		Multivariate model 4d Months 25+	
	OR	(95% CI)	OR	(95% CI)	OR	(95% CI)	OR	(95% CI)
I MFF CAs								
Parent psychopathology	0.7	(0.5–1.0)	1.1	(0.9–1.5)				
Parent substance misuse	1.1	(0.8–1.7)	0.7	(0.5–1.1)				
Parent criminality	1.0	(0.7–1.4)	1.0	(0.7–1.3)				
Family violence	2.0*	(1.5–2.7)	1.5*	(1.1–2.1)	1.9*	(1.4–2.5)	1.4*	(1.0–1.9)
Physical abuse	1.1	(0.8–1.6)	0.7*	(0.5–0.8)			0.6*	(0.5–0.8)
Sexual abuse	1.3	(0.9–1.9)	0.6*	(0.4–0.9)			0.6*	(0.4–0.8)
Neglect	0.6*	(0.4–0.8)	0.9	(0.7–1.2)	0.6*	(0.4–0.8)		
χ^{2b}_{7}	39.3*		36.9*		22.5*		37.5*	
χ^{2c}_{6}	33.5*		36.7*		19.7*		32.9*	
II Other CAs								
Parent death	1.0	(0.7–1.3)	1.2	(0.9–1.6)				
Parent divorce	0.9	(0.6–1.3)	1.2	(0.9–1.7)				
Other parent loss	0.7	(0.4–1.2)	0.9	(0.6–1.2)				

(cont.)

Table 16.4 *(cont.)*

	Multivariate model 4a Months 1–24		Multivariate model 4b Months 25+		Multivariate model 4c Months 1–24		Multivariate model 4d Months 25+	
	OR	(95% CI)	OR	(95% CI)	OR	(95% CI)	OR	(95% CI)
Serious physical illness	1.3	(0.8–2.0)	0.9	(0.6–1.3)				
Economic adversity	0.9	(0.5–1.4)	1.0	(0.8–1.4)				
χ^{2b}_5	5.2		5.6					
χ^{2c}_4	4.0		5.2					
χ^{2d}_{12}	44.9*		50.8*					

*Significant at the 0.05 level, two-sided test.
[a]Coefficients are based on multivariate discrete-time person-month survival models for early recovery (months 1–24) and later recovery (months 25–120) among the 1,575 respondents with PTSD associated with random traumas (a total of *n* = 111,355 person-months) controlling for number of follow-up person-months, survey, and all significant variables in Table 16.3, multivariate models 3c and 3d.
[b]The joint significance of the full set of ORs for CAs in the group.
[c]The significance of the differences among the ORs within the group.
[d]The joint significance of all CAs in the model.

Table 16.5 Associations between mental disorders prior to randomly selected trauma and recovery from DSM-IV/CIDI PTSD in the WMH surveys (*n* = 1,575)[a]

	Multivariate model 5a Months 1–24		Multivariate model 5b Months 25+		Multivariate model 5c Months 1–24		Multivariate model 5d Months 25+	
	OR	(95% CI)	OR	(95% CI)	OR	(95% CI)	OR	(95% CI)
I Mood Disorders								
MDD or dysthymic disorder	1.6*	(1.2–2.0)	0.6*	(0.4–0.7)			0.6*	(0.5–0.8)
BPD (broad definition)	1.2	(0.6–2.2)	1.3	(0.9–1.9)				
Number					1.4*	(1.1–1.7)		
χ^{2b}_2	18.7*		21.9*					
χ^{2c}_1	0.7		12.0*					
II Anxiety Disorders								
Panic disorder or agoraphobia	1.0	(0.7–1.5)	0.9	(0.6–1.2)				
GAD	1.0	(0.7–1.4)	1.4*	(1.0–1.9)			1.3	(1.0–1.7)
PTSD	0.8	(0.6–1.1)	0.4*	(0.3–0.6)			0.4*	(0.3–0.6)
Social phobia	0.7*	(0.6–0.9)	0.7*	(0.6–0.9)			0.8*	(0.6–0.9)
Specific phobia	1.1	(0.8–1.4)	1.2	(1.0–1.6)				
Separation anxiety disorder	0.5*	(0.3–0.7)	1.3*	(1.1–1.7)			1.5*	(1.2–1.8)
Number					0.8*	(0.8–0.9)		
χ^{2b}_6	21.5*		50.1*				$\chi^2_4 = 39.1$*	
χ^{2c}_5	10.4		50.1*				$\chi^2_3 = 38.9$*	
III Disruptive Behavioral Disorders								
ADHD	2.3*	(1.4–3.7)	1.6	(0.6–4.0)	1.9*	(1.2–3.0)		
CD	0.6	(0.3–1.2)	1.1	(0.7–1.9)				
IED	1.3	(0.6–2.6)	0.8	(0.5–1.3)				
ODD	0.9	(0.5–1.4)	0.8	(0.5–1.3)				
χ^{2b}_4	25.8*		2.2					
χ^{2c}_3	15.2*		2.2					
IV Substance Use Disorders								
Alcohol abuse or dependence	0.7	(0.5–1.1)	0.9	(0.6–1.4)				
Drug abuse or dependence	1.6*	(1.0–2.5)	1.1	(0.7–1.9)				

Table 16.5 *(cont.)*

	Multivariate model 5a Months 1–24		Multivariate model 5b Months 25+		Multivariate model 5c Months 1–24		Multivariate model 5d Months 25+	
	OR	(95% CI)	OR	(95% CI)	OR	(95% CI)	OR	(95% CI)
χ_2^{2b}	4.6		0.3					
χ_1^{2c}	4.0*		0.2					
χ_{14}^{2d}	66.3*		78.4*		$\chi_3^2 = 26.9$*		$\chi_5^2 = 52.9$*	

*Significant at the 0.05 level, two-sided test.
[a]Coefficients are based on multivariate discrete-time person-month survival models for early recovery (months 1–24) and later recovery (months 25–120) among the 1,575 respondents with PTSD associated with random traumas (a total of *n* = 111,355 person-months) controlling for number of follow-up person-months, survey location, and all significant variables in earlier models.
[b]The joint significance of the set of ORs for mental disorders in the group.
[c]The significance of the difference among the ORs within the group.
[d]The joint significance of all the mental disorders in the model.

in the early-recovery model, but not the later-recovery model. Substance use disorders were not significant as a set in either model. In the reduced early-recovery model (model 5c), number of mood disorders and ADHD were associated with significantly elevated odds of recovery (OR = 1.4–1.9) and number of anxiety disorders with significantly reduced odds (OR = 0.8). In the reduced later-recovery model (model 5d), prior separation anxiety disorder was associated with significantly elevated odds of recovery (OR = 1.5), whereas major depression-dysthymia, PTSD, and social phobia had significantly reduced odds (OR = 0.4–0.8).

Overall Model Performance

Each respondent was assigned 20 predicted probabilities of recovery in each person-month, based on the coefficients in 20 replicates of 10-fold cross-validated versions of models with the predictors in models 5c and 5d (i.e., the final models), but with coefficients allowed to vary across these replicates. The observations in these two sets of 20 replicates were then divided into three groups consisting of the cases in the top 25%, next 25%, and lowest 50% of *predicted* probabilities of recovery. Speed-of-recovery curves based on *observed* time to recovery in these subgroups were then generated to simulate the likely performance of the models in an independent dataset (see Figure 16.2).

The model distinguished well the two groups predicted to have highest probabilities of recovery (i.e., top 25% and next 25%) from the 50% with lowest predicted probability of recovery and less well between the top two groups. It took 3–4 months for 25% of respondents in the top two groups to recover compared to 12 months in the group predicted to have lowest probability of recovery (see Figure 16.2a). It took 12 months for 50% of respondents in the top group to recover, and 66% recovered by 24 months, compared to 55% in the middle group and 42% in the group with lowest predicted probability of recovery. Seventy-five percent of respondents with highest predicted probability of later recovery did, in fact, recover within 10 years of onset (25% within 3 years, 50% within 5 years), compared to 68% of those with intermediate predicted probabilities (25–50% within 5 years) and 39% of those with lowest predicted probabilities (25% within 5 years) (see Figure 16.2b).

Discussion

Despite substantial variation in the definition of "recovery" in prior studies of PTSD course (Steinert et al., 2015), our findings that 50% of WMH respondents with PTSD recovered within 2 years and roughly 25% had not recovered within 10 years are broadly consistent with previous epidemiological estimates of PTSD recovery after random traumas (Breslau et al., 1998). However, it should be noted that slightly lower and slower rates of recovery have been reported in epidemiological studies of PTSD based on "worst" traumas (Kessler et al., 1995; Chapman et al., 2012).

Our failure to find a sex difference in PTSD recovery is consistent with the results of a meta-analysis of predictors of PTSD recovery (Morina et al., 2014). Our finding of opposite-sign sex differences in early recovery (women higher recovery than men) and later recovery (women lower recovery than men) is new as no previous studies have examined interactions between predictors and timing of recovery. Nor are we aware of any

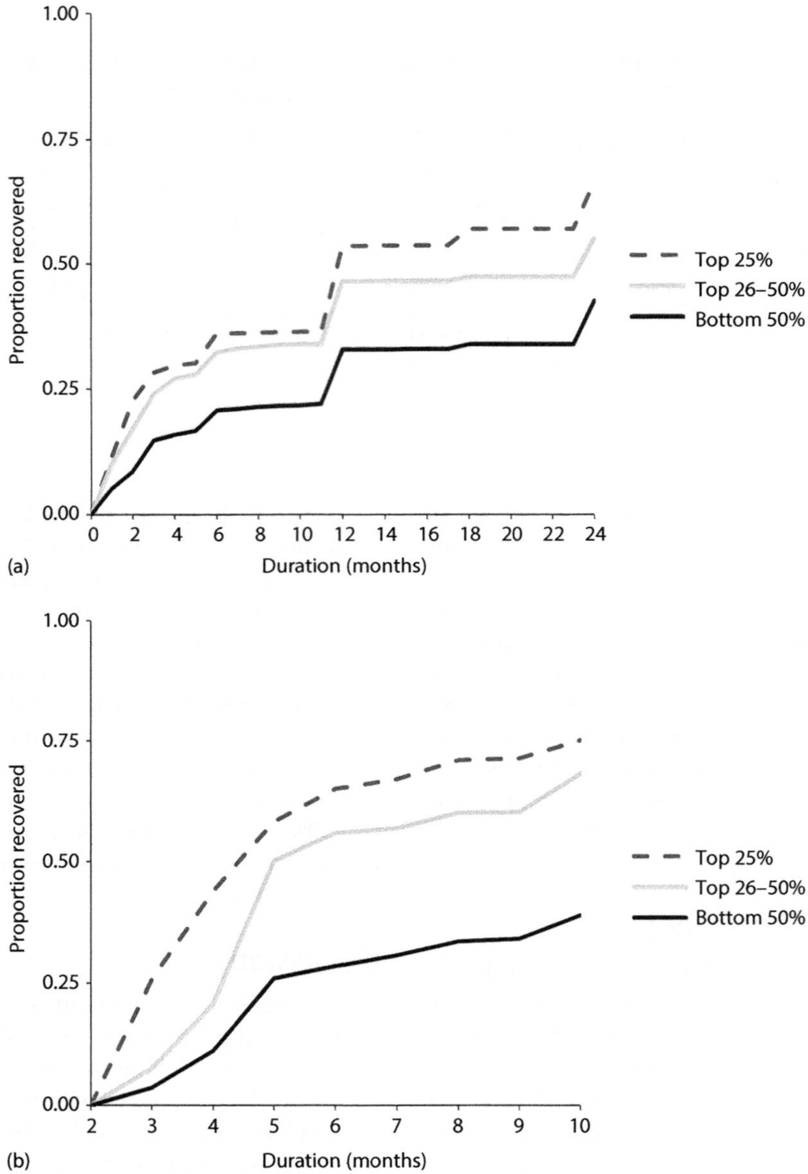

Figure 16.2 Speed of recovery from random trauma PTSD within subgroups defined by cross-validated final model predicted probability of recovery separately for early-recovery (a, 1–24 months) and later-recovery (b, 25–120 months) models

previous research that addresses the significant association we found between length of recall and retrospective reports about PTSD recovery. As noted earlier, this association is most plausibly interpreted as resulting from a recall bias related to length of the recall period. But this association was largely confined to later recovery, so our results regarding the predictors of early recovery may well have been less influenced by recall bias.

Very low relative odds of early recovery (OR = 0.0–0.3) were found for two trauma types (purposefully injuring/torturing/killing someone and witnessing atrocities) and of later recovery for another (being kidnapped). Very high odds of early recovery (OR = 3.0+) were found for no trauma types and of later recovery for two trauma types (accidentally causing injury/death, and human-made disaster). Other significant between-trauma differences in recovery were few in number and comparatively modest in magnitude. No trauma type was a significant predictor in both early-recovery and later-recovery models. These results are broadly consistent with prior research showing that between-trauma differences in recovery rates are for the most part nonsignificant (Morina et al., 2014). While the literature suggests there is an exception to this general pattern – that there is a significantly higher recovery rate from natural disasters than from other traumas – the WMH data did not replicate this finding.

We are unaware of previous epidemiological research on the associations of PTSD recovery with prior traumas or CAs, even though both factors have consistently been found to predict increased risk of *onset* of PTSD (Liu et al., 2017; McLaughlin et al., 2017). In the WMH data, history of being a refugee and of witnessing atrocities (early recovery) and accidentally causing serious injury/death (later recovery) were the only prior traumas associated with very low odds of recovery. No prior trauma type was associated with very high odds of recovery, and no CAs were associated either with very low or with very high odds of recovery. No prior trauma type other than witnessing death/dead body/serious injury, and no CA other than exposure to childhood family violence was a significant predictor in both the early-recovery and later-recovery models. However, the consistently significant ORs for these variables were not large (OR = 1.4–1.9).

Our finding that history of DSM-IV anxiety disorders (i.e., number of disorders, social phobia, and PTSD) was associated with decreased likelihood of PTSD recovery is broadly consistent with the results of both cohort (Pietrzak et al., 2014) and clinical (Zlotnick et al., 2004) studies that found comorbid prior anxiety disorders to be associated with a more chronic course of PTSD. It is noteworthy, though, that separation anxiety disorder was associated with decreased likelihood of early PTSD recovery, but increased likelihood of later recovery. Such divergent results may help explain why a summary measure of *any* pretrauma anxiety disorder was not significantly associated with PTSD recovery in the one prior general population epidemiological study that examined these associations using retrospective reports (Chapman et al., 2012). We are unaware of prior studies that examined the association of temporally primary ADHD with PTSD recovery.

Our finding that observed recovery curves differed substantially between the subgroups defined as having higher and lower predicted probabilities of recovery raises the possibility that a model such as the ones presented here could be developed at the time of trauma exposure to classify survivors into those with higher and lower probabilities of recovery. However, it is unclear how much value such a model would have for targeting interventions. After all, much more robust models that predict PTSD onset already exist (Kessler et al., 2014), and various post-trauma factors, such as initial treatment response, which are not available at the time of trauma exposure, have been found to predict recovery (Brackbill et al., 2009; North et al., 2011; Pietrzak et al., 2014). The receipt of an evidence-based treatment for PTSD, which we did not evaluate here, is also an important determinant of PTSD recovery (Courtois et al., 2017). Nonetheless, our results are noteworthy, given that the pretrauma predictors considered here as well as the random trauma type are associated with striking differences in the shape of speed-of-recovery curves.

A number of limitations of the analysis are noteworthy. First, the data were based on retrospective reports that are subject to recall bias. Second, PTSD was assessed with a fully structured diagnostic interview with a low sensitivity rather than with a semi-structured clinical interview, while recovery was defined using a relatively coarse dichotomous measure. Third, the predictors were limited to those available in the survey, namely, socio-demographics, CAs, prior (to the index trauma) traumas, and prior psychopathology. Fourth, we did not take into consideration treatment or other factors that occurred after the trauma. Within the context of these limitations, we analyzed a unique cross-national epidemiological sample. We focused on representative PTSD cases associated with randomly selected traumas. We replicated the findings in previous studies that a substantial minority of PTSD cases recover within a short period of time, that the majority of cases recover within 2 years, and that another substantial minority of cases do not recover even after many years. We found weak evidence for associations of socio-demographics, trauma types, and trauma history with recovery. We found that prior anxiety disorders predict recovery, but again with fairly modest magnitudes of association. Although our composite risk model discriminated well between the recovery trajectories within the 50% of patients predicted to have the highest and lowest probabilities of recovery, this recovery model was much weaker than models using the same kinds of pretrauma variables to predict PTSD onset, highlighting the importance of including information on post-trauma symptoms and experiences to develop robust models of PTSD recovery.

Acknowledgment

Portions of this chapter are based on Rosellini, A. J., Fayyad, J., Koenen, K. C. and Kessler, R. C. (2018). Recovery from DSM-IV post-traumatic stress disorder in the WHO World Mental Health surveys, *Psychological Medicine*, 48, 437–50 reproduced with permission.

References

Benjet, C., Bromet, E., Karam, E. G., et al. (2016). The epidemiology of traumatic event exposure worldwide: results from the World Mental Health Survey Consortium. *Psychological Medicine*, 46, 327–43.

Brackbill, R. M., Hadler, J. L., DiGrande, L., et al. (2009). Asthma and posttraumatic stress symptoms 5 to 6 years following exposure to the World Trade Center terrorist attack. *JAMA*, 302, 502–16.

Breslau, N., Kessler, R. C., Chilcoat, H. D., et al. (1998). Trauma and posttraumatic stress disorder in the community: the 1996 Detroit Area Survey of Trauma. *Archives of General Psychiatry*, 55, 626–32.

Chapman, C., Mills, K., Slade, T., et al. (2012). Remission from post-traumatic stress disorder in the general population. *Psychological Medicine*, 42, 1695–703.

Courtois, C. A., Sonis, J., Brown, L. S., et al. (2017). Clinical practice guideline for the treatment of Posttraumatic Stress Disorder (PTSD) in adults (online). Available at: www.apa.org/ptsd-guideline/ptsd.pdf (Accessed August 22, 2017).

Halli, S. S., & Rao, K. V. (1992). *Advanced Techniques of Population Analysis*. New York, NY: Springer US.

Kessler, R. C., Rose, S., Koenen, K. C., et al. (2014). How well can post-traumatic stress disorder be predicted from pre-trauma risk factors? An exploratory study in the WHO World Mental Health Surveys. *World Psychiatry*, 13, 265–274.

Kessler, R. C., Sonnega, A., Bromet, E., Hughes, M., & Nelson, C. B. (1995). Posttraumatic stress disorder in the National Comorbidity Survey. *Archives of General Psychiatry*, 52, 1048–60.

Kessler, R. C., & Üstün, T. B. eds. (2008). *The WHO World Mental Health Surveys: Global Perspectives on the Epidemiology of Mental Disorders*. New York, NY: Cambridge University Press.

Liu, H., Petukhova, M. V., Sampson, N. A., et al. (2017). Association of DSM-IV posttraumatic stress disorder with traumatic experience type and history in the World Health Organization World Mental Health surveys. *JAMA Psychiatry*, 74, 270–81.

McLaughlin, K. A., Koenen, K. C., Bromet, E. J., et al. (2017). Childhood adversities and post-traumatic stress disorder: evidence for stress sensitization in the World Mental Health Surveys. *British Journal of Psychiatry*, 211, 280–8.

Morina, N., Wicherts, J. M., Lobbrecht, J., & Priebe, S. (2014). Remission from post-traumatic stress disorder in adults: a systematic review and meta-analysis of long term outcome studies. *Clinical Psychology Review*, 34, 249–55.

North, C. S., Pfefferbaum, B., Kawasaki, A., Lee, S., & Spitznagel, E. L. (2011). Psychosocial adjustment of directly exposed survivors 7 years after the Oklahoma City bombing. *Comprehensive Psychiatry*, 52, 1–8.

Perkonigg, A., Pfister, H., Stein, M. B., et al. (2005). Longitudinal course of posttraumatic stress disorder and posttraumatic stress disorder symptoms in a community sample of adolescents and young adults. *American Journal of Psychiatry*, 162, 1320–7.

Pietrzak, R. H., Feder, A., Singh, R., et al. (2014). Trajectories of PTSD risk and resilience in World Trade Center responders: an 8-year prospective cohort study. *Psychological Medicine*, 44, 205–19.

Pietrzak, R. H., Goldstein, R. B., Southwick, S. M., & Grant, B. F. (2011). Prevalence and Axis I comorbidity of full and partial posttraumatic stress disorder in the United States: results from Wave 2 of the National Epidemiologic Survey on Alcohol and Related Conditions. *Journal of Anxiety Disorders*, 25, 456–65.

SAS Institute Inc. (2008). *SAS Software, Version 9.2*. Cary, NC: SAS Institute Inc.

SAS Institute Inc. (2010). *SAS/STATR Software. Version 9.3 for Unix*. Cary, NC: SAS Institute Inc.

Smith, G. C., Seaman, S. R., Wood, A. M., Royston, P., & White, I. R. (2014). Correcting for optimistic prediction in small data sets. *American Journal of Epidemiology*, 180, 318–24.

Steinert, C., Hofmann, M., Leichsenring, F., & Kruse, J. (2015). The course of PTSD in naturalistic long-term studies: high variability of outcomes. A systematic review. *Nordic Journal of Psychiatry*, 69, 483–96.

Tarrier, N., & Gregg, L. (2004). Suicide risk in civilian PTSD patients – predictors of suicidal ideation, planning and attempts. *Social Psychiatry and Psychiatric Epidemiology*, 39, 655–61.

Willett, J. B., & Singer, J. D. (1993). Investigating onset, cessation, relapse, and recovery: why you should, and how you can, use discrete-time survival analysis to examine event occurrence. *Journal of Consulting and Clinical Psychology*, 61, 952–65.

Wolter, K. M. (1985). *Introduction to Variance Estimation*. New York, NY: Springer-Verlag.

Zlotnick, C., Rodriguez, B. F., Weisberg, R. B., et al. (2004). Chronicity in posttraumatic stress disorder and predictors of the course of posttraumatic stress disorder among primary care patients. *Journal of Nervous and Mental Disease*, 192, 153–9.

Chapter 17

DSM-5 and ICD-11 Definitions of Posttraumatic Stress Disorder: Investigating "Narrow" and "Broad" Approaches

Dan J. Stein, Matthew J. Friedman, Katie A. McLaughlin, Kate M. Scott, and Ronald C. Kessler

As noted in Chapter 1, the diagnostic criteria for posttraumatic stress disorder (PTSD) have changed with each subsequent edition of the *Diagnostic and Statistical Manual of Mental Disorders* (DSM), including the latest edition, DSM-5, released in 2013, reflecting in part debates about the distinctions between normal versus maladaptive responses to traumatic stressors (Yehuda & McFarlane, 1995) and the potential for inappropriate medicalization of suffering (Stein et al., 2007). The diagnostic criteria for PTSD have also varied across editions of the International Classification of Diseases (ICD), with anticipated tightening of criteria in the forthcoming 11th edition in order to avoid the overdiagnosis of PTSD (Maercker et al., 2013a). These changes to the PTSD diagnosis, evident in DSM-5 and anticipated in ICD-11, have, in turn, reinvigorated debate about the appropriate criteria for PTSD and the implications of criteria differences across each of the diagnostic systems (Friedman et al., 2011; Friedman, 2013; Kilpatrick, 2013; Maercker & Perkonigg, 2013).

DSM-IV and ICD-10 criteria for PTSD differ in multiple ways. First, DSM-IV defined the potentially traumatic event (which we refer to in this volume simply as "trauma") as one that causes threat to the integrity of the person or others (A1 criterion), with the reaction of the individual characterized by intense fear, helplessness, or horror (A2 criterion) (American Psychiatric Association, 2000), whereas ICD-10 Diagnostic Criteria for Research (ICD-10-DCR) refer to an event that precipitates distress in almost anyone (World Health Organization, 1993). Second, although DSM-IV criteria included both avoidance and numbing symptoms, ICD-10-DCR includes only avoidance symptoms. Third, DSM-IV required the presence of clinically significant distress or impairment, while ICD-10-DCR does not. Fourth, DSM-IV required that symptoms continue for at least 1 month, whereas ICD-10-DCR emphasizes that symptoms begin within 6 months of the event and that some persist, but does not specify a minimum required duration.

Two important changes to the definition of a traumatic stressor and the associated symptoms needed to qualify for a PTSD diagnosis were made in DSM-5 (American Psychiatric Association, 2013). First, based on evidence that the A2 criterion had insufficient clinical utility, the requirement of a subjective response to the trauma of fear, helplessness, or horror was eliminated (Friedman et al., 2011) (see also Chapter 18). By eliminating A2, DSM-5 expanded the context of PTSD from an exclusively fear-based anxiety disorder to a disorder that also included anhedonic/dysphoric and externalizing phenotypes. Second, based on factor analyses of PTSD symptoms (Friedman et al., 2011), the number of clusters of PTSD symptoms required to qualify for a diagnosis was increased from three to four, with avoidance and numbing symptoms split into separate clusters and expanded to represent avoidance and persistent negative alterations in cognitions and mood. The expanded symptoms include persistent negative evaluation of self or others, elevated self-blame, a negative emotional state, and reckless or self-destructive behavior.

Anticipated revisions to the PTSD diagnosis in ICD-11 (Cloitre et al., 2013; Maercker et al., 2013a, 2013b) emphasize that the construct of PTSD should have both global applicability and clinical utility (International Advisory Group for the Revision of ICD-10 Mental and Behavioural Disorders, 2011), reflecting concerns about the potential overdiagnosis of PTSD in disaster-exposed populations (Tol et al., 2011). In keeping with previous recommendations (Spitzer et al., 2007; Brewin et al., 2009), the ICD-11 Workgroup has recommended including three core symptom clusters (re-experiencing, avoidance of traumatic reminders, and hyperarousal) and removing nonspecific symptoms that are also found in other conditions (e.g., trouble concentrating, sleep problems). Duration of required symptoms and degree of functional impairment are used to differentiate normal reactions to traumatic stressors from PTSD.

Several questions about these changes and differences deserve further consideration. First, what is the impact of changes in the diagnostic criteria sets on PTSD prevalence cross-nationally? Second, to what extent do the diagnostic criteria identify overlapping populations of individuals? Previous evidence suggests that prevalence estimates of DSM-IV and ICD-10 PTSD are similar, but that the systems identify somewhat distinct sets of individuals, although this research is based on data from only one country (Peters et al., 1999). Third, do individuals diagnosed with PTSD using each of the diagnostic criteria sets exhibit similar clinical characteristics, including distress, impairment, suicidality, and comorbidity? Given that ICD-10 does not require distress and impairment for diagnosis, it is likely that ICD-10 cases are associated with lower levels of such outcomes. Again, prior comparison of DSM-IV and ICD-10 PTSD has shown that the absence of the distress/impairment criterion results in higher PTSD prevalence in ICD-10 (Peters et al., 1999). Fourth, as part of a broader concern with implications of differences among systems, is PTSD differentially associated with socio-demographic factors, trauma types, and lifetime history of mental disorder across the systems?

Answering these questions is key to understanding the global impact of changes to the diagnostic criteria for PTSD. The World Mental Health (WMH) surveys provide an important opportunity for beginning to do so.

Methods

When this analysis was carried out, data were available from WMH surveys in 13 countries, including eight classified by the World Bank as high-income (Belgium, Germany, Italy, Japan, the Netherlands, New Zealand, Spain, and the United States), four upper-middle-income (São Paulo in Brazil, Bulgaria, Mexico, and Romania), and one lower-middle-income (Colombia). There were 34,321 Part II WMH survey respondents across these 13 surveys. Traumas and PTSD were assessed using the methods described in Chapter 2. A total of 23,936 Part II respondents across surveys reported one or more lifetime traumas, with 24.6% of those with traumas reporting exactly one and the others reporting a mean of 6.0 (range 2–160; interquartile range 3–6), for a total of approximately 114,000 traumas. The analyses reported here focused on PTSD assessed for the random trauma across these 23,936 respondents, with weighting to adjust for between-person differences in probability of the random trauma being selected based on number of lifetime traumas experienced by the respondent.

Both DSM-IV and ICD-10 criteria for PTSD were fully operationalized in the CIDI, as ICD-10 criteria B–D are a subset of the DSM-IV criteria. DSM-5 criteria (American Psychiatric Association, 2013) were approximated by fully operationalizing DSM-5 criteria B (one or more of five symptoms of intrusive recollection), C (one or both of two symptoms of avoidance), F (duration of more than one month), and G (clinically significant distress or impairment), and partially operationalizing criteria D (two or more of seven symptoms of negative alterations in cognitions and mood, three of which were not assessed in the CIDI) and E (two or more of six symptoms of marked alterations in arousal and reactivity, one of which was not assessed in the CIDI). Proposed ICD-11 diagnostic guidelines (Maercker et al., 2013a) were approximated by operationalizing the requirements of (1) avoidance of thoughts-memories of the trauma or of activities-situations reminiscent of the trauma, (2) excessive hypervigilance or enhanced startle reactions, and (3) significant impairment in functioning, while closely approximating the requirement of (4) re-experiencing the trauma in the form of either vivid intrusive memories, flashbacks, or nightmares accompanied by fear or horror. (A detailed description of coding rules is available on request.)

In addition to PTSD, the CIDI assessed five DSM-IV fear disorders (panic disorder without agoraphobia, specific phobia, social phobia, agoraphobia without history of panic disorder, and obsessive compulsive disorder), three distress disorders (major depressive disorder/dysthymia, generalized anxiety disorder, bipolar disorders [I–II and sub-threshold BPD]), three disruptive behavior disorders (oppositional-defiant disorder [ODD], and conduct disorder [CD], intermittent explosive disorder), and two substance disorders (alcohol and drug abuse with or without dependence). Age-of-onset of each disorder was assessed using special probing techniques shown experimentally to improve recall accuracy (Knäuper et al., 1999). DSM-IV organic exclusion rules and diagnostic hierarchy rules were used (other than for ODD, which was defined with or without CD, and substance abuse, which was defined with or without dependence). As detailed elsewhere (Haro et al., 2006), generally good concordance was found between these CIDI diagnoses and blinded clinical diagnoses based on clinical reappraisal interviews with the SCID (First et al., 1994).

Differential predictors of the different types of PTSD were investigated by focusing on the following predictors: sex, age at trauma exposure, trauma type (war-related, other interpersonal violence, intimate/sexual violence, accidents, death of loved one, other network traumas, and other traumas), number of temporally prior lifetime fear/distress disorders (anxiety and mood disorders), and number of temporally prior lifetime behavior/substance disorders. Four outcomes were considered: severe distress or impairment associated with symptoms of PTSD as assessed by CIDI questions requiring first lifetime onset of suicidal ideation in conjunction with the focal trauma in the subsample of respondents with no lifetime history of suicidality; and first lifetime onset of any fear disorder or any distress disorder in the subsample of respondents with no lifetime history of those disorders. Suicidality was assessed with the CIDI Suicidal Behavior module (Kessler & Üstün, 2004).

Multivariate additive associations among PTSD symptoms were examined with exploratory factor analysis of the tetrachoric correlation matrix between all logically possible pairs of dichotomously scored symptoms. The parallel analysis simulation method (Hayton et al., 2004) was used to select the number of factors to retain in the analysis, while promax rotation was used to improve our ability to interpret the solution. Prevalence estimates of PTSD based on each of the four diagnostic systems, on any of the four systems (referred to below as *broadly defined* PTSD), and on multisystem profiles were then estimated with cross-tabulations.

Regression analysis was then used to examine the associations of PTSD according to the different diagnostic systems with each of the four outcomes. As the cross-tabulations showed that the numbers of cases in some of the 15 logically possible multivariate profiles of diagnoses across the four systems (i.e., 2^4–1) were too small to allow completely disaggregated comparisons, we made only three comparisons for each of the four diagnostic systems for each outcome: (1) between *narrow* cases within the diagnostic system (i.e., cases that met criteria for PTSD according to the criteria of the system, but not according to the criteria of any of the other three systems) and broadly defined noncases (i.e., respondents that did not meet criteria for PTSD according to the criteria of any of the four systems); (2) between *total* cases within the diagnostic system (i.e., cases that met criteria for PTSD according to the criteria of the system whether or not they also meet criteria in any of the other three systems) and broadly defined non-cases; and (3) between *other* cases (i.e., cases that did not meet criteria for PTSD according to the criteria of the system, but did meet criteria for at least one of the other three systems) and broadly defined noncases.

The equations to predict comorbid fear and distress disorders predicted lifetime first onset of each such disorder in the year of trauma exposure in the subsample of respondents without a lifetime history of the outcome disorder. These equations were based on a combined person-disorder data array in which a separate sample of eligible respondents was defined for each disorder. For example, a separate sample was defined for each of the five fear disorders depending on lifetime history of that disorder. These five datasets were then combined and a single logistic regression equation was estimated in this combined dataset (with four dummy control variables to distinguish among the five disorders) to estimate a single set of predictor coefficients constrained to be equal across all five outcomes.

We then used logistic regression to examine differences in the socio-demographic, trauma-related, and psychopathological predictors of PTSD in the four different types of PTSD. This was done by estimating four logistic regression equations, one for PTSD diagnoses in each system, that used information about sex, age at trauma exposure, type of trauma (using the seven-category classification scheme described earlier with traumatic death of a loved one serving as the reference category), and (to the age of trauma exposure) lifetime history of fear/distress and behavior/substance disorders (dummy variables for exactly one and more than one disorder of each type) to distinguish between *total* cases according to the focal system and *other* cases. Logistic regression coefficients and their standard errors were exponentiated and are reported here as odds ratios (ORs) with 95% confidence intervals (CIs). Statistical significance was consistently evaluated using 0.05-level two-sided tests. The design-based Taylor series method implemented in the SAS software system (Wolter, 2007) was used to adjust for the weighting and clustering of observations.

Results

Exploratory Factor Analysis

Exploratory factor analysis was carried out on the matrix of tetrachoric correlations among the 17 DSM-IV criteria B–D symptoms of PTSD assessed in

Table 17.1 Rotated (promax) standardized regression coefficients based on exploratory factor analysis of DSM-IV/CIDI PTSD symptom questions ($n = 23{,}936$)[a]

	I	II	III	IV
I IRs				
Repeated unwanted memories of random trauma	0.84	0.11	0.00	0.03
Repeated unpleasant dreams about random trauma	0.79	0.06	−0.02	0.05
Flashbacks of random trauma happening	0.84	0.06	−0.07	0.05
Get very upset when reminded of random trauma	0.87	0.00	0.10	−0.05
Have physical reactions when reminded of random trauma	0.59	−0.05	0.16	0.20
II AV				
Try not to think about random trauma	0.13	0.82	−0.05	0.10
Purposely stay away from things that remind of random trauma	−0.03	0.75	0.28	0.05
III CM				
Unable to remember important parts of random trauma	−0.01	0.48	0.46	−0.10
Lose interest in things used to enjoy	0.14	0.09	0.84	−0.11
Feel emotionally distant/cut-off from people	0.08	0.14	0.84	−0.03
Trouble feeling love/happiness toward others	−0.06	0.12	0.87	0.08
Feel no reason to plan for the future	−0.07	0.09	0.79	0.11
IV AR				
Trouble falling asleep during random trauma	0.32	−0.12	0.18	0.50
More irritable than usual during random trauma	0.09	−0.17	0.37	0.55
More trouble concentrating during random trauma	0.21	−0.20	0.50	0.39
Much more alert/watchful with no real need	−0.03	0.22	−0.14	0.94
More easily startled by ordinary noises	0.08	0.11	−0.01	0.83

[a]Principal axis factor analysis of weighted (see the text for a discussion of weighting) tetrachoric correlation matrix of responses to dichotomous symptom question.

the WMH surveys. Parallel analysis showed that four meaningful factors existed in the data (see Table 17.1). Promax rotation led to a solution that corresponded closely to the DSM-5 symptom dimensions of re-experiencing, avoidance, numbing, and arousal.

Table 17.2 Prevalence of PTSD according to the criteria of each and any of the four diagnostic systems ($n = 23{,}936$)

	Total sample		Among respondents with broadly defined PTSD[a]	
	%	(SE)	%	(SE)
DSM-IV	3.3	(0.2)	58.4	(2.5)
DSM-5	3.0	(0.2)	53.5	(2.5)
ICD-10	4.4	(0.3)	79.4	(2.2)
ICD-11	3.2	(0.2)	57.4	(2.7)
Any	5.6	(0.3)	100.0	–
(*n*)	(23,936)		(1,581)	

[a]Broadly defined PTSD is PTSD according to the criteria of any of the four systems.

Prevalence

A total of 5.6% of respondents met criteria for PTSD in at least one of the four systems (see Table 17.2). We refer to these cases below as having broadly defined PTSD. The system with the highest prevalence (standard error in parentheses) was ICD-10 (4.4 [0.3]%, including 79.3% of all broadly defined cases), followed by DSM-IV and ICD-11 (each 3.2 [0.2]%, including 58.4% and 57.4%, respectively, of all broadly defined cases), and the lowest was DSM-5 (3.0 [0.2]%, including 53.4% of all broadly defined cases) (see Table 17.3). One-third of broadly defined cases (1.8% of all respondents) met criteria in all four systems, an additional one-third of broadly defined cases in either three (0.9% of all respondents) or two (an additional 0.9% of all respondents) systems, and the final one-third of broadly defined cases (1.9% of all respondents) in only one of the four systems. The much higher prevalence of cases based on ICD-10 than the other systems was reflected in the fact that narrow ICD-10 PTSD was the second most common profile (22.1% of all broadly defined cases), the most common being cases meeting criteria in all four systems, while the other narrowly defined types were quite uncommon (1.5–6.3% of all broadly defined cases).

Variation in Adverse Outcomes Associated with Different Types of PTSD

The vast majority (95%) of the 44 ORs that compared outcomes among respondents with PTSD to outcomes among respondents classified as broadly defined non cases were greater than 1.0 and statistically significant

Table 17.3 The cross-classification of PTSD prevalence across the four diagnostic systems ($n = 23{,}936$)

	Total sample		Among respondents with broadly defined PTSD	
	%	(SE)	%	(SE)
I Meets Criteria in All Four Systems				
DSM-IV, DSM-5, ICD-10, ICD-11	1.8	(0.2)	33.1	(2.2)
II Meets Criteria in Three Systems				
DSM-IV, DSM-5, ICD-10	0.4	(0.1)	7.7	(1.2)
DSM-IV, DSM-5, ICD-11	0.3	(0.1)	5.8	(1.3)
DSM-IV, ICD-10, ICD-11	0.1	(0.0)	2.6	(0.5)
DSM-5, ICD-10, ICD-11	0.0	(0.0)	0.8	(0.5)
Any three systems	0.9	(0.1)	16.8	(1.8)
III Meets Criteria in Two Systems				
DSM-IV, DSM-5	0.1	(0.0)	0.9	(0.3)
DSM-IV, ICD-10	0.2	(0.1)	2.8	(0.8)
DSM-IV, ICD-11	0.1	(0.1)	1.4	(1.1)
DSM-5, ICD-10	0.2	(0.1)	3.3	(1.0)
DSM-5, ICD-11	0.0	(0.0)	0.5	(0.3)
ICD-10, ICD-11	0.4	(0.1)	7.0	(1.2)
Any two systems	0.9	(0.1)	15.8	(1.8)
IV Meets Criteria in One System				
DSM-IV	0.2	(0.0)	4.4	(0.8)
DSM-5	0.1	(0.0)	1.5	(0.7)
ICD-10	1.2	(0.2)	22.1	(2.4)
ICD-11	0.4	(0.1)	6.3	(1.2)
Any one system	1.9	(0.2)	34.3	(2.4)
V Meets Criteria in Any of the Four Systems				
Any	5.6	(0.3)	100.0	–
(*n*)	(23,936)		(1,581)	

(89%) (see Table 17.4). The same was true of all four ORs associated with narrowly defined DSM-IV PTSD, all four of those associated with narrowly defined DSM-5 PTSD, three of the four ORs associated with narrowly defined ICD-10 PTSD, and one of the four ORs associated with narrowly defined ICD-11 PTSD. These results suggested that each of the four diagnostic systems detected at least some clinically significant cases that were missed by the three other systems. Narrowly defined DSM-IV cases tended to be more severe than DSM-IV cases that also met criteria for PTSD in any of the other systems. The opposite was true for narrowly defined ICD-10 and ICD-11 cases, both of which had consistently lower severity scores than total cases. The number of narrowly defined DSM-5 cases was so small that comparisons between narrowly defined and total DSM-5 cases could not be made. Total DSM-IV and DSM-5 cases were consistently more severe than other cases, while total ICD-10 and ICD-11 cases were for the most part less severe than other cases.

Differential Predictors

The associations of age of trauma exposure and sex with PTSD risk did not vary significantly across the four diagnostic systems (see Table 17.5). However, there was some variation in the differential risk of PTSD across trauma types, depending on the diagnostic system used to define PTSD. The most important source of this variation was that interpersonal violence was associated with significantly higher PTSD risk relative to the unexpected death of a loved one when PTSD was defined using ICD-11 criteria (which was true for 57.4% of respondents with broadly defined PTSD) rather than criteria based on any of the other diagnostic systems (which was true for the remaining 42.6% of respondents with broadly defined PTSD). There was also evidence that unexpected death of a loved one was associated with significantly higher PTSD risk relative to a number of other traumas when PTSD was defined using narrowly defined DSM-IV criteria rather than other criteria. However, given that only 4.4% of respondents with broadly defined PTSD had narrowly defined DSM-IV PTSD, these differences were not as important as those associated with ICD-11 PTSD. The associations of prior lifetime DSM-IV fear/distress and behavior/substance disorders with PTSD risk did not vary significantly across the four diagnostic systems other than for a greater importance of having exactly one prior externalizing disorder in the small proportion of cases where PTSD was defined using narrowly defined DSM-IV criteria rather than other criteria. Finally, predictors of broadly defined PTSD included female sex (OR = 1.8), sexual assault (OR = 2.6), and history of fear/distress (OR = 2.0–4.3) or behavior/substance (OR = 2.0–4.3) disorders.

Discussion

This analysis had four important limitations. First, PTSD was assessed using fully structured lay-administered interviews rather than semi-structured clinical interviews. Second, these interviews were based on retrospective reports about lifetime rather than recent traumas. Third, DSM-5 criteria were incompletely operationalized. Fourth, since the proposed ICD-11 diagnostic guidelines were not written as research criteria, they needed to be approximated. As a consequence, the results reported here were likely

Table 17.4 Associations of PTSD classified by only one ("narrow" cases) versus more than one ("all other" cases) diagnostic systems with indicators of clinical significance among respondents exposed to trauma

	Severe distress or impairment				Suicidality				Comorbid disorders: Distress				Comorbid disorders: Fear			
	%	(SE)	OR	(95% CI)	%	(SE)	OR	(95% CI)	%	(SE)	OR	(95% CI)	%	(SE)	OR	(95% CI)
I DSM-IV																
Narrow[a]	90.9	(3.7)	497.7*	(177.2 to >999)	15.5	(8.6)	12.9*	(3.5–47.9)	7.9	(2.2)	11.1*	(5.9–20.8)	2.9	(1.6)	13.7*	(4.3–44.0)
Total[a]	83.3	(2.9)	321.7*	(202.0–512.4)	7.4	(1.3)	4.5*	(2.7–7.5)	5.1	(0.7)	6.8*	(4.6–9.9)	1.8	(0.5)	5.1*	(2.6–9.9)
All others	62.0	(4.1)	96.1*	(63.4–145.5)	3.0	(1.7)	1.9	(0.6–6.1)	2.6	(0.7)	3.7*	(2.0–7.0)	1.3	(0.4)	4.4*	(2.2–8.6)
No PTSD	2.2	(0.4)	1.0	–	1.2	(0.1)	1.0	–	0.7	(0.1)	1.0	–	0.3	(0.0)	1.0	–
II DSM-5																
Narrow[a,b]	–	–	–	–	–	–	–	–	–	–	–	–	–	–	–	–
Total[a]	87.5	(2.4)	492.7*	(289.9–837.5)	8.2	(1.8)	5.3*	(2.9–9.4)	5.5	(0.8)	7.8*	(5.2–11.7)	2.0	(0.5)	5.6*	(3.0–10.4)
All others	59.4	(3.9)	82.1*	(56.7–118.8)	2.5	(0.9)	1.5	(0.6–3.5)	2.4	(0.5)	3.2*	(1.8–5.5)	1.1	(0.3)	3.8*	(1.9–7.4)
No PTSD	2.2	(0.4)	1.0	–	1.2	(0.1)	1.0	–	0.7	(0.1)	1.0	–	0.3	(0.03)	1.0	–
III ICD-10																
Narrow[a]	52.0	(6.1)	52.9*	(28.1–95.7)	1.6	(0.9)	1.0	(0.3–3.6)	2.4	(0.9)	3.6*	(1.5–8.5)	1.1	(0.5)	4.7*	(1.8–12.2)
Total[a]	73.4	(2.8)	164.3*	(114.2–236.3)	4.6	(0.8)	2.9*	(1.8–4.6)	4.0	(0.5)	5.4*	(3.7–7.9)	1.5	(0.4)	4.8*	(2.6–8.9)
All others	78.7	(6.1)	273.4*	(135.9–550.2)	8.6	(4.1)	5.2*	(1.7–15.4)	4.2	(1.2)	5.7*	(2.8–11.5)	1.7	(0.6)	4.8*	(2.4–9.5)
No PTSD	2.2	(0.4)	1.0	–	1.2	(0.1)	1.0	–	0.7	(0.1)	1.0	–	0.3	(0.03)	1.0	–
IV ICD-11																
Narrow[a]	57.2	(10.5)	89.1*	(32.9–241.4)	1.1	(1.0)	0.4	(0.1–3.0)	0.5	(0.2)	0.5	(0.2–1.5)	0.8	(0.4)	2.4	(0.7–8.0)
Total[a]	82.4	(3.1)	346.1*	(211.3–566.7)	5.5	(1.1)	3.1*	(1.8–5.4)	4.0	(0.6)	5.3*	(3.5–8.0)	1.6	(0.5)	4.2*	(2.0–8.9)
All others	63.8	(4.1)	93.3*	(61.5–141.6)	5.3	(2.0)	3.6*	(1.7–8.0)	4.0	(0.8)	5.8*	(3.5–9.4)	1.5	(0.4)	5.7*	(3.2–10.0)
No PTSD	2.2	(0.4)	1.0	–	1.2	(0.1)	1.0	–	0.7	(0.1)	1.0	–	0.3	(0.03)	1.0	–
(*n*)	(23,936)				(22,030)[c]				(79,836)[d]				(112,460)[e]			

*Significantly different from respondents who did not meet criteria for PTSD in any of the four diagnostic systems at the 0.05 level, two-sided test.

[a] *Narrow* cases are those that meet criteria for PTSD in the one diagnostic system represented in the subheading but in none of the other three systems. *Total* cases, in comparison, are all those who meet criteria for PTSD in the diagnostic system represented in the subheading whether or not they also meet criteria in one or more of the other three systems. *All other* cases, finally, are all those who do not meet criteria for PTSD in the diagnostic system represented in the subheading but do meet criteria in one or more of the three other systems. All three groups are contrasted with respondents who experienced a trauma but did not develop PTSD according to the criteria of any of the four systems.

[b] Respondents with narrow DSM-5 PTSD were excluded from analysis due to their small number.

[c] Respondents with a history of suicidal ideation at an earlier age than when they experienced the focal trauma were excluded.

[d] Four distress disorders were included in the analysis (MDD, BPD, GAD, and OCD). A separate observational file was created for each of these disorders excluding respondents with a lifetime history of this disorder at an earlier age than when they experienced the focal trauma. The four data files were then stacked and a single set of coefficients was estimated for the pooled within-disorder odds of onset in the year of trauma exposure. The sample size given here is for the stacked dataset. Disorder-specific samples ranged in size from 11,925 for OCD to 23,500 for BPD. The small sample size for OCD is due to the fact that OCD was assessed in only a subsample of cases in a subset of countries.

[e] Five fear disorders were included in the analysis (agoraphobia, panic disorder, separation anxiety disorder, social phobia, and specific phobia). A separate observational file was created for each of these disorders excluding respondents with a lifetime history of this disorder at an earlier age than when they experienced the focal trauma. The four data files were then stacked and a single set of coefficients was estimated for the pooled within-disorder odds of onset in the year of trauma exposure. The sample size given here is for the stacked dataset. Disorder-specific samples ranged in size from 20,429 for specific phobia to 23,629 for agoraphobia.

Table 17.5 Socio-demographic and trauma-related predictors of broadly defined PTSD and PTSD based on each of the diagnostic systems

	Broadly defined PTSD vs. noncases		Among respondents with broadly defined PTSD: Narrow[a] DSM-IV vs. others		Total[b] DSM-5 vs. others		Narrow[a] ICD-10 vs. others		Narrow[a] ICD-11 vs. others	
	OR	(95% CI)	OR	(95% CI)	OR	(95% CI)	OR	(95% CI)	OR	(95% CI)
I Socio-demographics										
Age of trauma exposure										
Age in decades	1.0	(0.9–1.1)	0.9	(0.7–1.1)	0.9	(0.7–1.0)	1.2	(1.0–1.5)	1.1	(0.8–1.5)
Sex										
Female	1.8*	(1.3–2.4)	1.7	(0.7–4.1)	0.9	(0.6–1.5)	0.8	(0.4–1.5)	1.2	(0.6–2.8)
Male	1.0	–	1.0	–	1.0	–	1.0	–	1.0	–
II Trauma Type										
War traumas	0.7	(0.3–1.4)	0.0*	(0.0–0.0)	0.4	(0.1–1.2)	1.3	(0.3–6.3)	6.1	(1.0–38.1)
Other interpersonal violence	0.9	(0.6–1.4)	0.1*	(0.0–0.4)	0.8	(0.4–1.7)	0.9	(0.4–2.4)	5.8*	(1.6–21.7)
Intimate/sexual violence	2.6*	(1.9–3.8)	0.0*	(0.0–0.2)	1.3	(0.6–2.5)	0.4	(0.2–1.1)	4.5*	(1.2–17.0)
Accidents/injuries	0.6*	(0.4–0.8)	0.0*	(0.0–0.2)	0.8	(0.4–1.6)	1.7	(0.4–6.4)	0.4	(0.1–1.9)
Network traumas	0.8	(0.5–1.2)	0.5	(0.2–1.5)	0.5*	(0.3–1.0)	1.5	(0.7–3.4)	0.8	(0.3–2.6)
Other	2.0*	(1.4–3.0)	0.1*	(0.0–0.4)	0.9	(0.4–2.0)	1.5	(0.5–4.6)	0.8	(0.2–3.3)
UD of loved one	1.0	–	1.0	–	1.0	–	1.0	–	1.0	–
χ^2_6	88.1*		913.3*		9.9		9.0		16.3*	
III Lifetime History of Mental Disorders										
Fear/distress disorders										
0	1.0	–	1.0	–	1.0	–	1.0	–	1.0	–
1	2.0*	(1.5–2.7)	0.7	(0.3–1.8)	1.3	(0.8–2.2)	1.2	(0.6–2.2)	0.6	(0.2–1.7)
2+	4.3*	(3.1–5.9)	1.6	(0.5–5.2)	1.2	(0.8–1.9)	1.0	(0.5–2.2)	1.1	(0.4–3.2)
χ^2_2	83.7*		2.5		1.7		0.3		1.4	
Disruptive behavioral/substance use disorders										
0	1.0	–	1.0	–	1.0	–	1.0	–	1.0	–
1	1.2	(0.8–1.8)	5.5*	(1.7–17.4)	1.1	(0.6–2.1)	0.8	(0.3–1.9)	0.6	(0.2–2.3)
2+	2.1*	(1.6–2.9)	1.1	(0.2–6.1)	1.6	(0.7–3.7)	1.4	(0.3–6.3)	0.2*	(0.0–1.0)
χ^2_2	24.1*		8.7*		1.0		0.5		4.2	
(*n*)	(23,936)		(728)		(1,581)		(669)		(796)	

*Significant difference between PTSD according to the diagnostic system indicated by the column heading and one or more of the other three diagnostic systems

[a]*Narrow* cases are those that meet criteria for PTSD in the one diagnostic system represented in the column heading but in none of the other three systems.

[b]*Total* cases are all those who meet criteria for DSM-5 PTSD whether or not they also meet criteria in one or more of the other three systems. Total cases were used instead of narrow cases of DSM-5 PTSD because of the rarity of narrow DSM-5 PTSD.

imprecise, and possibly biased. The fact that four (20%) DSM-5 symptoms were not assessed in the CIDI might account for our finding of lower prevalence of DSM-5 versus ICD-11 PTSD as this finding differs from other work comparing DSM-5 with ICD-11 PTSD prevalence (O'Donnell et al., 2014; Hansen et al., 2015; Hyland et al., 2016; Wisco et al., 2016; Hafstad et al., 2017). However, it is also noteworthy that at least one large epidemiological study found that DSM-5 PTSD criteria can be approximately closely with DMS-IV criteria due to the rarity of the new symptoms added in DSM-5 (Rosellini et al., 2015). Regardless of this limitation, the analysis was valuable insofar as these were the first large-scale cross-national data comparing DSM-IV, DSM-5, ICD-10, and ICD-11 PTSD.

Five findings are noteworthy. First, the exploratory factor analysis reported here found results consistent with DSM-5 in distinguishing four PTSD symptom clusters (American Psychiatric Association, 2013). Although a number of previous analyses have also yielded a four-factor solution (Yufik & Simms, 2010; Friedman et al., 2011), there has been debate about whether the fourth factor should be limited to numbing or should include nonspecific arousal symptoms

(King et al., 1998; Simms et al., 2002). The current findings were the first based on a large cross-national sample and supported a model in which the factors are re-experiencing, avoidance, numbing, and arousal.

Second, although 5.6% of respondents met criteria for "broadly defined" PTSD (in which PTSD criteria for any diagnostic system are met), a similar proportion of these broadly defined cases met criteria for DSM-5 (53.4%, or 3% of total sample) and ICD-11 (57.4%, or 3.2% of total sample). A larger proportion of respondents with broadly defined PTSD met ICD-10 diagnostic criteria, consistent with the more stringent, conservative approach to PTSD diagnosis taken by DSM-5 and ICD-11.

Third, the different diagnostic systems detected populations of PTSD that overlap only partially. One-third of broadly defined cases (1.8% of all respondents) met criteria in all four systems, an additional one-third in either three (0.9% of all respondents) or two (an additional 0.9% of all respondents) systems, and the final one-third (1.9% of all respondents) in only one of the four systems. Narrowly defined ICD-10 PTSD comprised 22.1% of all broadly defined cases, but other narrowly defined types were quite uncommon (1.5–6.3% of all broadly defined cases).

Fourth, while differences in associations with indicators of clinical severity were consistent with ICD-10 criteria being least strict and DSM-IV criteria most strict, the more striking result in this regard was that indicators of clinical significance were found even for narrowly defined cases across all four diagnostic systems. Thus, the use of any one diagnostic system will overlook many individuals who suffer from clinically significant symptoms, including distress and impairment.

Fifth, little evidence could be found in our results for significant differences in socio-demographic, trauma-related, or prior lifetime psychopathological (including both fear/distress and behavioral/substance disorders) predictors of PTSD across the different systems, indicating that there is a similar underlying risk profile for PTSD irrespective of the definition. This general pattern, and especially the finding that the associations of prior psychopathology with PTSD were indistinguishable across the four diagnostic systems, adds support to the argument above that all four definitions are providing information on unique clinically significant cases omitted from the other systems.

These findings extend previous work comparing different diagnostic criteria sets for PTSD (Peters et al., 1999; Zimmerman et al., 2004; Breslau & Alvarado, 2007; Forbes et al., 2011; van Ameringen et al., 2011) and are consistent with the argument that refinements to DSM-IV aimed at removing symptoms that overlap with those of other mood and anxiety disorders, are not associated with a major change in prevalence of PTSD, nor with evidence of a change in disability, comorbidity, or structural validity (Franklin & Zimmerman, 2001; Elhai et al., 2008; Grubaugh et al., 2010; van Emmerik & Kamphuis, 2011). Based on these findings, we suggest that broadly defined PTSD may be a particularly useful additional construct in future epidemiological studies of PTSD.

Acknowledgment

Portions of this chapter are based on Stein, D. J., McLaughlin, K. A., Koenen, K. C., et al. (2014). DSM-5 and ICD-11 definitions of post-traumatic stress disorder: investigating "narrow" and "broad" approaches. *Depression and Anxiety,* **31**, 494–505, by permission of Wiley-Blackwell.

References

American Psychiatric Association. (2000). *Diagnostic and Statistical Manual of Mental Disorders, Fourth Edition, Text Revision. DSM-IV-TR*. Washington, DC: American Psychiatric Association.

American Psychiatric Association. (2013). *Diagnostic and Statistical Manual of Mental Disorders, Fifth Edition. DSM-5*. Arlington, VA: American Psychiatric Association.

Breslau, N., & Alvarado, G. F. (2007). The clinical significance criterion in DSM-IV post-traumatic stress disorder. *Psychological Medicine*, 37, 1437–44.

Brewin, C. R., Lanius, R. A., Novac, A., Schnyder, U., & Galea, S. (2009). Reformulating PTSD for DSM-V: life after Criterion A. *Journal of Traumatic Stress*, 22, 366–73.

Cloitre, M., Garvert, D. W., Brewin, C. R., Bryant, R. A., & Maercker, A. (2013). Evidence for proposed ICD-11 PTSD and complex PTSD: a latent profile analysis. *European Journal of Psychotraumatology*, 4, 20706.

Elhai, J. D., Grubaugh, A. L., Kashdan, T. B., & Frueh, B. C. (2008). Empirical examination of a proposed refinement to DSM-IV posttraumatic stress disorder symptom criteria using the National Comorbidity Survey Replication data. *Journal of Clinical Psychiatry*, 69, 597–602.

First, M. B., Spitzer, R. L., Gibbon, M., & Williams, J. B. W. (1994). *Structured Clinical Interview for DSM-IV Axis I Disorders*. New York, NY: Biometrics Research Department, New York State Psychiatric Institute.

Forbes, D., Fletcher, S., Lockwood, E., et al. (2011). Requiring both avoidance and emotional numbing in DSM-V PTSD: will it help? *Journal of Affective Disorders*, 130, 483–6.

Franklin, C. L., & Zimmerman, M. (2001). Posttraumatic stress disorder and major depressive disorder: investigating the role of overlapping symptoms in diagnostic comorbidity. *Journal of Nervous and Mental Disease*, 189, 548–51.

Friedman, M. J. (2013). Finalizing PTSD in DSM-5: getting here from there and where to go next. *Journal of Traumatic Stress*, 26, 548–56.

Friedman, M. J., Resick, P. A., Bryant, R. A., & Brewin, C. R. (2011). Considering PTSD for DSM-5. *Depression and Anxiety*, 28, 750–69.

Grubaugh, A. L., Long, M. E., Elhai, J. D., Frueh, B. C., & Magruder, K. M. (2010). An examination of the construct validity of posttraumatic stress disorder with veterans using a revised criterion set. *Behaviour Research and Therapy*, 48, 909–14.

Hafstad, G. S., Thoresen, S., Wentzel-Larsen, T., Maercker, A., & Dyb, G. (2017). PTSD or not PTSD? Comparing the proposed ICD-11 and the DSM-5 PTSD criteria among young survivors of the 2011 Norway attacks and their parents. *Psychological Medicine*, 48, 1283–91.

Hansen, M., Hyland, P., Armour, C., Shevlin, M., & Elklit, A. (2015). Less is more? Assessing the validity of the ICD-11 model of PTSD across multiple trauma samples. *European Journal of Psychotraumatology*, 6, 28766.

Haro, J. M., Arbabzadeh-Bouchez, S., Brugha, T. S., et al. (2006). Concordance of the Composite International Diagnostic Interview Version 3.0 (CIDI 3.0) with standardized clinical assessments in the WHO World Mental Health Surveys. *International Journal of Methods in Psychiatric Research*, 15, 167–80.

Hayton, J. C., Allen, D. G., & Scarpello, V. (2004). Factor retention decisions in exploratory factor analysis: a tutorial on parallel analysis. *Organizational Research Methods*, 7, 191–205.

Hyland, P., Shevlin, M., McNally, S., Murphy, J., Hansen, M., & Elklit, E. (2016). Exploring differences between the ICD-11 and DSM-5 models of PTSD: does it matter which model is used? *Journal of Anxiety Disorders*, 37, 48–53.

International Advisory Group for the Revision of ICD-10 Mental and Behavioural Disorders. (2011). A conceptual framework for the revision of the ICD-10 classification of mental and behavioural disorders. *World Psychiatry*, 10, 86–92.

Kessler, R. C., & Üstün, T. B. (2004). The World Mental Health (WMH) Survey Initiative version of the World Health Organization (WHO) Composite International Diagnostic Interview (CIDI). *International Journal of Methods in Psychiatric Research*, 13, 93–121.

Kilpatrick, D. G. (2013). The DSM-5 got PTSD right: comment on Friedman (2013). *Journal of Traumatic Stress*, 26, 563–66.

King, D. W., Leskin, G. A., King, L. A., & Weathers, F. W. (1998). Confirmatory factor analysis of the Clinician-Administered PTSD Scale: evidence for the dimensionality of posttraumatic stress disorder. *Psychological Assessment*, 10, 90–6.

Knäuper, B., Cannell, C. F., Schwarz, N., Bruce, M. L., & Kessler, R. C. (1999). Improving accuracy of major depression age-of-onset reports in the US National Comorbidity Survey. *International Journal of Methods in Psychiatric Research*, 8, 39–48.

Maercker, A., Brewin, C. R., Bryant, R. A., et al. (2013a). Proposals for mental disorders specifically associated with stress in the International Classification of Diseases-11. *The Lancet*, 381, 1683–5.

et al. (2013b). Diagnosis and classification of disorders specifically associated with stress: proposals for ICD-11. *World Psychiatry*, 12, 198–206.

Maercker, A., & Perkonigg, A. (2013). Applying an international perspective in defining PTSD and related disorders: comment on Friedman (2013). *Journal of Traumatic Stress*, 26, 560–2.

O'Donnell, M. L., Alkemade, N., Nickerson, A., et al. (2014). Impact of the diagnostic changes to post-traumatic stress disorder for DSM-5 and the proposed changes to ICD-11. *British Journal of Psychiatry*, 205, 230–5.

Peters, L., Slade, T., & Andrews, G. (1999). A comparison of ICD10 and DSM-IV criteria for posttraumatic stress disorder. *Journal of Traumatic Stress*, 12, 335–43.

Rosellini, A. J., Stein, M. B., Colpe, L. J., et al. (2015). Approximating a DSM-5 diagnosis of PTSD using DSM-IV criteria. *Depression and Anxiety*, 32, 493–501.

Simms, L. J., Watson, D., & Doebbeling, B. N. (2002). Confirmatory factor analyses of posttraumatic stress symptoms in deployed and nondeployed veterans of the Gulf War. *Journal of Abnormal Psychology*, 111, 637–47.

Spitzer, R. L., First, M. B., & Wakefield, J. C. (2007). Saving PTSD from itself in DSM-V. *Journal of Anxiety Disorders*, 21, 233–41.

Stein, D. J., Seedat, S., Iversen, A., & Wessely, S. (2007). Post-traumatic stress disorder: medicine and politics. *The Lancet*, 369, 139–44.

Tol, W. A., Barbui, C., Galappatti, A., et al. (2011). Mental health and psychosocial support in humanitarian settings: linking practice and research. *The Lancet*, 378, 1581–91.

van Ameringen, M., Mancini, C., & Patterson, B. (2011). The impact of changing diagnostic criteria in posttraumatic stress disorder in a Canadian epidemiologic sample. *Journal of Clinical Psychiatry*, 72, 1034–41.

van Emmerik, A. A., & Kamphuis, J. H. (2011). Testing a DSM-5 reformulation of posttraumatic stress disorder: impact on prevalence and comorbidity among treatment-seeking civilian trauma survivors. *Journal of Traumatic Stress*, 24, 213–17.

Wisco, B. E., Miller, M. W., Wolf, E. J., et al. (2016). The impact of proposed changes to ICD-11 on estimates of PTSD prevalence and comorbidity. *Psychiatry Research*, 240, 226–33.

Wolter, K. (2007). *Introduction to Variance Estimation*. New York, NY: Springer New York.

World Health Organization. (1993). *The ICD-10 Classification of Mental and Behavioural Disorders: Diagnostic Criteria for Research*. Geneva, Switzerland: WHO.

Yehuda, R., & McFarlane, A. C. (1995). Conflict between current knowledge about posttraumatic stress disorder and its original conceptual basis. *American Journal of Psychiatry*, 152, 1705–13.

Yufik, T., & Simms, L. J. (2010). A meta-analytic investigation of the structure of posttraumatic stress disorder symptoms. *Journal of Abnormal Psychology*, 119, 764–76.

Zimmerman, M., Chelminski, I., & Young, D. (2004). On the threshold of disorder: a study of the impact of the DSM-IV clinical significance criterion on diagnosing depressive and anxiety disorders in clinical practice. *Journal of Clinical Psychiatry*, 65, 1400–5.

Chapter 18

The Role of Criterion A2 in the DSM-IV Diagnosis of Posttraumatic Stress Disorder

Elie G. Karam, Evelyn J. Bromet, Ayelet Meron Ruscio, Dan. J. Stein, and Ronald C. Kessler

As noted in Chapter 17, there has long been controversy over what should qualify as a trauma for posttraumatic stress disorder (PTSD), resulting in differences between the DSM and ICD systems as well as changes across the different editions of each of these systems. Some experts have favored a broader and others a narrower definition (Kilpatrick et al., 1998; Weathers & Keane, 2007). DSM-IV (American Psychiatric Association, 1994) tried to find a middle ground by including both an objective (criterion A1) and a subjective (criterion A2) component of the definition of a trauma. Criterion A1 was broader than favored by some, as it included any event a person "experienced, witnessed, or (was) confronted with" that involved "actual or threatened death or serious injury or a threat to the physical integrity of oneself or others." The inclusion of indirect exposure and the ambiguity of the phrase, "threat to physical integrity," were particular points of controversy (McNally, 2004; Creamer et al., 2005). Criterion A2, new to DSM-IV, was designed to restrict qualifying events to those where the immediate response involved "intense fear, helplessness, or horror" to prevent the overdiagnosis that might otherwise occur because of the broad scope of A1.

The few studies that focused specifically on A2 showed that a substantial proportion of individuals exposed to an A1 event met criterion A2 (Breslau & Kessler, 2001; Creamer et al., 2005). This meant that the inclusion of the A2 requirement in the criterion set reduced estimated prevalence only modestly (Kilpatrick et al., 1998; Schnurr et al., 2002). However, failure to meet A2 strongly predicted failure to meet other criteria (Breslau & Kessler, 2001), making assessment of A2 useful in two ways. First, as A2 was the only PTSD criterion that could be assessed near the time of exposure, early assessment of A2 could help predict subsequent PTSD, although a meaningful proportion of individuals who subsequently met all other criteria for PTSD failed to meet A2 at the time of trauma exposure (O'Donnell et al., 2010). Second, even when the assessment took place months or years after exposure, initial retrospective assessment of A2 could provide a quick rule-out (McNally, 2004). Nevertheless, the modest impact of the A2 requirement on PTSD diagnoses argued against retaining A2, based on the desire to simplify diagnoses by eliminating redundant criteria (Zimmerman et al., 2006; Andrews et al., 2007).

The empirical foundation on which these competing views were based was limited to a small number of American and Australian studies. Furthermore, only scant data existed on the relationship between A2 and other clinical correlates (Creamer et al., 2005), making it unclear whether the A2 requirement excluded clinically significant cases. Based on the fact that the World Mental Health (WMH) surveys operationalized both DSM-IV and ICD-10 criteria, we assessed A2, but continued questioning if the A2 criterion was not met. This allowed us to contribute information of unprecedented scope on the controversy about the A2 criterion.

This chapter reviews the results of the WMH analysis of the A2 criterion, based on which we concluded that the criterion was not useful in defining PTSD. Consistent with this conclusion, this criterion was subsequently dropped from DSM-5 (American Psychiatric Association, 2013).

Methods

At the time the WMH analysis of the A2 criterion was carried out, data were available from 21 WMH surveys: 10 high-income (Belgium, France, Germany, Israel, Italy, Japan, the Netherlands, New Zealand, Spain, and the United States), 6 upper-middle-income (Brazil, Bulgaria, Lebanon, Mexico, Romania, and South Africa) and 5 low- and lower-middle-income (Colombia, India, Nigeria, Beijing, and Shanghai in the People's Republic of China [PRC], and Ukraine) countries. The reader will note that India was not listed in Table 18.2 as India subsequently left the WMH collaboration and the Indian data were not included in the more recent WMH papers. There were a total of 52,826 respondents in the Part II surveys included in the analysis of A2. The weighted (by sample size) average response rate was 71.6%. The random trauma-level dataset was used in the analysis.

Criterion A2 was considered to be met if the respondent endorsed any of three questions about whether, at the time of the random trauma, he–she felt (i) terrified or very frightened, (ii) helpless, or (iii) shocked or horrified. The remaining DSM-IV criteria were then assessed whether or not A2 was endorsed with questions about re-experiencing DSM-IV (criterion B), avoidance-numbing (criterion C), arousal (criterion D), duration (criterion E), and clinically significant distress impairment (criterion F). A retrospective question asked respondents how many months or years the symptoms persisted.

The analysis investigated the extent to which prevalence and correlates of PTSD differed depending on whether criterion A2 was required for a diagnosis. Among the correlates considered were other lifetime DSM-IV/CIDI disorders and suicidal ideation (assessed with a single question that asked respondents if they ever seriously thought about killing themselves and, if so, the age when this first occurred).

Cross-tabulations examined frequency of individual traumas, conditional prevalence of DSM-IV PTSD with and without A2, and co-occurrence of criteria B–F. Logistic regression (Hosmer & Lemeshow, 2000) examined socio-demographic predictors of PTSD with and without A2. Discrete-time survival analysis (Efron, 1988) with person-year as the unit of analysis was used to examine association between PTSD with and without A2 and persistence as well as subsequent first onset of other DSM-IV disorders and suicidal ideation. All parameters were estimated using the Taylor series method (Wolter, 1985) in the SUDAAN software system (Research Triangle Institute, 2002). Significance was evaluated using 0.05-level two-sided Wald χ^2 tests.

Results

The Importance of Criterion A2 to DSM-IV PTSD

Approximately one-third (37.6%) of weighted lifetime traumas were reported as having resulted in peritraumatic reactions that met criterion A2 (see Table 18.1). This proportion was substantially lower in high-income than in upper-middle- or low- and lower-middle-income countries. Conditional prevalence of meeting all other DSM-IV/CIDI criteria for PTSD was dramatically higher in the presence (9.7%) than in the absence (0.1%) of A2. Conditional prevalence of PTSD given A2 was positively related to country income level. Conditional prevalence of all other requirements for PTSD in the absence of A2 was very low (0.0–0.1%), regardless of country income level. Similar results were found when we looked separately within countries (see Table 18.2) and within trauma types (see Table 18.3).

Table 18.1 Percentage of the representative sample of traumas assessed in the WMH sample that had criterion A2 and conditional prevalence of DSM-IV/CIDI PTSD in the presence versus absence of A2

	Percentage of traumas that had criterion A2			Conditional prevalence of PTSD in the presence of A2			Conditional prevalence of all other requirements for a diagnosis of PTSD in the absence of A2		
	%	(SD)	(*n*)[a]	%	(SD)	(*n*)[a]	%	(SD)	(*n*)[a]
Country Income Levels									
High-income	28.6	(1.1)	(17,815)	15.0	(1.2)	(6,341)	0.1	(0.0)	(11,474)
Upper-middle-income	52.2	(1.7)	(6,962)	6.3	(0.8)	(3,103)	0.1	(0.1)	(3,859)
Low- and lower-middle-income	49.5	(2.7)	(3,713)	3.8	(1.0)	(1,677)	0.0	(0.0)	(2,036)
Total	37.6	(0.9)	(28,490)	9.7	(0.7)	(11,121)	0.1	(0.0)	(17,369)

[a]The *n*s reported here are unweighted denominators of the number of traumas on which the prevalence estimates are based. For example, a weighted 36.7% of the 28,490 traumas reported (an observed 11,121 traumas) were classified as meeting the DSM-IV/CIDI A2 criterion, while a weighted 9.7% of these 11,121 traumas were classified as meeting all other DSM-IV/CIDI criteria for PTSD. The ratio of the number of respondents who reported at least one trauma to the total sample size (28,490/52,949 = 53.8%) is lower than the weighted 67.9% of respondents who reported a trauma because people with high rates of trauma exposure were somewhat under-represented in the samples.

Table 18.2 Prevalence of criterion A2 and conditional prevalence of broadly defined DSM-IV/CIDI PTSD in the presence versus absence of A2 separately for the random traumas assessed in each of the WMH surveys

	Prevalence of A2			Conditional prevalence of PTSD in the presence of A2			Conditional prevalence of PTSD in the absence of A2		
	%	(SE)	(*n*)[a]	%	(SE)	(*n*)[a]	%	(SE)	(*n*)[a]
I High-Income Countries									
Belgium	17.3	(2.5)	(698)	20.3	(9.9)	(220)	0.1	(0.1)	(478)
France	14.5	(3.0)	(1,054)	16.9	(4.3)	(335)	0.0	(0.1)	(719)
Germany	12.0	(1.6)	(913)	18.1	(5.0)	(252)	0.0	(0.0)	(661)
Israel	11.9	(1.5)	(1,493)	24.7	(8.6)	(290)	0.0	(0.0)	(1,203)
Italy	14.6	(2.2)	(1,048)	19.1	(5.5)	(315)	0.0	(0.0)	(733)
Japan	16.1	(1.7)	(1,138)	10.1	(2.5)	(321)	0.0	(0.0)	(817)
The Netherlands	18.6	(2.8)	(779)	32.2	(7.0)	(260)	0.0	(0.0)	(519)
New Zealand	24.7	(1.1)	(5,969)	16.3	(1.5)	(2,134)	0.1	(0.1)	(3,835)
Spain	16.6	(1.8)	(1,265)	24.4	(9.0)	(386)	0.1	(0.1)	(879)
United States	53.1	(2.6)	(3,458)	12.0	(1.5)	(1,828)	0.2	(0.1)	(1,630)
II Upper-Middle-Income Countries									
Brazil – São Paulo	31.1	(3.2)	(1,803)	11.8	(2.5)	(431)	0.1	(0.1)	(1,372)
Bulgaria	47.4	(5.3)	(447)	21.1	(4.8)	(203)	0.0	(0.0)	(244)
Lebanon	64.8	(8.8)	(451)	3.8	(1.4)	(310)	1.2	(0.9)	(141)
Mexico	15.7	(2.0)	(1,818)	13.6	(4.1)	(414)	0.0	(0.0)	(1,404)
Romania	39.2	(3.3)	(969)	12.6	(6.6)	(445)	0.1	(0.0)	(524)
South Africa	85.3	(2.5)	(1,474)	3.3	(0.9)	(1,300)	0.0	(0.0)	(174)
III Low- and Lower-Middle-Income Countries									
Colombia	12.4	(1.4)	(2,068)	19.3	(6.8)	(399)	0.0	(0.0)	(1,669)
India	86.1	(5.6)	(74)	0.7	(0.7)	(66)	0.0	(0.0)	(8)
Nigeria	61.8	(4.4)	(605)	0.0	(0.0)	(394)	0.0	(0.0)	(211)
PRC – Beijing/Shanghai	55.7	(6.2)	(216)	1.8	(1.0)	(138)	0.0	(0.0)	(78)
Ukraine	85.9	(5.5)	(750)	3.9	(1.5)	(680)	0.1	(0.1)	(70)

[a]The *n*'s reported here are unweighted denominators of the number of experiences on which the prevalence estimates are based. For example, a weighted 17.3% of the 698 experiences reported in Belgium (an observed 220 experiences) were classified as meeting the DSM-IV/CIDI A2 criterion, while a weighted 20.3% of these 220 experiences were classified as meeting all other DSM-IV/CIDI criteria for PTSD.

It was unclear whether these results, which involved retrospective reporting of A2 – in some cases, many years after the random trauma – accurately reflected the way that respondents would have characterized their short-term reactions at the time of the trauma. To the extent that they did, though, the results meant that an assessment of A2 shortly after trauma exposure could help predict subsequent PTSD. Indeed, when we compared the proportion of all random traumas that met full criteria for PTSD (by multiplying conditional prevalence of PTSD given A2 by the proportion of all traumas with A2) with the additional proportion that would meet criteria for PTSD if A2 was no longer required for diagnosis (by multiplying conditional prevalence of PTSD without A2 by the proportion of all traumas without A2), we found that only 1.4% of respondents who met all other requirements for PTSD would have been missed if follow-up assessment had been carried out only among people with A2. This estimated proportion was very similar in high-income, upper-middle-income, and low- and lower-middle-income countries (0.6–2.0%). More detailed examination found very few countries (see Table 18.4) or traumas (see Table 18.5) for which significantly more than 2% of respondents meeting all other requirements who would have been missed by focusing on A2-positives, although the proportions were notable for Lebanon (15.2%) and for life-threatening automobile accidents (9.1%). Furthermore, additional analyses found that the percent was even smaller (1.1%) among traumas for which professional treatment had been sought, demonstrating that the low percentage held for the most clinically relevant traumas.

As noted in the introduction, one other rationale for including A2 in DSM-IV was the claim that it provided a quick rule-out for noncases. However, our results suggested this was not true. Exclusion of traumas that failed A2 would have reduced by an estimated 62.4% (i.e., 100% minus the 37.6% of traumas that met

Table 18.3 Prevalence of criterion A2 and conditional prevalence of broadly-defined DSM-IV/CIDI PTSD in the presence versus absence of A2 separately for each type of trauma pooled across WMH surveys

	Prevalence of A2			Conditional prevalence of PTSD in the presence of A2			Conditional prevalence of PTSD in the absence of A2		
	%	(SE)	(*n*)[a]	%	(SE)	(*n*)[a]	%	(SE)	(*n*)[a]
I Exposure to Organized Violence									
Relief worker in war zone	24.3	(11.7)	(104)	1.6	(1.2)	(26)	0.0	(0.0)	(78)
Civilian in war zone	40.7	(4.5)	(656)	3.3	(1.6)	(246)	0.0	(0.0)	(410)
Civilian in region of terror	28.5	(4.3)	(246)	8.0	(4.7)	(71)	0.0	(0.0)	(175)
Refugee	53.0	(5.5)	(235)	16.5	(8.9)	(89)	0.0	(0.0)	(146)
Kidnapped	39.6	(6.8)	(107)	31.0	(8.8)	(45)	0.0	(0.0)	(62)
II Participation in Organized Violence									
Witnessed death/dead body/ serious injury	35.8	(3.2)	(3,135)	2.7	(0.7)	(993)	0.0	(0.0)	(2,142)
Accidentally caused serious injury/death	35.9	(7.3)	(158)	8.0	(3.5)	(57)	0.0	(0.0)	(101)
Combat experience	34.4	(5.7)	(377)	20.7	(7.4)	(119)	0.0	(0.0)	(258)
Purposefully injured/ tortured/killed someone	32.0	(10.0)	(55)	9.3	(7.9)	(11)	0.0	(0.0)	(44)
Witnessed atrocities	20.3	(4.0)	(295)	9.2	(4.6)	(83)	0.0	(0.0)	(212)
III Physical Violence Victimization									
Beaten by caregiver	36.0	(3.4)	(1,168)	13.4	(4.7)	(340)	0.0	(0.0)	(828)
Beaten by someone else	39.0	(4.3)	(685)	7.3	(2.3)	(246)	0.0	(0.0)	(439)
Witnessed physical fight at home	33.8	(3.5)	(1,137)	10.1	(3.0)	(340)	0.3	(0.3)	(797)
IV Sexual Violence Victimization									
Raped	56.0	(7.8)	(545)	34.1	(11.2)	(271)	0.3	(0.3)	(274)
Sexually assaulted	37.3	(3.0)	(911)	27.3	(4.2)	(370)	0.5	(0.5)	(541)
Stalked	38.6	(4.8)	(708)	21.4	(6.3)	(261)	0.0	(0.0)	(447)
Beaten by spouse/romantic partner	58.0	(3.1)	(853)	17.3	(2.9)	(403)	0.2	(0.2)	(450)
Trauma to loved one	43.6	(5.5)	(680)	9.7	(3.1)	(288)	0.0	(0.0)	(392)
Private trauma[b]	42.7	(2.7)	(1,419)	19.6	(3.5)	(682)	0.1	(0.1)	(737)
V Accidents/Injuries									
Natural disaster	24.6	(4.9)	(941)	0.8	(0.4)	(301)	0.0	(0.0)	(640)
Toxic chemical exposure	10.1	(2.4)	(439)	0.7	(0.6)	(66)	0.0	(0.0)	(373)
Automobile accident	32.0	(2.5)	(1,954)	8.5	(1.7)	(731)	0.4	(0.3)	(1,223)
Life-threatening illness	36.2	(2.9)	(1,884)	4.5	(1.1)	(719)	0.0	(0.0)	(1,165)
Child with serious illness	53.1	(5.2)	(1,272)	5.6	(1.5)	(660)	0.0	(0.0)	(612)
Other life-threatening accident	37.8	(4.8)	(704)	15.6	(8.7)	(245)	0.2	(0.1)	(459)
VI Other									
Mugged/threatened with a weapon	32.7	(2.7)	(1,886)	5.7	(1.5)	(649)	0.1	(0.1)	(1,237)
Human-made disaster	32.3	(5.3)	(378)	11.4	(5.5)	(126)	0.0	(0.0)	(252)
UD of a loved one	45.8	(1.7)	(5,558)	8.7	(1.2)	(2,683)	0.1	(0.1)	(2,875)

[a]The *n*s reported here are unweighted denominators of the number of experiences on which the prevalence estimates are based. For example, a weighted 24.3% of the 104 relief workers in a war zone (an observed 26 traumas) were classified as meeting the DSM-IV/CIDI A2 criterion, while a weighted 1.6% of these 26 traumas were classified as meeting all other DSM-IV/CIDI criteria for PTSD.

[b]A *private* event is a trauma that some individuals reported in response to a question asked at the very end of the trauma section that asked if they ever had some other very upsetting experience they did not tell us about already (and this includes in response to a prior open-ended question about "any other" trauma) because they were too embarrassed or upset to talk about it. Respondents were told, before they answered, that if they reported such a trauma we would not ask them anything about what it was, only about their age when the trauma happened.

Table 18.4 The percentage of cases of DSM-IV/CIDI PTSD that do not meet criterion A2 by country

	%	(SE)	(*n*)[a]
I High-Income Countries			
Belgium	1.6	(1.5)	(30)
France	3.0	(3.1)	(55)
Germany	0.0	(0.0)	(30)
Israel	0.0	(00)	(230)
Italy	0.3	(0.3)	(400)
Japan	0.0	(0.0)	(26)
The Netherlands	0.0	(0.0)	(48)
New Zealand	2.5	(1.5)	(352)
Spain	1.5	(1.9)	(59)
United States	1.2	(0.6)	(318)
II Upper-Middle-Income Countries			
Brazil – São Paulo	1.9	(1.9)	(73)
Bulgaria	0.0	(0.0)	(59)
Lebanon	15.2	(8.8)	(31)
Mexico	0.0	(0.0)	(36)
Romania	0.7	(0.6)	(25)
South Africa	0.0	(0.0)	(43)
III Low- and Lower-Middle-Income Countries			
Colombia	0.8	(0.9)	(36)
India	0.0		(1)
Nigeria			(0)
PRC – Beijing/Shanghai	0.0	(0.0)	(4)
Ukraine	0.4	(0.4)	(51)

[a]The *ns* reported here are unweighted denominators of the number of traumas on which the estimates of percentages are based. For example, a weighted 1.6% of the 30 respondents in Belgium who met DSM-IV/CIDI criteria for PTSD were classified as not meeting the A2 criterion.

criterion A2) the number who would have to be further assessed and would have missed only 1.4% who met all other criteria. Although this seemed like a very effective screening rule, higher conditional prevalence of A2 than other DSM-IV criteria meant that the proportion of noncases ruled out by A2 would have been considerably lower than those ruled out by assessing any other DSM-IV criterion. For example, beginning by assessing criterion F (clinically significant distress impairment) would have excluded 90.4% of noncases compared to 62.4% excluded by assessing A2.

The Clinical Significance of PTSD without Criterion A2

The aforementioned results showed that removing A2 from the criterion set had very little effect on the number of people who qualified for a diagnosis of PTSD. PTSD prevalence based on randomly selected traumas would have increased only from 3.64% to 3.69% (about a 2% increase on the base of 3.64%) if we had excluded

Table 18.5 The percentage of cases of DSM-IV/CIDI PTSD that do not meet criterion A2 by type of trauma pooled across WMH surveys

	Prevalence of A2		
	%	(SE)	(*n*)[a]
I Exposure to Organized Violence			
Relief worker in warzone	0.0	(0.0)	(4)
Civilian in war zone	0.0	(0.0)	(11)
Civilian in a region of terror	0.0	(0.0)	(4)
Refugee	0.0	(0.0)	(9)
Kidnapped	0.0	(0.0)	(16)
II Participation in Organized Violence			
Witnessed death/dead body/serious injury	0.0	(0.0)	(53)
Accidentally caused serious injury/death	0.0	(0.0)	(12)
Combat experience	0.0	(0.0)	(20)
Purposefully injured/tortured/killed someone	0.0	(0.0)	(2)
Witnessed atrocities	0.0	(0.0)	(7)
III Physical Violence Victimization			
Beaten by caregiver	0.0	(0.0)	(55)
Beaten by someone else	0.0	(0.0)	(20)
Witnessed physical fight at home	4.7	(4.7)	(39)
IV Sexual Violence Victimization			
Raped	0.7	(0.3)	(116)
Sexually assaulted	2.8	(2.3)	(97)
Stalked	0.0	(0.0)	(41)
Beaten by a spouse or romantic partner	0.9	(0.9)	(89)
Trauma to loved one	0.0	(0.0)	(38)
Private trauma[b]	0.9	(0.5)	(132)
V Accidents/Injuries			
Natural disaster	0.0	(0.0)	(4)
Toxic chemical exposure	0.0	(0.0)	(2)
Automobile accident	9.1	(7.0)	(56)
Life-threatening illness	1.0	(0.9)	(59)
Child with serious illness	0.0	(0.0)	(73)
Other life-threatening accident	1.6	(1.4)	(19)
VI Other			
Mugged or threatened with a weapon	4.9	(3.5)	(44)
Human-made disaster	0.0	(0.0)	(10)
UD of a loved one	1.0	(0.8)	(308)

[a]The *ns* reported here are unweighted denominators of the number of traumas on which the estimates of proportions are based. For example, a weighted 9.1% of the 56 respondents with life-threatening automobile accidents who met DSM-IV/CIDI criteria for PTSD were classified as not meeting the A2 criterion.

[b]A *private* event is a trauma that some individuals reported in response to a question asked at the very end of the trauma section that asked if they ever had some other very upsetting experience they did not tell us about already (and this includes in response to a prior open-ended question about "any other" trauma) because they were too embarrassed or upset to talk about it. Respondents were told, before they answered, that if they reported such a trauma we would not ask them anything about what it was, only about their age when the trauma happened.

Table 18.6 Logistic regression equations predicting whether random traumas led to criterion A2 symptoms in the sample of random traumas assessed in the WMH sample that satisfy all other criteria for a DSM-IV/CIDI diagnosis of PTSD

	Country income level							
	All		High		Upper-middle		Low and lower-middle	
	OR	(95% CI)	OR	(95% CI)	OR	(95% CI)	OR	(95% CI)
I Age at Trauma Exposure								
0–9	0.5	(0.1–3.3)	0.8	(0.1–6.9)	0.0	(0.0–0.3)	–[b]	–
10–19	0.7	(0.1–5.0)	0.9	(0.1–9.6)	0.4	(0.0–6.5)	–	–
20–29	0.5	(0.1–3.7)	0.6	(0.1–6.8)	0.1	(0.0–0.9)	–	–
30–39	1.7	(0.3–12.0)	1.2	(0.1–21.8)	1.0	(0.1–13.6)	–	–
40+	1.0	–	1.0	–	1.0	–	–	–
χ^2_4	1.9		0.4		8.9		–[b]	
II Sex								
Female	1.0	–	1.0	–	1.0	–	1.0	–
Male	5.1*	(1.6–16.5)	8.4*	(2.1–33.8)	0.8	(0.1–4.9)	12.1*	(1.1–129.4)
III History of Prior (to Age of Trauma Exposure) DSM-IV/CIDI Disorders								
Yes	0.2*	(0.1–1.0)	0.2	(0.0–1.5)	0.4	(0.0–3.4)	0.3	(0.1–1.1)
No	1.0	–	1.0	–	1.0	–	1.0	–
IV History of Prior (to Age of Occurrence of the Random Trauma) Trauma Exposure								
Yes	0.8	(0.2–2.9)	1.0	(0.2–5.8)	0.5	(0.1–2.4)	1.1	(0.1–9.1)
No	1.0	–	1.0	–	1.0	–	1.0	–
(*n*)	(1,340)[a]		(981)[a]		(267)[a]		(92)[a]	

*Significant at the 0.05 level, two-sided test.

[a] The *n*s reported here are the unweighted numbers of traumas on which the regression equations are based. These include all traumas in the representative sample of traumas that were judged to meet all other DSM-IV/CIDI criteria for a diagnosis of PTSD in the presence or absence of A2. The outcome is whether or not the trauma led to all other PTSD criteria but not A2.

[b] The number of observed cases of PTSD without A2 in this subsample was too small to estimate the association with this polychotomous variable.

A2, adding only 21 cases classified as meeting full criteria for PTSD out of the 28,490 cases in the weighted sample. In considering whether such a modest difference justifies inclusion of A2 in the DSM criterion set, it is relevant to know whether the few otherwise qualifying cases were so distinct in terms of low clinical significance that they should be excluded.

We addressed this question by examining whether PTSD differed in course, depending on presence–absence of A2. No such difference was found. The odds ratio (OR; 95% confidence interval [CI] in parentheses) of presence–absence of A2 predicting differential persistence of PTSD among cases with versus without A2 was nonsignificant (1.02 (0.42–2.47), $\chi^2_1 = 0.0, p = 0.97$). The OR of PTSD without A2 predicting subsequent first onset of other DSM-IV/CIDI disorders was actually higher, although not significantly so, for PTSD without than with A2: 9.9 (2.1–47.1) versus 4.4 (3.2–6.1). The same basic pattern held in predicting subsequent onset of suicidal ideation, with an OR (95% CI) of 3.6 (2.8–4.7) for PTSD with A2 and 4.4 (0.8–24.7) for PTSD without A2 ($\chi^2_1 = 0.1, p = 0.83$).

Compositional Differences between PTSD with and without A2

We investigated whether the composition of cases of PTSD differed depending on presence–absence of A2, using logistic regression where information about respondents' sex, age at time of trauma exposure, history of prior lifetime DSM-IV/CIDI disorders, and history of prior trauma exposures was used to distinguish PTSD with and without A2 (see Table 18.6). Men had significantly higher odds than women of PTSD with than without A2 (5.1). Respondents with a history of prior DSM-IV/CIDI disorders had significantly lower odds than others of PTSD with than without A2 (0.2). But otherwise the differences were unremarkable.

Discussion

We found that a much higher proportion of random traumas met criterion A2 than any other DSM-IV PTSD criterion, that conditional prevalence of meeting all other diagnostic criteria was significantly higher in the presence than in the absence of A2, and that only a small fraction of respondents who met these other diagnostic criteria failed to meet A2. The last of these results meant that the sample-specific prevalence of PTSD increases only very slightly when A2 is not required for a diagnosis. Furthermore, cases meeting all other PTSD criteria do not differ in persistence, subsequent suicidal ideation, or secondary disorders from PTSD cases. We concluded from these results that A2 should be reconceptualized as a risk factor for PTSD rather than as a diagnostic requirement as the retrospective data indirectly suggested that the presence of A2 symptoms shortly after the occurrence of a trauma is significantly predictive of subsequent PTSD, even though the inclusion of A2 as a requirement for diagnosis has little effect on case definition once other diagnostic requirements are met.

In fact, as mentioned in the introduction, A2 was removed from DSM-5 precisely because it had little clinical utility. In addition to our study, several subsequent studies (Friedman et al., 2011; Pereda & Forero, 2012) showed that the inclusion of A2 does not improve diagnostic accuracy. While DSM-5 also features a few other differences from DSM-IV such as an increase in the number of clusters of PTSD symptoms required to qualify for a diagnosis from three to four, at least one report suggests that the two criterion sets typically lead to the same diagnosis (Rosellini et al., 2015). As a result, there is now a consensus among researchers that DSM-IV symptoms can be used to approximate DSM-5 diagnoses of PTSD (Rosellini et al., 2015).

Our finding that a substantial minority of traumas were reported as causing intense fear, helplessness, or horror in countries throughout the world is consistent with previous studies in a narrower range of countries (Brewin et al., 2000; Breslau & Kessler, 2001; Schnurr et al., 2002; Creamer et al., 2005). It is unclear, though, why conditional prevalence of A2 is significantly lower in high-income (28.6%) than in lower-income (49.5–52.2%) countries. This could be due to traumas in lower-income countries being, on average, more extreme (either in terms of characteristics of or objective consequences of the events) than in high-income countries. Another possibility is that people in low-income countries are more likely than those in high-income countries to be shocked or horrified by the occurrence of a traumatic stressor. We are not aware of any cross-national research that addresses this second possibility, but it is indirectly inconsistent with research in the United States documenting that some traumas lead to more shock and horror among middle class than among lower class people since those in the middle class are more likely to have illusory world views about control and justice, which are shattered by exposure to traumas (Wortman & Silver, 1989; Janoff-Bulman & Frantz, 1996). The reason why we would find the opposite pattern in cross-national comparisons is perplexing. Another significant between-country difference is that conditional prevalence of PTSD given A2 is significantly higher in high-income (15.0%) than in lower-income (3.8–6.3%) countries. These differences might reflect between-country differences in coping resources that influence emotional reactions to trauma. This possibility was recently proposed as a posthoc explanation of between-country differences (Duckers et al., 2016), although the number of countries considered and the vast number of differences among these countries makes much a suggestion merely speculative.

Our finding that conditional prevalence of A2 among individuals exposed to traumas far exceeded conditional prevalence of any other DSM-IV criterion of PTSD suggests that it would be more efficient to use a criterion other than A2 for screening to provide a quick rule-out of a PTSD diagnosis. This is due to the high prevalence of A2 occurring not only among individuals with PTSD but also among individuals without PTSD. However, this suggestion would be of no value in a prospective screening effort carried out in an emergency department as other symptoms require at least 30 days to manifest. As a result, A2 might still be valuable to use for prediction of the subsequent onset of PTSD among individuals evaluated in the immediate aftermath of trauma exposure. We discuss this in more detail in Chapter 22, where we investigate the feasibility of developing a prediction algorithm for PTSD to guide targeting of preventive interventions that could be used in the immediate aftermath of trauma exposure to predict which patients are likely to develop PTSD.

Our finding that only about 1% of traumas without A2 are associated with all other DSM-IV requirements for PTSD is consistent with most (Kilpatrick et al., 1998; Breslau & Kessler, 2001; Schnurr et al., 2002; Creamer et al., 2005), but not all (O'Donnell et al., 2010), previous studies. This means that removal of A2 from the criterion set would lead to only a modest increase in the number of individuals diagnosed with PTSD. This small number of cases of PTSD without A2 in the WMH series had equal PTSD persistence and equally elevated risk of temporally secondary mental disorders and suicidal ideation as cases with

A2, suggesting that these otherwise qualifying cases should not be excluded from a diagnosis. This conclusion is reinforced by evidence from other research that A2 is often absent in patients who are amnesic to details of the trauma (O'Donnell et al, 2010) and in patients from high-risk occupations (e.g., military, police, fire fighters) who otherwise meet criteria for PTSD associated with traumas that occurred in the context of their occupation (Adler et al., 2008). Some of this reluctance to report fear, helplessness, or horror by patients in these high-risk occupations may also contribute to decreased reporting of A2 among males relative to females in the WMH surveys.

An especially intriguing finding was that conditional risk of PTSD with A2 was significantly lower among respondents with a history of other DSM-IV/CIDI disorders than among other respondents. This might have been caused by prior psychopathology creating stronger vulnerability for PTSD associated with less severe traumas, where the occurrence of A2 symptoms might have been a marker of trauma severity. This possibility is consistent with the general diathesis-stress model (Williams et al., 2005), which suggests that increased vulnerability to stress (as indicated here by history of psychopathology) reduces the amount of stress needed to promote onset of PTSD, whereas vulnerability factors become less important at high levels of stress exposure due to resistance resources becoming overwhelmed.

As noted in the introduction, one rationale for including A2 in DSM-IV was that expansion of criterion A1 in DSM-IV might lead to an inappropriate broadening of the definition of PTSD unless a new subjective A2 requirement was used to delimit the range of qualifying traumas (McNally, 2004; Creamer et al., 2005; Weathers & Keane, 2007). As it turns out, the WMH results show that A2 did not have this desired effect. A somewhat different version of this argument is that the definition of trauma needs to include a short-term subjective component to focus clinical attention in the immediate aftermath of trauma exposure on the subset of traumas most likely to lead to the other PTSD criteria. This view might make good sense when it comes to predicting subsequent onset of PTSD from information about short-term emotional reactions to traumas because conditional risk of PTSD is low in the absence of A2. Longitudinal studies have confirmed this predictive association (Zatzick et al., 2002; Ehring et al., 2008). Targeting preventive interventions consequently might make use of such information (Rauch et al., 2001).

This possible value of the assessment of A2 near the time of trauma exposure as a predictor of future PTSD should not be confused with the role of A2 as a requirement for a diagnosis of PTSD. The distinction is familiar in other areas of medicine. For example, detection of hypertension is clinically useful as a predictor of heart attack and usually triggers initiation of preventive interventions. It makes no sense, though, to require a history of hypertension for a diagnosis of myocardial infarction when a person has a heart attack. Similarly with PTSD: when a patient presents for treatment of reactions to a trauma that include DSM-IV criteria B–F, it would seem perverse to use the patient's retrospective report of not experiencing A2 at the time of the trauma exposure to rule out a diagnosis of PTSD.

Another argument for retaining A2 is that information about A2 can be valuable in making a differential diagnosis between PTSD and other syndromes, such as comorbid reactive depression with phobia, when a patient presents with a mixture of depression and anxiety related to a trauma. The question of whether to make a diagnosis of PTSD if the patient's current symptoms meet PTSD criteria B–F, even if the patient fails to recall A2 emotional reactions at the time of the trauma then has to be considered. The data presented here were unable to address this issue. Research that investigates this issue would be an important addition to other studies that have been called for to refine our understanding of differential treatment response in PTSD (Stein et al., 2009), especially if a differential treatment response could be found based on retrospective assessment of A2.

These findings should be interpreted in the context of several important limitations. First, WMH interviews were conducted by lay interviewers rather than clinicians. This was an especially important issue for the evaluation of retrospective reports of complex emotional responses like those involved in A2. Second, results may not generalize to trauma types that were not considered in the CIDI assessment or that were so rarely reported that few such traumas were represented in our randomly selected series. Third, PTSD was assessed in a lifetime framework, which introduced the possibility of recall bias. This limitation is especially important in light of the high proportion of respondents with other requirements for a diagnosis of PTSD who retrospectively reported that they met A2 at the time of trauma exposure (98.6%). This proportion exceeded the comparable proportion found in the one prospective general population study that examined this issue (89%) (Brewin et al., 2000), raising the possibility that A2 was recalled as being more prevalent than it actually was. If this was the case, then the small proportion of cases of estimated to be excluded from a PTSD diagnosis by the A2 requirement may constitute an underestimate. This possibility has to be considered in the context of the calls by some investigators to broaden A2 beyond a focus on fear, helplessness, and horror to include other strong emotions sometimes associated with PTSD, such as anger, shame, grief, and extreme emotional blunting (i.e., shock, dissociation) (Roemer et al., 1998; Brewin et al., 2000; Brunet et al., 2001). If A2 was broadened in these ways, then it would have been easy to imagine that virtually 100% of the people who met other requirements for PTSD would also have met the broadened definition of A2. This would have made A2 completely redundant with the other criteria, which would argue even more forcefully than the results reported here that A2 should be considered a risk factor rather than a diagnostic criterion for PTSD. Based on these results and observations, we excluded the A2 criterion in the substantive analyses of prevalence and correlates of DSM-IV PTSD in the WMH analyses reported in the remainder of this volume.

Acknowledgment

Portions of this chapter are based on Karam, E. G., Andrews, G., Bauch, E., et al. (2010). The role of Criterion A2 in the DSM IV Diagnosis of Post-Traumatic Stress Disorder. *Biological Psychiatry*, **68,** 465–73, by permission of Elsevier.

References

Adler, A. B., Wright, K. M., Bliese, P. D., Eckford, R., & Hoge, C. W. (2008). A2 diagnostic criterion for combat-related posttraumatic stress disorder. *Journal of Traumatic Stress*, 21, 301–8.

American Psychiatric Association. (1994). *Diagnostic and Statistical Manual of Mental Disorders, Fourth Edition. DSM-IV*. Washington, DC: American Psychiatric Association.

American Psychiatric Association. (2013). *Diagnostic and Statistical Manual of Mental Disorders, Fifth Edition. DSM-5*. Arlington, VA: American Psychiatric Association.

Andrews, G., Slade, T., Sunderland, M., & Anderson, T. (2007). Issues for DSM-V: simplifying DSM-IV to enhance utility: the case of major depressive disorder. *American Journal of Psychiatry*, 164, 1784–5.

Breslau, N., & Kessler, R. C. (2001). The stressor criterion in DSM-IV posttraumatic stress disorder: an empirical investigation. *Biological Psychiatry*, 50, 699–704.

Brewin, C. R., Andrews, B., & Rose, S. (2000). Fear, helplessness, and horror in posttraumatic stress disorder: investigating DSM-IV Criterion A2 in victims of violent crime. *Journal of Traumatic Stress*, 13, 499–509.

Brunet, A., Weiss, D. S., Metzler, T. J., et al. (2001). The Peritraumatic Distress Inventory: a proposed measure of PTSD criterion A2. *American Journal of Psychiatry*, 158, 1480–5.

Creamer, M., McFarlane, A. C., & Burgess, P. (2005). Psychopathology following trauma: the role of subjective experience. *Journal of Affective Disorders*, 86, 175–82.

Duckers, M. L., Alisic, E., & Brewin, C. R. (2016). A vulnerability paradox in the cross-national prevalence of post-traumatic stress disorder. *British Journal of Psychiatry*, 209, 300–5.

Efron, B. (1988). Logistic regression, survival analysis, and the Kaplan-Meier curve. *Journal of the American Statistical Association*, 83, 414–25.

Ehring, T., Ehlers, A., Cleare, A. J., & Glucksman, E. (2008). Do acute psychological and psychobiological responses to trauma predict subsequent symptom severities of PTSD and depression? *Psychiatry Research*, 161, 67–75.

Friedman, M. J., Resick, P. A., Bryant, R. A., & Brewin, C. R. (2011). Considering PTSD for DSM-5. *Depression and Anxiety*, 28, 750–69.

Hosmer, D. W., & Lemeshow, S. (2000). *Applied Logistic Regression*, 2nd edn. New York, NY: Wiley.

Janoff-Bulman, R., & Frantz, C. M. (1996). The loss of illusions: the potent legacy of trauma. *Journal of Personal and Interpersonal Loss*, 1, 133–50.

Kilpatrick, D. G., Resnick, H. S., Freedy, J. R., et al. (1998). The posttraumatic stress disorder field trial: evaluation of the PTSD construct – Criteria A through E. In T. A. Widiger, A. J. Frances, H. A. Pincus, et al., eds., *DSM-IV Sourcebook*, Volume 4. Washington, DC: American Psychiatric Press, pp. 803–44.

McNally, R. J. (2004). Conceptual problems with the DSM-IV criteria for posttraumatic stress disorder. In G. M. Rosen, ed., *Posttraumatic Stress Disorder: Issues and Controversies*. New York, NY: Wiley, pp. 1–14.

O'Donnell, M. L., Creamer, M., McFarlane, A. C., Silove, D., & Bryant, R. A. (2010). Should A2 be a diagnostic requirement for posttraumatic stress disorder in DSM-V? *Psychiatry Research*, 176, 257–60.

Pereda, N., & Forero, C. G. (2012). Contribution of criterion A2 to PTSD screening in the presence of traumatic events. *Journal of Traumatic Stress*, 25, 587–91.

Rauch, S. A., Hembree, E. A., & Foa, E. B. (2001). Acute psychosocial preventive interventions for posttraumatic stress disorder. *Advances in Mind-Body Medicine*, 17, 187–91.

Research Triangle Institute. (2002). *SUDAAN: Professional Software for Survey Data Analysis, Version 8.0.1.* Research Triangle Park, NC: Research Triangle Institute.

Roemer, L., Litz, B. T., Orsillo, S. M., Ehlich, P. J., & Friedman, M. J. (1998). Increases in retrospective accounts of war-zone exposure over time: the role of PTSD symptom severity. *Journal of Traumatic Stress*, 11, 597–605.

Rosellini, A. J., Stein, M. B., Colpe, L. J., et al. (2015). Approximating a DSM-5 diagnosis of PTSD using DSM-IV criteria. *Depression and Anxiety*, 32, 493–501.

Schnurr, P. P., Spiro, A., III, Vielhauer, M. J., Findler, M. N., & Hamblen, J. L. (2002). Trauma in the lives of older men: findings from the Normative Aging Study. *Journal of Clinical Geropsychology*, 8, 175–87.

Stein, D. J., Cloitre, M., Nemeroff, C. B., et al. (2009). Cape Town consensus on posttraumatic stress disorder. *CNS Spectrums*, 14, 52–8.

Weathers, F. W., & Keane, T. M. (2007). The Criterion A problem revisited: controversies and challenges in defining and measuring psychological trauma. *Journal of Traumatic Stress*, 20, 107–21.

Williams, N. L., Reardon, J. M., Murray, K. T., & Cole, T. M. (2005). Anxiety disorders: a developmental vulnerability-stress perspective. In B. L. Hankin, & J. R. Z. Abela, eds., *Development of Psychopathology: A Vulnerability-Stress Perspective*. Thousand Oaks, CA: Sage, pp. 289–327.

Wolter, K. M. (1985). *Introduction to Variance Estimation.* New York, NY: Springer-Verlag.

Wortman, C. B., & Silver, R. C. (1989). The myths of coping with loss. *Journal of Consulting and Clinical Psychology*, 57, 349–57.

Zatzick, D. F., Kang, S. M., Muller, H. G., et al. (2002). Predicting posttraumatic distress in hospitalized trauma survivors with acute injuries. *American Journal of Psychiatry*, 159, 941–6.

Zimmerman, M., Chelminski, I., McGlinchey, J. B., & Young, D. (2006). Diagnosing major depressive disorder X: can the utility of the DSM-IV symptom criteria be improved? *The Journal of Nervous and Mental Disease*, 194, 893–7.

Chapter 19

Threshold versus Subthreshold Posttraumatic Stress Disorder

Katie A. McLaughlin, Koen Demyttenaere, Karestan C. Koenen, José Posada-Villa, Ayelet Meron Ruscio, and Ronald C. Kessler

Many individuals exposed to traumas fail to meet full criteria for posttraumatic stress disorder (PTSD), but nonetheless develop subthreshold PTSD (Weiss et al., 1992; Schnurr et al., 1993; Stein et al., 1997, 2002; Schnurr et al., 2000; Breslau et al., 2004). These subthreshold cases, which are often clinically significant, may require therapeutic intervention (Carlier & Gersons, 1995; Naylor et al., 2013). Considerable research exists on subthreshold PTSD, despite concerns about possible overdiagnosis (McNally, 2003) and secondary gain (Jones & Wessely, 2007). Most prior studies of subthreshold PTSD (Stein et al., 2002; Zlotnick et al., 2002; Lai et al., 2004; Jakupcak et al., 2007) examine the levels of distress, impairment, suicidality, and comorbidity that are found among individuals who meet full PTSD criteria, most, but not all symptoms of PTSD, and no symptoms of PTSD (Favaro et al., 2006; Jakupcak et al., 2007; Cukor et al., 2010; Gellis et al., 2010). However, these studies are inconsistent in their definitions of subthreshold PTSD. The most common definitions are (i) at least one symptom of each DSM criterion (Schnurr et al., 1993, 2004; Stein et al., 1997, 2002; Schnurr et al., 2000; Breslau et al., 2004; Lai et al., 2004; Favaro et al., 2006; Pietrzak et al., 2012); (ii) all required symptoms of re-experiencing and one other DSM criterion (Schnurr et al., 1993, 2004; Blanchard et al., 1994, 1995; Schutzwohl & Maercker, 1999; Pietrzak et al., 2012); (iii) all required symptoms of re-experiencing and hyper-arousal and at least one avoidance symptom (Kulka et al., 1990; Lipschitz et al., 2000); and (iv) all required symptoms of at least one DSM criterion (Patterson et al., 1990; McLeer et al., 1992). Because the number of symptom criteria required for a PTSD diagnosis has increased from three to four in DSM-5, additional definitions of subthreshold DSM-5 PTSD are now also possible.

One consequence of these inconsistent definitions has been that lifetime prevalence estimates of subthreshold PTSD have varied widely across studies (Jeon et al., 2007; Naylor et al., 2013). The few studies that examined multiple definitions argued for creating a consensus definition that could be used as the foundation for future studies (Schutzwohl & Maercker, 1999; Marshall et al., 2001; Mylle & Maes, 2004). However, only a handful of studies have proposed such a definition (Schutzwohl & Maercker, 1999; Breslau et al., 2004), and they did so, based on a comparison of only two definitions. In contrast, in the World Mental Health (WMH) surveys, we considered all previously proposed definitions of subthreshold PTSD and compared estimates of prevalence and correlates across them. Our hope was that systematic comparison of results across the range of WMH surveys would be of value to the field in settling on a consensus definition of subthreshold PTSD.

Methods

When we carried out the WMH analysis of subthreshold PTSD, data were available for 13 surveys that assessed PTSD associated with random traumas: 8 in high-income countries (Belgium, Germany, Italy, Japan, the Netherlands, New Zealand, Spain, and the United States), 4 in upper-middle-income countries (São Paulo in Brazil, Bulgaria, Mexico, and Romania), and 1 in a lower-middle-income country (Colombia). The 23,936 respondents in those surveys who reported lifetime trauma exposure were the focus of analysis.

Based on preliminary analyses comparing DSM-IV and DSM-5 criteria in an independent sample (Rosellini et al., 2015), we used the DSM-IV/CIDI PTSD symptom assessment to approximate DSM-5 criteria (American Psychiatric Association, 2013) in the way described in Chapter 17. We fully operationalized DSM-5 criteria B (one of five symptoms of intrusive recollection), C (one of two symptoms of avoidance), F (duration more than 1 month), and G (clinically significant distress or impairment), and conservatively operationalized criteria D (two of the four symptoms of negative alterations in cognitions and mood assessed in the CIDI, whereas two of seven are required in DSM-5) and E (two of the five symptoms of marked alterations in arousal and reactivity assessed in the CIDI, whereas two of six are required in DSM-5) (see Table 19.1). Our approximation was conservative because it required the same number of criteria D and E symptoms as DSM-5, but from smaller sets. Preliminary evaluation of this approximation in the independent sample mentioned earlier suggests that it captures over 90% of DSM-5 PTSD cases (Rosellini et al., 2015). Given this high sensitivity in conjunction with perfect specificity, we determined that a focus on approximate DSM-5 criteria was preferable to a focus on DSM-IV criteria since the use of DSM-5 criteria would be more helpful to both researchers as well as to policy makers.

We created four definitions of subthreshold PTSD to reflect the most commonly used definitions in previous studies and to capture the changes in the number of criteria and required symptoms within each cluster in DSM-5. These include definitions of subthreshold PTSD requiring (i) at least one symptom from each of the four DSM-5 criteria B–E, (ii) fully meeting three of criteria B–E, (iii) fully meeting two of criteria B–E, and (iv) fully meeting one of criteria B–E.

Table 19.1 DSM-5 PTSD criteria and definitions of subthreshold PTSD

DSM-5 PTSD criteria	Symptoms required[a]
A. Exposure to actual or threatened death, serious injury, or sexual violence	
B. RE	1 of 4
C. AV	1 of 2
D. Negative alterations in CM	2 of 7
E. HA	2 of 6
F. Duration of at least 1 month	
G. Clinically significant distress or impairment	
H. Symptoms not due to physiological effects of a substance or medical condition	
Subthreshold PTSD definitions	**Definition**
1. One or more symptoms of each criterion B–E	1+ symptom in each of the four criteria B–E
2. Three of four criteria B–E	Exactly 3 of 4 criteria B–E
3. Two of four criteria B–E	Exactly 2 of 4 criteria B–E
4. One of four criteria B–E	Exactly 1 of 4 criteria B–E

[a]The number of symptoms required to meet each criterion is listed only for criteria B–E. The full list of symptoms that comprise each of these criteria can be found in the DSM-5.

Six outcomes were considered in the analysis: duration of PTSD symptoms (coded for symptoms with longest duration to allow comparison of threshold and subthreshold PTSD); clinically significant distress impairment associated with these symptoms; severe distress impairment associated with these symptoms; first lifetime onset of suicidal ideation in the wake of the focal trauma; first lifetime onset of any of five DSM-IV/CIDI fear disorders in the wake of the focal trauma among respondents with no history of these disorders (panic disorder with or without agoraphobia, agoraphobia without a history of panic disorder, specific phobia, social phobia, and obsessive compulsive disorder); and first lifetime onset of any of three DSM-IV/CIDI distress disorders (major depressive disorder/dysthymia, generalized anxiety disorder, and bipolar disorders [I–II and subthreshold]) in conjunction with the focal trauma among respondents with no history of these disorders.

Initial regression analyses focused on associations between the number of DSM-5 symptoms (0, 1, 2+) within each PTSD criterion and the six outcomes, to determine whether each symptom cluster was associated with these outcomes and to evaluate the implications of the DSM-5 thresholds requiring only one symptom from each of criteria B and C and two symptoms from each of criteria D and E. We then estimated the associations between the number of DSM-5 *criteria* (1, 2, 3, 4) and the six outcomes to select an optimal subthreshold PTSD definition. Once a definition was selected, we estimated parallel regression equations examining predictors of threshold PTSD, subthreshold PTSD, and PTSD symptoms falling short of our subthreshold definitions compared to respondents with no PTSD symptoms. The predictors included respondent sex, age at trauma exposure, type of trauma, and counts of four types of prior lifetime DSM-IV/CIDI disorders: the fear and distress disorders listed earlier as well as three disruptive behavior disorders (oppositional-defiant disorder, conduct disorder, and intermittent explosive disorder) and two substance use disorders (alcohol and drug abuse with or without dependence).

The regression equations were estimated using a logistic link function at the person level to study predictors of all outcomes other than symptom duration. Discrete-time survival analysis in a logistic regression framework using person-month as the unit of analysis was used to study predictors of symptom duration. Control variables included country, sex, type of trauma, and respondent age at occurrence of the focal trauma. The analyses predicting comorbid fear and distress disorders focused on first lifetime onset of each such disorder in the year of trauma occurrence, using a disorder-specific data array that was pooled across the five fear disorders and separately across the three distress disorders. Pooling was used because of the rarity of each comorbid disorder having first onset in the year of trauma occurrence. The equations used to predict these comorbid disorders included dummy predictor variables to distinguish the outcome disorders, thereby constraining coefficients to be constant across this range of outcomes. As in all other analyses reported in this volume, the logistic regression coefficients and their standard errors were exponentiated and are reported here as odds ratios (ORs) with 95% confidence intervals (CIs). Statistical significance was evaluated using 0.05-level two-sided tests. The design-based Taylor series method (Wolter, 1985) implemented in SAS (SAS Institute Inc., 2008) was used to adjust for weighting and clustering.

Results

Prevalence of PTSD Symptom Profiles

Prevalence of the CIDI approximation of DSM-5 PTSD was 3.0%, while an additional 4.6% of respondents met criteria for at least one definition of subthreshold PTSD (see Table 19.2). Prevalence of subthreshold PTSD was lowest for the definition requiring at least one symptom for each criterion B–E (0.7%) and highest for the definition requiring fully meeting symptoms for at least one of the four criteria B–E (4.6%). Only a small proportion of respondents (0.2%) reported at least one symptom in criteria B–E and failed to qualify for any definition of subthreshold PTSD.

Table 19.2 Distribution of threshold and subthreshold DSM-5/CIDI PTSD symptom profiles in the WMH representative sample of traumas

	%	(SE)	(*n*)[a]
I Threshold PTSD	3.0	(0.2)	(835)
II Subthreshold PTSD			
One or more symptoms of each criterion B–E	0.7	(0.1)	(248)
Three of the four criteria B–E	1.8	(0.1)	(621)
Two of the four criteria B–E	1.7	(0.4)	(1,085)
One of the four criteria B–E	4.6	(0.5)	(1,413)
Any subthreshold	4.6	(0.5)	(1,413)
III Others with any criterion B–E symptoms	0.2	(0.1)	(49)
IV No symptoms	92.2	(0.5)	(21,639)
V Total	100.0	–	(23,936)

[a]Sample sizes reported are the numbers of respondents in the numerators. The denominator for all calculations is 23,936.

Associations of DSM-5 PTSD Criteria B–E Symptoms with the Outcomes

Within-criterion symptom-level models found considerable variation across criteria in the associations between symptoms and outcomes (see Table 19.3). Criterion D symptoms were significantly associated with all six outcomes (χ^2_2 = 6.2–38.3, p = 0.045–<0.001), criterion E symptoms with four outcomes (χ^2_2=6.1–11.2, p=0.048–0.004), criterion B symptoms with two outcomes (χ^2_2= 10.0–10.4, p = 0.012–0.007), and criterion C symptoms with only one outcome (χ^2_2= 8.0, p = 0.018). The pattern of results for criteria B (re-experiencing) and C (avoidance) symptoms was largely consistent with the DSM-5 symptom threshold of 1+ symptom for each of these criteria. For models with globally significant effects of criteria B–C and at least one individually significant coefficient, ORs associated with 1 symptom (2.2 and 1.4, respectively) were virtually identical to those associated with 2+ symptoms (2.1 and 1.4, respectively). Both ORs in each pair were statistically significant. The results for criteria D (negative alterations in cognition and mood) and E (hyper-arousal) symptoms were also largely consistent with the DSM-5 symptom threshold of 2+ symptoms. Results for models with globally significant effects of criteria D–E showed ORs associated with 2+ symptoms (1.7–5.3) to be statistically significant and higher than the nonsignificant ORs associated with 1 symptom (0.7–2.7) in 9 of 10 comparisons.

Confounding due to Contemporaneous Comorbidity

Before concluding that the DSM-5 criteria B–E symptom thresholds were appropriate, we considered the possibility that the aforementioned results were due to uncontrolled contemporaneous comorbidity rather than to subthreshold PTSD. The analyses in Table 19.3 were consequently replicated after adding controls for the onset of fear and distress disorders in the same years as the focal traumas. Results were not affected by introducing these controls, arguing against the suggestion that these results were due to unmeasured comorbidity (see Appendix Tables 19.A1–19.A3).

Table 19.3 Associations of symptom counts across DSM-5/CIDI PTSD criteria B–E with a range of outcomes in the WMH sample of randomly selected traumas[a]

	Distress impairment						Suicidal ideation[b]			Comorbid disorders						Symptom duration[c]		
	Clinically significant[d]			Severe[e]						Fear[f]			Distress[f]					
	%	OR	(95% CI)	%	OR	(95% CI)	%	OR	(95% CI)	%	OR	(95% CI)	%	OR	(95% CI)	Mean duration	OR	(95% CI)
I Criterion B. IR																		
0	84.0	1.0	–	54.4	1.0	–	1.2	1.0	–	0.3	1.0	–	0.6	1.0	–	70.2	1.0	–
1	86.1	1.6	(0.6–4.4)	68.1	2.2*	(1.0–4.8)	3.6	1.5	(0.6–4.1)	0.1	0.4	(0.1–2.2)	3.9	1.7	(0.6–5.0)	66.2	1.1	(0.7–1.7)
2+	93.1	2.1	(1.0–4.5)	78.2	2.1*	(1.3–3.4)	5.2	1.1	(0.5–2.1)	1.4	2.3	(1.0–5.2)	3.9	1.1	(0.6–1.9)	89.9	0.9	(0.7–1.4)
χ^2_2		3.9			10.4*			0.8			10.0*†			1.1			0.4	
II Criterion C. AV																		
0	82.9	1.0	–	66.1	1.0	–	1.2	1.0	–	0.3	1.0	–	0.7	1.0	–	52.0	1.0	–
1	91.9	1.4	(0.7–3.1)	75.7	1.1	(0.6–2.0)	4.7	0.6	(0.2–1.8)	0.7	0.4	(0.2–1.1)	3.7	0.9	(0.4–1.7)	90.2	1.4*	(1.1–1.9)
2+	96.1	2.7*	(1.1–6.5)	75.8	0.7	(0.4–1.3)	5.4	0.6	(0.2–1.4)	1.7	0.7	(0.2–1.8)	4.0	0.8	(0.4–1.4)	103.1	1.4*	(1.1–2.0)
χ^2_2		5.2			2.4			1.6			3.7			0.9			8.0*	
III Criterion D. CM																		
0	81.7	1.0	–	60.9	1.0	–	1.2	1.0	–	0.3	1.0	–	0.6	1.0	–	49.1	1.0	–
1	92.5	1.7	(0.9–3.3)	55.4	0.9	(0.5–1.7)	1.0	0.7	(0.2–2.4)	0.8	2.7	(0.7–9.8)	1.8	0.9	(0.4–2.2)	81.1	1.3	(0.9–1.7)
2+	96.5	2.5*	(1.1–5.8)	85.2	4.2*	(2.4–7.1)	7.7	5.3*	(2.3–11.9)	1.8	3.9*	(1.5–10.3)	5.3	2.9*	(1.4–6.0)	106.5	1.7*	(1.2–2.0)
χ^2_2		6.2*			38.3*			24.8*			8.2*			28.9*			10.9*	

IV Criterion E. AR																		
0	76.0	1.0	–	54.1	1.0	–	1.2	1.0	–	0.3	1.0	–	0.6	1.0	–	67.6	1.0	–
1	79.3	1.9	(0.6–6.1)	55.0	1.1	(0.5–2.8)	2.2	1.2	(0.4–4.1)	0.2	0.3	(0.1–1.3)	1.8	1.7	(0.9–3.6)	53.0	1.7*	(1.1–2.6)
2+	95.0	5.0*	(1.5–16.1)	77.6	2.3*	(1.3–4.3)	5.2	1.5	(0.6–3.6)	1.3	1.0	(0.5–2.2)	4.2	3.3*	(1.6–6.8)	90.1	1.4	(0.9–2.0)
χ^2_2		7.8*			10.9*			0.8			3.2			11.2*			6.1*	
χ^2_8		41.8*			72.3*			55.7*			48.8*			152.3*			34.0*	
(*n*)	(2,499)[d]			(2,297)[e]			(22,030)[b]			(23,936)[f]			(23,908)[f]			(2,297)[c]		

*Significant at the 0.05 level, two-sided test.

[†]The coefficients are significant as a pair even though neither OR is individually significant. This occurs because there is a significant difference between the insignificantly elevated OR for 2+ symptoms and the insignificantly reduced OR for 1 symptom.

[a]See the section on Analysis Methods in the text for a description of the regression models.

[b]The sample is limited to cases where the respondent did not have a lifetime history of suicidal ideation prior to age of occurrence of the trauma, as first lifetime onset of suicidal ideation is the outcome. Presence of clinically significant distress or impairment associated with the trauma was not required in defining this sample, but criteria B–E symptoms were classified as present in defining the predictors only if the respondent reported clinically significant distress or impairment associated with these symptoms.

[c]The sample is limited to cases where the respondent reported one or more symptoms of at least one criterion B–E symptom lasting more than 1 month and reported clinically significant distress or impairment associated with this/these symptom(s), as these are the cases for which symptom duration was assessed. The predictors of symptom duration were estimated in a discrete-time survival framework with person-month the unit of analysis. Duration was censored at 60 months if symptoms persisted longer than 60 months in order to reduce the effects of extreme outliers. A total of 71,304 person-months were included in the analysis.

[d]The sample is limited to cases where the respondent reported one or more symptoms of at least one criterion B–E lasting more than 1 month, as clinically significant distress and impairment were assessed only when at least one such symptom was reported.

[e]The sample is limited to cases where the respondent reported one or more symptoms of at least one criterion B–E lasting more than 1 month and reported clinically significant distress or impairment associated with this/these symptom(s), as severe distress and impairment were assessed only in this subsample. Note that the outcome of severe distress impairment is conditionally independent of the outcome of serious distress impairment because all respondents in the sample used to predict severe distress impairment reported significant distress impairment.

[f]The ORs reported here are pooled across disorder-specific equations for each of the fear and distress disorders assessed in the surveys. The % estimates are averages across those pooled equations. Presence of clinically significant distress or impairment associated with the trauma was not required in defining these samples, but criteria B–E symptoms were classified as present in defining the predictors only if the respondent reported clinically significant distress or impairment associated with these symptoms. The 23,936 respondents included in the pooled person-disorder data array for the five fear disorders resulted in 112,460 observations, and the 23,908 respondents included in the pooled person-disorder data array for mood disorders resulted in 79,836 observations.

Associations of DSM-5 Subthreshold PTSD Profiles with the Outcomes

Subsequent analyses examined associations of each subthreshold definition with the outcomes based on dichotomous classifications for whether or not the DSM-5 symptom threshold was met for each criterion. We did not examine the subthreshold definition requiring at least one symptom in each criterion, given our results supporting the DSM-5 symptom thresholds and the low prevalence of this definition of subthreshold PTSD. A clear gradient was found across the aggregated number-of-criteria profiles for all six outcomes, with the highest outcome scores consistently associated with threshold PTSD, the next highest generally associated with the three-of-four criteria profile (with the exception of clinically significant distress impairment, which was somewhat higher in the two-of-four profile), and next highest with the two-of-four profiles (with the exception of suicidality, which was higher in the one-of-four profile than in the two-of-four profile) (see Table 19.4). The none-of-four profile, finally, had the lowest scores on all outcomes other than symptom duration. The number of respondents with the none-of-four profile whose symptom duration was estimated (i.e., those with clinically significant symptoms persisting more than 1 month) was very small ($n = 49$), though, making the estimate of mean duration unstable in this subgroup.

Leaving aside duration because of this instability, differences in all five other outcome scores were statistically significant among respondents with threshold PTSD and three-of-four criteria compared to the none-of-four, for four outcomes among respondents with two-of-four, and for one outcome among respondents with one-of-four. Significance tests comparing the outcomes of respondents with threshold PTSD versus subthreshold profiles found three significant differences with the three-of-four profiles (clinically significant and severe distress impairment and comorbid distress disorders; $\chi^2_1 = 4.0–17.3$, $p = 0.045$ to <0.001) and four each with the two-of-four (all outcomes other than comorbid fear disorders; $\chi^2_1 = 4.4–27.5$, $p = 0.036$ to <0.001) and one-of-four (all outcomes other than comorbid fear disorders; $\chi^2_1 = 4.0–39.5$, $p = 0.045$ to <0.001) profiles.

Differences in Outcomes within DSM-5 Subthreshold Profiles

The aforementioned analyses focused on differences between, but not within the three-of-four, two-of-four, and one-of-four DSM-5 subthreshold profiles. In order to investigate the latter distinctions, we estimated disaggregated versions of the models in Table 19.4 to consider different combinations of criteria within each of the subthreshold symptom profiles. There were 14 such profiles: 4 representing three-of-four criteria profiles, 6 two-of-four criteria profiles, and 4 one-of-four criteria profiles. The pattern of results from these models did not suggest any specific type or combination of symptoms of particular importance (see Appendix Table 19.A4).

Predictors of Threshold versus Subthreshold PTSD

Based on our finding that respondents with two-of-four criteria B–E exhibited consistently worse outcomes than those with one-of-four criteria B–E or less, we defined subthreshold PTSD as meeting at least two-of-four criteria B–E. A number of interesting similarities and differences were found in the predictors of threshold PTSD, subthreshold PTSD, and other symptoms of PTSD versus no symptoms among individuals exposed to traumas (see Table 19.5). Females had significantly elevated odds of all symptomatic outcomes compared to males (OR = 1.7–3.1). History of DSM-IV/CIDI fear and distress disorders predicted threshold (OR = 1.7–1.9) and subthreshold (OR = 1.5–1.7) PTSD, but not other symptoms of PTSD, whereas prior substance use disorder predicted threshold PTSD (OR = 1.4) but not the other two outcomes. Childhood trauma exposure was associated with elevated odds of threshold PTSD (OR = 3.1), but not the other symptomatic outcomes, while adolescent trauma exposure was associated with significantly reduced odds of other symptoms (OR = 0.4), but not of either threshold or subthreshold PTSD. Traumas involving intimate partner violence and sexual violence were associated with significantly elevated odds (relative to unexpected death of a loved one) of threshold PTSD (OR = 2.6), but not of the other outcomes, while traumas that occurred to a loved one were associated with significantly reduced relative odds of threshold PTSD (OR = 0.5), but not of the other outcomes. War-related traumas (OR = 0.3), accidents (OR = 0.5–0.6), and "other" traumas (OR = 2.1–2.5) were associated with significantly reduced relative odds of both threshold and subthreshold PTSD, but not of other PTSD symptoms.

Discussion

The data reported here were the first large-scale cross-national data on prevalence and correlates of

Table 19.4 Associations of different definitions of DSM-5 subthreshold PTSD with a range of outcomes in the WMH sample of randomly selected traumas[a]

	Distress impairment						Suicidal ideation[b]			Comorbid disorders						Symptom duration[c]		
	Clinically significant[d]			Severe[e]						Fear[f]			Distress[f]					
	%	OR	(95% CI)	%	OR	(95% CI)	%	OR	(95% CI)	%	OR	(95% CI)	%	OR	(95% CI)	Mean duration	OR	(95% CI)
I Threshold PTSD	98.0[g]	26.9*[g]	(6.7–108.0)	87.6	22.3*	(6.4–75.2)	8.2	5.4*	(3.0–9.8)	2.0	5.5*	(2.9–10.3)	5.5	8.6*	(5.6–13.0)	117	2.0	(1.0–3.6)
II Three of criteria B–E	93.4	8.6*	(2.4–30.4)	70.4	6.8*	(2.2–20.2)	3.6	2.3*	(1.0–5.1)	0.9	2.6*	(1.2–5.8)	3.6	4.9*	(2.8–8.4)	82.3	1.7	(0.8–3.2)
III Two of criteria B–E	92.9	9.7*	(2.2–42.7)	69.4	5.4*	(1.8–16.5)	1.4	1.0	(0.4–2.6)	0.5	2.8*	(1.3–5.9)	1.9	3.0*	(1.7–5.2)	47.3	1.1	(0.6–2.2)
IV One of criteria B–E	72.7	1.4	(0.4–5.2)	47.6	2.3	(0.8–7.2)	2.3	1.5	(0.5–4.9)	0.5	2.2	(0.8–6.0)	1.9	2.9*	(1.4–6.0)	58.9	0.9	(0.4–1.9)
V None of criteria B–E	68.0	1.0	–	30.7	1.0	–	1.2	1.0	–	0.3	1.0	–	0.6	1.0	–	69.1	1.0	–
VI Total	90.7			72.8			1.4			0.4			0.8			84.4		
(*n*)	(2,499)[d]			(2,297)[e]			(22,030)[b]			(23,936)[f]			(23,908)[f]			(2,297)[c]		

*Significant at the 0.05 level, two-sided test.
[a]See the section on Analysis Methods in the text for a description of the regression models.
[b]The sample is limited to cases where the respondent did not have a lifetime history of suicidal ideation prior to age of occurrence of the trauma, as first lifetime onset of suicidal ideation is the outcome. Presence of clinically significant distress or impairment associated with the trauma was not required in defining this sample, but criteria B–E symptoms were classified as present in defining the predictors only if the respondent reported clinically significant distress or impairment associated with these symptoms.
[c]The sample is limited to cases where the respondent reported one or more symptoms of at least one criterion B–E lasting more than 1 month and reported clinically significant distress or impairment associated with this/these symptom(s), as these are the cases for which symptom duration was assessed. The predictors of symptom duration are estimated in a discrete-time survival framework with person-month the unit of analysis. Duration was censored at 60 months if symptoms persisted longer than 60 months in order to reduce the effects of extreme outliers. A total of 71,304 person-months was included in the analysis.
[d]The sample is limited to cases where the respondent reported one or more symptoms of at least one criterion B–E lasting more than 1 month, as clinically significant distress and impairment were assessed only when at least one such symptom was reported.
[e]The sample is limited to cases where the respondent reported one or more symptoms of at least one criterion B–E lasting more than 1 month and reported clinically significant distress or impairment associated with this/these symptom(s), as severe distress and impairment were assessed only in this subsample. Note that the outcome of severe distress impairment is conditionally independent of the outcome of serious distress impairment because all respondents in the sample used to predict severe distress impairment reported clinically significant distress impairment.
[f]The ORs reported here are pooled across disorder-specific equations for each of the fear and distress disorders assessed in the surveys. The % estimates are averages across those pooled equations. Presence of clinically significant distress or impairment associated with the trauma was not required in defining these samples, but criteria B–E symptoms were classified as present in defining the predictors only if the respondent reported clinically significant distress or impairment associated with these symptoms. The 23,936 respondents included in the pooled person-disorder data array for the five fear disorders resulted in 112,460 observations, and the 23,908 respondents included in the pooled person-disorder data array for mood disorders resulted in 79,836 observations.
[g]The requirement of clinically significant distress or impairment was not operationalized in defining threshold cases for this outcome as this would have led to 100% of cases having the outcome and making it impossible to include them in the regression equation.

Table 19.5 Associations of socio-demographic variables, temporally prior mental disorders, and characteristics of traumas with DSM-5/CIDI PTSD, subthreshold PTSD, and PTSD symptoms in the WMH representative sample of traumas[a]

	Threshold PTSD		Subthreshold[b]		Others with symptoms[c]	
	OR	(95% CI)	OR	(95% CI)	OR	(95% CI)
I Age of Trauma Exposure						
0–12	3.1*	(1.4–6.5)	1.0	(0.8–4.0)	0.4	(0.1–1.4)
13–19	1.2	(0.5–2.6)	1.2	(0.5–2.1)	0.4*	(0.2–0.9)
20–29	1.3	(0.7–2.3)	1.1	(0.7–2.3)	0.5	(0.2–1.1)
30–44	0.9	(0.5–1.7)	1.0	(0.7–1.8)	1.1	(0.5–2.2)
45+ years	1.0	–	1.0	–	1.0	–
χ^2_4	24.6*		5.8		11.1*	
II Sex						
Female	1.7*	(1.1–2.6)	2.6*	(1.6–4.2)	1.8*	(1.1–3.1)
Male	1.0	–	1.0	–	1.0	–
III Prior Mental Disorders[d]						
Fear disorders	1.9*	(1.7–2.2)	1.5*	(1.3–1.8)	1.2	(0.9–1.7)
Distress disorders	1.7*	(1.4–2.0)	1.5*†	(1.2–1.9)	1.0	(0.7–1.4)
Disruptive behavioral disorders	1.1	(0.8–1.6)	0.8†	(0.5–1.5)	1.9*	(1.0–3.5)
Substance use disorders	1.4*	(1.0–1.8)	1.3†	(0.9–2.0)	0.7	(0.4–1.3)
χ^2_3	190.6*		35.9*		7.4	
IV Type of Trauma						
War-related traumas	0.3*	(0.2–0.7)	0.3*	(0.2–0.6)	1.0	(0.4–2.8)
Other interpersonal violence	0.7	(0.4–1.2)	0.9	(0.5–1.5)	0.6	(0.4–1.2)
Intimate/sexual violence	2.6*‡	(1.7–4.0)	1.2	(0.7–1.9)	1.5	(0.6–3.3)
Accidents/injuries	0.5*	(0.3–0.8)	0.6*	(0.4–0.9)	1.0	(0.5–1.8)
Other traumas to loved ones	0.5*‡	(0.3–0.8)	1.1	(0.7–1.9)	0.7	(0.4–1.3)
Other	2.1*	(1.3–3.3)	2.5*	(1.6–4.0)	3.1	(0.9–10.5)
UD of a loved one	1.0	–	1.0	–	1.0	–
χ^2_6	86.9*		53.9*		8.0	
(*n*)	(22,474)		(22,742)		(22,016)	

*Significant at the 0.05 level, two-sided test.
†Significant difference between the ORs for sub-threshold DSM-5 PTSD and some criteria B–E symptoms.
‡Significant difference between the ORs for threshold and sub-threshold DSM-5 PTSD.
[a]Based on logistic regression analysis controlling for country income group, marital status and education at the time of the random trauma, and traumas occurring prior to the random trauma, with the reference group equaling respondents with a random trauma who did not have any criterion B–E symptoms lasting at least 1 month.
[b]Subthreshold cases include all respondents meeting criteria for at least two of four criteria B–E.
[c]Others with symptoms includes all respondents with one or more criterion B–E symptoms lasting at least 1 month but not meeting criteria for threshold or subthreshold DSM-5 PTSD.
[d]Prior mental disorder variables represent counts of fear, distress, substance use, and behavior disorders with onsets prior to the occurrence of the random trauma.

subthreshold PTSD and provided the first comprehensive comparison of diverse subthreshold PTSD definitions. Before commenting on those results, though, we should mention that the associations between DSM-5 criteria B–E symptom counts and the outcomes considered here generally support the DSM-5 thresholds of one symptom each for criterion B (re-experiencing), criterion C (avoidance), and two symptoms each for criterion D (negative alterations in cognition and mood), and criterion E (hyper-arousal). A question could be raised, though, whether our use of a conservative approximation of DSM-5 criteria biased the data. We do not believe this was the case as our independent comparison of diagnoses based on our approximations with diagnoses based on full DSM-5 criteria suggested that any such bias was minimal (i.e., more than 90% of DSM-5 cases captured by our approximation) (Rosellini et al., 2015). Since the symptoms added in DMS-5 are much less common than those already in DSM-IV, the number of individuals with the new symptoms in the absence of the DSM-IV symptoms is small. Thus, the criterion-level thresholds considered here should be good approximations of DSM-5 thresholds, bolstering the validity of our empirical support for the DSM-5 thresholds.

As expected, we found threshold DSM-5 PTSD to be associated with distress impairment, and comorbidity at levels generally higher than subthreshold PTSD.

This result is broadly consistent with previous studies (Stein et al., 1997; Lipschitz et al., 2000; Schnurr et al., 2000; Breslau et al., 2004; Maia et al., 2007). However, the main focus of the analysis was on alternative subthreshold symptom profiles. We found that the subthreshold profiles requiring two or three criteria B–E are associated with more adverse outcomes than those associated with one-of-four criteria B–E, leading us to recommend that future epidemiological studies define subthreshold DSM-5 PTSD as meeting two or three criteria B–E.

It is noteworthy that our proposed definition focuses only on number of DSM-5 PTSD criteria, while previous studies made distinctions regarding specific symptoms, most notably regarding the particular importance of avoidance (Schutzwohl & Maercker, 1999), re-experiencing (Schnurr et al., 1993), and hyper-arousal (Schnurr et al., 2004). We found no evidence for the special importance of these or other specific symptoms. It is also noteworthy that wide variation was found in prevalence estimates of subthreshold PTSD across the range of definitions proposed in the literature, demonstrating that it is important to have a consensus definition to avoid wide variation in estimates of prevalence and correlates. The use of such a consistent definition could also promote the accumulation of data allowing valid comparisons of prevalence, predictors, and markers of clinical significance. Such evidence might subsequently lead to changes in the diagnostic threshold for PTSD or to the introduction of new traumatic stress disorders that are less severe than PTSD, yet still clinically significant (Strain & Friedman, 2011).

When using our preferred definition of subthreshold PTSD, the proportion of trauma-exposed individuals classified as having subthreshold DSM-5 PTSD (3.6%, see Table 19.2) was roughly comparable to the proportion classified as having threshold PTSD (3.0%). Although this finding is generally consistent with other studies (Marshall et al., 2001; Breslau et al., 2004; Lai et al., 2004), our additional finding of significant differences in relative prevalence of threshold versus subthreshold PTSD across trauma types showed that this comparability will vary, depending on the types of trauma under study.

The aforementioned results need to be interpreted in the context of three limitations in the WMH assessment of PTSD, all of which would be expected to introduce a conservative bias into the designation of respondents as having threshold DSM-5 PTSD. First, the assessment was based on a conservative approximation of DSM-5 criteria. Second, we used a fully structured lay interview rather than a semi-structured clinical interview. Third, focal traumas were selected randomly from all the traumas respondents ever experienced rather than from the traumas designated by respondents as their worst.

As noted earlier, we determined that the conservative bias associated with using DSM-IV symptom measures to approximate DSM-5 criteria reduced the prevalence estimate of DSM-5 PTSD by less than 10% (i.e., true DSM-5 prevalence might have been 3.3% compared to the 3.0% estimated with our approximation). The conservative bias associated with using the fully-structured CIDI was noted in Chapter 2, where we reported that the vast majority of CIDI PTSD cases were confirmed in blinded SCID clinical reappraisal interviews, while the SCID also found additional cases that were missed by the CIDI. The conservative bias associated with the focus on randomly selected traumas, in comparison, is related to the fact that roughly 15% of respondents reported that their randomly selected trauma was part of a linked trauma cluster. If the random trauma was not the central trauma in the cluster (e.g., the random trauma was a motor vehicle collision, whereas the linked trauma that caused the PTSD was the death of a loved one in that accident) and if the respondent answered the symptom questions with a narrow focus on the random trauma rather than on the entire cluster (e.g., nightmares about the crash rather than about the death), the presence of symptoms associated with the linked trauma might not have been reported, leading to a conservative bias in estimating threshold PTSD.

These conservative biases almost certainly led to an underestimation of the prevalence of threshold DSM-5 PTSD. It was less clear, though, whether they increased or decreased the estimated prevalence of subthreshold PTSD or the ORs reported here as the incorrect classification of true threshold cases as subthreshold would increase estimated subthreshold prevalence and severity, while the incorrect classification of true subthreshold cases as asymptomatic would reduce estimated subthreshold prevalence and severity. More fine-grained assessments than those in the WMH surveys would be needed to determine the relative importance of these competing types of bias and whether there is a more valid definition of subthreshold PTSD than the one proposed here. Until such data are available, we suggest that our proposed definition be used as a way to systematize comparisons across existing datasets and to provide a starting point for the evaluation of more refined definitions in new studies collecting more nuanced data.

Acknowledgment

Portions of this chapter are based on McLaughlin, K. A., Koenen, K. C., Friedman, M. J., et al. (2015). Sub-threshold post-traumatic stress disorder in the World Health Organization World Mental Health Surveys. *Biological Psychiatry*, 77, 375–84, by permission of Elsevier.

References

American Psychiatric Association. (2013). *Diagnostic and Statistical Manual of Mental Disorders, Fifth Edition.DSM-5*. Arlington, VA: American Psychiatric Association.

Blanchard, E. B., Hickling, E. J., Taylor, A. E., Loos, W. R., & Gerardi, R. J. (1994). Psychological morbidity associated with motor vehicle accidents. *Behaviour Research and Therapy*, 32, 283–90.

Blanchard, E. B., Hickling, E. J., Vollmer, A. J., et al. (1995). Short-term follow-up of post-traumatic stress symptoms in motor vehicle accident victims. *Behaviour Research and Therapy*, 33, 369–77.

Breslau, N., Lucia, V. C., & Davis, G. C. (2004). Partial PTSD versus full PTSD: an empirical examination of associated impairment. *Psychological Medicine*, 34, 1205–14.

Carlier, I. V., & Gersons, B. P. (1995). Partial posttraumatic stress disorder (PTSD): the issue of psychological scars and the occurrence of PTSD symptoms. *Journal of Nervous and Mental Disease*, 183, 107–9.

Cukor, J., Wyka, K., Jayasinghe, N., & Difede, J. (2010). The nature and course of subthreshold PTSD. *Journal of Anxiety Disorders*, 24, 918–23.

Favaro, A., Tenconi, E., Colombo, G., & Santonastaso, P. (2006). Full and partial post-traumatic stress disorder among World War II prisoners of war. *Psychopathology*, 39, 187–91.

Gellis, L. A., Mavandadi, S., & Oslin, D. W. (2010). Functional quality of life in full versus partial posttraumatic stress disorder among veterans returning from Iraq and Afghanistan. *Primary Care Companion to the Journal of Clinical Psychiatry*, 12, e1–6.

Jakupcak, M., Conybeare, D., Phelps, L., et al. (2007). Anger, hostility, and aggression among Iraq and Afghanistan war veterans reporting PTSD and subthreshold PTSD. *Journal of Traumatic Stress*, 20, 945–54.

Jeon, H. J., Suh, T., Lee, H. J., et al. (2007). Partial versus full PTSD in the Korean community: prevalence, duration, correlates, comorbidity, and dysfunctions. *Depression and Anxiety*, 24, 577–85.

Jones, E., & Wessely, S. (2007). A paradigm shift in the conceptualization of psychological trauma in the 20th century. *Journal of Anxiety Disorders*, 21, 164–75.

Kulka, R. A., Schlenger, W. E., Fairbank, J. A., et al. (1990). *Trauma and the Vietnam War Generation: Report of Findings from the National Vietnam Veterans Readjustment Study*. New York, NY: Bruner/Mazel.

Lai, T. J., Chang, C. M., Connor, K. M., Lee, L. C., & Davidson, J. R. (2004). Full and partial PTSD among earthquake survivors in rural Taiwan. *Journal of Psychiatric Research*, 38, 313–22.

Lipschitz, D. S., Rasmusson, A. M., Anyan, W., Cromwell, P., & Southwick, S. M. (2000). Clinical and functional correlates of posttraumatic stress disorder in urban adolescent girls at a primary care clinic. *Journal of the American Academy of Child & Adolescent Psychiatry*, 39, 1104–11.

Maia, D. B., Marmar, C. R., Metzler, T., et al. (2007). Post-traumatic stress symptoms in an elite unit of Brazilian police officers: prevalence and impact on psychosocial functioning and on physical and mental health. *Journal of Affective Disorders*, 97, 241–5.

Marshall, R. D., Olfson, M., Hellman, F., et al. (2001). Comorbidity, impairment, and suicidality in subthreshold PTSD. *American Journal of Psychiatry*, 158, 1467–73.

McLeer, S. V., Deblinger, E., Henry, D., & Orvaschel, H. (1992). Sexually abused children at high risk for post-traumatic stress disorder. *Journal of the American Academy of Child & Adolescent Psychiatry*, 31, 875–79.

McNally, R. J. (2003). Progress and controversy in the study of posttraumatic stress disorder. *Annual Review of Psychology*, 54, 229–52.

Mylle, J., & Maes, M. (2004). Partial posttraumatic stress disorder revisited. *Journal of Affective Disorders*, 78, 37–48.

Naylor, J. C., Dolber, T. R., Strauss, J. L., et al. (2013). A pilot randomized controlled trial with paroxetine for subthreshold PTSD in Operation Enduring Freedom/ Operation Iraqi Freedom era veterans. *Psychiatry Research*, 206, 318–20.

Patterson, D. R., Carrigan, L., Questad, K. A., & Robinson, R. (1990). Post-traumatic stress disorder in hospitalized patients with burn injuries. *Journal of Burn Care and Research*, 11, 181–4.

Pietrzak, R. H., Schechter, C. B., Bromet, E. J., et al. (2012). The burden of full and subsyndromal posttraumatic stress disorder among police involved in the World Trade Center rescue and recovery effort. *Journal of Psychiatric Research*, 46, 835–42.

Rosellini, A. J., Stein, M. B., Colpe, L. J., et al. (2015). Approximating a DSM-5 diagnosis of PTSD using DSM-IV criteria. *Depression and Anxiety*, 32, 493–501.

SAS Institute Inc. (2008). *SAS Software Version 9.2*. Cary, NC: SAS Institute Inc.

Schnurr, P. P., Ford, J. D., Friedman, M. J., et al. (2000). Predictors and outcomes of posttraumatic stress disorder in World War II veterans exposed to mustard gas. *Journal of Consulting and Clinical Psychology*, 68, 258–68.

Schnurr, P. P., Friedman, M. J., & Rosenberg, S. D. (1993). Premilitary MMPI scores as predictors of combat-related PTSD symptoms. *American Journal of Psychiatry*, 150, 479–83.

Schnurr, P. P., Lunney, C. A., & Sengupta, A. (2004). Risk factors for the development versus maintenance of posttraumatic stress disorder. *Journal of Traumatic Stress*, 17, 85–95.

Schutzwohl, M., & Maercker, A. (1999). Effects of varying diagnostic criteria for posttraumatic stress disorder are endorsing the concept of partial PTSD. *Journal of Traumatic Stress*, 12, 155–65.

Stein, M. B., Hofler, M., Perkonigg, A., et al. (2002). Patterns of incidence and psychiatric risk factors for traumatic events. *International Journal of Methods in Psychiatric Research*, 11, 143–53.

Stein, M. B., Walker, J. R., Hazen, A. L., & Forde, D. R. (1997). Full and partial posttraumatic stress disorder: findings from a community survey. *American Journal of Psychiatry*, 154, 1114–9.

Strain, J. J., & Friedman, M. J. (2011). Considering adjustment disorders as stress response syndromes for DSM-5. *Depression and Anxiety*, 28, 818–23.

Weiss, D. S., Marmar, C. R., Schlenger, W. E., et al. (1992). The prevalence of lifetime and partial post-traumatic stress disorder in Vietnam theatre veterans. *Journal of Traumatic Stress*, 5, 365–76.

Wolter, K. M. (1985). *Introduction to Variance Estimation.* New York, NY: Springer-Verlag.

Zlotnick, C., Franklin, L., & Zimmerman, M. (2002). Does "subthreshold" posttraumatic stress disorder have any clinical relevance? *Comprehensive Psychiatry*, 43, 413–19.

Appendix

Table 19.A1 The effects of controlling for contemporaneous comorbidity on associations of DSM-5/CIDI PTSD and subthreshold PTSD on clinically significant distress or impairment[a]

		Controls for contemporaneous comorbidity				
		Yes		No		
	%	OR	(95% CI)	OR	(95% CI)	(*n*)
I PTSD	98.0	4,846.7*	(1,952.7–12,030.0)	4,686.6*	(1,867.4–11,762.4)	(850)
II Three of Criteria B–E						
AV, RE, NM	99.0	9,650.1*	(2,583.0–36,052.4)	10,201.0*	(2,686.5–38,735.5)	(99)
AV, RE, HA	92.3	1,380.7*	(676.1–2,819.6)	1,332.9*	(664.2–2,674.7)	(351)
AV, NM, HA	98.3	5,405.3*	(1,325.0–22,051.6)	5,569.4*	(1,345.6–23,050.9)	(74)
RE, NM, HA	90.4	1,033.2*	(141.2–7,558.2)	897.0*	(126.9–6,339.7)	(132)
III Two of Criteria B–E						
AV, RE	86.7	588.6*	(220.1–1,573.8)	628.0*	(231.5–1,703.5)	(129)
AV, NM	88.7	671.3*	(216.6–2,080.7)	648.0*	(211.5–1,985.6)	(86)
AV, HA	93.8	1,690.6*	(477.9–5,980.2)	1,767.8*	(495.3–6,310.0)	(72)
RE, NM	98.7	7,418.7*	(704.0–78,172.9)	4,321.2*	(478.4–39,030.4)	(27)
RE, HA	95.3	1,695.8*	(369.6–7,780.2)	1,756.9*	(374.6–8,239.1)	(169)
NM, HA	95.0	2,258.6*	(489.0–10,431.9)	2,008.8*	(400.2–10,083.0)	(40)
IV One of Criteria B–E						
AV	76.7	322.0*	(114.9–902.0)	331.4*	(118.7–925.1)	(144)
RE	63.2	115.4*	(21.8–609.5)	120.9*	(23.3–626.4)	(125)
NM	63.6	126.5*	(24.1–663.4)	131.2*	(25.7–668.8)	(20)
HA	84.2	428.8*	(163.6–1,123.6)	420.4*	(159.2–1,109.8)	(117)
V None of Criteria B–E	1.2	1.0	–	1.0	–	(21,501)

*Significant at the 0.05 level, two-sided test.

[a]The requirement of having clinically significant distress or impairment was not operationalized in defining either threshold or subthreshold PTSD for purposes of carrying out this analysis as this would lead to the requirement that 100% of respondents with threshold and subthreshold PTSD were classified yes on the dichotomous outcome considered here.

Table 19.A2 The effects of controlling for contemporaneous comorbidity on associations of DSM-5/CIDI PTSD and subthreshold PTSD on severe distress or impairment[a]

		Controls for contemporaneous comorbidity				
		Yes		No		
	%	OR	(95% CI)	OR	(95% CI)	(*n*)
I PTSD	87.6	1,743.1*	(1,096.2–2,771.8)	1,693.7*	(1,063.5–2,697.2)	(835)
II Three of Criteria B–E						
AV, RE, NM	65.8	284.9*	(103.0–787.8)	300.7*	(106.4–850.4)	(95)
AV, RE, HA	62.3	359.4*	(205.8–627.6)	356.0*	(206.15–614.8)	(325)
AV, NM, HA	80.5	1,114.6*	(416.5–2,983.1)	1,113.6*	(407.9–3,040.6)	(70)
RE, NM, HA	92.6	2,884.2*	(1,131.3–7,353.0)	2,594.3*	(1,009.5–6,667.3)	(131)
III Two of Criteria B–E						
AV, RE	69.0	0.0*	(0.0–0.0)	0.0*	(0.0–0.0)	(105)
AV, NM	68.1	0.0*	(0.0–0.0)	0.0*	(0.0–0.0)	(74)
AV, HA	48.3	268.1*	(105.1–683.7)	275.5*	(109.0–696.2)	(63)
RE, NM	89.0	1,723.7*	(192.3–15,451.9)	1,518.7*	(167.1–13,806.1)	(26)
RE, HA	73.9	354.9*	(177.0–711.9)	359.0*	(177.3–727.1)	(160)
NM, HA	65.9	0.0	(0.0–1.8)	0.0	(0.0–1.8)	(36)
IV One of Criteria B–E						
AV	33.9	60.9*	(24.3–152.6)	61.6*	(24.1–157.7)	(109)
RE	46.0	173.3*	(46.2–649.7)	180.2*	(48.7–667.4)	(103)
NM	82.4	1,147.6*	(222.9–5,907.6)	1,204.3*	(228.4–6,349.5)	(17)
HA	55.2	196.9*	(81.2–477.2)	182.5*	(77.6–428.8)	(99)
V None of Criteria B–E	0.6	1.0	–	1.0	–	(21,688)

*Significant at the 0.05 level, two-sided test.
[a]The distribution of threshold and subthreshold cases differs here compared to Appendix Table 19A.1 due to the fact that these diagnoses were made requiring clinically significant distress or impairment here but not in Appendix Table 19A.1. See footnote a of Appendix Table 19A.1.

Table 19.A3 The effects of controlling for contemporaneous comorbidity on associations of DSM-5/CIDI PTSD and subthreshold PTSD on first lifetime onset of suicide ideation[a]

		Controls for contemporaneous comorbidity				
		Yes		No		
	%	OR	(95% CI)	OR	(95% CI)	(*n*)
I PTSD	8.2	5.4*	(3.0–9.8)	2.6*	(1.4–4.8)	(724)
II Three of Criteria B–E						
AV, RE, NM	7.8	5.5*	(1.4–21.0)	5.7*	(1.6–20.9)	(84)
AV, RE, HA	1.2	0.7	(0.2–2.0)	0.5	(0.2–1.5)	(280)
AV, NM, HA	0.8	0.4	(0.1–2.2)	0.4	(0.1–2.0)	(60)
RE, NM, HA	11.3	8.6*	(2.4–30.4)	3.3	(0.5–21.3)	(113)
III Two of Criteria B–E						
AV, RE	0.2	0.2	(0.0–1.2)	0.2	(0.0–1.3)	(99)
AV, NM	2.2	1.1	(0.2–6.6)	0.9	(0.2–4.6)	(64)
AV, HA	1.5	1.3	(0.2–6.8)	1.0	(0.2–7.0)	(56)
RE, NM	2.9	2.1	(0.2–18.3)	0.4	(0.0–4.6)	(23)
RE, HA	0.9	0.7	(0.1–4.1)	0.6	(0.1–3.0)	(146)
NM, HA	10.0	8.4*	(2.1–34.2)	3.4	(0.6–19.9)	(32)
IV One of Criteria B–E						
AV	0.8	1.0	(0.1–7.2)	0.8	(0.1–6.4)	(106)
RE	1.2	0.6	(0.1–3.4)	0.7	(0.2–2.9)	(98)
NM	0.0	0.0*	(0.0–0.0)	0.0*	(0.0–0.0)	(15)
HA	4.5	2.7	(0.5–14.1)	1.9	(0.5–7.0)	(90)
V None of Criteria B–E	1.2	1.0	–	1.0	–	(20,040)

*Significant at the 0.05 level, two-sided test.
[a]Among respondents without a lifetime history of suicide ideation prior to age of occurrence of the trauma.

Table 19.A4 Associations between multivariate profiles of proposed DSM-5/CIDI PTSD symptom criteria B–E with a range of outcomes in the WMH sample of randomly selected traumas[a]

	Distress impairment						Suicidal ideation[b]			Comorbidity						Symptom duration[c]		
	Clinically significant[d]			Severe[e]						Fear[f]			Distress[f]					
	%	OR	(95% CI)	%	OR	(95% CI)	%	OR	(95% CI)	%	OR	(95% CI)	%	OR	(95% CI)	Mean duration	OR	(95% CI)
I PTSD																		
AV, IR, CM, AR	98.0[g]	4.2*[g]	(1.6–11.0)	87.6	3.9*	(2.4–6.3)	8.2	6.4*	(3.6–11.5)	2.0	7.6*	(4.3–13.7)	5.5	2.5*	(1.8–3.7)	117.0	1.4*	(1.1–1.7)
II Three of Criteria B–E																		
AV, IR, CM	99.0	9.6*	(2.7–34.2)	65.8	0.7	(0.3–1.6)	7.8	6.5*	(1.9–22.9)	0.4	1.1	(0.3–4.9)	1.5	0.5	(0.2–1.6)	87.3	1.1	(0.7–1.6)
AV, IR, AR	92.3	1.1	(0.5–2.4)	62.3	0.8	(0.5–1.4)	1.2	0.8	(0.3–2.5)	0.7	2.9*	(1.1–7.8)	2.9	1.2	(0.6–2.6)	82.8	1.1	(0.8–1.6)
AV, CM, AR	98.3	4.3*	(1.1–17.5)	80.5	2.3	(1.0–5.6)	0.8	0.5	(0.1–2.7)	0.1	0.5	(0.1–3.5)	2.9	1.1	(0.4–3.1)	110.6	1.7	(0.7–3.6)
IR, CM, AR	90.4	0.9	(0.2–5.9)	92.6	6.5*	(2.8–15.4)	11.3	10.3*	(3.1–34.3)	2.3	13.0*	(4.3–39.0)	7.6	3.4*	(2.0–5.6)	58.6	1.1	(0.7–1.6)
III Two of Criteria B–E																		
AV, IR	86.7	0.6	(0.2–1.7)	69.0	0.7	(0.3–1.8)	0.2	0.2	(0.0–1.3)	0.4	2.3	(0.5–11.5)	0.7	0.3*	(0.1–0.8)	61.3	1.4	(0.9–2.3)
AV, CM	88.7	0.6	(0.2–1.8)	68.1	0.9	(0.4–2.2)	2.2	1.3	(0.2–7.2)	1.4	6.6*	(2.0–21.0)	2.6	1.1	(0.4–2.7)	78.6	1.4	(0.8–2.6)
AV, AR	93.8	1.1	(0.4–3.2)	48.3	0.6	(0.3–1.4)	1.5	1.5	(0.3–7.5)	0.2	0.8	(0.1–6.1)	1.1	0.6	(0.2–1.5)	68.9	0.9	(0.5–1.8)
IR, CM	98.7	6.9	(0.8–62.9)	89.0	3.9	(0.6–26.7)	2.9	2.5	(0.3–19.4)	4.4	28.5*	(12.5–65.1)	13.0	7.2*	(2.7–19.4)	105.4	2.0	(0.9–5.3)
IR, AR	95.3	3.2	(0.5–22.3)	73.9	1.0	(0.6–1.9)	0.9	0.8	(0.1–4.4)	0.4	3.7*	(1.0–13.8)	1.4	0.7	(0.3–1.6)	30.0	0.6*	(0.4–0.8)
CM, AR	95.0	1.8	(0.4–8.1)	65.9	0.8	(0.2–3.2)	10.0	10.0*	(2.6–38.0)	0.0	0.0*	(0.0–0.0)	7.5	3.1*	(1.1–8.9)	24.8	0.5*	(0.3–0.9)
IV One of Criteria B–E																		
AV	76.7	0.3*	(0.1–0.9)	33.9	0.1*	(0.1–0.4)	0.8	1.1	(0.2–7.6)	0.8	7.1*	(1.3–38.4)	1.2	0.6	(0.2–2.6)	25.4	0.5*	(0.3–0.8)
IR	63.2	0.2*	(0.1–0.5)	46.0	0.5	(0.2–1.3)	1.2	0.8	(0.2–3.7)	0.5	2.2	(0.6–7.6)	0.5	0.2*	(0.1–0.7)	55.9	0.5*	(0.3–0.9)
CM	63.6	0.1*	(0.0–0.6)	82.4	3.5	(0.7–16.9)	0.0	0.0*	(0.0–0.0)	0.0	0.0*	(0.0–0.0)	2.5	1.0	(0.2–4.4)	83.7	1.3	(0.5–3.7)
AR	84.2	0.3*	(0.1–0.8)	55.2	0.5	(0.2–1.1)	4.5	3.2	(0.7–15.5)	0.5	3.1	(0.9–10.5)	3.6	1.6	(0.6–4.4)	82.2	1.0	(0.6–1.8)

(cont.)

Table 19.A4 *(cont.)*

	Distress impairment						Suicidal ideation[b]			Comorbidity						Symptom duration[c]		
	Clinically significant[d]			Severe[e]						Fear[f]			Distress[f]					
	%	OR	(95% CI)	%	OR	(95% CI)	%	OR	(95% CI)	%	OR	(95% CI)	%	OR	(95% CI)	Mean duration	OR	(95% CI)
V Total	90.7	1.0	–	72.8	1.0	–	1.4	1.0	–	0.4	1.0	–	0.8	1.0	–	84.4	1.0	–
(*n*)		(2,499)[d]			(2,297)[e]			(22,030)[b]			(23,936)[f]			(23,908)[f]			(2,297)[c]	

*Significant at the 0.05 level, two-sided test.

[a]See the section on Analysis Methods in the text for a description of the regression models.

[b]The sample is limited to cases where the respondent did not have a lifetime history of suicidal ideation prior to age of occurrence of the trauma as first lifetime onset of suicidal ideation is the outcome. Presence of clinically significant distress or impairment associated with the trauma was not required in defining this sample, but criteria B–E symptoms were classified as present in defining the predictors only if the respondent reported clinically significant distress or impairment associated with these symptoms.

[c]The sample is limited to cases where the respondent reported one or more symptoms of at least one criterion B–E lasting more than 1 month and reported clinically significant distress or impairment associated with this/these symptom(s) as these are the cases for which symptom duration was assessed. The predictors of symptom duration are estimated in a discrete-time survival framework with person-month the unit of analysis. Duration was censored at 60 months if symptoms persisted longer than 60 months in order to reduce the effects of extreme outliers. A total of 71,304 person-months was included in the analysis.

[d]The sample is limited to cases where the respondent reported one or more symptoms of at least one criterion B–E lasting more than 1 month as clinically significant distress and impairment were assessed only when at least one such symptom was reported.

[e]The sample is limited to cases where the respondent reported one or more symptoms of at least one criterion B–E lasting more than 1 month and reported clinically significant distress or impairment associated with this/these symptom(s) as severe distress and impairment were assessed only in this subsample. Note that the outcome of severe distress impairment is conditionally independent of the outcome of serious distress impairment because all respondents in the sample used to predict severe distress impairment reported significant distress impairment.

[f]The ORs reported here are pooled across disorder-specific equations for each of the fear and distress disorders assessed in the surveys. The percent estimates are averages across those pooled equations. Presence of clinically significant distress or impairment associated with the trauma was not required in defining these samples, but criteria B–E symptoms were classified as present in defining the predictors only if the respondent reported clinically significant distress or impairment associated with these symptoms. The 23,936 respondents included in the pooled person-disorder data array for the five fear disorders resulted in 112,460 observations, and the 23,908 respondents included in the pooled person-disorder data array for mood disorders resulted in 79,836 observations.

[g]The requirement of clinically significant distress or impairment was not operationalized in defining threshold cases for this outcome as this would have led to 100% of cases having the outcome and making it impossible to include them in the regression equation.

Chapter 20

Dissociative versus Nondissociative Posttraumatic Stress Disorder

Dan J. Stein, Brendan Bunting, José Miguel Caldas de Almeida, Ayelet Meron Ruscio, David Spiegel, and Ronald C. Kessler

Clinicians have long documented a number of dissociative phenomena in trauma survivors, such as affect compartmentalization, disrupted memory encoding, time distortion, and fugue (Janet, 1907; Strachey, 1955). Two dissociative symptoms, flashbacks and psychogenic amnesia, were included in the DSM-IV diagnostic criteria for posttraumatic stress disorder (PTSD) (American Psychiatric Association, 2000). Furthermore, in DSM-5, a dissociative subtype of PTSD was operationalized (American Psychiatric Association, 2013). This subtype was based on a growing number of rigorous empirical studies of dissociative symptoms in PTSD, including the hallmark symptoms of derealization and depersonalization (Laniuset al., 2010a; Hansen et al., 2017). It was hoped that better recognition of dissociative symptoms could improve the diagnosis and treatment of PTSD (Putnam et al., 1996; Waelde et al., 2005; Lanius et al., 2010b; Wolf et al., 2012a).

Initial support for the dissociative subtype of PTSD included evidence that trauma and stress are linked to dissociation (Lanius et al., 2010b), that distinctive psychobiological mechanisms underlie dissociation (Ginzburg et al., 2006), that dissociation predicts poor treatment outcome (Spiegel et al., 2011; Lanius et al., 2012), and that dissociation has implications for PTSD treatment selection (Resick et al., 2012). However, these studies were based primarily on treatment-seeking samples in developed countries (Putnam et al., 1996; Waelde et al., 2005; Ginzburg et al., 2006; Zucker et al., 2006; Cloitre et al., 2012; Nugent et al., 2012; Steuwe et al., 2012; Wolf et al., 2012a, 2012b). As treatment seekers exhibit greater comorbidity and impairment than nontreatment seekers, clinical samples do not represent the full spectrum of PTSD in the population. Indeed, dissociation may prove especially sensitive to treatment selection bias, given that symptoms such as reduced awareness, fragmented memory, and affect compartmentalization could influence help-seeking. However, no large-scale population-based studies of dissociation in PTSD were available when the inclusion of this subtype in DSM-5 was being debated, leaving it unclear whether associations documented in clinical studies, such as those between the dissociative subtype and childhood adversities (CAs) or repeated exposure to traumas (Ginzburg et al., 2006; Cloitre et al., 2009; Dalenberg et al., 2012), generalize to the population. There was also a concern that dissociation might be highly sensitive to cultural bias, making it important to consider the possibility of cross-cultural variability in symptom expression and meaning (Brown & Lewis-Fernandez, 2011; Hinton & Lewis-Fernandez, 2011).

Based on these considerations, we carried out an analysis of the World Mental Health (WMH) survey data to examine the generalizability of previously reported results regarding the prevalence and correlates of PTSD with versus without dissociation. We focused on both predictors (characteristics of the trauma implicated in the PTSD, socio-demographics, CAs, prior traumas, and temporally primary comorbid disorders) and outcomes (PTSD symptom counts, role impairments, suicidality, and treatment) that we had reason to believe, based on previous studies (Ginzburg et al., 2006; Zucker et al., 2006; Cloitre et al., 2009; Lanius et al., 2010b; Nugent et al., 2012; Steuwe et al., 2012; Wolf et al., 2012a, 2012b), might distinguish between PTSD with and PTSD without dissociation.

Methods

At the time the analysis was carried out, 16 WMH surveys had been completed that featured an expanded assessment of dissociation in Part II of their samples. These included surveys in nine high-income countries (Belgium, France, Germany, Italy, Japan, Northern Ireland, Portugal, Spain, and the United States) and seven low- and middle-income countries (LMICs): São Paulo in Brazil, Bulgaria, Colombia, Lebanon, Mexico, Romania, and Beijing/Shanghai in the People's Republic of China (PRC). The assessment of dissociative symptoms was administered as an exploratory question series as part of a larger battery on nonspecific psychological distress in the 30 days before interview. The number of Part II respondents in this subsample ranged from 189 across five Western European countries (Belgium, France, Germany, Italy, and Spain) to 5,692 in the United States and totaled 25,018 across all countries.

DSM-5 defines the dissociative subtype as the subset of PTSD cases experiencing persistent or recurrent depersonalization or derealization. The 30-day nonspecific psychological distress series in the WMH surveys included two questions on depersonalization (*the experience of feeling as though they are standing next to themselves or watching themselves do something and they actually see themselves as if they were looking at another person*; and *the experience of feeling that their body does not seem to belong to them*) and one on derealization (*the experience of feeling that other people, objects, and the world around them are not real*) from the Dissociative Experiences Scale (Bernstein & Putnam, 1986). We defined respondents with 12-month DSM-IV/CIDI PTSD as having an approximation of the dissociative subtype if they reported having one or more of these experiences either *often* or *sometimes* (on a four-category response scale that also included the categories *rarely* and *never*).

The analysis focused on respondents with 12-month PTSD and compared correlates of PTSD with dissociation versus PTSD without dissociation. The correlates included (to the onset of PTSD) trauma history, CAs, current impairments due to PTSD, recent treatment, and temporally primary comorbid mental disorders. Trauma history was assessed by calculating the number of lifetime traumas the respondent reported experiencing before exposure to the index trauma implicated in their current PTSD. CAs were assessed with 12 measures, some overlapping with the traumas implicated in the PTSD, that included three types of interpersonal loss (parent death, parent divorce, and other parent–caregiver loss), four types of parent maladjustment (mental illness, substance abuse, criminality, and family violence), four types of maltreatment (physical, sexual, and emotional abuse as well as neglect), and family economic adversity. The assessment of these CAs is discussed in Chapter 10.

Impairment due to PTSD was assessed with separate questions about suicidality and role functioning. Suicidality was assessed with the CIDI Suicidal Behavior module (Nock et al., 2009), which asked about 12-month occurrence of suicide ideation, plans, and attempts. Role functioning was assessed with a modified version of the Sheehan Disability Scale (SDS) (Leon et al., 1997), which asked respondents to rate how much their PTSD interfered with each of four role domains (home management, ability to work, social life, and close relationships) using a 0–10 response scale of *none* (0), *mild* (1–3), *moderate* (4–6), *severe* (7–9), and *very severe* (10) interference. A global SDS score was created by assigning each respondent the highest SDS domain score across the four domains.

Recent treatment was assessed with questions administered to all Part II WMH respondents about treatment in the past 12 months *for problems with your emotions, nerves, or your use of alcohol or drugs* in each of four sectors: specialty mental health (psychiatrist, psychologist, or other healthcare provider in a mental health specialty setting), general medical (nonpsychiatrist healthcare provider not in a mental health specialty setting), human services (religious–spiritual advisor, social worker, or counselor not in a mental health specialty setting), and complementary-alternative medical (any other healer, Internet support group, or self-help group). In addition, respondents with 12-month PTSD were asked if they saw any professional in the past 12 months specifically for their PTSD.

The comorbid mental disorders considered included five anxiety disorders (separation anxiety disorder, panic disorder and/or agoraphobia, generalized anxiety disorder, specific phobia, and social phobia), two mood disorders (major depressive disorder/dysthymia, and bipolar disorder), four disruptive behavior disorders (attention-deficit/hyperactivity disorder [ADHD], oppositional-defiant disorder [ODD], conduct disorder [CD], and intermittent explosive disorder [IED]), and two substance use disorders (alcohol and drug abuse with/without dependence). Age-of-onset (AOO) reports were used to define temporally primary comorbid disorders to predict dissociation in 12-month PTSD.

Logistic regression analysis (Hosmer & Lemeshow, 2000) was used to examine correlates of dissociation among respondents with 12-month PTSD. As in other chapters, the logistic regression coefficients and their standard errors were exponentiated and are reported here as odds ratios (ORs) with design-based 95% confidence intervals.

Results

Prevalence

Twelve-month prevalence (standard error) of DSM-IV/CIDI PTSD in the total sample was 1.9% (0.1), with 14.4% (1.3) of these cases estimated to have the

Table 20.1 Prevalence of dissociative symptoms among respondents with 12-month DSM-IV/CIDI PTSD as a function of trauma type implicated in the PTSD[a]

	Percentage with dissociative symptoms[b]		
	%	(SE)	(*n*)[c]
War-related	17.5	(4.6)	(30)
Sexual violence victimization	19.9	(3.4)	(144)
Physical violence victimization	13.9	(3.1)	(102)
Accidents/injuries	16.2	(4.9)	(80)
UD of a loved one	13.0	(3.3)	(201)
Network trauma	12.0	(3.5)	(98)
Other/private trauma[d]	8.9	(2.6)	(92)
Total	14.4	(1.3)	(747)

[a]War-related traumas include combat experience, purposefully injuring or torturing or killing someone, relief worker in a war zone, civilian in a war zone, civilian in a region of terror, refugee, and seeing atrocities. Sexual violence traumas include rape, sexual assault, and stalked. Physical violence traumas include beaten by a parent or other childhood caregiver, beaten by a spouse or other romantic partner, beaten up by anyone else, mugged or threatened with a weapon, and kidnapped. Accident traumas include natural disaster, toxic chemical exposure, other human-made disaster, life-threatening automobile accident, other life-threatening accident or injury, and life-threatening illness. Network traumas include life-threatening illness, any other traumas experienced by a loved one, witnessing physical violence at home as a child, discovering or seeing a dead body or witnessing someone die or become seriously injured, and accidentally causing someone to have a serious injury or die.

[b]The percentage of cases with DSM-IV/CIDI PTSD who had dissociative symptoms does not differ significantly across trauma types ($\chi^2_6 = 8.5, p = 0.20$).

[c]The sample sizes reported represent the denominators (i.e., all respondents with the trauma type in the row; not the proportion of this total that had dissociative symptoms).

[d]"Other" traumas include all those reported in response to an open-ended question about exposure to traumas not on the prespecified WMH list that would not clearly be classified back into one of the more specific categories on that list. "Private" traumas include those reported in response to the following question: "Sometimes people have experiences they don't want to talk about in interviews. I won't ask you to describe anything like this, but, without telling me what it was, did you ever have a trauma that you didn't report to me because you didn't want to talk about it?"

dissociative subtype (see Table 20.1). The latter proportion did not differ significantly across the seven broad types of trauma assessed in the surveys ($\chi^2_6 = 8.5, p = 0.20$). This compared to a 2.8% (0.1) prevalence of these dissociative symptoms in the remainder of the sample.

PTSD Symptom Dimensions

Among respondents with 12-month DSM-IV/CIDI PTSD, presence of dissociation was significantly and positively associated with number of re-experiencing symptoms (criteria B1–B5), but not with number of avoidance (criteria C1–C3), emotional numbing (criteria C4–C7), or hyper-arousal (criteria D1–D5) symptoms (see Table 20.2). More detailed analyses found that criterion B3 (flashbacks; OR = 2.3, 95% CI = 1.3–4.2) accounted for the association of re-experiencing with dissociation, that the only other individual symptom significantly associated with dissociation was criterion C3 (psychogenic amnesia; OR = 1.6, 95% CI = 1.0–2.6), and that no significant differences existed by country income level in the associations of symptom with dissociation ($\chi^2_4 = 0.4, p = 0.82$).

Socio-Demographics, Trauma History, and PTSD Onset Duration

Controlling for type of trauma implicated in the PTSD, odds of dissociation among respondents with 12-month PTSD were significantly elevated among men (OR = 1.7), respondents whose PTSD started in childhood (OR = 2.8–4.1), and respondents who experienced prior traumas (OR = 2.0–4.7) (see Table 20.3). By contrast, the number of years since onset of PTSD and country income level, in comparison, was not significantly associated with dissociation. These patterns were largely unchanged with additional controls for number of re-experiencing, avoidance, emotional numbing, and hyper-arousal symptoms. More detailed analyses found a significant interaction of country income level with AOO of PTSD in predicting dissociation ($\chi^2_3 = 3.4, p = 0.022$). This interaction indicated that the elevated OR of dissociation associated with early AOO was confined to ages 0–12 in high-income countries and extended to ages 0–19 in LMICs. None of the other predictors in Table 20.3 had a significant interaction with country income level.

Childhood Adversities

Almost all CAs considered in the WMH surveys were associated with elevated odds of dissociation among respondents with 12-month PTSD in bivariate models (OR = 1.3–2.2). Four of these associations were significant (parent mental illness, parent substance use disorder, family violence, and parental divorce)

Table 20.2 Mean differences and multivariate associations of standardized DSM-IV/CIDI PTSD symptom counts among respondents with 12-month DSM-IV/CIDI PTSD in the presence versus absence of dissociative symptoms ($n = 747$)

	Dissociative symptoms present		Dissociative symptoms absent			
	Mean[a]	(SE)	Mean[a]	(SE)	OR[b]	(95% CI)
RE	0.39*	(0.15)	−0.07	(0.05)	1.3*	(1.1–1.7)
AV	0.22	(0.15)	−0.04	(0.07)	1.1	(0.9–1.4)
Numbing	0.20	(0.11)	−0.03	(0.05)	1.1	(0.9–1.4)
HA	0.16	(0.20)	−0.03	(0.05)	1.0	(0.8–1.3)
Total	0.38	(0.20)	−0.07	(0.05)	1.4	(1.0–1.9)
(*n*)	(126)		(621)			

*Significant at the 0.05 level, two-sided test.
[a]Symptom scores were standardized to a mean of 0 and variance of 1.
[b]Based on a multivariate logistic regression model with the four symptom counts predicting the presence versus absence of dissociative symptoms among respondents with 12-month DSM-IV/CIDI PTSD.

Table 20.3 Associations of socio-demographic variables and trauma characteristics with the presence versus absence of dissociative symptoms among respondents with 12-month DSM-IV/CIDI PTSD ($n = 747$)[a]

	No controls		With controls	
	OR	(95% CI)	OR	(95% CI)
I Country Income level				
High-income	1.0	–	1.0	–
Low- and middle-income	1.1	(0.6–1.9)	1.1	(0.6–2.0)
II AOO of PTSD[b]				
0–6	4.1*	(1.4–11.4)	4.2*	(1.4–12.6)
7–12	2.8*	(1.2–6.6)	2.7*	(1.1–6.4)
13–19	1.4	(0.7–2.5)	1.3	(0.7–2.5)
20+	1.0	–	1.0	–
χ^2_3	3.1*		3.0*	
III Sex				
Female	1.0	–	1.0	–
Male	1.7*	(1.0–2.5)	1.7*	(1.0–2.8)
IV Number of Years Since Onset of PTSD[b]				
0–4	1.5	(0.6–3.6)	1.7	(0.7–3.9)
5–12	0.7	(0.4–1.5)	0.8	(0.4–1.7)
13–24	1.3	(0.6–2.5)	1.2	(0.6–2.4)
25+	1.0	–	1.0	–
χ^2_3	2.4		2.4	
V Number of Prior Traumas[c]				
0	1.0	–	1.0	–
1–4	2.0*	(1.1–3.9)	1.8	(0.9–3.5)
5+	4.7*	(2.2–10.1)	3.8*	(1.6–8.7)
χ^2_2	8.4*		5.3*	

*Significant at the 0.05 level, two-sided test.
[a]Based on a multivariate logistic regression model predicting the presence versus absence of dissociative symptoms among respondents with 12-month DSM-IV/CIDI PTSD controlling for trauma type without and then with additional controls for numbers of RE, AV, NM, and HA symptoms.
[b]The predictor was divided to create roughly equal sample sizes in each category.
[c]The predictor was divided to capture the functional form detected by examining the association with a completely disaggregated version of the variable.

(see Table 20.4). These associations all attenuated in a multivariate additive model. An alternative model in which number of CAs rather than types of CAs was used as predictors found a significant dose–response relationship between number of maladaptive family functioning CAs and dissociation. The ORs of individual CAs all became nonsignificant when controls were introduced for number of CAs. The ORs in the number-of-CAs model remained significant when additional controls were introduced for number of re-experiencing, avoidance, emotional numbing, and hyper-arousal symptoms. More detailed analyses found no significant differences by country income level in the associations of CAs with dissociation.

Prior Disorders

All but 2 of the 13 temporally prior (to the onset of PTSD) lifetime comorbid DSM-IV/CIDI disorders considered here were associated with elevated odds of dissociation among respondents with 12-month PTSD in bivariate models (OR = 1.4–3.3). Six of these associations were significant (bipolar disorder, separation anxiety disorder, panic/agoraphobia, generalized anxiety disorder, specific phobia, and oppositional-defiant disorder) (see Table 20.5). An alternative model in which the number rather than types of comorbid disorders was used as predictors found that high comorbidity (i.e., four or more comorbid disorders) was associated with especially elevated odds of dissociation (10.0). The number-of-disorders coefficients became nonsignificant while the coefficients associated with separation anxiety disorder and specific phobia remained significant (OR = 3.0–3.6) in a model that included both types and number of comorbid disorders as predictors. The ORs in the most parsimonious model (i.e., the

Table 20.4 Bivariate and multivariate associations of CAs with the presence versus absence of dissociative symptoms among respondents with 12-month DSM-IV/CIDI PTSD ($n = 747$)[a]

	Bivariate		Multivariate additive		Number of CAs		Multivariate nonadditive		Number of CAs with controls	
	OR	(95% CI)	OR	(95% CI)	OR	(95% CI)	OR	(95% CI)	OR	(95% CI)
I MFF CAs										
Parent psychopathology	2.1*	(1.1–8.6)	1.8*	(1.0–3.3)			1.7	(0.9–3.2)		
Parent substance misuse	2.1*	(1.0–4.2)	1.6	(0.8–3.1)			1.3	(0.6–3.0)		
Parent criminality	1.8	(0.9–3.5)	1.2	(0.6–2.4)			1.2	(0.6–2.6)		
Family violence	2.2*	(1.4–3.6)	1.8*	(1.0–3.0)			1.5	(0.8–2.8)		
Physical abuse	1.3	(0.7–2.5)	1.0	(0.5–1.9)			0.8	(0.4–1.8)		
Sexual abuse	1.4	(0.7–3.0)	1.3	(0.7–2.5)			1.2	(0.6–2.3)		
Neglect	1.5	(0.9–2.5)	0.7	(0.4–1.4)			0.7	(0.4–1.3)		
χ^{2b}_{7}			2.1*				1.0			
II Other CAs										
Parent death	0.8	(0.4–1.7)	0.8	(0.4–1.8)			0.9	(0.4–2.2)		
Parent divorce	1.9*	(1.0–3.4)	1.5	(0.8–2.9)			1.6	(0.8–3.5)		
Other parent loss	1.5	(0.8–3.0)	1.3	(0.6–2.7)			1.6	(0.7–3.4)		
Serious physical illness	1.7	(0.9–3.2)	1.7	(0.9–3.2)			2.0	(0.9–4.3)		
Economic adversity	1.7	(1.0–3.0)	1.2	(0.7–2.2)			1.4	(0.7–3.0)		
χ^{2b}_{5}			1.6				1.0			
III Number of MFF CAs										
1					1.5	(0.8–3.0)	1.0	–	1.5	(0.7–3.1)
2					2.6*	(1.2–5.3)	1.6	(0.6–4.0)	2.5*	(1.2–5.1)
3+					3.3*	(1.5–7.2)	1.5	(0.4–5.5)	3.1*	(1.4–6.8)
χ^{2}_{3}					3.2*		$\chi^2_2 = 0.5$		2.9*	
IV Number of Other CAs										
1					1.2	(0.7–2.0)	1.0	–	1.2	(0.7–2.0)
2					1.7	(0.9–3.4)	0.9	(0.4–2.1)	1.7	(0.9–3.3)
3+					1.6	(0.6–4.6)	0.5	(0.1–2.4)	1.5	(0.5–4.5)
χ^{2}_{3}					1.0		$\chi^2_2 = 0.4$		0.9	

*Significant at the 0.05 level, two-sided test.

[a]Based on a series of logistic regression models controlling for trauma type and the predictor variables in Table 20.3 predicting the presence versus absence of dissociative symptoms among respondents with 12-month DSM-IV/CIDI PTSD. The "number of CAs with controls" model additionally controls for numbers of RE, AV, NM, and HA symptoms.

[b]The joint significance of the set of ORs for CAs in the group.

model using only number of disorders as predictors) were largely unchanged when additional controls were introduced for number of re-experiencing, avoidance, emotional numbing, and hyper-arousal symptoms. More detailed analyses found no significant differences by country income level in these associations of disorders with dissociation.

Impairment, Suicidality, and Treatment

Significantly higher proportions of respondents with rather than without dissociation reported severe 12-month role impairments due to their PTSD (see Table 20.6). ORs in bivariate models across the four SDS scales (OR = 1.8–3.6) were consistently significant and remained elevated (OR = 1.8–3.6) in models that controlled for PTSD symptom counts. Dissociation was also associated with significantly elevated odds of 12-month suicidality (OR = 3.4–6.1). These ORs remained elevated (OR = 3.2–5.0) in models that controlled for PTSD symptom counts. More detailed analyses found no significant interactions between country income level and dissociation in predicting either impairments or suicidality ($\chi^2_1 = 0.1$–1.9, $p = 0.17$–0.79).

The rate of 12-month treatment for any emotional problem was not significantly higher among respondents with PTSD in the presence versus PTSD in the absence of dissociative symptoms and remained

Table 20.5 Bivariate and multivariate associations of temporally primary lifetime DSM-IV/CIDI disorders with the presence versus absence of dissociative symptoms among respondents with 12-month DSM-IV/CIDI PTSD ($n = 747$)[a]

	Bivariate		Multivariate additive		Number of disorders		Multivariate nonadditive		Number of disorders with controls	
	OR	(95% CI)	OR	(95% CI)	OR	(95% CI)	OR	(95% CI)	OR	(95% CI)
I Mood Disorders										
MDD or dysthymic disorder	1.5	(0.9–2.7)	1.0	(0.5–2.0)			1.1	(0.6–2.1)		
BPD (broad definition)	2.5*	(1.1–5.8)	1.1	(0.4–2.8)			1.0	(0.3–2.8)		
χ^{2b}_{2}			0.0							
II Anxiety Disorders										
Panic disorder or agoraphobia	2.3*	(1.2–4.7)	1.2	(0.5–2.5)			1.1	(0.5–2.6)		
GAD	2.5*	(1.2–5.1)	1.8	(0.8–3.9)			2.0	(0.8–4.6)		
Social phobia	1.4	(0.7–2.8)	0.8	(0.4–1.8)			0.9	(0.5–1.9)		
Specific phobia	3.3*	(2.1–5.3)	3.0*	(1.9–4.8)			3.6*	(1.8–7.1)		
Separation anxiety disorder	3.2*	(1.9–5.6)	2.7*	(1.5–4.7)			3.0*	(1.5–6.1)		
χ^{2b}_{5}			8.0*				3.7*			
III Disruptive Behavioral Disorders										
ADHD	1.7	(0.8–3.8)	1.4	(0.6–3.3)			1.4	(0.5–3.7)		
CD	2.2	(0.8–6.5)	1.5	(0.5–4.7)			1.6	(0.5–5.2)		
IED	1.8	(0.9–3.3)	1.7	(0.9–3.4)			1.9	(0.9–4.3)		
ODD	2.4*	(1.0–5.5)	1.4	(0.5–3.7)			1.5	(0.6–4.1)		
χ^{2b}_{4}			1.2				1.2			
IV Substance Use Disorders										
Alcohol abuse or dependence	0.8	(0.4–1.6)	0.6	(0.3–1.4)			0.7	(0.3–1.8)		
Drug abuse or dependence	1.0	(0.4–2.9)	0.8	(0.2–2.6)			0.7	(0.2–2.4)		
χ^{2b}_{2}			1.1				0.8			
V Number of Disorders										
1					3.6*	(1.4–9.2)	1.0	–	3.7*	(1.4–9.7)
2					2.6	(1.0–6.8)	0.5	(0.2–1.6)	2.6*	(1.0–6.7)
3					2.2	(0.7–7.4)	0.3	(0.1–1.2)	2.1	(0.6–7.2)
4+					10.0*	(3.8–26.3)	0.7	(0.1–3.5)	9.3*	(3.4–25.3)
χ^{2}_{4}					6.7*		$\chi^{2}_{3} = 1.4$		5.8*	

*Significant at the 0.05 level, two-sided test.
[a]Based on a series of multivariate logistic regression models controlling for the variables in Table 20.3 predicting the presence versus absence of dissociative symptoms among respondents with 12-month DSM-IV/CIDI PTSD. The "number of disorders with controls" model additionally controls for numbers of RE, AV, NM, and HA symptoms.
[b]The joint significance of the set of ORs for mental disorders in the group.

unchanged when we controlled for PTSD symptom counts. The rate of 12-month treatment specifically for PTSD was not meaningfully higher in the presence versus in the absence of dissociative symptoms, despite the higher rates of severe role impairment and suicidality associated with dissociation. More detailed analyses found no significant interactions between country income level and dissociation in predicting either type of treatment ($\chi^2_1 = 1.0$–2.0, $p = 0.16$–0.31).

Discussion

Several study limitations should be considered when interpreting these results. The number of WMH respondents with 12-month PTSD was too small to allow country-specific analyses. PTSD assessment was based on a fully structured lay-administered interview rather than on a semi-structured clinician-administered interview, introducing the possibility of misdiagnosis. Furthermore, dissociation items were chosen post

Table 20.6 Mean differences and multivariate associations of 12-month impairment and treatment among respondents with 12-month DSM-IV/CIDI PTSD in the presence versus absence of dissociative symptoms[a]

	Dissociative symptoms present		Dissociative symptoms absent		No controls		With controls	
	%	(SE)	%	(SE)	OR	(95% CI)	OR	(95% CI)
I Severe Impairment in Role Functioning								
Home	43.2*	(5.8)	29.3	(3.1)	1.8*	(1.0–3.3)	1.8	(1.0–3.1)
Work	45.0*	(5.8)	28.2	(3.1)	2.1*	(1.2–3.7)	2.0*	(1.1–3.5)
Close relationships	61.9*	(5.7)	30.9	(3.2)	3.6*	(2.2–6.0)	3.6*	(2.2–6.0)
Social life	61.5*	(7.4)	36.8	(3.5)	2.7*	(1.4–5.2)	2.8*	(1.4–5.4)
Any	79.4*	(4.9)	50.0	(3.3)	3.9*	(2.0–7.4)	3.8*	(2.0–7.4)
II Suicidality								
Ideation	29.2*	(5.1)	10.9	(1.7)	3.4*	(1.9–6.1)	3.2*	(1.8–5.7)
Plan	13.9*	(3.5)	3.1	(0.7)	5.0*	(2.3–10.9)	4.0*	(1.8–8.9)
Attempt	11.5*	(3.3)	2.1	(0.6)	6.1*	(2.6–14.3)	5.0*	(2.1–11.7)
III Treatment								
For any emotional problem	57.7	(6.1)	44.8	(2.8)	1.7	(1.0–2.9)	1.6	(0.9–2.8)
For PTSD	31.8	(5.0)	30.6	(3.3)	1.1	(0.6–1.8)	0.9	(0.5–1.6)
(*n*)[b]	(126)		(621)					

*Significant at the 0.05 level, two-sided test.

[a]Based on a series of logistic regression models in each of which one of the impairment, suicidality or treatment items predicted the presence versus absence of dissociative symptoms among respondents with 12-month DSM-IV/CIDI PTSD. The "with controls" model additionally controls for numbers of RE, AV, NM, and HA symptoms.

[b]The results for severe impairment and treatment of PTSD are based on the smaller subsample of 429 respondents (89 with and 340 without dissociative symptoms) who met full criteria for DSM-IV/CIDI PTSD for at least 1 month in the past year. The other 318 (747–429) respondents met full criteria for DSM-IV/CIDI PTSD prior to the past year but either had full symptoms for less than 1 month in the past year or had partial but not full symptoms for at least 1 month in the past year.

hoc rather than developed specifically to operationalize DSM-5 criteria, which were still only in draft form when the analysis was carried out. This limited assessment, the potential overlap of dissociation with a range of distinct symptoms (e.g., in mood, anxiety, and psychotic disorders) (van Ijzendoorn & Schuengel, 1996; Waller et al., 1996; Lochner et al., 2004), and the fact that dissociative symptoms were assessed in a separate part of the interview and for a different time frame (past 30 days) should all lead to caution in interpreting results. Likewise, our use of a simple yes–no dichotomy to differentiate cases of PTSD with dissociation from cases of PTSD without dissociation, while consistent with the DSM-5 formulation, also failed to consider either the more fine-grained differentiations among dissociative symptoms called for in some studies (van der Hart et al., 2004; Bryant, 2007) or the possibility that dissociation might be better characterized as being on a continuum rather than as constituting a distinct dichotomous subtype of PTSD (Watson, 2003). These refinements could not be investigated due to the small number of dissociative symptoms assessed.

Nevertheless, the results presented here provide the first cross-national population-level epidemiological data on the distribution and correlates of dissociative symptoms in PTSD. A number of key findings are noteworthy. The most fundamental finding is that 14.4% of PTSD cases in the community met criteria for the dissociative subtype. Since this proportion, which is within the range found in previous studies (Putnam et al., 1996; Waelde et al., 2005; Nugent et al., 2012; Wolf et al., 2012a, 2012b), did not differ significantly across the diverse set of countries considered here, our study demonstrates clearly that the dissociative subtype is not confined to developed countries. Furthermore, the fact that the prevalence of dissociative symptoms was five times higher among those with PTSD than the rest of the sample (14.4% vs. 2.8%) provides further evidence that trauma elicits dissociation (Dalenberg et al., 2012).

Only one of our findings was inconsistent with previously observed correlates of dissociation in PTSD: that the proportion of cases meeting criteria for a dissociative subtype was significantly higher among males than females. Previous clinical studies either found dissociation more common among women than men (Putnam et al., 1996; Steuwe et al., 2012; Wolf et al., 2012a) or found no difference between sexes (Wolf et al., 2012b). Yet the elevated OR of dissociation among males versus females was quite stable in the WMH data in both high-income countries and LMICs. Given this consistency, further investigation is warranted to evaluate possible methodological versus substantive explanations for the association, consider reasons for the opposite pattern observed in clinical settings, and determine the psychological or biological mechanisms involved.

An especially intriguing set of findings was that dissociation among respondents with PTSD was associated with childhood onset, exposure to prior traumas (especially to a high number [5+] of prior traumas), and CAs. When considered in conjunction with the finding that dissociation was not related to trauma type, this implies that early age of exposure and repeated exposure are more critical than the content of exposure in promoting dissociative symptoms among individuals with PTSD. Clinical research shows that dissociative symptoms in PTSD can be found across a wide range of trauma types (Bremner et al., 1992; Ginzburg et al., 2006). A number of studies have also found that dissociation might be more common in early-onset PTSD associated with exposure to a complicated series of traumas (e.g., Evren et al., 2011; Kamen et al., 2012; Wolf et al., 2012b). This pattern is consistent with discussions in clinical studies about "complex PTSD" and "Disorders of Extreme Stress Not Otherwise Specified" (DESNOS) (Herman, 1992; Friedman et al., 2011) (see Chapter 21). However, these formulations suggest that such individuals also exhibit behavioral difficulties (such as impulsivity, aggression, sexual acting out, alcohol/drug abuse, and self-destructive actions), emotional difficulties (such as affective lability, rage, depression, and panic), cognitive difficulties (such as dissociation and pathological changes in personal identity), interpersonal difficulties, somatization, and deficits in regulating emotional distress (Cloitre et al., 2005). These broader sets of symptoms were not assessed in the WMH surveys, leaving it for future investigators to determine the relationship between the dissociative subtype and complex PTSD.

Our findings that dissociation was associated with elevated PTSD symptom counts, high role impairment, and suicidality are consistent with clinical evidence that dissociation is related to severity of PTSD (Foote et al., 2008; Lanius et al., 2012; Wolf et al., 2012a). It is striking in light of this that we failed to find evidence that respondents whose PTSD featured dissociation were more likely than those without dissociation to obtain treatment for their PTSD. This finding appears to highlight an unmet need for a particularly impaired subset of individuals with PTSD and, together with earlier studies pointing to treatment implications of dissociation in this disorder (Resick et al., 2012), may suggest the need for differential screening and treatment strategies for individuals whose PTSD includes dissociative symptoms (Cloitre et al., 2002; Lanius et al., 2010b).

These results help to characterize the dissociative subtype of PTSD in community samples by showing clearly that dissociation exists in a meaningful and roughly equal proportion of PTSD cases throughout a diverse set of countries. We found that the dissociative subtype operationalization distinguishes a meaningful proportion of PTSD cases and that these cases have a distinct clinically meaningful set of predictors and consequences that are roughly equivalent across countries. We also found that this subtype is associated with a particularly impairing form of PTSD. Dissociation might turn out to be a marker of a complex form of PTSD characterized not only by early onset and exposure to multiple childhood traumas adversities, but also by multiple comorbidities and other clinical features not assessed in the WMH surveys. While evaluation of this possibility goes beyond the scope of the WMH data, the results presented here suggest that it deserves future empirical investigation.

Acknowledgment

Portions of this chapter are based on Stein, D. J., Koenen, K. C., Friedman, M. J., et al. (2013). Dissociation in PTSD: evidence from the World Mental Health Surveys. *Biological Psychiatry*,**73**, 302–12, by permission of Elsevier.

References

American Psychiatric Association. (2000). *Diagnostic and Statistical Manual of Mental Disorders, Fourth Edition, Text Revision. DSM-IV-TR*. Washington, DC: American Psychiatric Association.

American Psychiatric Association. (2013). *Diagnostic and Statistical Manual of Mental Disorders, Fifth Edition.DSM-5*. Arlington, VA: American Psychiatric Association.

Bernstein, E. M., & Putnam, F. W. (1986). Development, reliability, and validity of a dissociation scale. *The Journal of Nervous and Mental Disease*, 174, 727–35.

Bremner, J. D., Southwick, S., Brett, E., et al. (1992). Dissociation and posttraumatic stress disorder in Vietnam combat veterans. *The American Journal of Psychiatry*, 149, 328–32.

Brown, R. J., & Lewis-Fernandez, R. (2011). Culture and conversion disorder: implications for DSM-5. *Psychiatry*, 74, 187–206.

Bryant, R. A. (2007). Does dissociation further our understanding of PTSD? *Journal of Anxiety Disorders*, 21, 183–91.

Cloitre, M., Koenen, K. C., Cohen, L. R., & Han, H. (2002). Skills training in affective and interpersonal regulation followed by exposure: a phase-based treatment for PTSD related to childhood abuse. *Journal of Consulting and Clinical Psychology*, 70, 1067–74.

Cloitre, M., Miranda, R., Stovall-McClogh, K. C., & Han, H. (2005). Beyond PTSD: emotion regulation and interpersonal problems as predictors of functional impairment in survivors of childhood abuse. *Behavior Therapy*, 36, 119–24.

Cloitre, M., Petkova, E., Wang, J., & Lu Lassell, F. (2012). An examination of the influence of a sequential treatment on the course and impact of dissociation among women with PTSD related to childhood abuse. *Depression and Anxiety*, 29, 709–17.

Cloitre, M., Stolbach, B. C., Herman, J. L., et al. (2009). A developmental approach to complex PTSD: childhood and adult cumulative trauma as predictors of symptom complexity. *Journal of Traumatic Stress*, 22, 399–408.

Dalenberg, C. J., Brand, B. L., Gleaves, D. H., et al. (2012). Evaluation of the evidence for the trauma and fantasy models of dissociation. *Psychological Bulletin*, 138, 550–88.

Evren, C., Sar, V., Dalbudak, E., et al. (2011). Lifetime PTSD and quality of life among alcohol-dependent men: impact of childhood emotional abuse and dissociation. *Psychiatry Research*, 186, 85–90.

Foote, B., Smolin, Y., Neft, D. I., & Lipschitz, D. (2008). Dissociative disorders and suicidality in psychiatric outpatients. *The Journal of Nervous and Mental Disease*, 196, 29–36.

Friedman, M. J., Resick, P. A., Bryant, R. A., et al. (2011). Classification of trauma and stressor-related disorders in DSM-5. *Depression and Anxiety*, 28, 737–49.

Ginzburg, K., Koopman, C., Butler, L. D., et al. (2006). Evidence for a dissociative subtype of post-traumatic stress disorder among help-seeking childhood sexual abuse survivors. *Journal of Trauma & Dissociation*, 7, 7–27.

Hansen, M., Ross, J., Armour, C. (2017). Evidence of the dissociative PTSD subtype: a systematic literature review of latent class and profile analytic studies of PTSD. *Journal of Affective Disorders*, 213, 59–69.

Herman, J. L. (1992). Complex PTSD: a syndrome in survivors of prolonged and repeated trauma. *Journal of Traumatic Stress*, 5, 377–91.

Hinton, D. E., & Lewis-Fernandez, R. (2011). The cross-cultural validity of posttraumatic stress disorder: implications for DSM-5. *Depression and Anxiety*, 28, 783–801.

Hosmer, D. W., & Lemeshow, S. (2000). *Applied Logistic Regression*, 2nd edn. New York, NY: Wiley & Sons.

Janet, P. (1907). *The Major Symptoms of Hysteria: Fifteen Lectures Given in the Medical School of Harvard University*. New York, NY: MacMillan.

Kamen, C., Bergstrom, J., Koopman, C., Lee, S., & Gore-Felton, C. (2012). Relationships among childhood trauma, posttraumatic stress disorder, and dissociation in men living with HIV/AIDS. *Journal of Trauma & Dissociation*, 13, 102–14.

Lanius, R. A., Frewen, P. A., Vermetten, E., & Yehuda, R. (2010a). Fear conditioning and early life vulnerabilities: two distinct pathways of emotional dysregulation and brain dysfunction in PTSD. *European Journal of Psychotraumatology*, 1, 5467.

Lanius, R. A., Vermetten, E., Loewenstein, R. J., et al. (2010b). Emotion modulation in PTSD: clinical and neurobiological evidence for a dissociative subtype. *The American Journal of Psychiatry*, 167, 640–7.

Lanius, R. A., Brand, B., Vermetten, E., Frewen, P. A., & Spiegel, D. (2012). The dissociative subtype of posttraumatic stress disorder: rationale, clinical and neurobiological evidence, and implications. *Depression and Anxiety*, 29, 701–8.

Leon, A. C., Olfson, M., Portera, L., Farber, L., & Sheehan, D. V. (1997). Assessing psychiatric impairment in primary care with the Sheehan Disability Scale. *International Journal of Psychiatry in Medicine*, 27, 93–105.

Lochner, C., Seedat, S., Hemmings, S. M., et al. (2004). Dissociative experiences in obsessive-compulsive disorder and trichotillomania: clinical and genetic findings. *Comprehensive Psychiatry*, 45, 384–91.

Nock, M. K., Hwang, I., Sampson, N., et al. (2009). Cross-national analysis of the associations among mental disorders and suicidal behavior: findings from the WHO World Mental Health Surveys. *PLOS Medicine*, 6, e1000123.

Nugent, N. R., Koenen, K. C., & Bradley, B. (2012). Heterogeneity of posttraumatic stress symptoms in a highly traumatized low income, urban, African American sample. *Journal of Psychiatric Research*, 46, 1576–83.

Putnam, F. W., Carlson, E. B., Ross, C. A., et al. (1996). Patterns of dissociation in clinical and nonclinical samples. *The Journal of Nervous and Mental Disease*, 184, 673–9.

Resick, P. A., Suvak, M. K., Johnides, B. D., Mitchell, K. S., & Iverson, K. M. (2012). The impact of dissociation on PTSD treatment with cognitive processing therapy. *Depression and Anxiety*, 29, 718–30.

Spiegel, D., Loewenstein, R. J., Lewis-Fernandez, R., et al. (2011). Dissociative disorders in DSM-5. *Depression and Anxiety*, 28, E17–45.

Steuwe, C., Lanius, R. A., & Frewen, P. A. (2012). Evidence for a dissociative subtype of PTSD by latent profile

and confirmatory factor analyses in a civilian sample. *Depression and Anxiety*, 29, 689–700.
Strachey, J. (1955). *The Standard Edition of the Complete Psychological Works of Sigmund Freud, Volume II (1893–1895): Studies on Hysteria*. London, England: The Hogarth Press and the Institute of Psycho-Analysis.
van der Hart, O., Nijenhuis, E., Steele, K., & Brown, D. (2004). Trauma-related dissociation: conceptual clarity lost and found. *The Australian and New Zealand Journal of Psychiatry*, 38, 906–14.
van Ijzendoorn, M. H., & Schuengel, C. (1996). The measurement of dissociation in normal and clinical populations: meta-analytic validation of the Dissociative Experiences Scale (DES). *Clinical Psychology Review*, 16, 365–82.
Waelde, L. C., Silvern, L., & Fairbank, J. A. (2005). A taxometric investigation of dissociation in Vietnam veterans. *Journal of Traumatic Stress*, 18, 359–69.
Waller, N., Putnam, F. W., & Carlson, E. B. (1996). Types of dissociation and dissociative types: a taxometric analysis of dissociative experiences. *Psychological Methods*, 1, 300–21.
Watson, D. (2003). Investigating the construct validity of the dissociative taxon: stability analyses of normal and pathological dissociation. *Journal of Abnormal Psychology*, 112, 298–305.
Wolf, E. J., Lunney, C. A., Miller, M. W., et al. (2012a). The dissociative subtype of PTSD: a replication and extension. *Depression and Anxiety*, 29, 679–88.
Wolf, E. J., Miller, M. W., Reardon, A. F., et al. (2012b). A latent class analysis of dissociation and posttraumatic stress disorder: evidence for a dissociative subtype. *Archives of General Psychiatry*, 69, 698–705.
Zucker, M., Spinazzola, J., Blaustein, M., & van der Kolk, B. A. (2006). Dissociative symptomatology in posttraumatic stress disorder and disorders of extreme stress. *Journal of Trauma & Dissociation*, 7, 19–31.

Appendix

Table 20.A1 WMH sample characteristics by World Bank income categories[a]

Country by income category	Survey[b]	Sample characteristics[c]	Field dates	Age range	Sample size		Response rate[e]
					Part I	Part II[d]	
I Low- and Lower-Middle-Income Countries							
Colombia	NSMH	All urban areas of the country (approximately 73% of the total national population)	2003	18–65	4,426	2,381	87.7
PRC – Beijing/ Shanghai	B-WMH/S-WMH	Beijing and Shanghai metropolitan areas	2002–3	18–70	5,201	1,628	74.7
(Total)					(9,627)	(4,009)	
II Upper-Middle-Income Countries							
Brazil – São Paulo	São Paulo Megacity	São Paulo metropolitan area	2005–7	18–93	5,037	2,942	81.3
Bulgaria	NSHS	Nationally representative	2003–7	18–98	5,318	2,233	72.0
Lebanon	LEBANON	Nationally representative	2002–3	18–94	2,857	1,031	70.0
Mexico	M-NCS	All urban areas of the country (approximately 75% of the total national population)	2001–2	18–65	5,782	2,362	76.6
Romania	RMHS	Nationally representative	2005–6	18–96	2,357	2,357	70.9
(Total)					(21,351)	(10,925)	
III High-Income Countries							
Japan	WMHJ 2002–2006	Eleven metropolitan areas	2002–6	20–98	4,129	1,655	55.1
Northern Ireland	NISHS	Nationally representative	2004–7	18–97	4,340	1,986	68.4
Portugal	NMHS	Nationally representative	2008–9	18–81	3,849	562	57.3
United States	NCS-R	Nationally representative	2002–3	18–99	9,282	5,692	70.9

(cont.)

Table 20.A1 *(cont.)*

Country by income category	Survey[b]	Sample characteristics[c]	Field dates	Age range	Sample size		Response rate[e]
					Part I	Part II[d]	
Western Europe (Total)	ESEMeD[f]	Nationally representative	2001–3	18–100	19,053 (40,653)	189 (10,084)	64.4
IV Total					(71,631)	(25,018)	69.0

[a]The World Bank. (2008). Data and Statistics. Accessed May 12, 2009 at: http://go.worldbank.org/D7SN0B8YU0.
[b]NSMH (The Colombian National Study of Mental Health); B-WMH (The Beijing World Mental Health Survey); S-WMH (The Shanghai World Mental Health Survey); NSHS (Bulgaria National Survey of Health and Stress); LEBANON (Lebanese Evaluation of the Burden of Ailments and Needs of the Nation); M-NCS (The Mexico National Comorbidity Survey); RMHS (Romania Mental Health Survey); WMHJ2002–2006 (World Mental Health Japan Survey); NISHS (Northern Ireland Study of Health and Stress); NMHS (Portugal National Mental Health Survey); NCS-R (The US National Comorbidity Survey Replication); ESEMeD (The European Study of the Epidemiology of Mental Disorders).
[c]Most WMH surveys are based on stratified multistage clustered area probability household samples in which samples of areas equivalent to counties or municipalities in the United States were selected in the first stage followed by one or more subsequent stages of geographic sampling (e.g., towns within counties, blocks within towns, households within blocks) to arrive at a sample of households, in each of which a listing of household members was created and one or two people were selected from this listing to be interviewed. No substitution was allowed when the originally sampled household resident could not be interviewed. These household samples were selected from Census area data in most countries. One of the ESEMeD Western European countries (France) used telephone directories to select households; while other ESEMeD countries, including Belgium, Germany and Italy, used municipal resident registries to select respondents without listing households. The Japanese sample is the only unclustered sample with households randomly selected in each of the 11 metropolitan areas and one random respondent selected in each sample household. Seven of the 14 surveys are based on nationally representative household samples.
[d]Sample size of individuals assessed for dissociative PTSD.
[e]The response rate is calculated as the ratio of the number of households in which an interview was completed to the number of households originally sampled, excluding from the denominator households known not to be eligible either because of being vacant at the time of initial contact or because the residents were unable to speak the designated languages of the survey. The weighted average response rate is 70.1%.
[f]There are six countries in the Western Europe ESEMeD (European Study of the Epidemiology of Mental Disorders) series (Belgium, France, Germany, Italy, the Netherlands, and Spain). Although these six surveys include a total of 21,425 respondents, only a tiny fraction of these respondents (and none in the Netherlands) were administered the 30-day symptom scale that contained the dissociation questions analyzed here.

Table 20.A2 Distribution of responses to depersonalization and derealization questions among respondents with 12-month DSM-IV/CIDI PTSD ($n = 747$)[a]

	%	(SE)
Feeling as though standing next to self	8.5	(1.1)
Feeling as though body does not belong to self	6.3	(0.9)
Feeling other people, objects, world are not real	6.5	(1.1)
Any of the above	14.4	(1.3)

[a]See the text for complete wording of questions.

Table 20.A3 Associations of individual CIDI symptoms of DSM-IV PTSD with the presence versus absence of dissociative symptoms among respondents with 12-month DSM-IV/CIDI PTSD ($n = 747$)

	Prevalence of symptom among respondents with 12-month PTSD with dissociation		Prevalence of symptom among respondents with 12-month PTSD without dissociation			
	%	(SE)	%	(SE)	OR	(95% CI)
I AV						
Try not to think about trauma	82.5	(4.2)	78.1	(2.3)	1.3	(0.7–2.5)
Purposely stay away from things that remind of trauma	74.7	(6.2)	72.3	(2.1)	1.1	(0.6–2.3)
Unable to remember important parts of trauma	50.2	(5.0)	38.5	(2.7)	1.6*	(1.0–2.6)

(cont.)

Table 20.A3 *(cont.)*

	Prevalence of symptom among respondents with 12-month PTSD with dissociation		Prevalence of symptom among respondents with 12-month PTSD without dissociation			
	%	(SE)	%	(SE)	OR	(95% CI)
II NM						
Lose interest in things used to enjoy	85.0	(3.2)	80.7	(1.8)	1.4	(0.8–2.4)
Feel emotionally distant/cut-off from people	78.0	(4.7)	82.9	(2.3)	0.7	(0.4–1.4)
Trouble feeling love/happiness toward others	82.3	(3.8)	74.4	(2.3)	1.6	(0.9–2.8)
Feel no reason to plan for the future	63.0	(5.5)	51.4	(2.5)	1.6	(1.0–2.6)
III RE						
Repeated unwanted memories of trauma	96.0	(2.7)	87.9	(1.8)	3.3	(0.8–14.4)
Repeated unpleasant dreams of trauma	75.8	(5.5)	71.4	(2.2)	1.3	(0.7–2.4)
Flashbacks of trauma happening	81.7	(4.0)	65.7	(2.5)	2.3*	(1.3–4.2)
Get very upset when reminded of trauma	89.6	(3.8)	86.6	(1.8)	1.3	(0.6–3.2)
Have physical reactions when reminded of trauma	79.5	(5.2)	67.7	(2.7)	1.9	(0.9–3.8)
IV HA	100.0	(0.0)	100.0	(0.0)		
Trouble falling asleep during trauma	85.3	(4.1)	89.6	(1.7)	0.7	(0.3–1.4)
More irritable than usual during trauma	73.2	(4.4)	66.3	(2.5)	1.4	(0.9–2.2)
More trouble concentrating during trauma	88.6	(4.0)	83.9	(1.9)	1.5	(0.7–3.4)
Much more alert/watchful with no real need	79.1	(5.7)	74.0	(2.4)	1.3	(0.6–2.8)
More easily startled by ordinary noises	78.4	(6.9)	75.5	(2.4)	1.2	(0.5–2.8)

*Significant at the 0.05 level, two-sided test.

Table 20.A4 Interactions of country income level with socio-demographic variables and trauma characteristics in predicting presence versus absence of dissociative symptoms among respondents with 12-month DSM-IV/CIDI PTSD (*n* = 747)[a]

	Marginal effects in high-income countries		Interactions comparing LMICs to high-income countries	
	OR	(95% CI)	OR	(95% CI)
I Country Income Level				
High-income	1.0	–		
Low- and middle-income	0.1	(0.0–3.7)		
II Sex				
Female	1.0	–	1.0	–
Male	1.4	(0.9–2.5)	2.5	(0.7–10.0)
III AOO of PTSD[b]				
0–6	3.2*	(1.1–9.7)	6.5	(0.1–643.1)
7–12	2.0	(0.8–5.0)	4.8	(0.3–72.3)
13–19	0.9	(0.4–1.9)	8.6*	(2.0–36.5)
20+	1.0	–	1.0	–
χ^2_3	1.6		3.4*	
IV Number of Years Since Onset of PTSD[b]				
0–4	1.3	(0.5–3.5)	2.6	(0.2–33.7)
5–12	0.6	(0.3–1.3)	2.9	(0.2–34.6)
13–24	0.9	(0.4–2.0)	6.3	(0.6–69.9)
25+	1.0	–	1.0	–
χ^2_3	2.3*		0.9	

(cont.)

Table 20.A4 *(cont.)*

	Marginal effects in high-income countries		Interactions comparing LMICs to high-income countries	
	OR	(95% CI)	OR	(95% CI)
V Number of Prior Traumas[c]				
0	1.0	–	1.0	–
1–4	1.6	(0.8–3.2)	6.8	(0.3–147.9)
5+	4.7*	(2.0–11.2)	2.6	(0.1–72.7)
χ^2_2	7.1*		1.3	

*Significant at the 0.05 level, two-sided test.
[a]Based on a multivariate logistic regression model with interactions between country income level and all other predictors.
[b]The predictor was divided to create roughly equal sample sizes in each category.
[c]The predictor was divided to capture the functional form detected by examining the association with a completely disaggregated version of the variable.

Table 20.A5 Interactions of country income level with number of MFF CAs in predicting presence versus absence of dissociative symptoms among respondents with 12-month DSM-IV/CIDI PTSD (*n* = 747)[a]

	Marginal effects in high-income countries		Interactions comparing low- and middle- to high-income countries	
	OR	(95% CI)	OR	(95% CI)
Number of MFF CAs				
0	1.0	–	1.0	–
1	1.2	(0.7–2.0)	5.5	(1.0–31.4)
2	2.5*	(1.1–5.5)	1.2	(0.2–6.9)
3+	2.4*	(1.0–5.6)	3.4	(0.6–18.3)
χ^2_3	2.2		1.7	

*Significant at the 0.05 level, two-sided test.
[a]Based on a multivariate logistic regression model with interactions between country income level and all other predictors controlling for the predictors in Table 20.3. The best-fitting model was one that included as predictors only a count of MFF CAs. The coefficients from that model are reported here.

Table 20.A6 Interactions of country income level with number of temporally primary DSM-IV/CIDI disorders in predicting presence versus absence of dissociative symptoms among respondents with 12-month DSM-IV/CIDI PTSD (*n* = 747)[a]

	Marginal effects in high-income countries		Interactions comparing low- and middle- to high-income countries	
	OR	(95% CI)	OR	(95% CI)
Number of Prior DSM-IV/CIDI Disorders				
0	1.0	–	1.0	–
1	2.6	(0.8–8.9)	2.7	(0.4–17.9)
2	2.4	(0.9–6.6)	1.1	(0.1–8.9)
3	2.0	(0.6–7.2)	1.0	(0.1–14.2)
4+	9.7*	(3.6–26.1)	1.0	(0.2–6.6)
χ^2_3	6.5*		0.6	

*Significant at the 0.05 level, two-sided test.
[a]Based on a multivariate logistic regression model with interactions between country income level and all other predictors controlling for the predictors in Table 20.4. The best-fitting model was one that included as predictors only a count of prior disorders. The coefficients from that model are reported here.

Chapter 21

Simple versus Complex Posttraumatic Stress Disorder

Elie G. Karam, Evelyn J. Bromet, Ronald C. Kessler, Maria Carmen Viana, and Karestan C. Koenen

In accordance with diagnostic criteria, epidemiological studies have typically assessed posttraumatic stress disorder (PTSD) only in relation to an index trauma. However, as we saw in Chapter 3, exposure to multiple traumas is common in the general population. And we know from clinical experience that many of the patients who present for treatment of PTSD do so after exposure to complex trauma clusters and histories. There has been some suggestion in the literature that individuals with PTSD whose symptoms are rooted in multiple types of trauma or repeated exposures to a single type of trauma (e.g., chronic childhood abuse) have greater morbidity and dysfunction than those exposed to only one instance of one trauma (Herman, 1992; Cloitre et al., 2002, 2009, 2010, 2011). However, these studies were based largely on treatment-seeking samples in which there may have been a referral bias (Cohen & Cohen, 1984). The few community epidemiological studies that examined this issue have been limited mostly to adolescent samples in the United States or Europe (Follette et al., 1996; Suliman et al., 2009; McLaughlin et al., 2010; Turner et al., 2010).

We investigated this issue in the World Mental Health (WMH) survey data by focusing on respondents who experienced an episode of PTSD during the 12 months before interview. These recent cases were asked to refer back to the traumas that they had circled in their lifetime trauma list and to specify those traumas that were implicated in their recent symptoms. We analyzed these responses to determine the proportion of 12-month PTSD cases in the general population that were rooted in exposure to complex traumas and the associations of this complexity with a variety of characteristics of 12-month PTSD.

Methods

When this analysis was carried out, we had WMH surveys in 11 high-income countries (Belgium, France, Germany, Italy, Israel, Japan, the Netherlands, New Zealand, Northern Ireland, Spain, and the United States) and 9 upper-middle-income (São Paulo in Brazil, Bulgaria, Lebanon, Mexico, Romania, and South Africa) or low- and lower-middle-income countries (Colombia, Ukraine, and Beijing as well as Shanghai in the People's Republic of China [PRC]). We examined the associations of trauma complexity among cases of recent PTSD with the other DSM-IV disorders assessed in the survey: five anxiety disorders (separation anxiety disorder, panic disorder and/or agoraphobia, generalized anxiety disorder [GAD], specific phobia, and social phobia), two mood disorders (major depressive disorder [MDD]/dysthymia and bipolar disorder), four disruptive behavior disorders (attention-deficit/hyperactivity disorder [ADHD], oppositional-defiant disorder [ODD], conduct disorder, and intermittent explosive disorder [IED]), and two substance use disorders (alcohol and drug abuse with/without dependence).

We also examined the association of trauma complexity among 12-month cases with role functioning using a modified version of the Sheehan Disability Scale (SDS) (Leon et al., 1997). This scale was operationalized by asking respondents with 12-month PTSD how much their PTSD interfered with their functioning in each of four role domains (home management, ability to work, social life, and close relationships) during the one month in the past 12 months when this interference was greatest. Responses were on a 0–10 response scale with labels of none (0), mild (1–3), moderate (4–6), severe (7–9), and very severe interference (10). A global SDS score was also created by assigning each respondent the highest SDS domain score reported across the four domains.

A hierarchy of logistic regression models was used to analyze responses. The first model examined the association of number of trauma types involved in the episode with severity of functional impairment, controlling for age, sex, country, age of onset (AOO), and duration (defined as time since AOO) of the recent PTSD episode. The second model then added

Table 21.1 Overall prevalence of 12-month DSM-IV/CIDI PTSD in each WMH survey

	%	(SE)	$(n_1)^a$	$(n_2)^a$
I High-Income Countries				
Belgium	0.6	(0.1)	(16)	(1,043)
France	1.4	(0.3)	(33)	(1,436)
Germany	0.5	(0.2)	(19)	(1,323)
Italy	0.4	(0.1)	(17)	(1,779)
Israel	0.4	(0.1)	(15)	(4,859)
Japan	0.4	(0.2)	(9)	(1,682)
The Netherlands	1.2	(0.3)	(31)	(1,094)
New Zealand	2.1	(0.2)	(304)	(7,312)
Northern Ireland	3.8	(0.5)	(96)	(1,986)
Spain	0.4	(0.1)	(29)	(2,121)
United States	2.5	(0.2)	(227)	(5,692)
Total	1.5	(0.1)	(797)	(30,327)
II Upper-Middle-Income Countries				
Brazil – São Paulo	1.0	(0.2)	(52)	(2,942)
Bulgaria	0.9	(0.2)	(35)	(2,233)
Lebanon	1.6	(0.6)	(22)	(1,031)
Mexico	0.3	(0.1)	(19)	(2,362)
Romania	0.4	(0.2)	(11)	(2,357)
South Africa	0.4	(0.1)	(21)	(4,315)
Total	0.7	(0.1)	(159)	(15,240)
III Low- and Lower-Middle-Income Countries				
Colombia	0.3	(0.1)	(10)	(2,381)
PRC – Beijing/ Shanghai	0.2	(0.1)	(7)	(1,628)
Ukraine	2.0	(0.4)	(69)	(1,719)
Total	0.8	(0.2)	(86)	(5,728)
IV Total	1.1	(0.0)	(1,042)	(51,295)
χ^{2b}_{2}		53.7*		
χ^{2c}_{19}		354.6*		

*Significant at the 0.05 level, two-sided test.
[a] n_1 is the number of respondents with 12-month DSM-IV/CIDI PTSD. n_2 is the total sample size of the survey.
[b] The significance of the differences in prevalence by country income.
[c] The significance of the differences in prevalence between all countries.

information about trauma types, and the third model added information about prior lifetime DSM-IV/CIDI disorders to determine whether these variables explained the observed association between number of trauma types involved in the episode and the outcomes. As in other chapters in this book, the logistic regression coefficients and their standard errors were exponentiated and are reported here as odds ratios (ORs) with design-based 95% confidence intervals (CIs).

Prevalence

Twelve-month prevalence (standard error) of DSM-IV/CIDI PTSD in the total sample was 1.1% (see Table 21.1). The three highest country-specific prevalence estimates were in Northern Ireland (3.8%), the United States (2.5%), and New Zealand (2.1%), whereas the lowest were in Beijing and Shanghai in the PRC (0.2%), Colombia (0.3%), and Mexico (0.3%). Prevalence varied significantly across the total subsamples of respondents in low- and lower-middle- (0.8%), upper-middle- (0.7%), and high- (1.5%) income countries ($\chi^2_2 = 53.7, p < 0.001$).

Symptoms associated with more than one trauma type were reported by 19.8% of respondents with 12-month PTSD. Severe role impairment associated with PTSD in at least one of the four SDS role domains was reported by 42% of respondents with 12-month PTSD, including 23.2% who reported severe impairment in the domain of work, 24.2% in home maintenance, 26.8% in close relationships, and 28.9% in social life (see Table 21.2). Functional impairment was significantly higher among cases where four or more trauma types were implicated in the PTSD, but no significant

Table 21.2 Functional impairment and 12-month DSM-IV/CIDI PTSD associated with three or fewer versus four or more traumas

	Total		3–/PTSD		4+/PTSD		
	Severe (%)	(SE)	Severe (%)	(SE)	Severe (%)	(SE)	χ^{2a}_{1}
Severe Impairment[b]							
Work	23.2	(2.0)	22.1	(1.8)	54.78	(8.6)	13.8*
Home maintenance	24.2	(2.0)	23.5	(1.8)	44.10	(8.6)	5.8*
Close relationships	26.8	(2.0)	25.1	(2.0)	75.20	(7.8)	22.2*
Social life	28.9	(2.0)	27.7	(2.1)	63.21	(8.8)	12.9*
Global	42.0	(2.0)	40.6	(2.1)	80.67	(6.8)	14.0*

*Significant at the 0.05 level, two-sided test.
[a] Based on a logistic regression controlling for age, sex, and country.
[b] Severe impairment is defined by having a score of 7–10 on the Sheehan impairment scale.

Table 21.3 The associations between number of trauma types implicated in PTSD and severe functional impairment in four domains of role functioning among respondents with 12-month DSM-IV/CIDI PTSD based on three different models ($n = 1{,}042$)[a]

	Number of traumas		Number and types of traumas		Number and types of trauma and comorbidity	
	OR	(95% CI)	OR	(95% CI)	OR	(95% CI)
I Work						
2 traumas	1.3	(0.7–2.4)	1.3	(0.7–2.3)	1.3	(0.7–2.6)
3 traumas	1.4	(0.6–3.7)	1.3	(0.5–2.9)	1.2	(0.5–2.8)
4+ traumas	5.2*	(2.3–11.4)	5.1*	(1.6–15.8)	4.7*	(1.4–16.0)
χ^2_3	17.4*		8.3*		6.8	
II Home Maintenance						
2 traumas	0.6	(0.3–1.1)	0.6	(0.3–1.1)	0.6	(0.3–1.1)
3 traumas	0.7	(0.2–1.9)	0.6	(0.2–1.7)	0.6	(0.2–1.9)
4+ traumas	2.6*	(1.2–5.7)	1.8	(0.6–5.7)	1.8	(0.5–5.8)
χ^2_3	9.6*		6.1		4.4	
III Close Relationships						
2 traumas	1.0	(0.6–1.9)	0.9	(0.4–1.7)	0.8	(0.4–1.8)
3 traumas	1.2	(0.6–2.5)	0.9	(0.4–2.2)	0.9	(0.4–2.0)
4+ traumas	7.6*	(3.1–18.3)	8.8*	(2.7–28.9)	7.4*	(2.1–26.7)
χ^2_3	20.8*		16.0*		11.2*	
IV Social Life						
2 traumas	1.0	(0.5–1.2)	1.0	(0.5–1.7)	1.0	(0.5–1.9)
3 traumas	1.6	(0.4–2.9)	1.2	(0.5–2.8)	1.2	(0.5–2.7)
4+ traumas	4.2*	(2.5–14.9)	3.8*	(1.3–11.3)	3.2	(0.9–10.7)
χ^2_3	14.3*		6.3		3.7	
V Global						
2 traumas	0.7	(0.5–1.2)	0.7	(0.4–1.2)	0.6	(0.3–1.2)
3 traumas	1.1	(0.4–2.9)	0.9	(0.4–2.2)	0.8	(0.3–1.9)
4+ traumas	6.0*	(2.5–14.9)	7.3*	(2.2–24.2)	6.2*	(1.9–20.0)
χ^2_3	16.4*		14.9*		12.0*	

*Significant at the 0.05 level, two-sided test.

[a]All models include controls for sex, country, AOO, and duration (defined as time since AOO). They are run on the subset of respondents with 12-month PTSD. Comorbidity is defined by dummies for other 12-month DSM-IV/CIDI disorders including MDD or dysthymic disorder, BPD, panic disorder or agoraphobia, GAD, adult separation anxiety, social phobia, specific phobia, IED, CD, ODD, ADHD, alcohol abuse or dependence, drug abuse, or dependence.

differences in functional impairment were observed among the remaining 95.2% of cases with 12-month PTSD as a function of number of associated trauma types in the range 1–3 (see Table 21.3). These elevated ORs remained significant after controlling for number and type of traumas and comorbid disorders, with ORs of severe functional impairment of 4.7 for work, 7.4 for close relationships, and 6.2 overall. However, only 4.8% of 12-month PTSD cases were associated with four or more trauma types.

Socio-demographic Correlates

In multivariable models, odds of PTSD cases being associated with 4+ trauma types were significantly elevated among individuals who were not married or cohabitating (OR = 2.5) and not employed (OR = 2.5). Women with PTSD had increased odds of 4+ trauma types compared to men (OR = 2.2), but the difference was not statistically significant. Education was unrelated to having 4+/PTSD.

Trauma Types

As one would expect, each of the trauma types considered here (which we collapsed to 15 because of sparseness of data) was more likely to be implicated in cases with 4+ trauma types than in cases with 1–3 trauma types. More interestingly, though, 5 of the 15 trauma types had significantly higher proportions among cases of 4+ trauma types than among cases of 1–3 trauma types(see Table 21.4). These included physical abuse

Table 21.4 Distributions of trauma types implicated in cases of 12-month DSM-IV/CIDI PTSD by number of implicated trauma types

	Percentage of people with each trauma type among cases with 1–3 types		Percentage of people with each trauma type among cases with 4+ types		Percentage of traumas among cases with 1–3 trauma types		Percentage of traumas among cases with 4+ trauma types	
	%	(SE)	%	(SE)	%	(SE)	%	(SE)
I War-Related Trauma								
Combat experience	0.8	(0.3)	6.0	(4.7)	0.6	(0.3)	1.1	(0.8)
Other war experience	2.5	(0.9)	16.8	(6.7)	2.0	(0.8)	3.0	(1.2)
II Physical Violence								
Physically abused as child	5.6*	(0.9)	44.0	(8.3)	4.6	(0.8)	7.9	(1.6)
Physically abused by spouse/partner	5.6*	(0.8)	56.2	(8.2)	4.6*	(0.7)	10.1	(1.4)
Physically assaulted or threatened	9.0*	(1.0)	67.5	(7.9)	7.3*	(0.8)	12.1	(1.4)
III Sexual Violence Victimization								
Sexually assaulted	13.5*	(1.2)	78.4	(6.6)	11.1	(1.0)	14.1	(1.3)
IV Accidents/Injuries								
Automobile accident	6.7*	(1.2)	28.7	(7.4)	5.5	(1.0)	5.2	(1.2)
Other life-threatening accident	3.9	(0.8)	11.6	(4.0)	3.2	(0.7)	2.1	(0.7)
Natural disaster	0.7	(0.3)	9.2	(4.4)	0.6	(0.2)	1.7	(0.8)
Life-threatening illness	8.5	(1.2)	21.9	(7.4)	7.0	(1.0)	4.0	(1.3)
V UD of a Loved One	31.6*	(2.2)	68.4	(8.5)	25.9*	(1.8)	12.3	(1.6)
VI Network/Witnessing								
Other trauma to a loved one	15.1*	(1.9)	39.1	(7.4)	12.4*	(1.5)	7.0	(1.3)
Witnessed family violence as a child	1.3*	(0.4)	41.8	(8.1)	1.1*	(0.3)	7.5	(1.4)
Witnessed a traumatic injury or death	3.8*	(0.8)	35.6	(8.0)	3.1*	(0.6)	6.4	(1.3)
VII Other Traumas	13.6	(1.6)	30.7	(7.9)	11.2*	(1.2)	5.5	(1.3)
(*n*)	(991)		(51)		(991)		(51)	

*Significant at the 0.05 level, two-sided test.

in childhood, physical abuse by a spouse or partner, physical assault, witnessing family violence as a child, and witnessing a traumatic injury or death. In contrast, sudden unexpected death of a loved one and network events comprised a larger proportion of all traumas associated with cases involving 1–3 trauma types than in cases involving 4+ trauma types.

AOO and Duration

Cases involving 4+ trauma types had significantly earlier AOO than cases involving 1–3 traumas. The earlier AOO can be seen in the cumulative AOO curves for the different subsets of cases (see Figure 21.1). Mean AOO of cases with 4+ trauma types was significantly lower – 16.2 years of age (SE = 1.5) compared to 31.7 years of age (SE = 0.7) – than for cases with 1–3 trauma types ($\chi^2_1 = 45.59, p < 0.001$). Duration of cases with 4+ trauma types was also significantly longer than for cases with 1–3 trauma types: mean duration 284.0 months (SE = 25.7) versus 147.1 months (SE = 5.4) ($\chi^2_1 = 45.59, p < 0.001$).

Comorbid Mental Disorders

In total, 5 of 15 12-month comorbid mental disorders considered here were significantly more common among PTSD cases involving 4+ than among cases involving 1–3 trauma types: bipolar disorder (OR = 2.6), GAD (OR = 2.9), adult separation anxiety

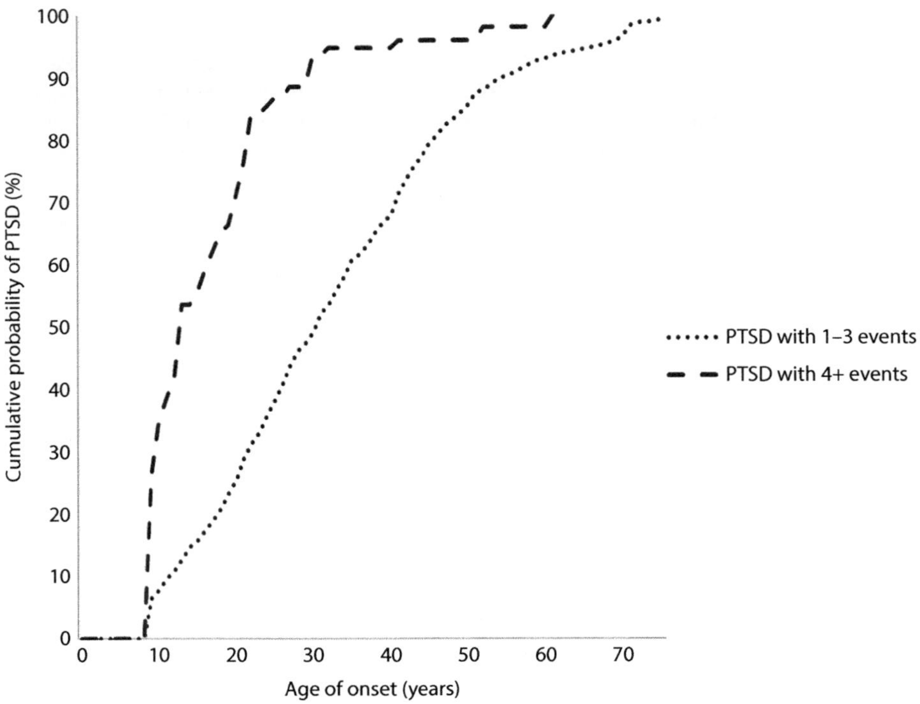

Figure 21.1 Cumulative probability of 4+/PTSD versus 3–/PTSD by age of onset in the WMH surveys

(OR = 3.6), social phobia (OR = 2.4), and specific phobia (OR = 2.1) (see Table 21.5). Prevalence of conduct disorder, drug abuse, and drug dependence was higher among respondents with 3–/PTSD, but the differences were not statistically significant.

PTSD Symptom Profiles

Mean number of total lifetime PTSD symptoms was significantly higher for 12-month cases involving with 4+ than for those involving 1–3 trauma types (see Table 21.6). This difference was driven largely by a significantly higher number of symptoms in the hyperarousal cluster.

Discussion

These results are limited by the fact that the number of cases with 4+ trauma types was too small for country-specific analyses. The total number of respondents with 12-month PTSD across all the surveys considered here was only 1,042, with 3.3% reporting 4+ traumas associated with their 12-month symptoms. Although our sample was larger than most treatment-seeking samples, the small number of cases with 4+ trauma types both limited the ability to detect effects and led to large standard errors in some cases. Another limitation was that we focused on trauma types rather than trauma frequency, as we did not have information on frequency of recent exposures within individual trauma types. As noted in the introduction, debate exists as to whether PTSD related to chronic exposure to a specific trauma type, such as often occurs with partner violence or childhood abuse, is more "complex" than from PTSD related to a single incident trauma (Cloitre et al., 2009 2011; Resick et al., 2012). The results presented here did not speak to this debate. A third limitation was that these results applied specifically to 12-month PTSD. Given that prevalent cases are more likely than others to be chronic, it is possible that our findings are more characteristic of chronic PTSD than of PTSD that remits. Further research is needed to examine this issue.

Notwithstanding the above limitations, the analysis had a number of noteworthy findings. While the majority of 12-month PTSD cases reported experiencing four or more trauma types over their lifetime, only 19% associated their 12-month symptoms with more than one trauma type. Although prior epidemiological

Table 21.5 Association between number of implicated trauma types and comorbidity of other 12-month DSM-V/CIDI disorders among respondents with 12-month PTSD ($n = 1{,}042$)

	Percentage of respondents with each comorbid disorder among cases with 1–3 trauma types		Percentage of respondents with each comorbid disorder among cases with 4+ trauma types		Associations between number of trauma types and comorbid disorders	
	%	(SE)	%	(SE)	OR[a]	(95% CI)
I Mood Disorders						
MDD or dysthymic disorder	40.9	(2.1)	60.8	(8.5)	2.1	(1.0–4.7)
BPD (broad definition)	8.2	(1.0)	26.2	(7.2)	2.6*	(1.1–6.2)
Any	42.6	(2.1)	68.8	(8.3)	2.7*	(1.2–6.3)
II Anxiety Disorders						
Panic disorder or agoraphobia	15.5	(1.4)	32.1	(7.9)	2.0	(0.9–4.2)
GAD	18.2	(1.4)	42.7	(8.9)	2.9*	(1.4–5.9)
Social phobia	17.5	(1.3)	41.7	(8.1)	2.4*	(1.3–4.7)
Specific phobia	25.0	(1.7)	49.9	(8.6)	2.1*	(1.1–4.1)
Separation anxiety disorder	3.8	(0.5)	16.6	(6.0)	3.6*	(1.4–9.3)
Any	46.2	(2.1)	85.8	(5.6)	5.2*	(2.2–12.5)
III Disruptive Behavior Disorders						
ADHD[b]	6.5	(1.6)	18.3	(8.6)	3.6	(0.7–17.9)
CD[b]	2.3	(0.9)	1.2	(1.2)	0.5	(0.1–4.0)
IED	5.6	(0.8)	14.1	(5.9)	2.3	(0.7–7.8)
ODD[b]	4.0	(0.9)	4.3	(3.1)	0.6	(0.1–3.4)
Any	14.5	(2.1)	18.3	(8.6)	1.1	(0.3–4.8)
IV Substance Use Disorders						
Alcohol abuse	6.3	(1.0)	11.2	(4.9)	1.7	(0.6–5.0)
Alcohol dependence	5.0	(0.8)	10.3	(4.8)	2.4	(0.8–6.9)
Drug abuse	2.3	(0.5)	1.7	(1.7)	0.7	(0.1–5.6)
Drug dependence	1.9	(0.5)	1.7	(1.7)	0.8	(0.1–6.3)
Any	7.7	(1.1)	14.1	(5.3)	1.8	(0.7–4.9)
χ^2_{15} [c]					69.2*	
χ^2_{14} [d]					23.2	

*Significant at the 0.05 level, two-sided test.
[a]Based on a logistic regression model controlling for country, age, and sex.
[b]Among the 1,042 individuals with 12-month PTSD, this represents a subgroup of 540 individuals who were no more than 44 years old at the time of interview.
[c]The joint significance of all mental disorders in the model.
[d]The significance of the differences among all mental disorders in the model.

studies have shown that exposure to multiple traumas is associated with increased risk of PTSD (Bromet et al., 1998; Darves-Bornoz et al., 2008; Roberts et al., 2010; Nelson et al., 2011), these data provide the first epidemiological evidence on the proportion of PTSD cases that are associated with multiple traumas. In addition, the small number of cases with symptoms related to 4+ trauma types had more severe functional impairments across all domains than other cases. Interestingly, the more severe functional impairment in work and close relationship domains observed among cases with 4+ trauma types was not explained by differences in trauma types or comorbid disorders.

Also noteworthy is that the types of traumas most commonly found in cases with 4+ trauma types turned out to be different from those found in other cases, with witnessing parent violence, physical abuse by a spouse or partner, and other physical assault comprising significantly higher proportions of the traumas among cases with 4+ trauma types. Unexpected death of a close friend or relative and network events comprised higher proportions of cases with 1–3 trauma types. Because trauma types, particularly interpersonal violence, tracked closely with number of traumas types, we cannot determine from our data whether there are differences by trauma types, after controlling for trauma number. However, it is noteworthy that cases with 4+ trauma types had higher proportion of traumas involving violence. Physical and sexual assault in childhood and adolescence are risk factors for re-victimization,

Table 21.6 Associations between number of implicated traumas and symptoms predicting 12 month DSM-IV/PTSD: multivariate symptom profile associations (no controls)

	3–/PTSD		4+/PTSD			
	Mean[a]	(SE)	Mean[a]	(SE)	OR	(95% CI)
Symptom Counts						
RE	−0.01	(0.04)	0.34	(0.18)	1.1	(0.8–1.5)
AV	0.00	(0.04)	−0.16	(0.18)	0.9	(0.7–1.1)
NM	−0.02	(0.05)	0.47	(0.18)	1.3	(0.9–1.8)
HA	−0.02	(0.05)	0.61	(0.14)	1.5*	(1.1–2.1)
Total	−0.02	(0.05)	0.52	(0.19)	1.4*	(1.1–1.9)
χ^{2b}_4					2.4*	
χ^{2c}_3					2.7*	

*Significant at the 0.05 level, two-sided test.
[a]Means are expressed in SD units.
[b]The joint significance of all symptoms in the model.
[c]The significance of the differences among all symptoms in the model.

including partner violence, in adulthood (Arata, 2000; Smith et al., 2003). Re-victimization may both lead some individuals to be exposed to multiple types of violence and contribute to the higher proportion of these traumas among cases with 4+ trauma types.

Finally, cases with 4+ trauma types, in contrast to cases with 1–3 trauma types, also had a significantly earlier AOO, longer duration, higher comorbidity with mood and anxiety disorders, and elevated level of hyperarousal symptoms. These patterns are all consistent with those in clinical samples, which have shown that PTSD associated with multiple traumas has a more "complex" presentation than other cases of PTSD (Briere et al., 2008; Cloitre et al., 2009, 2011). This broad pattern is also consistent with our finding in Chapter 20 that number and type of traumas are associated with a dissociative subtype of PTSD. However, discussions about a possible "complex PTSD" subtype have included characteristics such as emotional regulation deficits, identity disturbances, and interpersonal problems. That's because these symptoms are not systematically assessed in the CIDI. Future research is needed to explore the relationship between multiple trauma exposures and complex PTSD.

These findings have practical implications. Among individuals with 12-month PTSD, the small number whose episodes include symptoms associated with 4+ trauma types are the most severely impaired and thus may require disproportionate resources from the healthcare system. But, if so, then clinical research is needed to determine what kinds of treatment might be of particular value. Trauma-focused cognitive-behavioral therapies, including prolonged exposure therapy (Foa et al., 2005; Schnurr et al., 2007) and cognitive processing therapy (Resick et al., 2002), are effective for approximately 70% of persons with PTSD. However, according to the expert consensus treatment guidelines for "complex PTSD," individuals with PTSD related to multiple and chronic trauma exposure might require therapy that also includes skills training in areas such as interpersonal relationships and emotional regulation so that they can effectively engage in trauma-focused work (Cloitre et al., 2011). Finally, when considering the dissociative subtype of PTSD, which is associated with complex trauma presentation, augmentation of prolonged exposure therapy along with skills training in emotional and interpersonal regulation (Cloitre et al., 2012) or cognitive processing therapy along with both exposure and cognitive components (Lanius et al., 2010) might be of particular value. Further research is needed to determine whether the number of traumas implicated in symptoms is an important marker of this differential treatment response.

Acknowledgment

Portions of this chapter are based on Karam, E. G., Friedman, M. J., Hill, E. D., et al., (2014). Cumulative trauma and risk thresholds: 12-month PTSD in the World Mental Health (WMH) surveys. *Depression and Anxiety*, **31**, 130–42, by permission of Wiley-Blackwell.

References

Arata, C. M. (2000). From child victim to adult victim: a model for predicting sexual revictimization. *Child Maltreatment*, 5, 28–38.

Briere, J., Kaltman, S., & Green, B. L. (2008). Accumulated childhood trauma and symptom complexity. *Journal of Traumatic Stress*, 21, 223–6.

Bromet, E., Sonnega, A., & Kessler, R. C. (1998). Risk factors for DSM-III-R posttraumatic stress disorder: findings from the National Comorbidity Survey. *American Journal of Epidemiology*, 147, 353–61.

Cloitre, M., Koenen, K. C., Cohen, L. R., & Han, H. (2002). Skills training in affective and interpersonal regulation followed by exposure: a phase-based treatment for PTSD related to childhood abuse. *Journal of Consulting and Clinical Psychology*, 70, 1067–74.

Cloitre, M., Stolbach, B. C., Herman, J. L., et al. (2009). A developmental approach to complex PTSD: childhood and adult cumulative trauma as predictors of symptom complexity. *Journal of Traumatic Stress*, 22, 399–408.

Cloitre, M., Stovall-McClough, K. C., Nooner, K., et al. (2010). Treatment for PTSD related to childhood abuse: a randomized controlled trial. *American Journal of Psychiatry*, 167, 915–24.

Cloitre, M., Courtois, C. A., Charuvastra, A., et al. (2011). Treatment of complex PTSD: results of the ISTSS expert clinician survey on best practices. *Journal of Traumatic Stress*, 24, 615–27.

Cloitre, M., Petkova, E., Wang, J., & Lu, F. (2012). An examination of the influence of a sequential treatment on the course and impact of dissociation among women with PTSD related to childhood abuse. *Depression and Anxiety*, 29, 709–17.

Cohen, P., & Cohen, J. (1984). The clinician's illusion. *Archives of General Psychiatry*, 41, 1178–82.

Darves-Bornoz, J. M., Alonso, J., de Girolamo, G., et al. (2008). Main traumatic events in Europe: PTSD in the European study of the epidemiology of mental disorders survey. *Journal of Traumatic Stress*, 21, 455–62.

Foa, E. B., Hembree, E. A., Cahill, S. P., et al. (2005). Randomized trial of prolonged exposure for posttraumatic stress disorder with and without cognitive restructuring: outcome at academic and community clinics. *Journal of Consulting and Clinical Psychology*, 73, 953–64.

Follette, V. M., Polusny, M. A., Bechtle, A. E., & Naugle, A. E. (1996). Cumulative trauma: the impact of child sexual abuse, adult sexual assault, and spouse abuse. *Journal of Traumatic Stress*, 9, 25–35.

Herman, J. L. (1992). Complex PTSD: a syndrome in survivors of prolonged and repeated trauma. *Journal of Traumatic Stress*, 5, 377–91.

Lanius, R. A., Vermetten, E., Loewenstein, R. J., et al. (2010). Emotion modulation in PTSD: clinical and neurobiological evidence for a dissociative subtype. *American Journal of Psychiatry*, 167, 640–7.

Leon, A. C., Olfson, M., Portera, L., Farber, L., & Sheehan, D. V. (1997). Assessing psychiatric impairment in primary care with the Sheehan Disability Scale. *International Journal of Psychiatry in Medicine*, 27, 93–105.

McLaughlin, K. A., Fairbank, J. A., Gruber, M. J., et al. (2010). Trends in serious emotional disturbance among youths exposed to Hurricane Katrina. *Journal of the American Academy of Child and Adolescent Psychiatry*, 49, 990–1000.

Nelson, C., Cyr, K. S., Corbett, B., et al. (2011). Predictors of posttraumatic stress disorder, depression, and suicidal ideation among Canadian Forces personnel in a National Canadian Military Health Survey. *Journal of Psychiatric Research*, 45, 1483–8.

Resick, P. A., Nishith, P., Weaver, T. L., Astin, M. C., & Feuer, C. A. (2002). A comparison of cognitive-processing therapy with prolonged exposure and a waiting condition for the treatment of chronic posttraumatic stress disorder in female rape victims. *Journal of Consulting and Clinical Psychology*, 70, 867–79.

Resick, P. A., Bovin, M. J., Calloway, A. L., et al. (2012). A critical evaluation of the complex PTSD literature: implications for DSM-5. *Journal of Traumatic Stress*, 25, 241–51.

Roberts, A. L., Austin, S. B., Corliss, H. L., Vandermorris, A. K., & Koenen, K. C. (2010). Pervasive trauma exposure among US sexual orientation minority adults and risk of posttraumatic stress disorder. *American Journal of Public Health*, 100, 2433–41.

Schnurr, P. P., Friedman, M. J., Engel, C. C., et al. (2007). Cognitive behavioral therapy for posttraumatic stress disorder in women: a randomized controlled trial. *JAMA*, 297, 820–30.

Smith, P. H., White, J. W., & Holland, L. J. (2003). A longitudinal perspective on dating violence among adolescent and college-age women. *American Journal of Public Health*, 93, 1104–9.

Suliman, S., Mkabile, S. G., Fincham, D. S., et al. (2009). Cumulative effect of multiple trauma on symptoms of posttraumatic stress disorder, anxiety, and depression in adolescents. *Comprehensive Psychiatry*, 50, 121–7.

Turner, H. A., Finkelhor, D., & Ormrod, R. (2010). Poly-victimization in a national sample of children and youth. *American Journal of Preventive Medicine*, 38, 323–30.

Chapter 22

Data Mining to Predict Posttraumatic Stress Disorder Onset in the Wake of Trauma Exposure

Ronald C. Kessler, Sherri Rose, Paul Stang, and Alan M. Zaslavsky

Given that victims of trauma often come to the attention of the criminal justice and/or health-care systems shortly after trauma exposure, these individuals could easily be targeted for early preventive interventions. As a result, an emerging body of research has evaluated early preventive interventions for PTSD. While the interventions developed for delivery in the first few hours after trauma exposure have so far proven ineffective (Forneris et al., 2013), there are very promising new possibilities (Qi et al., 2016; Iyadurai et al., 2017). Furthermore, treatments delivered within a few weeks such as cognitive-behavioral therapy (Kliem & Kroger, 2013) and prolonged exposure therapy (Shalev et al., 2012) have been shown to be moderately effective in preventing chronic PTSD. In addition, ongoing research suggests that other potentially cost-effective preventive interventions might become available in the future (Ostrowski & Delahanty, 2014). However, most of these preventive interventions for PTSD are both labor-intensive and expensive, making it infeasible to offer them to all individuals exposed to trauma, although recent studies have raised the possibility that early interventions involving the use of video games might help prevent PTSD by reducing the consolidation of traumatic memories (Robin, 2012; James et al., 2015). Given that only a small minority of trauma victims tend to develop PTSD (Kessler, 2000), prediction rules that successfully identify those at highest PTSD risk shortly after trauma exposure could consequently improve intervention targeting and cost-effectiveness.

Meta-analyses (Brewin et al., 2000; Ozer et al., 2003; Tolin & Foa, 2006) and reviews (Breslau, 2002; DiGangi et al., 2013; Heron-Delaney et al., 2013) point to five especially promising predictor classes that could be assessed in the immediate aftermath of trauma exposure, all of which have been examined in the World Mental Health (WMH) surveys: type-severity of trauma (Ozer et al., 2003; Roberts et al., 2011); socio-demographics (Brewin et al., 2000; Breslau, 2002; Tolin & Foa, 2006); cumulative prior trauma exposure, including exposure to childhood adversities (CAs) (Brewin et al., 2000; Ozer et al., 2003; DiGangi et al., 2013); prior mental disorders (DiGangi et al., 2013; Heron-Delaney et al., 2013); and acute emotional and biological responses. Our focus with regard to the last of these predictor sets was the DSM-IV A1 criterion, but research has shown that more nuanced dimensions of peritraumatic emotional and biological reactions are more important than the A1 criterion (Brewin et al., 2000; Ozer et al., 2003; Heron-Delaney et al., 2013; van Zuiden et al., 2013). Other research has shown that social factors and secondary stressors occurring in the days and weeks *after* trauma exposure (e.g., low social support, heightened life stress) also predict onset of PTSD (Brewin et al., 2000; Ozer et al., 2003), although these post-trauma variables were not assessed in the WMH surveys.

Until recently, this literature has offered no guidance on how to combine information about these predictors into an optimal PTSD risk algorithm. Machine learning methods have been used to develop similar algorithms in other areas of medicine (Baca-Garcia et al., 2006; Connor et al., 2007). However, most studies using information obtained shortly after trauma exposure to predict PTSD are based on samples too small (typically $n = 100$–300) to apply these methods. This limitation could be overcome if future prospective studies were either much larger or used much more consistent measures (to allow individual-level data pooling for secondary analysis) than studies carried out up to now.

But a preliminary PTSD risk algorithm could be developed using the first four classes of predictors enumerated earlier (i.e., socio-demographics, type of focal trauma, prior trauma exposure, and prior psychopathology) based on an analysis of the WMH data. Although limited by being cross-sectional and relying on retrospective reports to examine associations of putative predictors with subsequent PTSD, such a preliminary prediction algorithm, if successful, could be validated in small prospective studies that are themselves too small for algorithm development and used as composite risk scores in future prospective studies to borrow strength from the large WMH series.

Given these assumptions, we developed a machine learning PTSD risk model from the WMH data. Our published work in this area (Kessler et al., 2014) coincided with two reports of analyses attempting to develop similar models that were based on much smaller prospective samples using methods of questionable validity (Galatzer-Levy et al., 2014; Karstoft et al., 2015). Based in part on the results of these initial studies, a much larger prospective study currently underway (the AURORA study) aims to build a more definitive prediction model. In this chapter, we review the results of the PTSD risk algorithm developed from cross-sectional data in the WMH surveys.

Methods

The analysis made use of data from all 26 of the WMH surveys described in Chapter 2. In order to increase statistical power, we combined reports of PTSD associated with random traumas and with worst traumas among respondents with a lifetime history of exposure to multiple traumas. Observations of worst traumas were assigned a trauma weight of 1.0 (i.e., PTSD associated with worst traumas was assessed for all respondents), while observations of random traumas were assigned a weight representing the inverse of the probability of selection of the one random trauma for a given respondent.

Three broad classes of predictors were included in the analysis: socio-demographics, traumas, and history of mental disorders. Childhood adversities (CAs) were not included because, as noted in Chapter 10, several important CAs were omitted from some surveys. The measures of socio-demographics in the analysis included sex along with three measures defined as of the time the focal trauma occurred – respondent age, education, and marital status. The trauma measures in the analysis included separate dummy variables for prior (to the focal trauma) lifetime exposure to each of the trauma types assessed in the surveys, dummy variables for the type of focal trauma, count variables for number of prior lifetime traumas in each of the trauma factors reported in Chapter 3, and nested dichotomies for each of these counts (e.g., exposure to one or more trauma types in the factor, two or more, and three or more). The prior (to respondent age at the time of the focal trauma) lifetime mental disorders included in the analysis were the same as those in Chapter 11.

The statistical analysis methods used were different from those used in other chapters. We used five separate algorithms to predict PTSD. While the first algorithm was the standard logistic regression modeling approach used in several other chapters in this volume, which included all of the predictors described earlier, the other four were machine learning algorithms. The machine learning algorithms included random forests (Breiman, 2001) and three elastic net penalized logistic regressions (Friedman et al., 2010). These algorithms were used to address two problems in conventional multiple regression: that coefficients are unstable when high correlations exist among predictors, as is the case with the predictors considered here, leading to low replication of predictions in independent samples (Berk, 2008); and that conventional regression assumes additivity, whereas the predictors considered here might have non-additive effects (Ozer et al., 2003; Tolin & Foa, 2006; DiGangi et al., 2013).

Random forests is an ensemble machine learning method that generates many regression trees to detect interactions, each of which is based on a separate bootstrapped pseudo-sample to protect against overfitting, and assigns individual-level predicted probabilities of outcomes based on modal values across replicates (Breiman, 2001). The algorithm was implemented in R-package randomForest (Liaw & Wiener, 2002). The R-package r-part (Thernau et al., 2012) was also used to examine the distribution of higher-order interactions underlying the data.

Elastic net penalized regression is an approach that trades off bias to decrease standard errors of estimates, reducing instability caused by high correlations among predictors, using a mixing parameter penalty (MPP) that varies in the range 0 to 1. The three penalties we used included: the lasso penalty (MPP = 1.0), which favors sparse models that force coefficients for all but one predictor in each strongly correlated set to zero; the ridge penalty (MPP = 0), which uses proportional coefficient shrinkage to retain all predictors; and an intermediate elastic net (MPP = 0.5), which combines both approaches. Internal cross-validation was used to select the coefficient in front of the penalty. The algorithms were implemented in the R-package *glmnet* (Friedman et al., 2010).

Finally, we used an ensembling method known as Super Learner (van der Laan et al., 2007; van der Laan

& Rose, 2011) to generate an optimally weighted composite prediction algorithm averaged across the five individual algorithms, using internal cross-validation implemented in the R-package Super Learner (Polley & van der Laan, 2011).

It is important to note that the internal cross-validation used in the penalized regressions improve on a more conventional approach that fits a model in a discovery sample and then tests the model fit in a hold-out sample in two ways. First, the internal cross-validation used the 10-fold cross-validation technique, which divides the sample into 10 equal subsamples and estimates a model for each of a large number of fixed coefficients in front of the penalty 10 times, in each of which one of the subsamples is held out and then the coefficients are applied to the hold-out sample. Model fit is then estimated across the 10 hold-out subsamples to evaluate model fit for the fixed value of the coefficient in front of the penalty. The value of that coefficient is then selected to maximize cross-validated model fit. Second, MPP itself was varied, which leads to variation in the number of predictors in the model. Super Learner applied a separate 10-fold cross-validation to this entire set of procedures to assign differential weights to the models with different MPP values as well as to the other algorithms.

Individual-level predicted PTSD probabilities based on the separate algorithms and super learner were created, receiver operating characteristic (ROC) curves generated, and area under the curve (AUC) calculated to evaluate prediction accuracy. Super learner predicted probabilities were then discretized into ventiles (20 groups of equal size ordered by predicted probabilities of PTSD) and cross-classified with observed PTSD. As prior PTSD was a dominant predictor in all algorithms, analysis was replicated for the 45,556 trauma exposures that occurred to respondents without a history of prior PTSD.

Results

Overall Prediction Accuracy

ROC curves showed that Super Learner substantially outperformed the individual algorithms other than random forests (AUC = 0.96 vs. 0.90 in the total sample; 0.97 vs. 0.85 in the subsample with no prior PTSD) (see Figure 22.1). Inspection of observed PTSD distributions across ventiles of predicted risk based on super learner shows 95.6% of observed PTSD cases occurred after the 10% of traumas having highest predicted probabilities of PTSD (see Figure 22.2). Conditional PTSD risk was 56.3% in the highest ventile, 20.0% in the second highest ventile, and 0.0–1.3% in the remaining 18 ventiles. In the subsample with no history of prior PTSD, 91.9% of observed PTSD occurred after the 10% of traumas having highest predicted probabilities of PTSD. Conditional PTSD risk was 32.2% for the highest ventile, 13.0% for the second highest ventile, and 0.0–1.2% in the remaining 18 ventiles.

Stability of Results

Results were found to be stable across subsamples defined by individual-level characteristics (sex, age, and income) and country-level characteristics (economic development, recent history of war or sectarian violence) (see Table 22.1). Between 94.3% and 97.6% of observed PTSD cases in each subsample were found among the 10% of cases having highest predicted probabilities (92.6–96.4% in the subsample with no prior PTSD). PTSD prevalence in these high-risk subsamples was 33.9–52.6% (20.5–33.2% in the subsample with no prior PTSD).

Components of Risk

It is hazardous to interpret individual machine learning model coefficients because the algorithms maximize overall prediction accuracy at the expense of individual coefficient accuracy. Nonetheless, an understanding of important predictors can be useful. We used a two-part approach to achieve this understanding. We first examined multivariate predictor profiles in 100 bootstrapped *rpart* trees to determine which interactions were important. These profiles all involved history of prior PTSD interacting either with history of prior unexpected death of a loved one and/or with history of prior sexual assault victimization (either rape or other sexual assault). We then included dummy predictor variables for those multivariate profiles in modified lasso regressions and compared ORs $\geq$1.5 or $\leq$1.5 in this model with those in additive lasso models.

Socio-demographic differences in PTSD risk were restricted to elevated odds-ratios (ORs) among women (OR = 1.5–1.6) and the previously married (OR = 1.5) (see Table 22.2). Nine trauma types also had elevated ORs, all but one of which (the exception being exposure to a life-threatening accident, with ORs of 1.4–1.8) involved interpersonal violence: rape (OR = 3.2–3.5), kidnap (OR = 1.8–3.4), childhood physical abuse (OR = 1.5–1.8), witnessing atrocities (OR = 1.4), and

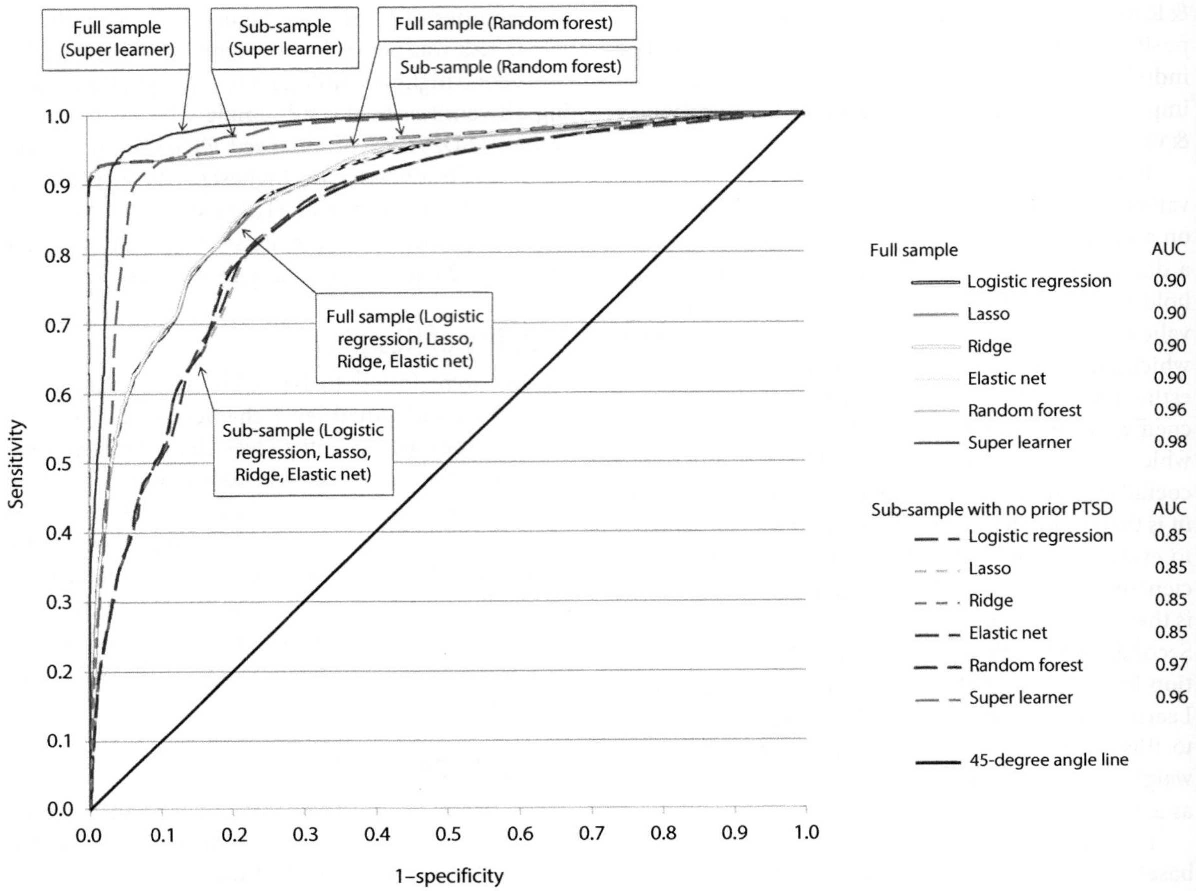

Figure 22.1 ROC curves for predicted probability of DSM-IV/CIDI PTSD after trauma exposure based on the different algorithms in the total sample ($n = 47{,}466$) and the subsample of exposures occurring to respondents with no history of prior PTSD ($n = 45{,}556$)

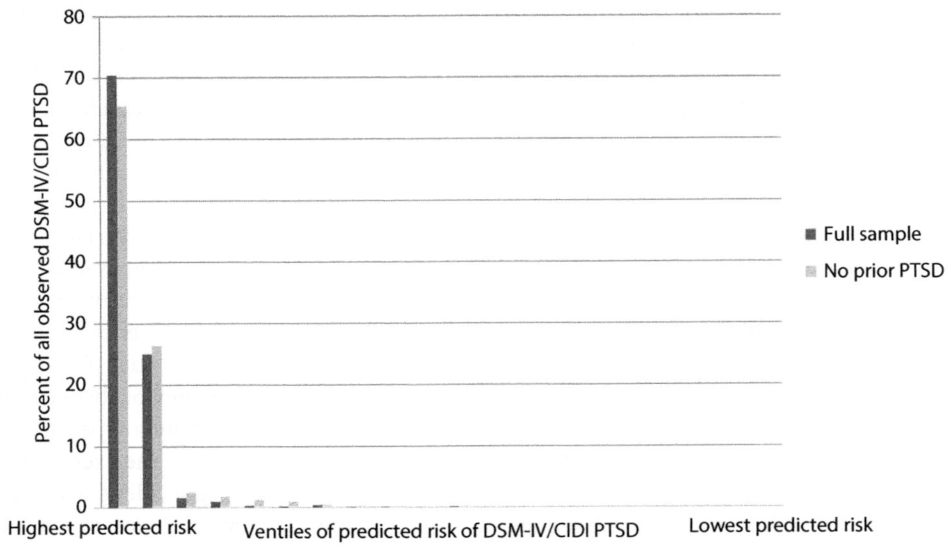

Figure 22.2 Concentration of risk for DSM-IV/CIDI PTSD

Table 22.1 Concentration of observed DSM-IV/CIDI PTSD in the 10% of exposures having highest predicted risk based on the Super Learner algorithm across subsamples

	Percentage of all PTSD associated with the 10% of exposures having highest predicted risk				Conditional observed PTSD risk in the 10% of exposures having highest predicted risk versus other exposures							
	Total sample		Respondents with no prior PTSD		Total sample				Respondents with no prior PTSD			
					Top 10%		Other 90%		Top 10%		Other 90%	
	%	(SE)	%	(SE)	%	(SE)	%	(SE)	%	(SE)	%	(SE)
I Country Income												
High-income	95.5	(0.6)	94.3	(0.8)	34.3	(1.5)	0.26	(0.03)	20.5	(1.2)	0.20	(0.03)
Low- and middle-income	95.3	(2.0)	92.6	(3.2)	52.6	(3.6)	0.14	(0.06)	33.2	(4.2)	0.13	(0.06)
II Age (Years)												
<25	95.2	(0.9)	93.3	(1.4)	41.5	(2.4)	0.22	(0.04)	23.0	(2.3)	0.18	(0.03)
≥25	95.8	(1.2)	94.6	(1.8)	33.9	(2.0)	0.18	(0.05)	23.3	(1.6)	0.16	(0.06)
III Sex												
Female	94.3	(1.0)	92.6	(1.4)	35.9	(1.4)	0.40	(0.07)	21.4	(1.1)	0.34	(0.07)
Male	97.6	(0.6)	96.4	(1.1)	43.4	(3.8)	0.06	(0.01)	27.7	(4.2)	0.05	(0.01)
IV Education[a]												
Low/low-average	94.7	(0.8)	92.6	(1.2)	37.5	(1.8)	0.24	(0.04)	21.0	(1.4)	0.20	(0.03)
High/high-average	96.9	(1.4)	96.1	(2.1)	39.5	(3.1)	0.13	(0.06)	28.2	(2.9)	0.11	(0.06)
V Country Involved in War or Sectarian Violence[b]												
Yes	95.9	(1.7)	94.4	(2.5)	44.4	(5.2)	0.13	(0.05)	28.8	(5.2)	0.13	(0.05)
No	95.3	(0.8)	93.6	(1.2)	36.6	(1.3)	0.23	(0.04)	21.6	(1.0)	0.19	(0.04)

[a]Educational level relative to others in the same country.
[b]Countries classified *yes* include Colombia, Israel, Lebanon, Nigeria, Northern Ireland, and South Africa.

Table 22.2 Lasso penalized logistic regression coefficients to predict onset of DSM-IV/CIDI PTSD after exposure to a focal trauma[a]

	Total sample	Subsample without prior PTSD	Total sample with interaction
	OR	OR	OR
I Focal Trauma			
Exposure to organized violence			
Witnessed atrocities	1.4	1.4	1.4
Witnessed death/dead body/serious injury	0.6	0.7	0.6
Kidnapped	3.0	1.8	3.4
Physical violence victimization			
Beaten by caregiver	1.5		
Sexual violence victimization			
Raped	3.2	3.5	3.5
Sexually assaulted			1.5
Beaten by spouse/romantic partner	1.8	1.5	1.7
Private trauma[b]	1.8	1.5	1.8
Some other trauma	1.6		1.5
Other			
Toxic chemical exposure	0.5	0.6	0.5
Natural disaster	0.4		0.5
Other life-threatening accident	1.8	1.4	1.6

(cont.)

Table 22.2 (*cont.*)

	Total sample	Subsample without prior PTSD	Total sample with interaction
	OR	OR	OR
II Collateral Traumas			
Multiple (2+) participants in organized violence	2.5	3.8	2.7
High (3+) exposure to physical violence	6.8	11.5	9.3
Any exposure to sexual violence	1.6	1.7	1.6
Multiple (2+) exposures to sexual violence	4.0	3.2	3.5
UD of a loved one	2.1	2.1	2.2
III Socio-demographics			
Female		1.6	1.5
Previously married	1.5		1.5
IV Lifetime Prior Traumas			
Witnessed atrocities	1.6	1.8	1.6
Raped		2.3	1.6
Sexually assaulted			1.4
UD of a loved one			1.6
V Lifetime Prior DSM-IV/CIDI Disorders			
GAD	2.2	2.5	2.2
PTSD	27.2		
Specific phobia			1.5
Separation anxiety disorder	2.0	1.7	1.9
ADHD	1.6		1.7
VI Interactions of Lifetime Prior PTSD with Lifetime Prior…			
Sexual violence and UD of a loved one			5.4
Sexual violence but no UD of a loved one			12.9
UD of a loved one but no sexual violence			5.7
Neither sexual violence nor UD of a loved one			134.7
(*n*)	(47,466)	(45,556)	(47,466)

[a]Based on Lasso penalized regression models. The model with interactions included the dominant interactions found in the *rpart* simulations. No CIs are reported because SEs are biased when predictors are selected from a larger set using machine learning methods.
[b]A *private* event is a trauma that some individuals reported in response to a question asked at the very end of the trauma section that asked if they ever had some other very upsetting experience they did not tell us about already (and this includes in response to a prior open-ended question about "any other" trauma) because they were too embarrassed or upset to talk about it. Respondents were told, before they answered, that if they reported such a trauma we would not ask them anything about what it was, only about their age when the trauma happened.

four other (than rape) trauma types in the relationship-sexual violence factor (OR = 1.5–1.8). Three trauma types had meaningfully reduced ORs: witnessing death/injury, toxic chemical spill, and natural disasters (OR = 0.4-0.7).

Five summary measures of collateral trauma types occurring in the same year as the focal trauma had meaningful ORs. Four of these five (the exception being unexpected death of a loved one) involved violence: 2+ traumas in the organized violence factor, 3+ traumas in the interpersonal violence factor, and any as well as 2+ traumas in the relationship-sexual violence factor. The collateral traumas involving single exposures (sexual or death) had ORs of 1.6–2.2, while those involving 2–3+ exposures had ORs of 2.5–11.5.

Also, 4 of the 29 prior lifetime trauma types had meaningful ORs, all of them elevated: witnessing atrocities (OR = 1.6–1.8), being raped (OR = 1.6–2.3) or sexually assaulted (OR = 1.4), and experiencing the unexpected death of a loved one (OR = 1.6).

In total, 5 of the 14 prior lifetime DSM-IV/CIDI disorders had meaningful ORs: attention-deficit/hyperactivity disorder (OR = 1.6–1.7), separation anxiety disorder (OR = 1.7–2.0), specific phobia (OR = 1.5), generalized anxiety disorder (OR = 2.2–2.5), and PTSD (OR = 27.2). The high OR for prior PTSD was due to the 3.5% of exposures occurring to respondents with prior PTSD accounting for 40.5% of all episodes of PTSD. Disaggregation into underlying multivariate profiles showed that this strong effect of prior PTSD was limited to individuals marked as vulnerable by virtue of having past PTSD after exposure to traumas generally not associated with high PTSD risk.

Discussion

Although caution is needed in interpreting these results because the WMH data were based on retrospective reports and fully structured lay-administered diagnostic interviews, it is nonetheless striking that we were able to produce a prediction algorithm in which the vast majority of PTSD cases were associated with the 10% of trauma exposures having highest predicted risk. By far the most powerful predictor in the algorithm was history of prior PTSD, but several other prior lifetime mental disorders were also significant predictors along with a number of measures of prior lifetime trauma exposure as well as socio-demographic factors and characteristics of the focal trauma.

Limitations introduced by the retrospective nature of the data could have led to upward bias in ORs if respondents defined as having a history of PTSD were more likely than others to recall prior lifetime trauma exposures and/or mental disorders. Importantly, the literature shows that this type of bias does, in fact, exist in retrospective reports among individuals with PTSD (Roemer et al., 1998; Harvey & Bryant, 2000; Zoellner et al., 2000). In addition, the concentration-of-risk estimates could have been upwardly biased compared to those that would be found among individuals who sought help in the immediate aftermath of trauma exposure in criminal justice or healthcare settings to the extent that this help-seeking predicted subsequent PTSD.

Despite these limitations, the results suggest that a PTSD risk algorithm based on machine learning methods might help improve the cost-effectiveness of preventive interventions for PTSD by pinpointing the small proportion of trauma-exposed individuals having high PTSD risk who account for most subsequent cases of PTSD. Our study is much larger than all other previous attempts to predict onset of PTSD from information about trauma types and pretrauma predictors. We showed that a composite risk score can be constructed from such data that classifies the vast majority of individuals who go on to develop PTSD into a high-risk segment of the population.

However, external validation of the risk algorithms in prospective samples is needed. A number of such prospective studies exist. All these studies are much smaller than the WMH database and not all assessed the full range of predictors considered in our analysis. Nonetheless, the strong results found here suggest that it would be valuable to carry out replications in these prospective studies. We are currently involved in several collaborative replication analyses of this sort and are eager to work with other researchers to evaluate the extent to which our algorithm fits in independent prospective samples. In addition, we are interested in collaborating with other groups to apply the methods used here to determine the predictive accuracy of algorithms based on data involving an expanded set of predictors, including biomarkers that might strengthen the algorithm. If the results of this ongoing work are encouraging, subsequent prospective studies should be designed so that they include the full range of predictors found to be important in these studies. This would advance the agenda of creating broadly useful PTSD risk algorithms (and subsequent algorithms to predict other psychopathological responses to trauma exposure) to target preventive interventions across a wide range of settings.

It is important to note that different predictors will almost certainly be found to be important in different populations (e.g., military personnel, first responders in disaster situations, civilians in less developed countries), in predicting PTSD associated with different traumas (e.g., sectarian violence in war zones or regions of terror, large-scale natural disasters), and screening settings (e.g., temporary emergency clinics established at the site of natural or manmade disasters, medical clinics in war zones, trauma units, emergency departments) (Brewin et al., 2000; Ozer et al., 2003; Heron-Delaney et al., 2013; van Zuiden et al., 2013). This means that an expansion of the current line of work will ultimately lead either to the development of a family of risk prediction algorithms or to a consolidated master algorithm that allows for complex interactions across populations, traumas, and screening settings. Developing such algorithms will require sensitivity to the variation in the costs of collecting different types of data (e.g., self-reports versus biomarkers), even data ostensibly assessing the same underlying constructs (e.g., self-reports of impulsivity versus neurocognitive tests of impulsivity), as well as the burdens of administering detailed risk factors assessments (both the time and the awkwardness associated with asking patients detailed questions of a sensitive nature in the immediate aftermath of trauma exposure). Thoughtful analysis will be needed of the cost–benefit trade-offs of including or excluding expensive and burdensome elements of the assessments, depending on strength of predictions. A consideration of the staging of assessments will doubtlessly be important here both to determine individual differences and the extent to which expensive or burdensome assessments might or might not be pivotal in determining clinical responses in light of the strength of provisional predictions, based on predictors that can be obtained inexpensively and without undue patient burden.

Acknowledgment

Portions of this chapter are based on Kessler, R. C., Rose, S., Koenen, K. C., et al. (2014). How well can post-traumatic stress disorder be predicted from pre-trauma risk factors? An exploratory study in the WHO World Mental Health Surveys. *World Psychiatry*, **13**, 265–74, by permission of Wiley-Blackwell.

References

Baca-Garcia, E., Perez-Rodriguez, M. M., Basurte-Villamor, I., et al. (2006). Using data mining to explore complex clinical decisions: a study of hospitalization after a suicide attempt. *Journal of Clinical Psychiatry*, 67, 1124–32.

Berk, R. A. (2008). *Statistical Learning from a Regression Perspective*. New York, NY: Springer.

Breiman, L. (2001). Random forests. *Machine Learning*, 45, 5–32.

Breslau, N. (2002). Epidemiologic studies of trauma, posttraumatic stress disorder, and other psychiatric disorders. *The Canadian Journal of Psychiatry. La Revue Canadienne de Psychiatrie*, 47, 923–9.

Brewin, C. R., Andrews, B., & Valentine, J. D. (2000). Meta-analysis of risk factors for posttraumatic stress disorder in trauma-exposed adults. *Journal of Consulting and Clinical Psychology*, 68, 748–66.

Connor, J. P., Symons, M., Feeney, G. F., Young, R. M., & Wiles, J. (2007). The application of machine learning techniques as an adjunct to clinical decision making in alcohol dependence treatment. *Substance Use and Misuse*, 42, 2193–206.

DiGangi, J. A., Gomez, D., Mendoza, L., et al. (2013). Pretrauma risk factors for posttraumatic stress disorder: a systematic review of the literature. *Clinical Psychology Review*, 33, 728–44.

Forneris, C. A., Gartlehner, G., Brownley, K. A., et al. (2013). Interventions to prevent post-traumatic stress disorder: a systematic review. *American Journal of Preventive Medicine*, 44, 635–50.

Friedman, J., Hastie, T., & Tibshirani, R. (2010). Regularization paths for generalized linear models via coordinate descent. *Journal of Statistical Software*, 33, 1–22.

Galatzer-Levy, I. R., Karstoft, K. I., Statnikov, A., & Shalev, A. Y. (2014). Quantitative forecasting of PTSD from early trauma responses: a Machine Learning application. *Journal of Psychiatric Research*, 59, 68–76.

Harvey, A. G., & Bryant, R. A. (2000). Memory for acute stress disorder symptoms: a two-year prospective study. *Journal of Nervous and Mental Disease*, 188, 602–7.

Heron-Delaney, M., Kenardy, J., Charlton, E., & Matsuoka, Y. (2013). A systematic review of predictors of posttraumatic stress disorder (PTSD) for adult road traffic crash survivors. *Injury*, 44, 1413–22.

Iyadurai, L., Blackwell, S. E., Meiser-Stedman, R., et al. (2018). Preventing intrusive memories after trauma via a brief intervention involving Tetris computer game play in the emergency department: a proof-of-concept randomized controlled trial. *Molecular Psychiatry*, 23, 674–82.

James, E. L., Bonsall, M. B., Hoppitt, L., et al. (2015). Computer game play reduces intrusive memories of experimental trauma via reconsolidation-update mechanisms. *Psychological Science*, 26, 1201–15.

Karstoft, K. I., Galatzer-Levy, I. R., Statnikov, A., Li, Z., & Shalev, A. Y. (2015). Bridging a translational gap: using machine learning to improve the prediction of PTSD. *BMC Psychiatry*, 15, 30.

Kessler, R. (2000). Posttraumatic stress disorder: the burden to the individual and to society. *Journal of Clinical Psychiatry*, 61, 4–12; discussion 13–4.

Kessler, R. C., Rose, S., Koenen, K. C., et al. (2014). How well can post-traumatic stress disorder be predicted from pre-trauma risk factors? An exploratory study in the WHO World Mental Health Surveys. *World Psychiatry*, 13, 265–74.

Kliem, S., & Kroger, C. (2013). Prevention of chronic PTSD with early cognitive behavioral therapy. A meta-analysis using mixed-effects modeling. *Behaviour Research and Therapy*, 51, 753–61.

Liaw, A., & Wiener, M. (2002). Classification and regression by randomForest. *R News*, 2, 18–22.

Ostrowski, S. A., & Delahanty, D. L. (2014). Prospects for the pharmacological prevention of post-traumatic stress in vulnerable individuals. *CNS Drugs*, 28, 195–203.

Ozer, E. J., Best, S. R., Lipsey, T. L., & Weiss, D. S. (2003). Predictors of posttraumatic stress disorder and symptoms in adults: a meta-analysis. *Psychological Bulletin*, 129, 52–73.

Polley, E. C., & van der Laan, M. J. (2011). *SuperLearner: Super Learner Prediction, Package Version 2.0-4*. Vienna, Austria: R Foundation for Statistical Computing.

Qi, W., Gevonden, M., & Shalev, A. (2016). Prevention of post-traumatic stress disorder after trauma: current evidence and future directions. *Current Psychiatry Reports*, 18, 20.

Roberts, A. L., Gilman, S. E., Breslau, J., Breslau, N., & Koenen, K. C. (2011). Race/ethnic differences in exposure to traumatic events, development of post-traumatic stress disorder, and treatment-seeking for post-traumatic stress disorder in the United States. *Psychological Medicine*, 41, 71–83.

Robin, N. (2012). Tetris shown to lessen PTSD and flashbacks (online). Available at: www.scientificamerican.com/article/tetris-shown-to-lessen-ptsd-and-flashbacks/ (Accessed April 30, 2017).

Roemer, L., Litz, B. T., Orsillo, S. M., Ehlich, P. J., & Friedman, M. J. (1998). Increases in retrospective accounts of war-zone exposure over time: the role of PTSD symptom severity. *Journal of Traumatic Stress*, 11, 597–605.

Shalev, A. Y., Ankri, Y., Israeli-Shalev, Y., et al. (2012). Prevention of posttraumatic stress disorder by early treatment: results from the Jerusalem Trauma Outreach and Prevention study. *Archives of General Psychiatry*, 69, 166–76.

Thernau, T., Atkinson, B., & Ripley, B. (2012). rpart: Recursive Partitioning. R Package 4.1-0.

Tolin, D. F., & Foa, E. B. (2006). Sex differences in trauma and posttraumatic stress disorder: a quantitative review of 25 years of research. *Psychological Bulletin*, 132, 959–92.

van der Laan, M. J., Polley, E. C., & Hubbard, A. E. (2007). Super learner. *Statistical Applications in Genetics and Molecular Biology*, 6, Article 25.

van der Laan, M. J., & Rose, S. (2011). *Targeted Learning: Causal Inference for Observational and Experimental Data*. New York, NY: Springer.

Van Zuiden, M., Kavelaars, A., Geuze, E., Olff, M., & Heijnen, C. J. (2013). Predicting PTSD: pre-existing vulnerabilities in glucocorticoid-signaling and implications for preventive interventions. *Brain, Behavior, and Immunity*, 30, 12–21.

Zoellner, L. A., Foa, E. B., Brigidi, B. D., & Przeworski, A. (2000). Are trauma victims susceptible to "false memories"? *Journal of Abnormal Psychology*, 109, 517–24.

Chapter 23

The Population Burden of Posttraumatic Stress Disorder

Ronald C. Kessler, Sergio Aguilar-Gaxiola, Jordi Alonso, Sing Lee, and Karestan C. Koenen

As noted in Chapter 2, the population burden of posttraumatic stress disorder (PTSD) is most directly represented either as the point prevalence of the disorder or as the number of years in episode of the disorder per capita in the population. It is clear from the results reported so far that the magnitude of the associations of any predictor of 30-day prevalence will be a joint function of its strength in predicting exposure to specific trauma types, onset of PTSD among those exposed to these trauma types, and persistence of PTSD among the latter cases. Relative prevalence of the separate trauma types is also a critical aspect of these burden calculations. In this chapter, we trace out these pathways to examine the relative importance of different trauma types in accounting for the overall societal burden of PTSD.

Prevalence and Distribution of Trauma Exposure

We saw in Chapter 3 that 70.4% of World Mental Health (WMH) respondents experienced at least one trauma in their lifetimes. Mean number of lifetime trauma types among those with any was 2.0, for 1.4 trauma types for capita (i.e., 0.704 × 2.0) (see Table 23.1). By far the most common trauma types at the respondent-level (i.e., whether or not this type of trauma ever occurred to the respondent, ignoring how many times it occurred) were unexpected death (UD) of a loved one (reported by 31.4% of respondents) and direct exposure (i.e., witnessing or discovering) to death or serious injury (23.7%). The next most common trauma types at the respondent level were muggings (14.4%), life-threatening automobile accidents (14.0%), and life-threatening illnesses (11.8%). "Private" traumas were reported by 4.9% of respondents. When considered in terms of broader categories, the most common traumas at the respondent level were those that either occurred to a loved one or were witnessed (35.7% of respondents), those involving accidents (34.3%), and death of a loved one (31.49%) followed by physical violence (22.9%), intimate partner-sexual violence (14.0%), war-related traumas (13.1%), and "other" traumas (8.4%).

The aforementioned results did not take into consideration that the mean number of exposures varied significantly across trauma types for the 18 traumas that were assessed for frequency ($\chi^2_{17} = 1{,}528.4$, $p < 0.001$). (The other trauma types were not assessed for frequency because they represented ongoing situations rather than discrete events.) When we multiplied the proportion of respondents with any lifetime exposure to a given trauma type by mean number of exposures among those with any, we found a mean number of exposures to any trauma among those with any of 4.6. This translates into 3.2 lifetime trauma exposures per capita (i.e., 704 with any exposure × 4.6). The societal burden of these traumas is concentrated among traumas that happen to others, either death of a loved one (16.5% of all traumas) or other traumas that happened to a loved one or that the respondent witnessed (25.0%), collectively accounting for over 40% of all trauma exposures. Another 24.6% of traumas were accidents and another roughly one-fourth either intimate partner-sexual violence (9.8%) or physical violence (13.8%). The remaining categories of war-related (7.4%) and "other" (2.8%) traumas were much less common.

Differential Risk of PTSD Depending on Trauma Type

As detailed in Chapter 5, conditional risk of DSM-IV/CIDI PTSD after trauma exposure was 4.0% overall and varied significantly by trauma type (see Table 23.2). The highest conditional risk was associated with being raped (19.0%), physically abused by a romantic partner (11.7%), kidnapped (11.0%), and sexually assaulted other than rape (10.5%). In terms of broader categories, the traumas associated with the highest PTSD risk

Table 23.1 Prevalence and distribution of lifetime traumas in the WMH surveys ($n = 68{,}894$)

	Person-level lifetime prevalence[a]		Mean exposures given any[b]		Number of exposures per 100 people[c]		Each trauma type as a percentage of all traumas[d]	
	%	(SE)	Mean	(SE)	Est	(SE)	%	(SE)
I War-Related Trauma								
Relief worker in war zone	1.0	(0.1)	–	–	1.0	(0.1)	0.3	(0.0)
Civilian in war zone	4.4	(0.1)	–	–	4.4	(0.1)	1.4	(0.0)
Civilian in region of terror	3.4	(0.1)	–	–	3.4	(0.1)	1.1	(0.0)
Refugee	2.2	(0.1)	–	–	2.2	(0.1)	0.7	(0.0)
Combat experience	3.1	(0.1)			3.1	(0.1)	1.0	(0.0)
Purposely injured/tortured/killed someone	0.9	(0.1)	2.5	(0.1)	2.1	(0.1)	0.7	(0.0)
Witnessed atrocities	3.7	(0.1)	2.1	(0.0)	7.6	(0.2)	2.4	(0.1)
Any	13.1	(0.2)	1.8	(0.0)	23.9	(0.5)	7.4	(0.1)
II Physical Violence Victimization								
Beaten by caregiver	7.9	(0.2)	–	–	7.9	(0.2)	2.5	(0.0)
Beaten by someone else	5.9	(0.1)	2.0	(0.0)	11.5	(0.3)	3.6	(0.1)
Mugged/threatened with a weapon	14.5	(0.2)	1.6	(0.0)	23.7	(0.4)	7.4	(0.1)
Kidnapped	1.1	(0.1)	1.1	(0.0)	1.2	(0.1)	0.4	(0.0)
Any	22.9	(0.3)	1.9	(0.0)	44.3	(0.6)	13.8	(0.2)
III Sexual Violence Victimization								
Raped	3.2	(0.1)	1.8	(0.0)	5.8	(0.2)	1.8	(0.1)
Sexually assaulted	5.8	(0.1)	2.0	(0.0)	11.7	(0.3)	3.6	(0.1)
Stalked	5.3	(0.1)	1.8	(0.0)	9.5	(0.2)	3.0	(0.1)
Beaten by spouse/romantic partner	4.5	(0.1)	–	–	4.5	(0.1)	1.4	(0.0)
Any	14.0	(0.2)	2.3	(0.0)	31.5	(0.6)	9.8	(0.2)
IV Accidents/Injuries								
Automobile accident	14.0	(0.2)	1.4	(0.0)	19.6	(0.3)	6.1	(0.1)
Other life-threatening accident	6.2	(0.1)	1.5	(0.0)	9.4	(0.2)	2.9	(0.1)
Natural disaster	7.4	(0.2)	1.8	(0.0)	13.1	(0.5)	4.1	(0.1)
Toxic chemical exposure	4.2	(0.1)	2.7	(0.1)	11.5	(0.4)	3.6	(0.1)
Human-made disaster	4.0	(0.1)	1.7	(0.0)	6.9	(0.2)	2.1	(0.1)
Accidentally caused serious injury/death	1.4	(0.1)	1.6	(0.1)	2.2	(0.1)	0.7	(0.0)
Life-threatening illness	11.8	(0.2)	1.4	(0.0)	16.5	(0.3)	5.1	(0.1)
Any	34.3	(0.3)	2.3	(0.0)	79.2	(1.1)	24.6	(0.2)
V UD of a Loved One	31.4	(0.3)	1.7	(0.0)	53.2	(0.7)	16.5	(0.2)
VI Other Traumas of Loved Ones or Witnessed								
Child with serious illness	7.9	(0.1)	1.3	(0.0)	10.1	(0.2)	3.1	(0.1)
Trauma to loved one	5.6	(0.1)	1.5	(0.0)	8.5	(0.3)	2.7	(0.1)
Witnessed parent violence	7.9	(0.2)	–	–	7.9	(0.2)	2.5	(0.0)
Witnessed death/dead body/serious injury	23.7	(0.3)	2.3	(0.0)	53.9	(0.9)	16.8	(0.2)
Any	35.7	(0.3)	2.2	(0.0)	80.4	(1.0)	25.0	(0.2)
VII Other Traumas								
Some other trauma	4.2	(0.1)	–	–	4.2	(0.1)	1.3	(0.0)
Private trauma[e]	4.9	(0.1)	–	–	4.9	(0.1)	1.5	(0.0)
Any	8.4	(0.2)	1.1	(0.0)	9.1	(0.2)	2.8	(0.1)
VIII Any	70.4	(0.3)	4.6	(0.0)	321.5	(2.9)	100.0	(0.0)

[a]The percent of all respondents who reported ever in their lifetime experiencing the trauma type indicated in the row heading. For example, 3.1% of respondents across surveys reported a history of combat experience.
[b]The mean number of lifetime occurrences of the trauma type indicated in the row heading among those who reported ever experiencing that trauma type. "–" entries indicate that we did not assess number of occurrences for the trauma type. For example, the respondents who reported ever in their life purposely injuring, torturing, or killing someone reported a mean of 2.5 such occurrences.
[c]The number of lifetime occurrences of the trauma type indicated in the row heading per 100 respondents, which equals the product of the two earlier row entries. For example, the 2.5 lifetime occurrences of purposely injuring, torturing, or killing someone reported by 0.9% of respondents results in 2.1 (0.9 × 2.5) lifetime occurrences of such a trauma for every 100 respondents in the sample.
[d]The ratio of the entry in the cell of the previous column to the 321.5 total lifetime traumas for every 100 respondents. For example, the 3.1 instances of combat experience represent approximately 1.0% of the 321.5 total.
[e]A *private* event is a trauma that some individuals reported in response to a question asked at the very end of the trauma section that asked if they ever had some other very upsetting experience they did not tell us about already (and this includes in response to a prior open-ended question about "any other" trauma) because they were too embarrassed or upset to talk about it. Respondents were told, before they answered, that if they reported such a trauma we would not ask them anything about what it was, only about their age when the trauma happened.

Table 23.2 Conditional risk of DSM-IV/CIDI PTSD by trauma category in the WMH surveys

	PTSD risk given trauma exposure[a]		Number of PTSD episodes per 100 people[b]		Percentage of all PTSD episodes for each trauma type[c]		
	%	(SE)	Est	(SE)	%	(SE)	(n)
I War-Related Trauma							
Relief worker in war zone	0.8	(0.7)	0.0	(0.0)	0.1	(0.1)	(139)
Civilian in war zone	1.3	(0.5)	0.1	(0.0)	0.5	(0.2)	(1,050)
Civilian in region of terror	1.6	(0.6)	0.1	(0.0)	0.4	(0.1)	(634)
Refugee	4.5	(2.0)	0.1	(0.0)	0.8	(0.3)	(406)
Combat experience	3.6	(0.8)	0.1	(0.0)	0.9	(0.2)	(535)
Purposely injured/tortured/killed someone	4.0	(3.1)	0.1	(0.1)	0.7	(0.5)	(102)
Witnessed atrocities	5.4	(4.1)	0.4	(0.3)	3.2	(2.2)	(533)
Any	3.5	(1.4)	0.8	(0.3)	6.4	(2.3)	(3,399)
II Physical Violence Victimization							
Beaten by caregiver	5.0	(1.0)	0.4	(0.1)	3.1	(0.6)	(2,082)
Beaten by someone else	2.5	(0.6)	0.3	(0.1)	2.2	(0.6)	(1,201)
Mugged/threatened with a weapon	1.8	(0.4)	0.4	(0.1)	3.4	(0.7)	(3,277)
Kidnapped	11.0	(3.0)	0.1	(0.0)	1.0	(0.3)	(216)
Any	2.8	(0.4)	1.3	(0.2)	9.7	(1.2)	(6,776)
III Sexual Violence Victimization							
Raped	19.0	(2.2)	1.1	(0.1)	8.6	(1.0)	(1,246)
Sexually assaulted	10.5	(1.5)	1.2	(0.2)	9.5	(1.3)	(1,574)
Stalked	7.6	(2.0)	0.7	(0.2)	5.6	(1.4)	(1,160)
Beaten by spouse/romantic partner	11.7	(1.3)	0.5	(0.1)	4.1	(0.5)	(1,675)
Any	11.4	(1.0)	3.6	(0.3)	27.8	(2.0)	(5,655)
IV Accidents/Injuries							
Automobile accident	2.6	(0.4)	0.5	(0.1)	4.0	(0.7)	(3,428)
Other life-threatening accident	4.9	(2.4)	0.5	(0.2)	3.5	(1.6)	(1,205)
Natural disaster	0.3	(0.1)	0.0	(0.0)	0.3	(0.1)	(1,669)
Toxic chemical exposure	0.1	(0.0)	0.0	(0.0)	0.1	(0.0)	(622)
Human-made disaster	2.9	(1.3)	0.2	(0.1)	1.5	(0.7)	(726)
Accidentally caused serious injury/death	2.8	(1.0)	0.1	(0.0)	0.5	(0.1)	(251)
Life-threatening illness	2.0	(0.3)	0.3	(0.1)	2.5	(0.4)	(3,249)
Any	2.0	(0.3)	1.6	(0.3)	12.4	(1.9)	(11,150)
V UD of a Loved One	5.4	(0.5)	2.9	(0.3)	22.2	(1.8)	(10,714)
VI Other Traumas of Loved Ones or Witnessed							
Child with serious illness	4.8	(0.6)	0.5	(0.1)	3.8	(0.5)	(2,452)
Trauma to loved one	5.1	(1.3)	0.4	(0.1)	3.4	(0.8)	(1,173)
Witnessed parent violence	3.8	(0.7)	0.3	(0.1)	2.4	(0.4)	(2,000)
Witnessed death/dead body/serious injury	1.3	(0.3)	0.7	(0.1)	5.5	(1.0)	(5,114)
Any	2.4	(0.2)	1.9	(0.2)	15.0	(1.4)	(10,739)
VII Other Traumas							
Some other trauma	9.1	(1.0)	0.4	(0.0)	3.0	(0.3)	(1,260)
Private trauma[d]	9.2	(1.1)	0.5	(0.1)	3.5	(0.4)	(1,503)
Any	9.2	(0.7)	0.8	(0.1)	6.5	(0.5)	(2,763)
VIII Any	4.0	(0.2)	12.9	(0.7)	100	(0.0)	(51,196)

[a]The conditional risk of PTSD associated with the trauma type indicated in the row heading. For example, 3.6% of combat experiences resulted in DSM-IV/CIDI PTSD.

[b]The mean number of lifetime episodes of PTSD associated with the trauma type indicated in the row heading per 100 respondents. For example, the 3.5% of lifetime war-related traumas that led to PTSD reported in the first column of Table 23.2, when multiplied by the 23.9 lifetime occurrences of such traumas per 100 respondents reported in the third column of Table 23.1, translates into 0.8 lifetime episodes of PTSD due to this category of traumas per 100 respondents.

[c]The ratio of the entry in the cell of the previous column to the total of 12.9 lifetime episodes of PTSD per 100 respondents. For example, the 0.8 cases of PTSD associated with war-related traumas represents 6.4% of the 12.9 total.

[d]A *private* event is a trauma that some individuals reported in response to a question asked at the very end of the trauma section that asked if they ever had some other very upsetting experience they did not tell us about already (and this includes in response to a prior open-ended question about "any other" trauma) because they were too embarrassed or upset to talk about it. Respondents were told, before they answered, that if they reported such a trauma we would not ask them anything about what it was, only about their age when the trauma happened.

were those involving intimate partner-sexual violence (11.4%), with aggregate conditional risk much lower in the other broad trauma categories (2.4–5.4%).

Prevalence of trauma exposure and conditional risk of PTSD both need to be considered in evaluating the trauma-specific population burden of PTSD. Given that 4.6 trauma exposures occurred per capita in the population, the 4.0% aggregate conditional risk of PTSD would translate into 18.4 lifetime episodes of PTSD per 100 people in the population. The trauma type associated with by far the highest number of these PTSD cases based on these calculations was UD of a loved one (2.9 episodes of PTSD/100 population; 22.2% of all lifetime episodes of PTSD), with rape (1.1 episodes of PTSD/100 population; 8.6% of all lifetime episodes) and sexual assault other than rape (1.2 episodes of PTSD/100 population; 9.5% of all lifetime episodes) together accounting for another 18.1% of lifetime episodes. As noted earlier, UD is a very common type of trauma (53.2/100 population; 16.5% of all lifetime traumas) with a high-average conditional risk of PTSD (5.4%), whereas rape and other sexual assault are less common (5.8–11.7 lifetime occurrences/100 population; 1.8–3.6% of all lifetime traumas) with much higher condition risks of PTSD (19.0–10.5%).

Four of the six trauma types associated with highest population proportions of lifetime PTSD episodes were in the category of intimate partner-sexual violence. These included 4.1% of all lifetime PTSD episodes associated with physical abuse by a romantic partner, 8.6% with rape, 9.5% with other sexual assault, and 5.6% with being stalked, for a total of 27.8% of all lifetime episodes of PTSD. Intimate partner-sexual traumas accounted for 9.8% of all lifetime trauma exposures and were associated with comparatively high conditional risk of PTSD. The only other trauma types accounting for as many cases of PTSD were the two most commonly occurring traumas considered here: UD of a loved one (22.2% of all cases of PTSD), which, as noted earlier, was the second most common trauma (16.5% of all traumas) associated with high-average conditional risk of PTSD, and direct exposure to death or serious injury (5.5% of all cases of PTSD), which was the most common trauma (16.8% of all traumas) and was associated with a comparatively low risk of PTSD (1.3%).

It is also relevant that the results in Chapter 9 showed that the vast majority of prior trauma types were significantly and positively associated with subsequent trauma exposure, the strongest of these associations (OR = 2.0–2.5) being for one type of physical violence (e.g., physical abuse in childhood) predicting other types of subsequent physical violence (e.g., being mugged) and intimate partner-sexual violence. It is especially important in light of this fact that we found in Chapter 9 that individuals with a history of prior trauma exposure were more likely than others to develop PTSD after exposure to subsequent traumas.

Persistence of PTSD Symptoms

As noted in Chapter 16, mean duration of PTSD varies widely across cases. The longest median duration was 5 years for PTSD symptoms associated with war-related traumas followed by 3 years for traumas involving physical or intimate partner-sexual violence. Median durations were only 1–2 years, in comparison, for PTSD due to the other broad trauma categories (see Table 23.3). Total population burden of PTSD associated with each trauma type was then calculated by multiplying these episode duration estimates by trauma-specific episode frequency estimates. When trauma-specific products were summed across all trauma types, we estimated that there were 77.7 lifetime person-years of PTSD in the population per 100 respondents. The four trauma types with the highest proportions of these person-years were rape (13.1%), other sexual assault (15.1%), being stalked (9.8%), and UD of loved one (11.6%). The broad category of intimate partner-sexual violence accounted for nearly 42.7% of all person-years with PTSD in the population.

Discussion

As noted in other chapters, the WMH results are limited in a number of ways. First, lifetime prevalence estimates of trauma exposure are likely to be conservative due to recall error. Second, diagnoses of lifetime PTSD are based on retrospective reports obtained in a cross-sectional survey using a fully structured lay-administered diagnostic interview rather than a semi-structured clinician-administered diagnostic interview. Third, the WMH clinical reappraisal study showed that PTSD prevalence was underestimated in the CIDI compared to blinded semi-structured clinical interviews, but that the vast majority of CIDI cases were confirmed in these clinical reappraisal interviews (Haro et al., 2006), suggesting that the WMH prevalence estimates are conservative. Finally, WMH results regarding PTSD persistence, in comparison, are anti-conservative because they assess persistence of any

Table 23.3 Mean duration and years in episode of DSM-IV/CIDI PTSD by trauma type in the WMH surveys

	Mean PTSD episode duration (in months) by trauma type[a]		Number of years with PTSD per 100 people[b]		Percentage of all years with PTSD for each trauma type[c]		
	Mean	(SE)	Est	(SE)	%	(SE)	(n)
I War-Related Trauma							
Relief worker in war zone	95.3	(45.8)	0.1	(0.0)	0.1	(0.1)	(2)
Civilian in war zone	62.9	(26.7)	0.3	(0.1)	0.4	(0.2)	(29)
Civilian in region of terror	38.5	(15.6)	0.2	(0.0)	0.2	(0.0)	(20)
Refugee	44.7	(20.2)	0.4	(0.1)	0.5	(0.2)	(20)
Combat experience	161.7	(23.3)	1.5	(0.3)	1.9	(0.5)	(54)
Purposely injured/tortured/killed someone	79.3	(8.9)	0.6	(0.4)	0.7	(0.5)	(7)
Witnessed atrocities	78.3	(22.1)	2.7	(1.6)	3.5	(2.0)	(29)
Any	82.0	(11.8)	5.7	(1.8)	7.3	(2.2)	(161)
II Physical Violence Victimization							
Beaten by caregiver	138.6	(25.7)	4.6	(0.7)	5.9	(1.0)	(174)
Beaten by someone else	22.7	(4.6)	0.5	(0.1)	0.7	(0.2)	(62)
Mugged/threatened with a weapon	115.0	(47.5)	4.2	(2.3)	5.4	(2.8)	(119)
Kidnapped	115.9	(38.1)	1.3	(0.5)	1.6	(0.7)	(40)
Any	101.4	(18.6)	10.6	(2.6)	13.6	(3.0)	(395)
I Sexual Violence Victimization							
Raped	110.3	(14.1)	10.2	(1.4)	13.1	(1.9)	(443)
Sexually assaulted	114.2	(18.5)	11.7	(2.1)	15.1	(2.7)	(280)
Stalked	127.1	(84.2)	7.6	(6.0)	9.8	(6.5)	(103)
Beaten by spouse/romantic partner	82.7	(9.0)	3.6	(0.5)	4.7	(0.7)	(318)
Any	110.9	(18.0)	33.2	(6.5)	42.7	(4.9)	(1,144)
IV Accidents/Injuries							
Automobile accident	52.5	(15.0)	2.2	(0.7)	2.9	(0.9)	(170)
Other life-threatening accident	28.6	(6.4)	1.1	(0.6)	1.4	(0.8)	(41)
Natural disaster	12.9	(4.3)	0.0	(0.0)	0.0	(0.0)	(22)
Toxic chemical exposure	40.4	(22.2)	0.0	(0.0)	0.1	(0.0)	(9)
Human-made disaster	41.3	(8.4)	0.7	(0.3)	0.9	(0.4)	(31)
Accidentally caused serious injury/death	54.5	(27.7)	0.3	(0.1)	0.4	(0.1)	(24)
Life-threatening illness	41.3	(9.0)	1.1	(0.3)	1.4	(0.3)	(152)
Any	41.2	(5.7)	5.5	(1.0)	7.1	(1.4)	(449)
V UD of a Loved One	37.7	(3.9)	9.0	(0.9)	11.6	(1.5)	(1,158)
VI Other Traumas of Loved Ones or Witnessed							
Child with serious illness	44.7	(8.7)	1.8	(0.4)	2.3	(0.5)	(225)
Trauma to loved one	45.7	(12.8)	1.7	(0.5)	2.1	(0.6)	(101)
Witnessed parent violence	107.1	(15.0)	2.7	(0.5)	3.5	(0.7)	(135)
Witnessed death/dead body/serious injury	45.4	(9.8)	2.7	(0.8)	3.5	(1.0)	(140)
Any	55.0	(5.1)	8.9	(1.1)	11.4	(1.6)	(601)
VII Other Traumas							
Some other trauma	62.1	(12.1)	2.0	(0.4)	2.5	(0.6)	(201)
Private trauma[d]	79.5	(13.1)	3.0	(0.4)	3.9	(0.6)	(248)
Any	71.5	(6.8)	5.0	(0.6)	6.4	(0.9)	(449)
VIII Any	72.3	(6.0)	77.7	(7.5)	100.0	(0.0)	(4,357)

[a]The mean duration (in months) of PTSD episodes associated with the trauma type indicated in the row heading. Recovery was defined as the number of months until the respondent stopped having any symptoms. For example, respondents with a history of PTSD due to combat experience reported that symptoms continued for a mean of 161.7 months (13.5 years).

[b]The number of lifetime episodes of PTSD due to the trauma type indicated in the row heading per 100 respondents from the second column in Table 23.2 multiplied by the mean duration (in years) from the first column of Table 23.3. For example, the 0.8 lifetime episodes of PTSD due to war-related traumas per 100 respondents multiplied by the mean 6.8 years per episode results in 5.7 (0.8 × 6.8) years of PTSD due to this category of traumas per 100 respondents.

[c]The ratio of the entry in the cell of the previous column to the total 77.7 years of PTSD due to any trauma for every 100 respondents. For example, the 5.7 years of war-related PTSD represent 7.3% of the 77.7 total.

[d]A *private* event is a trauma that some individuals reported in response to a question asked at the very end of the trauma section that asked if they ever had some other very upsetting experience they did not tell us about already (and this includes in response to a prior open-ended question about "any other" trauma) because they were too embarrassed or upset to talk about it. Respondents were told, before they answered, that if they reported such a trauma we would not ask them anything about what it was, only about their age when the trauma happened.

symptom rather than persistence of the full PTSD syndrome.

Within the context of these limitations, as we noted in Chapter 3, our finding that 70.4% of respondents were exposed to one or more traumas in their lifetimes is broadly consistent with previous research. However, the WMH surveys went beyond previous studies in assessing frequency of exposure, documenting that trauma exposure is even more common than previously known, with a per capita mean lifetime average of 2.0 trauma types and 4.6 trauma exposures. But these estimates are conservative, as they are based on calculations in which some ongoing traumas, such as physical abuse at the hands of a caregiver during childhood, are counted as only "one occurrence," even though these traumas might have persisted over many years.

Regarding the most common types of trauma, WMH results are consistent with previous research showing that UD of a loved one and automobile accidents are the two most common types of trauma in the general population. We also found, though, that traumas occurring to others account for over 40% of all reported traumas (16.5% involving UD of a loved one and an additional 25.0% other traumas that either occurred to a loved one or were witnessed), that accidents are the most common type of directly experienced trauma (24.6%), and that traumas involving intimate partner-sexual violence (9.8%) and physical violence (13.8%) account for the bulk of other traumas. It is noteworthy that the number of traumas that occurred to loved ones is clearly underreported by WMH respondents. That's because though we would expect the loved ones of each respondent to have as many traumas as the respondent, this is not the case in respondent reports. This discrepancy suggests that reports about traumas occurring to loved ones are limited to the traumas that are most psychologically salient.

We also found that trauma exposure is not distributed randomly in the population. Our results are consistent with the literature on basic socio-demographic correlates of trauma exposure (Hatch & Dohrenwend, 2007) and previous research showing that traumas involving violence and accidents are more likely to occur in adolescence and early adulthood than at other stages of the life course. We also found that trauma exposures are correlated over time, with individuals exposed to earlier traumas at significantly increased risk of being exposed to subsequent traumas. The latter pattern presumably reflects individual differences in predispositions, coping resources, life circumstances, and lifestyles. The WMH data were too coarse to search for modifiable risk factors that might be targeted to prevent future trauma exposure, but the strong inter-temporal patterning of exposure suggests that such an investigation might make sense. Given that preventive interventions can already address recurrences of drunk driving (Miller et al., 2015), intimate partner violence (Ramsay et al., 2009), and sexual violence (Marques et al., 2005), our results raise the possibility of also developing risk models to target broader types of secondary preventive interventions.

Our estimates of conditional PTSD risk among those exposed to traumas were mostly lower than in previous studies due to our focus on representative samples of traumas in comparison to the worst traumas examined in most other community epidemiological studies and in samples that overrepresent help-seekers focused on particular trauma types (e.g., Campbell et al., 2009; Goldmann & Galea, 2014). Our finding that conditional PTSD risk was elevated after traumas involving violence is broadly consistent with the results reported in reviews (Ozer et al., 2003; Atwoli et al., 2015). We also found that prior exposure to some traumas involving violence was associated with *generalized vulnerability* to subsequent PTSD. Although ongoing research is investigating pathways leading to such generalized vulnerability (Rutter, 2012; Daskalakis et al., 2013; Levy-Gigi et al., 2016), we know of no work on the differential effects of trauma types. However, suggestive related evidence exists on differences in associations of childhood adversities with adult mental disorders across different childhood adversity types (Pirkola et al., 2005; Kessler et al., 2010) and profiles (Putnam et al., 2013; McLafferty et al., 2015).

Finally, our results regarding persistence are broadly consistent with previous studies showing that a substantial minority of PTSD cases remit within months, but that a substantial minority of cases persist for many years. As shown in Chapter 16, we found much less evidence for systematic pre-onset predictors of course of illness than we found for the predictor of onset. This means that we would have no way to target the subset of patients at high risk of *chronic* PTSD for preventive interventions at the time of trauma exposure based on the variables considered in the WMH surveys. This presumably reflects the importance of factors that could not be assessed until after PTSD onset on the course of illness. We had no way to study these variables with the WMH data. This is a main focus of the new prospective AURORA study mentioned in Chapter 24. Taken together, these results demonstrate that there are a number of potential intervention points to reduce the population burden of PTSD, a topic covered in Chapter 24.

Acknowledgment

Portions of this paper are based on Kessler, R. C., Aguilar-Gaxiola, S., Alonso, J., et al. (2017). Trauma and PTSD in the WHO World Mental Health Surveys. *European Journal of Psychotraumatology*, 8 1353383.

References

Atwoli, L., Stein, D. J., Koenen, K. C., & McLaughlin, K. A. (2015). Epidemiology of posttraumatic stress disorder: prevalence, correlates and consequences. *Current Opinion in Psychiatry*, 28, 307–11.

Campbell, R., Dworkin, E., & Cabral, G. (2009). An ecological model of the impact of sexual assault on women's mental health. *Trauma, Violence & Abuse*, 10, 225–46.

Daskalakis, N. P., Bagot, R. C., Parker, K. J., Vinkers, C. H., & de Kloet, E. R. (2013). The three-hit concept of vulnerability and resilience: toward understanding adaptation to early-life adversity outcome. *Psychoneuroendocrinology*, 38, 1858–73.

Goldmann, E., & Galea, S. (2014). Mental health consequences of disasters. *Annual Review of Public Health*, 35, 169–83.

Haro, J. M., Arbabzadeh-Bouchez, S., Brugha, T. S., et al. (2006). Concordance of the Composite International Diagnostic Interview Version 3.0 (CIDI 3.0) with standardized clinical assessments in the WHO World Mental Health surveys. *International Journal of Methods in Psychiatric Research*, 15, 167–80.

Hatch, S. L., & Dohrenwend, B. P. (2007). Distribution of traumatic and other stressful life events by race/ethnicity, gender, SES and age: a review of the research. *American Journal of Community Psychology*, 40, 313–32.

Kessler, R. C., McLaughlin, K. A., Green, J. G., et al. (2010). Childhood adversities and adult psychopathology in the WHO World Mental Health Surveys. *British Journal of Psychiatry*, 197, 378–85.

Levy-Gigi, E., Richter-Levin, G., Okon-Singer, H., Keri, S., & Bonanno, G. A. (2016). The hidden price and possible benefit of repeated traumatic exposure. *Stress*, 19, 1–7.

Marques, J. K., Wiederanders, M., Day, D. M., Nelson, C., & van Ommeren, A. (2005). Effects of a relapse prevention program on sexual recidivism: final results from California's Sex Offender Treatment and Evaluation Project (SOTEP). *Sexual Abuse*, 17, 79–107.

McLafferty, M., Armour, C., McKenna, A., et al. (2015). Childhood adversity profiles and adult psychopathology in a representative Northern Ireland study. *Journal of Anxiety Disorders*, 35, 42–8.

Miller, P. G., Curtis, A., Sonderlund, A., Day, A., & Droste, N. (2015). Effectiveness of interventions for convicted DUI offenders in reducing recidivism: a systematic review of the peer-reviewed scientific literature. *American Journal of Drug and Alcohol Abuse*, 41, 16–29.

Ozer, E. J., Best, S. R., Lipsey, T. L., & Weiss, D. S. (2003). Predictors of posttraumatic stress disorder and symptoms in adults: a meta-analysis. *Psychological Bulletin*, 129, 52–73.

Pirkola, S., Isometsa, E., Aro, H., et al. (2005). Childhood adversities as risk factors for adult mental disorders: results from the Health 2000 study. *Social Psychiatry and Psychiatric Epidemiology*, 40, 769–77.

Putnam, K. T., Harris, W. W., & Putnam, F. W. (2013). Synergistic childhood adversities and complex adult psychopathology. *Journal of Traumatic Stress*, 26, 435–42.

Ramsay, J., Carter, Y., Davidson, L., et al. (2009). Advocacy interventions to reduce or eliminate violence and promote the physical and psychosocial well-being of women who experience intimate partner abuse. *The Cochrane Database of Systematic Reviews*, Issue 3, Cd005043.

Rutter, M. (2012). Resilience as a dynamic concept. *Development and Psychopathology*, 24, 335–44.

Chapter 24

Conclusions and Future Directions

Evelyn J. Bromet, Elie G. Karam, Karestan C. Koenen, and Dan J. Stein

Introduction

Since the first consensus operational definition of PTSD was published (American Psychiatric Association, 1980), there has been increasing recognition of the wide-ranging, detrimental effects of the disorder on health and well-being both in the scientific literature and in the mass media. This volume documents the prevalence, antecedents, consequences, symptom characteristics, and treatment patterns of this relatively common mental health disorder by examining a wealth of data on respondents with PTSD included in the World Mental Health (WMH) surveys. The interviews took place between 2001 and 2012 in 24 high-, middle-, and low-income countries. In this chapter, we first summarize our key findings on the global epidemiology and phenomenology of trauma and PTSD and then discuss their implications for future research and public health policy.

Key Findings of the WMH Surveys on Trauma and PTSD

One of the crucial findings of the WMH studies is that trauma exposure was common in almost all countries throughout the world, rich and poor alike, with nearly 70% of all WMH respondents reporting at least one trauma and one-third of exposed respondents reporting three or more. In four low- and middle-income countries (Colombia, Lebanon, Peru, and Ukraine) and one high-income country (the United States), more than 80% of respondents experienced at least one trauma during their lifetime. The average number of traumas in the WMH sample was 3.2, while the average among respondents with at least one exposure was 4.6. Overall, the two most frequently reported traumas were accidents/injuries (36.3%) and unexpected death of a loved one (23.7%). However, the proportion of respondents reporting specific types of trauma often varied considerably by country. For example, in half of the countries, 20% to 29% of respondents reported exposure to sexual violence victimization, a set of seven exposures ranging from rape to being beaten up by spouse/romantic partner. However, the proportions ranged from under 10% in China and Spain to more than 30% in New Zealand and the United States. Most traumas occurred early in life, and prior exposure itself was a significant risk factor for future traumas in all countries. Other universally consistent risk factors for trauma exposure included being unmarried, experiencing childhood adversities, and having a history of psychopathology (Chapter 4). The latter two risk factors were particularly strongly associated with subsequent exposure to traumas involving physical and sexual violence.

The second set of unique findings pertained to the magnitude, variability, and burden of PTSD around the globe. In contrast to other epidemiological surveys that assess PTSD for a respondent-identified worst trauma, the WMH surveys assessed PTSD for a randomly selected trauma, enabling us to provide unbiased estimates of lifetime prevalence. The overall lifetime prevalence of PTSD was 3.9% and was higher in the high- (5.0%) compared to the upper-middle- (2.3%) and low- and lower-middle- (2.1%) income sites. The lifetime prevalence among the trauma-exposed subgroup (conditional prevalence) was 5.6% overall and was also higher in high- (6.9%) compared to upper-middle- (3.6%) and low- and lower-middle- (3.0%) income countries. Consistent with prior studies, 50.5% of respondents with PTSD developed persistent symptoms although the rate varied from 31.7% for respondents in WMH sites in Africa to 60.7% for those living in Eastern Europe. Trauma involving sexual violence victimization was associated with the greatest risk of PTSD. Onset, but not persistence, was also consistently associated with female sex, being unmarried, unemployment, low education, and low household income. Childhood adversities and prior psychopathology (especially prior PTSD) were typically the most robust risk factors for the development of PTSD. Moreover, these risk factors remained significant and strong predictors in a series of trauma-specific analyses on sexual assault (Chapter 12), life-threatening motor vehicle collisions (Chapter 13), unexpected death of a loved one (Chapter 14), and disasters (Chapter 15) that also adjusted for trauma severity characteristics.

The considerable societal burden of PTSD resulted from a combination of several factors: high prevalence of traumas; meaningful, although generally not high, conditional prevalence of PTSD after trauma exposure; an early age of onset of PTSD found in many countries (such as the mid-20s in high-income countries); high PTSD persistence; ensuing impairment in multiple domains of life, such as marriage and employment; and the frequent occurrence of suicidal ideation as well as numerous mental and physical health conditions in conjunction with PTSD. In spite of PTSD's severe consequences, only a small proportion of affected respondents received any treatment, even in high-income countries where mental health care is typically available.

Another set of important WMH findings addressed several nosological controversies that directly impact future research on PTSD. First and foremost, we considered the possibility that the WMH epidemiological portrait of PTSD built on the DSM-IV diagnostic criteria might differ under either DSM-5 or ICD-11. However, as shown in Chapter 17, the population prevalence rates in these three diagnostic systems (as well as in ICD-10) were remarkably similar (3–4%), as were the clinical and demographic risk factors and the levels of impairment, suicidality, and distress associated with the diagnosis. Moreover, consistent with the WMH risk profiles for DSM-IV PTSD, two of the strongest risk factors for broadly defined PTSD (meeting criteria in any of the four systems) were female sex and intimate partner sexual violence. Second, the decision by DSM-5 to eliminate the A2 criterion (which referred to an immediate response to the qualifying trauma involving intense fear, hopelessness, or horror) was specifically informed by analyses of WMH data. As discussed in Chapter 18, its removal from the DSM-IV diagnostic criteria resulted only in a slight increase in the prevalence of trauma, but had little effect on the prevalence and correlates of PTSD.

Third, given the growing attention to subthreshold PTSD in the literature, we tested alternative definitions with the goal of constructing an optimal operational definition. Several prior studies of subthreshold PTSD have shown that individuals who do not meet the full diagnostic criteria still exhibit considerable impairment and would benefit from treatment. However, these studies lacked a consensus definition of subthreshold PTSD. The WMH analyses led us to recommend that meeting full criteria for 2–3 of the four DSM-5 symptom clusters (intrusion, avoidance, negative alterations in cognition and mood, and alterations in arousal and reactivity) was the preferred method for categorizing the syndrome. Fourth, DSM-5 added a new category of dissociative subtype of PTSD based in part on studies indicating that patients with co-occurring dissociative symptoms benefit from different types of treatment compared to patients without these symptoms (Friedman, 2016). The evidence base for this research, however, involved a mix of special populations, particularly samples of veterans (Ozer et al., 2003). In the WMH, 14.4% of respondents with 12-month PTSD had dissociative symptoms. Chapter 17 thus examined whether there were demographic or risk factor differences between PTSD cases with and without co-occurring dissociative symptoms. Importantly, we confirmed the potential value of distinguishing a dissociative subgroup from other cases of PTSD by finding that significantly more dissociative than other cases were male, had a childhood onset of PTSD, and reported exposure to childhood adversities. Fifth, one of the most important findings of the WMH nosological analyses concerned the validity of the proposed subtype of complex PTSD, or PTSD emanating from multiple traumas. As part of the WMH CIDI, respondents with 12-month PTSD were asked whether any of their other lifetime traumas were implicated in their recent symptoms. One in five respondents raised at least one other trauma. Notably, we found a dose response relationship between the number of contributing traumas and the degree of impairment associated with PTSD. Thus, compared to respondents whose PTSD was associated with a single trauma, those implicating four or more traumas were six times more likely to exhibit global impairment, independent of type of trauma and comorbidity.

Lastly, near the end of this book, we turned our attention to developing a universally relevant, predictive model that could best classify trauma-exposed respondents at risk of developing PTSD. Accomplishing this goal has both theoretical and practical implications for directing the scarce resources available for prevention and treatment (Qi et al., 2016). Chapter 22 shows that almost all cases of PTSD occurred among the 10.0% of respondents classified by a machine learning algorithm as having the highest predicted risk. Moreover, these novel and exciting findings were stable across demographic and geographic subpopulations of the WMH. Although the specific index would need to be revised and customized in short-term prospective studies in relevant populations in which the index would be used (e.g., survivors of natural disasters; patients seeking treatment in emergency departments in the aftermath of traumas), and may differ in military, treatment, and other unique cohorts, this analytic strategy could ultimately lead to findings that translate into better triaging of high-risk individuals and more cost-effective prevention and intervention programs.

Future Research on PTSD

In spite of the comprehensive reach of this volume, many important epidemiological questions about PTSD remain to be answered. Four that we consider most relevant to future extensions of the WMH work involve (1) resilience and remission in vulnerable samples; (2) aging-related mental and physical impairments; (3) biological substrates underlying its course and comorbidities; and (4) patterns of help-seeking.

Resilience and Remission in Vulnerable Samples

The WMH surveys confirm and extend the findings of numerous prior studies documenting the substantial risk of future traumas and PTSD among children exposed to maltreatment, particularly physical and sexual abuse along with neglect. Fortunately, some children exposed to these early traumas remain resilient throughout their lives. There is thus an urgent need to better understand the protective mechanisms that promote resilience even when these children encounter new traumas later in life (Walsh et al., 2010). Recent studies have shown that in addition to personal and socioenvironmental factors, resilience has biological and genetic roots (Bowes & Jaffee, 2013; Averill et al., 2017), indicating that self-report data by itself are insufficient to address this issue. A related and perplexing WMH finding was that among respondents with PTSD, childhood adversities were not significantly related to remission. However, our analyses were limited to environmental and familial risk factors. It is now clear from recent studies that a complex set of interacting environmental, biopsychosocial and genetic variables play a determinative role in predicting resilience (Cicchetti, 2013), onset of PTSD (e.g., Shalev et al., 2014), and remission (Baumeister et al., 2014).

The best methodological approach to identifying potential biopsychosocial antecedents of resilience and remission is a prospective study design in which a longitudinal cohort of healthy individuals is followed to predetermined endpoints. In this case, the endpoints are exposure to first trauma, first onset of PTSD (or other form of psychopathology), time to remission, and duration of remission. The prospective design is the most powerful naturalistic means of separating causes from consequences. Two prominent examples of multipurpose population-based prospective cohort studies of health outcomes are the National Survey of Health and Development, which followed 5,362 babies born in March 1946, in England, Scotland and Wales into adulthood (Wadsworth et al., 2006) and the Dunedin Multidisciplinary Health and Development Study, which followed 1,037 children born in a hospital in New Zealand who resided in the health district at age 3 (e.g., Goldman-Mellor et al., 2014). Cross-sectional surveys of adult cohorts, such as the Nurses' Health Study and the National Comorbidity Survey, have also been used as a baseline for launching follow-up evaluations, including studies focused specifically on PTSD and its consequences (e.g., Sumner et al., 2017). In treatment samples, prospective studies of new onset cases are also a powerful, naturalistic method for examining illness course and identifying prognostic factors (Bromet et al., 2011).

Given that the CIDI used unique methods to facilitate accurate recall of critical information such as age of onset of both risk factors and prior mental health disorders, the WMH surveys provide an excellent baseline for prospective studies of resilience and remission. Such studies would also broaden our understanding geographically since as shown in Chapter 1, most prior cross-sectional and longitudinal studies of community, high-risk, and treatment samples were conducted in North America and Europe. While the expense of launching new large-scale epidemiological studies can be prohibitive, nested studies targeting specific WMH subgroups would be a cost-effective way to advance our understanding of the determinants of resilience and remission, especially because the WMH respondents were extremely well-characterized. One such design might involve a nested follow-up study of demographically matched WMH respondents with and without adverse childhood exposures and with and without lifetime PTSD at initial interview. This design would allow a reverse risk model based on prospective analyses to be calculated from prospective data.

Until recently, prospective and longitudinal studies were not only expensive, but tracking individuals in countries such as the United States was difficult, leading to high rates of attrition. Future studies, however, can incorporate new mobile technologies and web-based methods to maintain samples and collect follow-up data at far less expense. More complex prospective studies could be modeled on the multicenter, multidisciplinary AURORA study launched by the National Institute of Mental Health (NIMH) in 2016 (National Institute of Mental Health, 2016). Led by researchers at the University of North Carolina and Harvard and carried out in samples selected from 16 emergency departments from around the United States, this study is following 5,000 trauma-exposed Americans for 1 year after an initial emergency department screening. The types of data included in the AURORA study could also be considered in WMH follow-up surveys, namely, blood and urine specimens, mood and activity levels, and sleep measures from mobile apps, in-depth psychological and neuropsychological examinations, and neuroimaging.

Aging-Related Mental and Physical Impairments Associated with PTSD

Across all regions of the world, in high-, middle-, and low-income countries alike, the proportion of the population over 65 is rapidly increasing. Because the WMH sampled adults, and life expectancy and adequacy of financial entitlements varied by country income level, current WMH respondents over the age of 65 constitute a highly select sample in several countries. In spite of this potential bias, the WMH found that PTSD was a significant risk factor for physical health problems associated with aging (e.g., arthritis, heart disease, stroke). Other research has shown that PTSD is a significant predictor of dementia (Yaffe et al., 2010). In the decades since the WMH was initiated, new evidence has shown that PTSD is also associated with prodromal signs of accelerated aging, including mild cognitive impairment (Clouston et al., 2016; Sumner et al., 2017) as well as impaired physical functioning (Clouston et al., in press).

The WMH interview did not administer objective measures of prodromal symptoms of late-life impairments. However, nested, longitudinal case–control follow-ups of carefully selected WMH subpopulations could test whether PTSD increases the risk of mild cognitive impairment and mild functional deficits as well as the speed of decline of these domains. Such studies could also include comprehensive neuropsychological evaluations, medical examinations, neuroimaging, and measures comprising the Research Domain Criteria (Roberts et al., 2017). Depending on the WMH site, a broader approach to assessing the rate of decline could also include ambulatory blood pressure monitoring, wearable activity trackers, ecological momentary assessments of daily functioning and symptoms, and serial blood samples for fine-grained analyses of changes in biological risk factors, like methylation patterns and gene expression. Recent studies of veterans with PTSD and a sample of middle-aged workers strongly support the feasibility of including daily measurement devices in longitudinal research of adult populations (Possemato et al., 2015; Schwartz et al., 2016). A nested follow-up of WMH respondents to assess cognitive and physical decline could also include collateral information from family or friends with knowledge about the respondents' daily functioning.

Lastly, as individuals develop aging-related health problems, they become high utilizers of medical services (although not necessarily psychiatric services) and are at increased risk of death. A WMH protocol to examine the effects of PTSD on accelerated aging should include, where possible, access to medical and death records. In this way, respondents could be passively as well as directly monitored for the onset of aging-related changes. Medical records could also be used to cross-check self-reports about the onset, treatment, and course of the chronic conditions. Thus, because of the richness of the initial assessments, the baseline WMH data could serve as an extraordinary platform for subsequent studies of aging-related changes. While the specific measures would depend on the research questions and the resources available in the different sites (across and within countries), respondents in understudied regions of the world could play an important part in filling in gaps in knowledge about the effects of PTSD on aging-related changes outside of the high-income, urban settings where clinical research is typically conducted.

Biological Substrates Underlying the Course and Comorbidities of PTSD

The WMH data confirmed the high comorbidity and bidirectional relationships of PTSD with other mental disorders. That is, temporally prior psychiatric disorders were associated with an elevated risk of PTSD onset, and PTSD was associated with an elevated risk of the onset of numerous other mental disorders. In Chapter 5, Kessler et al. attribute these associations to latent internalizing and externalizing factors, a hypothesis shared by other investigators (Miller et al., 2008, 2010; Wolf et al., 2010). PTSD was also associated with the onset of numerous physical conditions. The role of PTSD in the onset and course of medical conditions in patient populations is an active area of investigation, particularly in relation to cardiovascular disease (Boscarino & Chang, 1999; Boscarino, 2006, 2008; Kubzansky et al., 2007, 2009; Scherrer et al., 2010; Jordan et al., 2011; Vaccarino et al., 2013; Chen et al., 2015; Gradus et al., 2015; Roy et al., 2015; Sumner et al., 2015; Beristianos et al., 2016), type 2 diabetes (Boyko et al., 2010; Vaccarino et al., 2014; Roberts et al., 2015), and respiratory conditions (Kotov et al., 2015). These studies focus on shared lifestyle risk factors (e.g., smoking, heavy alcohol and drug use, disparities in use of health services), physiological variables (e.g., inflammation, dysregulation of the HPA axis, gene expression), and biomedical indices (e.g., heart rate variability, infectious disease history) as potential mechanisms that could explain the links between these disorders and PTSD. Few definitive conclusions can yet be drawn in part because of the small and select samples included in many published studies, the lack of pretrauma psychophysiological and neurobiological data, variability in the time interval between onset of PTSD and data collection, inadequate control groups, and differences across studies in the PTSD symptom profiles, stage of illness, and specific comorbidities (McFarlane & Bryant, 2017). Future WMH studies, both new sites and follow-up studies of current cohorts, have the potential to address many of the shortcomings of these recent studies of PTSD comorbidity by providing large and clinically targeted case groups, appropriate controls, and data on the time interval from onset of PTSD to the point of data collection.

In this volume, we focused only on PTSD after a randomly selected trauma, but the CIDI also assessed PTSD for the respondent-nominated worst trauma if it differed from the random trauma. Thus, the pool of cases for fine-grained biological studies can be enriched by including these additional cases. Overall, the WMH's large, carefully characterized samples would allow researchers to drill down and test hypotheses about differential pathways underlying different types and patterns of mental and physical comorbidities at the symptom as well as diagnostic levels. We note that to date four WMH surveys (Mexico, Colombia-Medellin, Murcia, and Portugal) collected DNA samples that, together with the phenotypic data on mental and physical health, were shared with the Psychiatric Genomics Consortium-PTSD Working Group mentioned in Chapter 1. (While the Brazil survey has also collected DNA samples, it did not contribute them to this effort.)

Patterns of Help-Seeking

The WMH findings in Chapter 8 show unequivocally that PTSD is undertreated in all regions of the world. As noted in Chapter 8, fewer than half of respondents with 12-month PTSD in high-income countries and just one-quarter of participants in low- and middle-income countries received minimally adequate treatment. Thus, most WMH respondents received either inadequate treatment or no treatment at all. Interestingly, female sex was the only demographic variable associated with treatment-seeking for PTSD. Of note, the WMH survey evaluated a broad set of structural and attitudinal barriers to care in relation to help-seeking for emotional problems in general, but not for PTSD symptoms per se. In addition, like most other studies of help-seeking behavior, the WMH did not explicitly assess facilitators of accessing care (Kantor et al., 2017).

In order to extend our knowledge about facilitators of help-seeking, sex-specific analyses can be conducted with existing WMH data focused on the subsequent mental health and role functioning trajectories of WMH respondents who did and did not seek help for PTSD, adjusting for pretreatment risk factors for poor outcomes. From a clinical perspective, trajectory patterns found among help-seekers could provide useful prognostic information and shed light, albeit indirectly, on why the WMH analyses failed to identify antecedent factors that are significantly associated with remission. From a public health perspective, the trajectories of non-help-seekers offer clues for designing new interventions. Specifically, these analyses could test hypotheses about differences between non-help-seekers who remit spontaneously and those who develop chronic PTSD and/or a fluctuating course of illness. Conceivably, the answers to these questions will vary by region and by type of trauma.

A second potentially valuable avenue of analyses entails a more explicit focus on comorbidity. It is long established that people with multiple conditions are more likely to seek help from medical providers than those with a single condition. While this poses a bias for clinical research, it has potential value for WMH research on the pathways to care. Is there a breaking point, as mental and physical disorders accumulate across the life span, where treatment becomes more likely? Is there a risk profile based on the timing and patterns of onset, duration, remission, and recurrence of mental and physical disorders that could identify respondents with a high likelihood of seeking care? Much more work is needed toward this end. The epidemiological focus has been on lack of treatment and inadequate treatment. Based on the findings of this volume and the psychiatric and medical antecedents and consequences of PTSD, along with the careful dating of each risk factor and outcome, the WMH offers a unique opportunity to initiate a new generation of studies on help-seeking that can illuminate trauma- and geographic-specific patterns of treatment for PTSD beyond what has been learned from high-income countries.

Lastly, given the small numbers of respondents with PTSD who sought care, more fine-grained approaches to understanding the barriers and facilitators of treatment seeking should be explored. Traditional qualitative and quantitative studies of barriers to care analyze responses to preset questions. We propose a different approach, namely, recording the life stories of WMH respondents with PTSD, as was done in the Schizophrenia Oral History Project. These oral histories can be gathered in-person or remotely by trained interviewers (Atkinson, 2002). State-of-the-art analysis strategies of language-based assessments are capable of capturing a range of factors related to trauma and PTSD, as well as sources of support, personal and public stigma, disabilities, and resilience. Cognitive appraisals of the level of threat and ability to cope with the trauma and post-traumatic growth (Ursano et al., 2017) – two areas not covered in the WMH surveys – can also be captured in the oral histories of respondents with PTSD and linked back to treatment-seeking behaviors. Most importantly, the WMH clinical and risk factor database combined with variables derived from the language-based assessments provide a unique analytic resource. A repository of oral histories, assuming proper consenting procedures, would also constitute a valuable addendum to the data contained in the WMH surveys.

The various future studies suggested earlier could make full use of the richness of the WMH surveys for understanding PTSD. The well-characterized respondents who participated in the initial interview are an extraordinary resource for follow-up studies aimed at understanding psychophysiological and neurobiological pathways underpinning the onset and course of PTSD in conjunction with environmental risk factors, and can shed light on pathways and facilitators of care. Each of the areas of research described in this section can and should be examined by studies outside the WMH initiative as well. Indeed, emerging research on PTSD in combat soldiers, veterans, refugees, victims of assault, emergency department patients, and population-based samples of all ages are incorporating all or parts of the multimodal approaches described earlier, and some are testing longitudinal hypotheses. To the extent that findings are confirmed across samples from different parts of the world, these fully integrated, longitudinal studies will greatly advance our understanding of the onset, course, and consequences of PTSD and ultimately reduce its burden on patients and society.

Public Health Policy Implications

The high prevalence of PTSD around the globe and disruptive nature of this disorder stand in stark contrast to the inadequate resources available for its prevention and treatment. Public health measures and improved recognition by medical and ancillary providers of health and mental health care, including knowledge of trauma-informed practices, are needed to reduce the population burden of PTSD (Lowe et al., 2015). As Shalev et al. (2011) point out, effective prevention and treatment of PTSD "requires accurate case identification, efficacious interventions, accessible services, and acceptance of care by trauma survivors at risk" (p. 765).

Because PTSD occurs in the wake of exposure to a trauma, primary prevention programs designed to reduce such exposures, especially early childhood adversities and sexual assault, would serve to decrease the prevalence of PTSD. Examples of primary prevention programs include the Child and Family Traumatic Stress Intervention (Berkowitz et al., 2011), the National Child Traumatic Stress Network, programs conducted by the US Centers for Disease Control and Prevention (Niolon et al., 2017), as well as school-based programs, such as Support for Students Exposed to Trauma and the university-based Bystander Interventions and similar programs aimed at reducing sexual violence on college campuses around the world (e.g., Coker et al., 2016; Adinew & Hagos, 2017).

PTSD is one of the most preventable mental disorders, as many individuals exposed to trauma come to clinical attention in first response settings, such as disaster triage locations, emergency rooms, intensive care units, and trauma centers. Some controlled clinical trials show that in the immediate aftermath of a trauma, PTSD risk can be significantly reduced (Foa et al., 1995; Kearns et al., 2012; Shalev et al., 2012). However, these interventions are expensive, and relatively few therapists have been trained to administer them reliably. Moreover, their real-world effectiveness has also not yet been demonstrated (Goldmann & Galea, 2014). Empirical support for the effectiveness of Psychological First Aid, one of the most recognizable and common interventions, is also lacking (Dieltjens et al., 2014). In the absence of evidenced-based consensus interventions, Hobfoll et al. (2007) recommended that five empirically supported principles be followed in the immediate aftermath of a trauma. These involve promoting a sense of safety, calming, perceived self- and community efficacy, connectedness, and hope. We also note here that medications reduce symptom severity, but there is little evidence that they are effective in preventing full-blown PTSD after trauma exposure (e.g., Amos et al., 2014). As shown in this book, the development of consensus post-trauma programs is also limited by the inability to predict who will be part of the small minority to develop PTSD (Kessler et al., 1995; Kessler, 2000; Roberts et al., 2010). The risk profiles described in Chapter 22 and the PsySTART screen described in Chapter 15 are designed to target trauma survivors who will benefit the most from mental health treatment and thus potentially lead to an evidence-based set of personalized, multi-layered, primary prevention programs (Hobfoll et al., 2007).

Secondary prevention efforts target cases in their early phase, before symptoms worsen and fully fledged PTSD sets in. This presumes the ability to identify individuals who sustained trauma exposure and are exhibiting mild or prodromal PTSD symptoms. The difficulty is that trauma history and PTSD symptoms are not typically part of routine screening in either primary care settings, where the majority of patients with mental health and psychosomatic symptoms seek care (Regier et al., 1978; Goldberg, 2003; Wang et al., 2005), or psychiatric outpatient clinics (Posner et al., 2008). In a review of research on PTSD in primary care, Greene et al. (2016) found that the rate of detection of PTSD by physicians ranged from 0% to 52%. Thus, even if general medical professionals are provided with documents like the American Psychiatric Association Practice Guidelines or the Australian Guidelines for the Treatment of Acute Stress Disorder and Posttraumatic Stress Disorder, the patients who might benefit from such treatments are hidden in the shadows of most medical facilities (Lecrubier, 2004). In addition to structural barriers to identifying patients with trauma and early symptoms of PTSD, patients often do not connect their current symptoms with trauma, are reluctant to disclose highly personal information, and may be unwilling to accept psychological treatment. The latter has led to research testing whether collaborative care models, in which mental health care is an integral component of overall care, improve detection and treatment visits for common mental disorders. Several such models have been tested successfully for comorbid depression and anxiety (e.g., Archer et al., 2012; Katon et al., 2012), but the evidence for PTSD is mixed (Schnurr, 2016; Watts, 2016). However, one positive example includes a study of patients presenting with traumatic injuries (Malcoun et al., 2010), most of whom were willing to accept psychological help as well. Thus, the context of the medical visit appears to play an important role in the success of collaborative care models for PTSD (Watts, 2016).

Tertiary prevention involves stopping the progression of PTSD symptoms in individuals with the diagnosis and reducing its multiple negative consequences. Although treatment of PTSD in primary settings has been shown to be effective (Roy-Byrne et al., 2010), most medical providers have no training in diagnosing and treating PTSD or other common forms of psychopathology. A generation ago, a similar situation existed with respect to depression. As a result, the National Institute of Mental Health created the Depression, Awareness, Recognition, and Treatment program (DART) (Regier et al., 1988). One of its primary goals was to raise the level of knowledge about depression and its treatment among the general medical providers. To this end, DART offered courses on depression at general and specialty medical association meetings directed at both detection and treatment. This model could also be followed for PTSD. To be maximally effective, PTSD education programs should clarify the distinction between normal responses to stressors and PTSD symptoms in need of treatment (Stein et al., 2007). Organizations like the International Society for Traumatic Stress Studies and the Veterans Affairs' National Center for PTSD have online materials tailored to health professionals.

For settings where professional mental health treatment is unavailable, clinician-assisted web-based programs may be able to deliver cognitive behavioral therapy to diagnosed PTSD patients at a low cost (Newman et al., 1999; Klein et al., 2010) although in theory, web-based programs are best considered as an adjunct to live treatment rather than as stand-alone treatments (Cohen et al., 2016). Mobile apps such as PTSD coach (ptsd.va.gov) are also available in several dozen countries. In low- and middle-income countries, another approach to treating patients identified in medical facilities with limited resources is task shifting from physicians to nonphysician healthcare workers; task shifting may be cost-effective (Joshi et al., 2014) as well as cost-saving for common mental disorders (Buttorff et al., 2012).

Final Thoughts

This book offers multiple insights into the nature and consequences of PTSD based on the WMH surveys. We hope that the current findings will serve as a springboard for future prospective and case–control studies of PTSD by WMH and other epidemiological investigators. While PTSD is by definition one of the most preventable mental disorders, worldwide efforts to reduce traumatic stress have yet to have much of an impact on its prevalence. Moreover, the outlook for both children and adults exposed to severe traumas is similar now to what it was decades ago. There is a clear need for further research and new and more effective treatments that can reduce the burden of PTSD in both high- and low-income countries. In the short run, this requires a deeper understanding of the mechanisms underlying the onset and course of PTSD, as well as resilience. A collaborative structure like that of the WMH can provide a research base for basic scientists who can build on the current surveys and ultimately achieve results that are generalizable as well as theoretically and practically valuable.

References

Adinew, Y. M., & Hagos, M. A. (2017). Sexual violence against female university students in Ethiopia. *BMC International Health and Human Rights*, 17, 19.

American Psychiatric Association. (1980). *Diagnostic and Statistical Manual of Mental Disorders, Third Edition. DSM-III*. Washington, DC: American Psychiatric Association.

Amos, T., Stein, D. J., & Ipser, J. C. (2014). Pharmacological interventions for preventing post-traumatic stress disorder (PTSD). *The Cochrane Database of Systematic Reviews*, CD006239.

Archer, J., Bower, P., Gilbody, S., et al. (2012). Collaborative care for depression and anxiety problems. *The Cochrane Database of Systematic Reviews*, 10, CD006525.

Atkinson, R. (2002). The life story interview. In J. F. Gubrium & J. A. Holstein, eds., *Handbook of Interview Research: Context and Method*. Thousand Oaks, CA: SAGE, pp. 121–40.

Averill, L. A., Smith, R. P., Katz, C. L., Charney, D. S., & Southwick, S. M. (2017). Neurobiology of disaster exposure. In R. J. Ursano, C. S. Fullerton, L. Weisaeth, & B. Raphael, eds., *Textbook of Disaster Psychiatry*. Cambridge, England; New York, NY: Cambridge University Press, pp. 44–59.

Baumeister, D., Lightman, S. L., & Pariante, C. M. (2014). The interface of stress and the HPA axis in behavioural phenotypes of mental illness. *Current Topics in Behavioral Neurosciences*, 18, 13–24.

Beristianos, M. H., Yaffe, K., Cohen, B., & Byers, A. L. (2016). PTSD and risk of incident cardiovascular disease in aging veterans. *The American Journal of Geriatric Psychiatry: Official Journal of the American Association for Geriatric Psychiatry*, 24, 192–200.

Berkowitz, S. J., Stover, C. S., & Marans, S. R. (2011). The child and family traumatic stress intervention: secondary prevention for youth at risk of developing PTSD. *Journal of Child Psychology and Psychiatry, and Allied Disciplines*, 52, 676–85.

Boscarino, J. A. (2006). Posttraumatic stress disorder and mortality among U.S. army veterans 30 years after military service. *Annals of Epidemiology*, 16, 248–56.

(2008). A prospective study of PTSD and early-age heart disease mortality among Vietnam veterans: implications for surveillance and prevention. *Psychosomatic Medicine*, 70, 668–76.

Boscarino, J. A., & Chang, J. (1999). Electrocardiogram abnormalities among men with stress-related psychiatric disorders: implications for coronary heart disease and clinical research. *Annals of Behavioral Medicine: A Publication of the Society of Behavioral Medicine*, 21, 227–34.

Bowes, L., & Jaffee, S. R. (2013). Biology, genes, and resilience: toward a multidisciplinary approach. *Trauma, Violence & Abuse*, 14, 195–208.

Boyko, E. J., Jacobson, I. G., Smith, B., et al. (2010). Risk of diabetes in U.S. military service members in relation to combat deployment and mental health. *Diabetes Care*, 33, 1771–7.

Bromet, E. J., Kotov, R., Fochtmann, L. J., et al. (2011). Diagnostic shifts during the decade following first admission for psychosis. *The American Journal of Psychiatry*, 168, 1186–94.

Buttorff, C., Hock, R. S., Weiss, H. A., et al. (2012). Economic evaluation of a task-shifting intervention for common mental disorders in India. *Bulletin of the World Health Organization*, 90, 813–21.

Chen, M. H., Pan, T. L., Li, C. T., et al. (2015). Risk of stroke among patients with post-traumatic stress disorder: nationwide longitudinal study. *The British Journal of Psychiatry: the Journal of Mental Science*, 206, 302–7.

Cicchetti, D. (2013). Annual research review: resilient functioning in maltreated children – past, present, and future perspectives. *Journal of Child Psychology and Psychiatry, and Allied Disciplines*, 54, 402–22.

Clouston, S. A. P., Kotov, R., Pietrzak, R. H., et al. (2016). Cognitive impairment among World Trade Center responders: long-term implications of re-experiencing the 9/11 terrorist attacks. *Alzheimer's & Dementia*, 4, 67–75.

Clouston, S. A. P., Guralnik, J., Kotov, R., Bromet, E. J., & Luft, B. J. (2017). Functional limitations in World Trade Center responders 14 years after the disaster: implications of chronic posttraumatic stress disorder. *Journal of Traumatic Stress*. 30, 443–52.

Cohen, J. A., Mannarino, A. P., Jankowski, K., et al. (2016). A randomized implementation study of trauma-focused cognitive behavioral therapy for adjudicated teens in residential treatment facilities. *Child Maltreatment*, 21, 156–67.

Coker, A. L., Bush, H. M., Fisher, B. S., et al. (2016). Multi-college bystander intervention evaluation for violence prevention. *American Journal of Preventive Medicine*, 50, 295–302.

Dieltjens, T., Moonens, I., Van Praet, K., De Buck, E., & Vandekerckhove, P. (2014). A systematic literature search on psychological first aid: lack of evidence to develop guidelines. *PLoS One*, 9, e114714.

Foa, E. B., Hearst-Ikeda, D., & Perry, K. J. (1995). Evaluation of a brief cognitive-behavioral program for the prevention of chronic PTSD in recent assault victims. *Journal of Consulting and Clinical Psychology*, 63, 948–55.

Friedman, M. J. (2016). Deconstructing PTSD. In E. J. Bromet, ed., *Long-Term Outcomes in Psychopathology Research: Rethinking the Scientific Agenda*. Oxford, England; New York, NY: Oxford University Press.

Goldberg, D. (2003). Psychiatry and primary care. *World Psychiatry: Official Journal of the World Psychiatric Association*, 2, 153–7.

Goldman-Mellor, S., Gregory, A. M., Caspi, A., et al. (2014). Mental health antecedents of early midlife insomnia: evidence from a four-decade longitudinal study. *Sleep*, 37, 1767–75.

Goldmann, E., & Galea, S. (2014). Mental health consequences of disasters. *Annual Review of Public Health*, 35, 169–83.

Gradus, J. L., Farkas, D. K., Svensson, E., et al. (2015). Associations between stress disorders and cardiovascular disease events in the Danish population. *BMJ Open*, 5, e009334.

Greene, T., Neria, Y., & Gross, R. (2016). Prevalence, detection and correlates of PTSD in the primary care setting: a systematic review. *Journal of Clinical Psychology in Medical Settings*, 23, 160–80.

Hobfoll, S. E., Watson, P., Bell, C. C., et al. (2007). Five essential elements of immediate and mid-term mass trauma intervention: empirical evidence. *Psychiatry*, 70, 283–315; discussion 316–69.

Jordan, H. T., Miller-Archie, S. A., Cone, J. E., Morabia, A., & Stellman, S. D. (2011). Heart disease among adults exposed to the September 11, 2001 World Trade Center disaster: results from the World Trade Center health registry. *Preventive Medicine*, 53, 370–6.

Joshi, R., Alim, M., Kengne, A. P., et al. (2014). Task shifting for non-communicable disease management in low and middle income countries – a systematic review. *PLoS One*, 9, e103754.

Kantor, V., Knefel, M., & Lueger-Schuster, B. (2017). Perceived barriers and facilitators of mental health service utilization in adult trauma survivors: a systematic review. *Clinical Psychology Review*, 52, 52–68.

Katon, W., Russo, J., Lin, E. H., et al. (2012). Cost-effectiveness of a multicondition collaborative care intervention: a randomized controlled trial. *Archives of General Psychiatry*, 69, 506–14.

Kearns, M. C., Ressler, K. J., Zatzick, D., & Rothbaum, B. O. (2012). Early interventions for PTSD: a review. *Depression and Anxiety*, 29, 833–42.

Kessler, R. C. (2000). Posttraumatic stress disorder: the burden to the individual and to society. *The Journal of Clinical Psychiatry*, 61 (Suppl 5), 4–12; discussion 13–14.

Kessler, R. C., Sonnega, A., Bromet, E., Hughes, M., & Nelson, C. B. (1995). Posttraumatic stress disorder in the national comorbidity survey. *Archives of General Psychiatry*, 52, 1048–60.

Klein, B., Mitchell, J., Abbott, J., et al. (2010). A therapist-assisted cognitive behavior therapy internet intervention for posttraumatic stress disorder: pre-, post- and 3-month follow-up results from an open trial. *Journal of Anxiety Disorders*, 24, 635–44.

Kotov, R., Bromet, E. J., Schechter, C., et al. (2015). Posttraumatic stress disorder and the risk of respiratory problems in World Trade Center responders: longitudinal test of a pathway. *Psychosomatic Medicine*, 77, 438–48.

Kubzansky, L. D., Koenen, K. C., Jones, C., & Eaton, W. W. (2009). A prospective study of posttraumatic stress disorder symptoms and coronary heart disease in women. *Health Psychology: Official Journal of the Division of Health Psychology, American Psychological Association*, 28, 125–30.

Kubzansky, L. D., Koenen, K. C., Spiro, A., III, Vokonas, P. S., & Sparrow, D. (2007). Prospective study of posttraumatic stress disorder symptoms and coronary heart disease in the normative aging study. *Archives of General Psychiatry*, 64, 109–16.

Lecrubier, Y. (2004). Posttraumatic stress disorder in primary care: a hidden diagnosis. *The Journal of Clinical Psychiatry*, 65 (Suppl 1), 49–54.

Lowe, S. R., Blachman-Forshay, J., & Koenen, K. C. (2015). Trauma as a public health issue: epidemiology of trauma and trauma-related disorders. In U. Schnyder & M. Cloitre, eds., *Evidence Based Treatments for Trauma-Related Psychological Disorders*. Cham, Switzerland: Springer, pp. 11–40.

Malcoun, E., Houry, D., Arndt-Jordan, C., et al. (2010). Feasibility of identifying eligible trauma patients for posttraumatic stress disorder intervention. *The Western Journal of Emergency Medicine*, 11, 274–8.

McFarlane, A. C., & Bryant, R. A. (2017). PTSD: the need to use emerging knowledge to improve systems of care and clinical practice in Australia. *Australasian Psychiatry: Bulletin of Royal Australian and New Zealand College of Psychiatrists*, 25, 329–31.

Miller, M. W., Fogler, J. M., Wolf, E. J., Kaloupek, D. G., & Keane, T. M. (2008). The internalizing and externalizing structure of psychiatric comorbidity in combat veterans. *Journal of Traumatic Stress*, 21, 58–65.

Miller, M. W., Wolf, E. J., Harrington, K. M., et al. (2010). An evaluation of competing models for the structure of PTSD symptoms using external measures of comorbidity. *Journal of Traumatic Stress*, 23, 631–8.

National Institute of Mental Health (2016). NIMH-funded study to track the effects of trauma (online). Available at: www.nimh.nih.gov/news/science-news/2016/nimh-funded-study-to-track-the-effects-of-trauma.shtml (Accessed September 11, 2017).

Newman, M. G., Consoli, A. J., & Taylor, C. B. (1999). A palmtop computer program for the treatment of generalized anxiety disorder. *Behavior Modification*, 23, 597–619.

Niolon, P. H., Kearns, M., Dills, J., et al. (2017). *Preventing Intimate Partner Violence across the Lifespan: A Technical Package of Programs, Policies, and Practices*. Atlanta, GA: National Center for Injury Prevention and Control.

Ozer, E. J., Best, S. R., Lipsey, T. L., & Weiss, D. S. (2003). Predictors of posttraumatic stress disorder and symptoms in adults: a meta-analysis. *Psychological Bulletin*, 129, 52–73.

Posner, J., Eilenberg, J., Friedman, J. H., & Fullilove, M. J. (2008). Quality and use of trauma histories obtained from psychiatric outpatients: a ten-year follow-up. *Psychiatric Services*, 59, 318–21.

Possemato, K., Maisto, S. A., Wade, M., et al. (2015). Ecological momentary assessment of PTSD symptoms and alcohol use in combat veterans. *Psychology of Addictive Behaviors: Journal of the Society of Psychologists in Addictive Behaviors*, 29, 894–905.

Qi, W., Gevonden, M., & Shalev, A. (2016). Prevention of post-traumatic stress disorder after trauma: current evidence and future directions. *Current Psychiatry Reports*, 18, 20.

Regier, D. A., Goldberg, I. D., & Taube, C. A. (1978). The de facto US mental health services system: a public health perspective. *Archives of General Psychiatry*, 35, 685–93.

Regier, D. A., Hirschfeld, R. M., Goodwin, F. K., et al. (1988). The NIMH depression awareness, recognition, and treatment program: structure, aims, and scientific basis. *The American Journal of Psychiatry*, 145, 1351–7.

Roberts, A. L., Agnew-Blais, J. C., Spiegelman, D., et al. (2015). Posttraumatic stress disorder and incidence of type 2 diabetes mellitus in a sample of women: a 22-year longitudinal study. *JAMA Psychiatry*, 72, 203–10.

Roberts, A. L., Austin, S. B., Corliss, H. L., Vandermorris, A. K., & Koenen, K. C. (2010). Pervasive trauma exposure among US sexual orientation minority adults and risk of posttraumatic stress disorder. *American Journal of Public Health*, 100, 2433–41.

Roberts, A. L., Koenen, K. C., Chen, Q., et al. (2017). Posttraumatic stress disorder and accelerated aging: PTSD and leukocyte telomere length in a sample of civilian women. *Depression and Anxiety*, 34, 391–400.

Roy-Byrne, P., Craske, M. G., Sullivan, G., et al. (2010). Delivery of evidence-based treatment for multiple anxiety disorders in primary care: a randomized controlled trial. *JAMA*, 303, 1921–8.

Roy, S. S., Foraker, R. E., Girton, R. A., & Mansfield, A. J. (2015). Posttraumatic stress disorder and incident heart failure among a community-based sample of US veterans. *American Journal of Public Health*, 105, 757–63.

Scherrer, J. F., Chrusciel, T., Zeringue, A., et al. (2010). Anxiety disorders increase risk for incident myocardial infarction in depressed and nondepressed veterans administration patients. *American Heart Journal*, 159, 772–9.

Schnurr, P. P. (2016). Extending collaborative care for posttraumatic mental health. *JAMA Internal Medicine*, 176, 956–7.

Schwartz, J. E., Burg, M. M., Shimbo, D., et al. (2016). Clinic blood pressure underestimates ambulatory blood pressure in an untreated employer-based US population: results from the masked hypertension study. *Circulation*, 134, 1794–1807.

Shalev, A. Y., Ankri, Y., Israeli-Shalev, Y., et al. (2012). Prevention of posttraumatic stress disorder by early treatment: results from the Jerusalem trauma outreach and prevention study. *Archives of General Psychiatry*, 69, 166–76.

Shalev, A. Y., Ankri, Y. L., Peleg, T., Israeli-Shalev, Y., & Freedman, S. (2011). Barriers to receiving early care for PTSD: Results from the Jerusalem trauma outreach and prevention study. *Psychiatric Services*, 62, 765–73.

Shalev, I., Moffitt, T. E., Braithwaite, A. W., et al. (2014). Internalizing disorders and leukocyte telomere erosion: a prospective study of depression, generalized anxiety disorder and post-traumatic stress disorder. *Molecular Psychiatry*, 19, 1163–70.

Stein, D. J., Seedat, S., Iversen, A., & Wessely, S. (2007). Post-traumatic stress disorder: medicine and politics. *Lancet*, 369, 139–44.

Sumner, J. A., Hagan, K., Grodstein, F., et al. (2017). Posttraumatic stress disorder symptoms and cognitive function in a large cohort of middle-aged women. *Depression and Anxiety*, 34, 356–66.

Sumner, J. A., Kubzansky, L. D., Elkind, M. S., et al. (2015). Trauma exposure and posttraumatic stress disorder symptoms predict onset of cardiovascular events in women. *Circulation*, 132, 251–9.

Ursano, R. J., Fullerton, C. S., Weisaeth, L., & Raphael, B. (2017). Individual and community responses to disasters. In R. J. Ursano, C. S. Fullerton, L. Weisaeth, & B. Raphael, eds., *Textbook of Disaster Psychiatry*. Cambridge, England; New York, NY: Cambridge University Press, pp. 1–25.

Vaccarino, V., Goldberg, J., Magruder, K. M., et al. (2014). Posttraumatic stress disorder and incidence of type-2 diabetes: a prospective twin study. *Journal of Psychiatric Research*, 56, 158–64.

Vaccarino, V., Goldberg, J., Rooks, C., et al. (2013). Post-traumatic stress disorder and incidence of coronary heart disease: a twin study. *Journal of the American College of Cardiology*, 62, 970–8.

Wadsworth, M., Kuh, D., Richards, M., & Hardy, R. (2006). Cohort profile: the 1946 national birth cohort (MRC national survey of health and development). *International Journal of Epidemiology*, 35, 49–54.

Walsh, W. A., Dawson, J., & Mattingly, M. J. (2010). How are we measuring resilience following childhood maltreatment? Is the research adequate and consistent? What is the impact on research, practice, and policy? *Trauma, Violence & Abuse*, 11, 27–41.

Wang, P. S., Lane, M., Olfson, M., et al. (2005). Twelve-month use of mental health services in the United States: results from the national comorbidity survey replication. *Archives of General Psychiatry*, 62, 629–40.

Watts, B. V. (2016). Current evidence does not support the widespread use of collaborative care for PTSD, but it is limited by not evaluating context. *Evidence Based Medicine*, 21, 176.

Wolf, E. J., Miller, M. W., Krueger, R. F., et al. (2010). Posttraumatic stress disorder and the genetic structure of comorbidity. *Journal of Abnormal Psychology*, 119, 320–30.

Yaffe, K., Vittinghoff, E., Lindquist, K., et al. (2010). Posttraumatic stress disorder and risk of dementia among US veterans. *Archives of General Psychiatry*, 67, 608–13.

Index